Screening and Surveillance in General Practice

For Jenny and Rupert

For Churchill Livingstone:
Publisher: Georgina Bentliff
Project Editor: Lucy Gardner
Editorial Co-ordination: Editorial Resources Unit
   Copy Editor: Eleanor Flood
   Indexer: Brian Armitage
Production Controller: Nancy Henry
Design: Design Resources Unit
Sales Promotion Executive: Marion Pollock

Screening and Surveillance in General Practice

Edited by

Cyril R. Hart MA MB DLitt FRCGP
Formerly General Practitioner, Yaxley, Peterborough, UK

Peter Burke MRCPI MRCGP DCH DObst
General Practitioner, St Bartholomew's Medical Centre, Oxford;
Formerly Senior Lecturer in Primary Medical Care,
University of Southampton, Southampton, UK

Foreword by
Sir Michael Drury OBE FRCP FRCGP FRACGP
Emeritus Professor of General Practice,
University of Birmingham, Birmingham, UK;
Past President, Royal College of General Practitioners, UK

CHURCHILL LIVINGSTONE
EDINBURGH LONDON MADRID MELBOURNE NEW YORK AND TOKYO 1992

CHURCHILL LIVINGSTONE
Medical Division of Longman Group UK Limited

Distributed in the United States of America by Churchill
Livingstone Inc., 650 Avenue of the Americas, New York, N.Y. 10011, and
by associated companies, branches and representatives
throughout the world.

First published 1992

ISBN 0-443-04160-1

British Library Cataloguing in Publication Data
A catalogue record for this book is available from the British Library.

Library of Congress Cataloging in Publication Data
Screening and surveillance in general practice/edited by Cyril R.
   Hart, Peter Burke.
      p. cm.
   Includes index.
   1. Medical screening. 2. Family medicine. I. Hart, C. R. (Cyril
R.) II. Burke, Peter.
   [DNLM: 1. Family Practice. 2. Mass Screening-methods. 3. Mass
Screening–organization & administration. 4. Preventive Medicine–
methods. WA 245 S433]
RA427.5.S36 1992
616-dc2C
DNLM/DLC
for Library of Congress   91-26577
                                                     CIP

The
publisher's
policy is to use
**paper manufactured
from sustainable forests**

Produced by Longman Singapore Publishers (Pte) Ltd
Printed in Singapore

Foreword

In his preface to *Screening in General Practice* published in 1975 Dr Cyril Hart described screening as a discipline still in its infancy. It has grown since then into a healthy child even if there is still much to be learnt before the parameters are defined. It is a rapidly changing subject and new data to help identify the balance between the cost of what we do and the benefits that accrue come thick and fast and sometimes add to confusion rather than clarifying. This is one reason why I particularly welcome and wish to commend this successor to that earlier volume.

During the 16 years that have elapsed an equally great change has taken place in our attitudes. This runs right across the spectrum of general practice and the opportunities for prevention are now seen as an important component of every consultant and every management plan. Ethical issues and matters of principle derive from this and these at any rate can provide important beacons in otherwise uncharted seas. This book identifies and discusses these.

The organisation of general practice is being transformed by the computerisation of data. This allows us to identify at risk groups with ease and introduce reliable follow-up in a way that was not possible even five years ago. Whilst much of our surveillance work may continue to be opportunistic in the future, as the authors point out, we shall need 'aides memoires' and prompts to work in a reliable way.

The authors collected by Cyril Hart and Peter Burke are an impressive collection. They have the intellectual range for a book of this nature but they are also largely general practitioners with experience of the real world of practice from the inner city to more comfortable middle-class residential life. I believe this book should be one of the most thumbed volumes in the practice library and I am delighted to be associated with it in this small way.

Birmingham, 1992   Professor Sir Michael Drury

Acknowledgements

We have received help and advice from numerous sources. In listing the following we inevitably omit others, and trust that they will not be offended.

Our thanks go to Professor J. Butler, Professor Ian Kennedy, Dr Sophie Botros, Mrs Sally Richards, Dr Linda Stanton, Dr Barry Keaton, Dr Sarah Peters, Mr J. G. Jackson, Dr A. Strahan and Dr P. Skrabanek.

Last, but not least, we would like to thank our wives for their patience and forbearance.

Cyril Hart and Peter Burke

Preface

Over the 17 years since this book's predecessor, *Screening in General Practice* appeared, there have been vast changes in primary medical care in the United Kingdom as in other countries. Prevention, management and teamwork have, for example, become important parts of our vocabulary. In the wake of the 1990 GP contract, the pace of change has increased dramatically. This book looks at the opportunities as well as the challenges which change brings.

From its title it will be clear that this book concerns prevention. The greatest emphasis is on screening or secondary prevention, the identification and management of pre-symptomatic health problems. However, the inclusion of the word 'surveillance' in the title is no accident: we have set ourselves wider terms of reference. Where appropriate we have moved into the area of primary prevention, in particular disease prophylaxis by early action against known risk factors. Similarly there is discussion of tertiary prevention, i.e. the prevention of complications arising from established disease. Screening and surveillance march hand-in-hand; neither should be practised in isolation.

We have tried to cover a very wide range of topics in a reasonable degree of depth. We do not expect that each chapter will be of interest to every reader. For this reason chapters can be read independently of each other. We have accepted the inevitability of some duplication, though we have used cross-reference as much as possible.

A multi-disciplinary authorship is essential given the breadth of our aims. The authors are predominently GPs, but also include academics, hospital specialists, community physicians, a practice manager, and a health economist. Although inevitably this results in variations of style and emphasis, we hope that the flavour is complementary rather than dissonant. Our policy has been to give weight in accordance not only with the current, but also with the anticipated importance of a topic. We have not shied away from controversy, and there are many views expressed with which readers may find themselves at odds. We have tried to ensure that sufficient evidence—with reference to the original sources—is provided to allow readers to make up their own minds.

We have divided the book into seven sections. The first is general, while the second covers organisational implications, as well as some of the tools available and their use. The next four sections review screening and surveillance techniques. They follow what is broadly an age-based structure. Though convenient, this is often of necessity arbitrary. For example, ischaemic heart disease falls under the heading of the 'younger adult', though it is not suggested that its prevention should stop the day a patient reaches the age of 65. The final section of the book covers groups of people who, for reasons of lifestyle, require special consideration.

The 'iceberg of illness' has been much discussed. Primarily, this comprises medical conditions, such as cervical carcinoma in situ, of which both doctor and patient are unaware until they are detected on a screening test. However, it also includes many other problems and risk factors, such as alcohol dependency, which are known to one or both parties but have never been brought openly onto the agenda. Identifying and confronting such 'hidden needs' is perhaps becoming an increasingly important part of our task, and the inclusion of chapters on lifestyle issues reflects this fact.

In dealing with each activity, we have tried to identify potential benefits and disadvantages, and to dwell also upon the broader resource implications of a screening programme. These include the secondary assessment services which must be provided in order to respond to its findings. Furthermore, no screening programme has completed its task once every eligible person has been through the net. Decisions must be made as to how soon the health benefits of the screen have worn off sufficiently to justify re-screening. A screening programme, therefore, is a little like the painting of the Forth Bridge: once the programme appears to have reached its natural conclusion, it is already time to return to the other end and start again. This will be a great deal easier if appropriate systems and methods have been set up on the first occasion. In many chapters, therefore, administrative issues feature prominently.

No book on screening today would be complete unless it mentioned 'opportunistic', or consultation-based screening, sometimes referred to as case finding. In a country where 70% of the population consult their general practitioner in the space of one year, case finding is at the very least a valuable adjunct to screening.

Finally, it is not our intention to proselytize. For any individual practice the screening programme adopted will ideally reflect local resources and needs. There is always a balance between the costs—economic and otherwise—and benefits of the screening programme. It is in no way a function of this book to dictate the perfect balance. There is no chapter in which the message is that 'every good practice must...'. Rather the book puts forward a series of ideas and options, adding to choice rather than restricting it. The catalogues of 'musts' in the medical literature do not need to be added to yet further.

Peterborough and Oxford
January 1992   Cyril Hart and Peter Burke

Contributors

Colin P. Bradley MD MRCGP
Lecturer in General Practice, University of Manchester, Manchester, UK

E. Graham Buckley MD FRCP(Edin) FRCGP
General Practitioner, Howden Health Centre, Livingston, UK; Formerly Editor, British Journal of General Practice

Peter Burke MRCPI MRCGP DCH DObst
General Practitioner, St Bartholomew's Medical Centre, Oxford; Formerly Senior Lecturer in Primary Medical Care, University of Southampton, Southampton, UK

Ralph H. Burton MB BS MRCGP
Senior Tutor in General Practice, St George's Hospital Medical School, London; General Practitioner, Ewell, Epsom, UK

Peter Campion FRCGP MRCP(UK) DCCH
Senior Lecturer in General Practice, Department of General Practice, University of Liverpool, Liverpool, UK

Carol Church MB BS DCH
Senior Clinical Medical Officer, Central Health Clinic, Southampton, UK

Nicholas M.P. Clarke ChM FRCS FRCS(Ed)
Consultant Orthopaedic Surgeon, Southampton General Hospital, Lymington Hospital and Lord Mayor Treloar Hospital, Alton, UK

John Coope MB MRCGP
General Practitioner, Bollington, Macclesfield, UK

Gay Davies
Practice Manager, Yaxley Group Practice, Yaxley, Peterborough, UK

Nicholas R. Dennis MB FRCP
Senior Lecturer in Clinical Genetics, University of Southampton, Southampton, UK

Peter Ellis MA MB BChir DCH DGM DRCOG Dip Med Ed MRCGP
General Practitioner, Harrow, UK

Charles B. Freer MB ChB MClSci MRCGP
General Practitioner, Glasgow, UK

A. Ward Gardner MD (Glas) FRCPI FFOM(Ireland) FFOM(Lond) DIH
Consultant Occupational Physician, Eling, Totton, Southampton, UK

Cyril R. Hart MA MB DLitt FRCGP
Formerly General Practitioner, Stilton, Peterborough, UK

Christopher Hinton MD
Consultant Surgeon, Princess Royal Hospital, Telford and Shropshire Breast Screening Service, Telford, UK

Tom Hutchison MRCP DCH
Consultant Community Paediatrician, Nottingham Health Authority, Nottingham, UK

Sanjeebit J. Jachuck BSc MBBS MRCP MRCGP AFOM
General Practitioner, Newcastle upon Tyne, UK

David Jewell MA MB BChir MRCGP
Consultant Senior Lecturer in General Practice, University of Bristol, Bristol, UK

Jacqueline Jolleys BA MB ChB MRCGP
Medical Director, Nottinghamshire Family Health Services Authority; Lecturer in General Practice, University of Nottingham, Nottingham, UK

Kevin Jones MB MRCP MRCGP DM FRCGP
Senior Lecturer in Primary Medical Care, University of Southampton; General Practitioner, Aldermoor Health Centre, Southampton, UK

Roger Jones MA DM FRCGP MRCP
Professor of Primary Health Care, University of Newcastle upon Tyne, Newcastle upon Tyne, UK

Katharine Orton MBBS MRCGP DCH DRCOG
Principal, General Practice, Hatfield Heath, Bishops
Stortford, UK

Calum R. Paton MA(Oxon) MPP(Harvard) DPhil(Oxon)
Director, MBA (Health Executive) Programme, Senior
Lecturer, Centre for Health Planning and
Management, University of Keele, UK

Leon Polnay FRCP DCH
Reader in Child Health, University of Nottingham;
Honorary Consultant Community Paediatrician,
Nottingham Health Authority, UK

Elizabeth M.E. Poskitt MA MB BChir FRCP
Senior Lecturer in Child Health, University of
Liverpool, Institute of Child Health, Royal Liverpool
Children's Hospitals (Alder Hey), Liverpool, UK

Bashir Qureshi FRCGP DCH AFOM (RCP) FRSH MICGP
FRIPHH
General Practitioner, Hounslow, London, UK; Author
of *Transcultural Medicine*; Member of the Council of
the RCGP and its International Committee; Member
of the Editorial Board of *Health Trends*

Ian Redhead MD FRCGP
Formerly General Practitioner, Yaxley, Peterborough;
Hospital Practitioner, Department of Genitourinary
Medicine, Peterborough District Hospital,
Peterborough, UK

Leone Ridsdale BA MSc(Econ) FRCPC
Senior Lecturer in General Practice, United Medical
and Dental Schools, Guy's and St Thomas's Hospitals,
London, UK

Lewis D. Ritchie BSc MSc MBChB MRCGP MFPHM MBCS
DRCOG
General Practitioner, Peterhead Health Centre,
Peterhead; Consultant in Public Health Medicine,
Grampian Health Board; Lecturer in General Practice,
University of Aberdeen, Aberdeen, UK

James Roy Robertson MBChB BSc FRCGP
General Practitioner, Muirhouse Medical Group,
Edinburgh, UK

John Robson MD MRCGP
General Practitioner, Chrisp Street Health Centre,
London, UK

Simon Smail MA BM BCh FRCGP DCH DRCOG
Senior Lecturer in General Practice, University of
Wales College of Medicine, Cardiff, UK

Nicki Spiegal BSc RGN HVCert
Primary Care Facilitator, Department of Primary
Medical Care, Aldermoor Health Centre,
Southampton, UK

Donald Thomson FRCP FRCGP
Senior Lecturer, Department of General Practice,
University of Edinburgh, Edinburgh, UK

Keith Thompson FRCGP
Formerly General Practitioner, Croydon, UK

Peter Tomson FRCGP
General Practitioner, Watford, UK

John Tuke MB MRCGP DCH
Consultant in Public Health Medicine, West Suffolk
Health Authority, Suffolk, UK

Alastair J. Tulloch MD FRCGP DObstRCOG
Formerly General Practitioner; Research Officer, Unit
of Clinical Epidemiology, University of Oxford,
Oxford, UK

Paul Wallace MSc MRCGP
Senior Lecturer, Department of General Practice, St
Mary's Hospital Medical School, London, UK

John Wilmot MB ChB FRCGP DCH DRCOG
General Practitioner, Leamington Spa, Warwickshire;
Senior Lecturer in General Practice, School of
Postgraduate Medical Education, University of
Warwick, Coventry, UK

Alastair F. Wright MD FRCGP
General Practitioner, Glenrothes, UK; Editor, British
Journal of General Practice

Contents

Principles

1. The history of screening

Cyril Hart

If preventable, why not prevented?

King Edward VII

THE ICEBERG OF DISEASE

It is a truism that in medical science, as in other departments of organised knowledge, the great wars of the past century have acted as catalysts for the development and application of fresh ideas. Just as the nursing profession was born from the horrors of the Crimea, so the very high rejection rate following medical examination of army volunteers during the Boer War led to the first realisation in this country of the extent of occult disease in the community. This experience was repeated in the two World Wars, not only in military medicine, but also in the examination of the civilian population in connection with evacuation and rationing (Davidson et al 1943).

Whenever circumstances result in the medical examination of a large number of people, no matter what the initial purpose, clinical interest in the detection of hitherto unrecognised disorders develops, and a screening situation exists. Routine examinations of schoolchildren, workers in industry and applicants for insurance have been a feature of medical practice in this country since Victorian times, and to these have been added more recently antenatal examinations, medical tests for drivers of lorries and public service vehicles and the examination of immigrants. In the past two decades millions of examinations have been carried out on disabled applicants for Mobility and Attendance Allowances. All these involve some form of screening.

At the turn of the present century, the prevalence of such conditions as deafness, valvular heart disease, hernia, tuberculosis, trachoma and favus in immigrants at the port of Boston, USA was commented upon (see Wilson 1966). One doubts whether the health of the existing population there was in much better shape; with few exceptions, no-one had occasion to examine them. It was about this time, however, that the US doctor, G M Gould, introduced the concept of the periodic health examination (Gould 1900). Not surprisingly, this idea commended itself to the American Medical Association, and was soon taken up throughout the country. In 1923 the National Health Council encouraged Americans to have an annual physical examination with the slogan 'Have a Health examination on your Birthday'. There was quite a good response, but the numbers were insufficient to warrant the setting up of any special organisation at that time, and the additional workload was absorbed by the existing medical facilities.

Many of these early examinations were hit-or-miss affairs, but in 1926 a survey instituted in the London Borough of Peckham enabled the health of a particular community to be monitored in an unhurried fashion over a period of years (Williamson and Pearse 1938, Pearse and Crocker 1943, Pearse 1970). I well remember spending a day at the Peckham Health Centre in about 1949 as a raw medical student. There we were introduced to the concept of the 'iceberg of disease'. This revelation of the staggering amount of undetected and untreated disease and defect in the population made such an impression on myself and my contemporaries of the early post-ward period, that it motivated much of our subsequent activity.

In 1963 J M Last, of the Social Medicine Research Unit of the Medical Research Council, attempted to quantify the iceberg by listing the unrecognised diseases in an average general practice. His estimates, extended slightly by R F Logan and C L Sharp, are reproduced in Table 1.1. As an indication of the size of the problem, the figures of this fundamental survey still have more than a purely historical value, because to a significant extent, they remain applicable to large sections of British general practice today.

Table 1.1   The iceberg of disease. Estimate of unrecognised diseases in an average general practice of 2250 patients in England and Wales in 1962 (from Last 1963; Logan 1964; Sharp 1968)

Disorder	Known to practitioner	Total in practice
Anaemia		
Males age 15–64	2	32 (Hb below 12 g%)
Males age 65+	1	24 (Hb below 12 g%)
Females age 15–64	19	132 (Hb below 11.5 g%)
Females age 65+	5	30 (Hb below 11.5 g%)
Cancer		
Cervix	1/2	3 invasive; 9 *in situ*
Breast	1	10 (lumps)
Chronic bronchitis (age 45–64)		
Males	24	47
Females	19	24
Diabetes mellitus	14	31 (glycosuria + diabetic GTT)
Epilepsy	8	14
Glaucoma (age 45+)	3	27 (early chronic)
Hypertensive disease (age 45+)	32	161 (diastolic 100+ mmHg)
Psychiatric disorders (age 15+)		
Males	32	91 (conspicuous morbidity)
Females	72	144
Psychotic depression	12	125
Rheumatoid arthritis (age 15+)	11	25
Suicide attempts (annually)	3	6
Urinary infections (age 15+)		
Females	25	140 (bacilluria)

THE FIRST SCREENING TECHNIQUES AND DETECTION DRIVES

It was soon realised that more than simple clinical examination was required if the earliest stages of many of the most common disorders were to be uncovered, and progress in the past half-century has been characterised by the development of a large number of screening techniques applicable to particular diseases. A few early examples may be given. Mass radiography for pulmonary tuberculosis, which started in the UK soon after D'Abreu introduced the photofluorographic technique in 1939, has proved one of the most successful of all screening procedures. From infectious diseases, attention then switched to the early detection of malignant neoplasms and in 1943 Papanicolaou published his classic paper on the diagnosis of cervical cancer by exfoliative cytology (Papanicolaou and Traut 1943). A spatula for scraping the cervix to obtain specimens was developed a few years later and it

remains in general use today (Ayre 1947). There was an immediate demand for laboratory facilities, and the first laboratory to be equipped for cervical cancer was opened in 1949 in British Columbia, Canada.

Interest in the early detection of metabolic disorders was stimulated by the publication in 1953 of a recommended diet for phenylketonuria, which for the first time offered hope to children born with this rare but devastating error in the metabolism of phenylalanine (Bickel et al 1953). As a result of this paper, the ferric chloride test on urine, first used by Folling when he discovered the disease in 1934, began to be adopted more widely. A test using a paper strip impregnated with the solution, after the style of litmus paper, was developed (Phenistix), later to be superseded by the Guthrie test on a drop of blood obtained by pricking the baby's heel (Guthrie 1966a).

In another sphere, large-scale investigation of the early stages of asthma and obstructive airways disease was made possible by the development of simple ventilatory function tests using the Wright Peak Flow Meter and the Vitalograph Spirometer, first marketed in 1959 and 1963, respectively. Technological advances of widespread application continued to be made at a remarkable rate. A dip-slide technique for culturing urinary pathogenic bacteria was first described by Guttmann and Naylor (1967). Increasing use of the dip-slide from 1970 onwards revolutionised the early detection of occult urinary infection (Arneil 1972).

The spread of knowledge of these and other techniques was one of the most potent factors that led to the era of 'detection drives' for individual diseases, or 'mass monophasic screening', as some preferred to call it. The first diabetes survey in the USA was reported by Wilkerson and Krall (1947), and a mass screening programme for glaucoma was described by Brav and Kirber (1951). In 1955 it was decided to introduce a cervical cytology screening service based on the aforementioned British Columbian laboratory (Kaiser et al 1960). A few years later, routine physical examination for asymptomatic breast cancer was first advocated, to be followed rapidly by mass soft-tissue X-ray detection of non-palpable breast tumours (Holleb et al 1960, Gershon-Cohen et al 1961).

THE TREND TOWARDS MULTIPHASIC SCREENING

Until quite recently, health screening of a community has been regarded as something of a luxury, and it is not surprising that its early development occured largely in those countries where the standard of living was high — at least for some sections of the population. Specialised health checks on businessmen started in the USA in about 1947, and in 1951 the Kaiser Permanente organisation began to utilise screening methods as part of a periodic health examination. This was made available on a prepayment basis to a large population on the western seaboad of the USA. As individual (monophasic) screening techniques were developed, they were incorporated piecemeal into the existing service, which was soon built up into a comprehensive multiphasic screening programme. By 1957 the Commission on Chronic Illness in the USA was able to list eight conditions for which it was considered that screening tests were applicable (Commission on Chronic Illness 1957). The impact of multiphasic screening on periodic medical examinations in the USA was reviewed by Breslow (1959).

Meanwhile, in Sweden the brothers Gunner and Ingmar Jungner were experimenting with automatic mass analytical methods for quantitative estimation of the main constituents of blood serum. By 1961 they had developed a battery of ten chemical tests, which was used straightaway in a large scale multiphasic screening project mounted by the National Board of Health, to cover a population of 100 000 in the county of Värmland. The programme, completed in 1969, was highly successful, and vindicated the concept of automated chemical screening (Jungner 1965, Engel 1968). Later, the Swedes perfected a computerised 'Auto-Chemist', which gave reliable results for a wide range of tests, and was capable of a very heavy workload (Jungner and Jungner 1968).

The Americans were quick to see the revolutionary implications of this new development, and by 1964 chemical screening had been integrated with the rest of the programme in two automated test laboratories run by the Permanente organisation (Collen 1965, 1968). By this time, the advantages of computerising the whole screening programme had been realised, and a year later the first textbook to deal with this new branch of medicine was published (Collen et al 1965). The result was an explosion of activity throughout the USA and computerised units for automated multiphasic screening (AMPS) were set up in many universities and hospitals. The early stages of this movement were admirably described by Dr Charles Hodes, a British general practitioner who spent 6 weeks studying these developments as a WHO Fellow in the autumn of 1968 (Hodes 1969). The movement continued to spread at an astonishing pace and it was not long before a network of screening clinics was established throughout the USA (Gelman 1971, Hsieh et al 1971, Branson and Constantine 1972).

Before long, other developed countries were experiencing the birth-pangs of similar programmes. In West Germany, for example, the first commercially-run screening clinic was set up at Weisbaden in 1970, followed soon afterwards by others at Frankfurt and Munich. These did not prove viable propositions, but the trade unions then moved into the field, and two more clinics were established in hospitals in Hessen (Sault 1973). The first venture on these lines in Japan was the multiphasic screening centre opened for employees of the Toshiba Electric Company in 1970. This company had a commercial interest in automated screening techniques and pioneered the automation of respirometry, sphygmomanometry and cervical smear testing in its own clinic (Yoshisuke 1973). The pace of development in Japan was such that, by 1973, AMPS was already common there (WMA Computer Panel 1973).

In London, a health screening clinic was started by the Institute of Directors as early as 1964, and in 1970 a similar unit was set up by BUPA, the British United

Provident Assocation (Wright 1971). Two years later the screening services of these two organisations were merged to form a Medical Centre at King's Cross. Here a fully computerised automated unit, modelled on the latest American pattern, started health checks for subscribers at the rate of 15 000 examinations a year.

Within the medical centre, individual screening tests were performed at a number of 'stations', each with its own specialised equipment and specially trained staff. These were visited in turn by the individual under test, starting with a comprehensive health questionnaire projected onto a visual display unit (VDU) (the Americans had already discovered that individuals will confide in a computer, trusting it with details of their personal lives that they would not dream of telling their physicians in the consulting room). Blood and urine samples were taken for automated chemical tests; the individual then moved on to automated checks of weight, height, blood pressure, electrocardiogram (ECG), visual fields and acuity, audiogram, spirometry, chest film and so on. As each test was completed, the results were transmitted automatically to the final station, where a physician monitored them and discussed the results with the subscriber, whose GP was provided with a print-out if the subscriber consented.

Similar but smaller units were started in the provinces, the first being at Manchester, Nottingham and Glasgow. By 1980 these were providing comprehensive health checks for 40 000 men and women each year. By 1988 BUPA screening centres had been established in all the large towns throughout the UK, and the annual number of individuals undergoing evaluation at these centres had risen to over 100 000. Over the years the content of the screening programme has been refined in range and quality of the tests performed; different scales of testing are available according to what the applicant is perceived to require and is able to afford, but the basic organisation of the programme remains much the same as that described above.

Other private screening organisations began to compete in a smaller way. Most of them centred their activities on medium-sized industries, the larger industrial concerns having quite often made in-house arrangements. In 1973 an organisation known as Health Care started a private biochemical screening service, using multichannel autoanalysers capable of determining 12 blood constituents, plus haematological and lipid analyses. This was made available to British industrial firms wishing their employees to be screened, the blood being collected within the factory.

Similar private facilities have since been created at several other centres throughout the country, and in 1987 BUPA moved into the occupational health care market with a number of mobile screening units set up in specially fitted lorries.

THE INITIATION OF SCREENING IN BRITAIN

One very important advantage that the medical care organisation in this country has over the United States, is the concept of general practice as a clear-cut mandate, as a responsibility for the health of families...The organisation of your services, subject as it is to improvement, at least provides for physicians who have responsibility for populations and for people whom they know, and with whom they can deal,... and in relation to whom they can initiate action.

C G Sheps (1966)

The words are those of an American professor of preventive medicine, when attending a symposium on screening in general practice held at Edinburgh in 1964. For better or for worse, the creation of the National Health Service in 1948 delayed the proliferation in the UK of the subscriber-orientated hospital-based multiphasic screening clinics that had become so characteristic a feature of the North American scene, and by the middle 1960s had already been extended through much of Europe and the more developed countries of the Near and Far East.

Because of the priority rightly given since the inception of the NHS to the development and coordination of therapeutic medicine, early screening activities in this country proceeded on a very patchy ad hoc basis, being regarded for the most part as a luxurious optional extra than as a basic necessity, and as something supplemental to existing preventive measures, rather than integral with them.

Initially, experiments in screening within the NHS were conducted as often by medical personnel of hospital and public health departments as by general practitioners. A classic early example was the survey by Dr Arthur Exton-Smith, a consultant geriatrician, of 215 elderly patients whom he visited in their own homes in the Borough of St Pancras in 1952 (Exton-Smith 1952). In the same year, a rather more ambitious but differently organised geriatric programme was initiated at Rutherglen Consultative Health Centre in Scotland. Here the Local Health Authority and the Departments of Psychology and of Geriatric Medicine at Glasgow University combined to offer a comprehensive health screen to older people who, although feeling well, desired a medical assessment or who, because of illness, were referred to the centre by their general practitioner. By 1972, over 1000 people aged 60 and over had been screened (Andrews et al 1971,

Cowan 1972). It should be noted, however, that the Rutherglen programme was essentially a research project, and the screen was offered only on a selective basis.

Other surveys were started by consultant geriatricians working in conjunction with general practitioners. The trend was set in a scheme mounted in Dr Roger Meyrick's practice at Hither Green, South East London in 1962, when patients were seen at a hospital clinic after a home visit by the general practitioner (Meyrick 1962). Occasionally, consultants in specialities other than geriatrics worked jointly on a programme with the public health authorities, notably in the screening of phenylketonuria and diabetes (Sharp 1964, Guthrie 1966b). On the whole, however, the number of hospital-based screening surveys of any kind on the general population of this country has not been large, and like the Rutherglen project they have been research-oriented.

PUBLIC HEALTH SCREENING

The 1960s and early 1970s witnessed an attempt to build up a tradition of public health participation in screening in spheres other than preventive geriatrics. The pioneering work of Dr J L Burns, the Medical Officer of Health for Salford, has been inadequately reported; between 1960 and 1962 he organised a unique multiphasic clinic in the town (Ferrer 1968). Better known are the Bedford surveys into diabetes and glaucoma, held between 1962 and 1966 (Sharp 1964, Wright 1966). Further screening in Bedford was brought to an end by the untimely death of Dr C L Sharp, who had initiated the venture. Meanwhile, interest had spread to Rotherham, where after some preliminary experiments the Medical Officer of Health, Dr R J Donaldson, conducted a 9-day multiphasic screen in 1966, attended by 5500 people (Rotherham Report 1969).

The results from Rotherham were found to be invaluable for statistical purposes and were often quoted, but perhaps of greater interest for our present review is the following description of the administrative arrangements, which were evidently run on a shoestring. They appear decidedly primitive by modern standards, and illustrate vividly the drawbacks of short-term detection drives:

We think the 'open door' clinic with no appointments gives us a better representation of the population than if we had appointment clinics...we stress to them the limitations of the service. ...The clinic itself is held in a large dance hall, and nine of the 11 test stations are around the hall. The other two, for breast cancer and cervical cytology, are in side rooms. The people coming in, after having registered, more or less choose their own test. ...The staff are mainly from our own department, and work with a tremendous amount of energy and enthusiasm, and find it an exhausting but exhilarating experience. After the clinic has closed comes the tedious sentence of hard labour in getting the data ready for processing and despatch to the general practitioner. (Donaldson 1968, see also Donaldson and Howell 1965).

Based on these and similar activities (developmental screening of infants, for example) a case was argued that 'screening procedures are the special prerogative of the Medical Officer of Health', but it received little support (Ferrer 1968). Valuable though these early public health surveys undoubtedly were, they did not form satisfactory models for a nationwide screening programme. Adequate staffing, resources and expertise were all lacking. With this realisation, Dr I A MacDougal, the County Medical Officer of Health for Hampshire, suggested that local authority doctors might conduct screening clinics from health centres (MacDougal 1970). It soon became obvious that if this idea was to become a reality, their most useful work would be in child health surveillance, but in fact even in this sphere most local health authority activity has taken place outside health centres. Apart from a dwindling amount of paediatric surveillance in the larger cities and conurbations (Chapter 12), such screening by district health authority staff as survives is almost entirely in the hands of nurses and health visitors, and increasingly their activities take place within the ambit of the primary care team. At the time of writing, it appears that the era of public health screening in Britain is fast coming to an end.

EARLY SCREENING IN BRITISH GENERAL PRACTICE

The inception of the National Health Service in 1948 had a profound effect on the organisation of general practice in the UK. In the early years of service, GPs were too busy accustoming themselves to working in the new regime to wish to take on extra responsibilities in preventive medicine and it was not until 1954 that the foundation of the Darbishire House Health Centre as a teaching unit of the Manchester Medical School enabled some experimental work to be undertaken. Dr H W Ashworth, the first general practitioner appointed there, began to investigate the incidence of anaemia among his patients as soon as the health centre opened (Ashworth 1963). In 1958, routine multiphasic health testing of the 45–54 age group was undertaken in the practice. At this date many of the more useful screening techniques had still to be developed, and Dr Ashworth was sceptical as to the value of his investigations (Ashworth 1959, 1964).

In the same year — 1958 — Dr Ian Redhead carried out a diabetes detection drive on 2000 patients in his Newcastle practice — the first practice-based survey of the incidence of diabetes in this country (Redhead 1960). This was a larger undertaking than one might think, it still being the test tube era for chemical tests on urine. The following decade witnessed many such drives, mostly for the detection of diabetes and carcinoma of the cervix, within the framework of general practice. Before long, multiphasic detection drives were being held in rural practices in Lincolnshire and Derbyshire (Cope & Smith 1967, 1972, Evans et al 1969). The description of the arrangements for the Derbyshire survey deserves to go on record here, both for comparison with the Rotherham survey and also as a classic contribution to the literature of screening in general practice:

The screening clinic was held in our surgery headquarters on two half-days only, and coincided with a visit from the Mobile Mass X-ray Unit a few hundred yards away. The only publicity was a circular letter which we sent to each household registered with the practice under the National Health Service. Patients under 15 years of age were not permitted to attend, and the elderly were gently discouraged from doing so.

With much help from varied sources it was possible to provide a wide range of tests. We crowded into our waiting room, registration, tests for anaemia and glycosuria, the measurement of weight, blood pressure, and Wright Peak Flow Meter reading, a history of cough and sputum and smoking, and a personality adjustment rating. The small examination room housed the electro-cardiograph and its technicians. One consulting room had observers examining for goitre (endemic in Derbyshire) and technicians taking venous blood for biochemical estimations. Another separate consulting room was used for breast examinations and for cervical cytology. Working conditions were noisy, tiring and very crowded.

In the two half-days 791 patients were screened — about a quarter of those eligible. The total was made up of 355 males and 436 females. The average age of men attending was 47, of women 48 years. In the same two days, the Mobile Mass X-ray Unit took over 1000 chest X-rays.

The enthusiasm of the patients was indeed obvious. We attempted to spread the load by asking patients to attend in an alphabetical sequence, but we offered them only a queue in the open air. Despite a staff of about 25 people, this queue was usually 10 or 20 yards long, and on one of our two days it was raining. The patients had relied on a tear-off strip telling us how many were intending to come. We catered for about 800 on the basis of their replies. We could not have coped with more. (Evans et al 1969)

Short term detection drives of this nature, or 'health fairs' as they were picturesquely described in the USA, served to alert GPs to the usefulness of multiphasic screening and during the 1960s there was a quiet but steady development of more lasting practice-based experiments, many of which remain unrecorded in the literature.

In my own practice at Yaxley, near Peterborough, for example, (where I had been joined as partner by Dr Ian Redhead from Newcastle late in 1959) we screened patients for diabetes from the outset. It soon became obvious that screening had to be a continuous process, partly to ensure long-term surveillance of the patients and partly to spread the workload so that it did not interfere too much with other routine practice activities. We also discovered that screening had to be a team effort, and in the late 1960s and early 1970s I carried out a complete geriatric screen of the practice, with the aid of Mrs Susan Jackson, our practice nurse/receptionist, and Mrs Sheila Ganeri, our health visitor. Another discovery in those early pioneering days was the importance of adequate documentation and systems of recall. An age/sex register was started and special recording cards were designed and printed, suitable for subsequent filing in the patient's records. All this was before the era of practice computers, but we had the rare advantage of a purpose-built surgery with adequate space and equipment. No funding was available from outside the practice; we paid for the screening out of the profits from dispensing (Hart 1975).

Ours was by no means the only practice involved in such developments. All over the country GPs were meeting in small groups, usually under the aegis of the College of General Practitioners, to discuss ways and means of introducing preventive medicine in their practices, and screening ventures were being started. An early pioneer was Dr Ian Gregg, who carried out screening tests between 1962 and 1965 using the Wright Peak Flow Meter to detect symptomless airways obstruction in chronic bronchitics in his practice at Kingston upon Thames (Gregg 1966). Thompson (1975) listed eight general practice geriatric screening surveys, which were reported in the British literature during the period 1968–73. Early screening programmes for hypertension were carried out in their practices by Tudor Hart at Glyncorrwg, South Wales, in 1968–9 (Hart 1980) and by Coope at Macclesfield, Cheshire, in the early 1970s (Coope 1974). At the same time, Pike was screening middle-aged men in his Birmingham practice (Pike 1972) and Wookey and Kerr were running 'well-women clinics' at Boston and Ashton-under-Lyne (Wookey 1971, Kerr 1972). The first accounts of screening by cervical smears in British general practice were by Ashworth and Rivett in 1964 (Ashworth 1964, Rivett 1965) followed by Freeling (1965) and Lloyd (1967). Developmental screening of infants was started a year or two later by several pioneers, notably Hooper in the Isle of Wight (Hooper 1965, 1971), Starte in Guildford, Surrey (Starte 1974, 1976), Curtis Jenkins in Ashford, Middlesex (Curtis Jenkins et al 1978) and Bain in Edinburgh (Bain 1977). Less obviously, but no less significantly, GPs were beginning to separate antenatal care from their routine surgeries, and to introduce to their practices screening procedures from hospital clinics to monitor the health of the mother and the development of the fetus.

All this, and much else besides, was reported in a multiauthor work, *Screening in General Practice*, which I had the honour to edit in 1975. The great majority of the contributors were ordinary GPs from all over the country and were representative of a much larger, anonymous group of practices whose dedication to the development of preventive medicine in NHS general practice was remarkable. They were not usually from academic departments (indeed at that time not many of these had been founded); their resources were minimal, with primitive practice organisations and tiny ancillary staffs. In spite of official exhortations, most areas of preventive medicine remained outside the GPs' contract, and they practised it to their financial detriment; their activities for the most part were funded from their own pockets and recorded and reported in their own spare time. Nearly all drew their inspiration from the College of General Practitioners.

What these screening programmes lacked in academic rigour, they more than made up for in enthusiasm. And whatever their deficiencies, they taught us all one lesson of lasting value: general practice is the natural *locus* for medical screening and surveillance in this country, and the primary care team are the best people to carry it out, *because of the on-going responsibility accepted by practitioners for monitoring the health care of their practice population.*

THE FIRST STEPS TOWARDS A PLANNED SCREENING PROGRAMME

On 7 July 1965 an important colloquium was held at Magdalen College, Oxford under the auspices of the Office of Health Economics, to discuss surveillance and early diagnosis in general practice. It was attended by members of the faculties of medicine of various British universities, by medical officers of health, representatives of the Medical Research Council and of the Ministry of Health, by a number of leading members of the College of General Practitioners and by distinguished visitors from Sweden and the USA; everyone, in fact, except those who would be actually doing the job (Wilson 1966).

The contrast between the proceedings of this august assembly and the hectic activities of the detection drives currently being held in Rotherham and Derbyshire could not have been more marked. Nevertheless, the colloquium proved just as decisive an event as the detection drives in the history of medical screening in this country. The discussion centred around such topics as: Who should be screened? Who should do it? Why should they do it? How is it to be organised? What procedures should be used? What are the long-term benefits? What is the cost? Can any list of priorities be given (i) for individual clinical practice and (ii) for social policy?

One of the many valuable contributions to the colloquium was that of Dr J M Wilson, then a Senior Medical Officer at the Ministry of Health, who listed the set of principles of case finding that became known as Wilson's Screening Criteria (see Table 2.2, p. 17). These criteria were difficult to meet then, and remain so today. Editorials appeared in the *Lancet* and *British Medical Journal* counselling caution, and recommending that carefully designed research studies should evaluate programmes of prescriptive screening before their general introduction as a branch of preventive medicine. A number of long-term screening investigations were put in hand in the newly established departments of general practice of universities in the national capitals of Cardiff (Winter et al 1972), Belfast (Irwin and Neill 1970) and Edinburgh (Scott and Robertson 1968, Illingworth 1970, Percy-Robb et al 1971).

The most ambitious of these was the South East London Screening Survey, in which long-term multiphasic screening was offered to the middle-aged patients of two group practices, the sessions being conducted in the evening in Local Health Authority clinics. The study, by far the most elaborate of its kind, was organised by the Department of Clinical Epidemiology and Social Medicine at St Thomas's Medical School, under the direction of Professor W W Holland and with support from the (then) Ministry of Health. Designed as a 5-year longitudinal study, it was commenced in November 1967 and the full results of the survey were not made available until the end of 1974. Unfortunately, the methodology was poor and the results disappointing. Its conclusions were overtaken by events. Revolutionary advances in screening techniques made during the period of the survey, particularly in the fields of data processing and computing, and in the involvement of primary care teams, rendered its results obsolete before their publication.

At the same time, however, the country's economy moved into a period of recession and retrenchment, in which the climate was not conducive to a widespread extension of screening activity. During these years the gap widened substantially between what had become feasible technically and what was affordable in practice. Improvements in our standard of preventive care did not keep up with what was happening in the rest of Europe.

TRENDS IN THE 1980s AND EARLY 1990s

As the standard of living rose during the 1980s there was a corresponding rise in public expectation of better preventive care. During the same period a number of trends, which had been discernible for some time as increasing the potential for screening in British general practice, began to exert mutual reinforcement, so that in aggregate their effect became far more significant. These were:

1. *Increase in practice size.* The average practice had more patients, and more staff to deal with them, than was the case in earlier decades. There was an increasing use of secretaries, receptionists and nurses, and they were better trained.
2. *Improvement in premises and resources.* General practice became less of a cottage industry.
3. *The computer revolution.* Computerisation extended patchily but inexorably into practices throughout the country, both internally within the practices and externally in record linkage with local health authorities and with hospitals. Practice staffs became better informed about the capabilities of computers. The pace of this trend increased dramatically with the GP contract of 1990.
4. *Better record keeping.* There was a slow but steady improvement in practice record keeping. More and more practices started to maintain age/sex and disease and recall registers, and the accuracy and quality of existing registers also improved. Individual record cards of patients were better kept and were updated more regularly. Variability between individual practices in the quality of record keeping was still huge, but less so than formerly. A consensus began to develop as to what records should be kept, and how they should be updated. The Royal College of General Practitioners deserves credit for encouraging much of this.
5. *Consumerism.* Patients expected more help from GPs, and of a higher standard. They were better informed; they expected to be kept informed and they became more critical and litigously minded. Patients' associations and self-help groups sprang up.
6. *The preventive approach.* In response to patient demand, more practices swung towards an interventionist policy.
7. *Development of protocols.* A number of initiatives were taken by the Royal College of General Practitioners, alone or in collaboration with other royal colleges and organisations of health professionals, to draw up provisional protocols for screening and surveillance in British general practice (RCGP Reports from General Practice 1981–9). In March 1989 these culminated in the first nationally agreed programme for child health surveillance in this country, drawn up by a joint working party formed by representatives of the principle professional bodies concerned (RCGP et al 1989). In other screening areas, however, national protocols were not finalised; furthermore they were all, of course, dependent for their implementation on governmental approval and effective funding.
8. *The political impetus.* The 1990 GP contract (see below) has increased the emphasis on preventive medicine and all political parties have declared their support for this aim, although offering widely varying means to achieve it.

The effect of all this has been a substantial increase in general practice screening and surveillance of all kinds since the early 1980s. However, there was virtually no corresponding increase in public funding for these activities, apart from cervical cytology and paediatric surveillance; so for the most part, each individual practice continued to do its own thing. Some screening initiatives, most notably the national breast screening programme, involve GPs but are organised mainly from within the secondary care sector (see Chapter 23).

THE NATIONAL HEALTH SERVICE REFORMS

We are now entering a radically new phase in the history of screening. The White paper, *Promoting Better Health*, appeared in 1987 (DHSS 1987) and proposed an ambitious package of preventive primary care. It received a mixed reception from the profession, although at the time it was cautiously welcomed by the Royal College of General Practitioners (RCGP 1988).

The proposals have subsequently been crystallised into the new contract for general practitioners (DHSS 1989), and this has now become reality. The crucial ingredients, from the point of view of this book, are the imposition of certain mandatory screening tasks, together with incentives for others. Specifically, the mandatory tasks are invitations for annual assessments of patients over 75, and invitations for screening to all those aged 15–65 who have not been seen for 3 years. The incentives include payments for surveillance of preschool children, and target payments for achieving specified levels of cover for immunisations and cervical cytology. There are also payments for holding special clinics for the purpose of health promotion.

The new contract has undoubtedly affected the workload and morale of general practitioners. There is a widespread feeling of having to work harder, or indeed to manipulate the system, to maintain income. There is a widespread view that an opportunity has been lost. Despite pleas to the contrary, a large number of untried innovations have arrived simultaneously, with little time being allowed for acclimatisation and no mechanism for evaluation. It has been argued that the contract concentrates on process to the exclusion of outcome, and on quantity to the exclusion of quality. While early indications are that the uptake of cervical cytology at least has risen, it remains to be seen whether there are other more substantial benefits to patient care, and whether these will be outweighed by the possible penalties (Lancet 1989).

Hot on the heels of the new contract has come the National Health Service reorganisation, with a purchaser–provider split, and the advent of the fund-holding practice. The arguments for and against these changes have been rehearsed too often to repeat here, and many of them are based on speculation and economic theory, rather than on hard evidence. The issues are discussed further in Chapter 3.

In principle, the new system should give rise to opportunities for innovative screening programmes but at the time of writing it is too soon to say whether this promise will be fulfilled. Without doubt, however, screening and surveillance have been placed very firmly on the political agenda.

In June 1991, in a significant departure from previous policy, the Department of Health published a consultative document, *The Health of the Nation* (DoH 1991), in which targets were proposed for the curtailment of preventable causes of mortality and morbidity, particularly cardiovascular disease, cancers, accidents, mental illness, diabetes and asthma. These targets are based on measurable outcomes rather than solely on process, and therefore set the scene for audit, on a national scale, of preventive health measures, including screening programmes. What impact this will have on general practice it is difficult to predict at the time of writing. While some commentators have remarked that it is more significant for what it omits than for what it includes, it can at least be viewed as a further step in the right direction.

After a long and painful gestation, screening and surveillance have at last arrived in general practice. It is now up to us to do all we can to keep the infant healthy. It is likely to prove to be an expensive and time-consuming business; but if successful, the dividends will be enormous.

REFERENCES

Andrews G R, Cowan N R, Anderson W F 1971 The practice of geriatric medicine in the community. In: MacLachlan G (ed) Problems and progress in medical care. Nuffield Provincial Hospitals Trust London

Arneil G C 1972 Urinary tract infections in children. Update. 1115

Ashworth H W 1959 Routine medical examination. Medical World. 90

Ashworth H W 1963 An experiment in presymptomatic diagnosis. Journal of the Royal College of General Practitioners 6: 71

Ashworth H W 1964 Presymptomatic diagnosis of carcinoma of the cervix. Medical World. August

Ayre J E 1947 Selective cytology smear for diagnosis of cancer. American Journal of Obstetrics and Gynaecology 53: 609–617

Bain D J 1977 Methods employed by general practitioners in developmental screening of preschool children. British Medical Journal 2: 363–365

Bickel H, Gerrard J, Hickmans E M 1953 Influence of phenylalamine intake on phenylketonuria. Lancet ii: 812–813

Branson M H, Constantine H P 1972 Designing multiphasic screening. Hospitals 46/9: 47

Brav S S, Kirber H P 1951 Mass screening for glaucoma. Journal of the American Medical Association 147: 1127

Breslow L 1959 Periodic health examinations and multiple screening. American Journal of Public Health 49: 1151

Collen M F 1965 A multiphasic screening programme. In: Teeling-Smith G (ed) Surveillance and early diagnosis in general practice. Office of Health Economics, London

Collen M F 1968 Automated multiphasic screening. In: Sharp C L, Keen H (eds) Presymptomatic detection and early diagnosis. Pitman, London

Collen M F, Rubin L, Davis L 1965 Computers in multiphasic screening. In: Stacey R W, Waxman B D (eds) 2 vols. Computers in biomedical research, Academic Press, New York: vol 1, p 339

Commission on Chronic Illness 1957 Chronic illness in the United States of America. Harvard University Press, Cambridge, Massachusetts

Cope J T, Smith D H 1967 A health week in rural general practice. British Medical Journal 2: 756

Cope J T, Smith D H 1972 A second multiple screening clinic in a rural general practice. Journal of the Royal College of General Practitioners 22: 113

Coope J 1974 A screening clinic for hypertension in general practice. Journal of the Royal College of General Practitioners 24: 161

Cowan N R 1972 The early recognition of disease in older people. In: Symposia on Geriatric Medicine. 1, 41–49.

West Midland Institute of Geriatric Medicine and Gerontology

Curtis Jenkins G H, Collins C, Andren S 1978 Surveillance in general practice. British Medical Journal 1: 1537–1540

Davidson L S, Donaldson G M, Lindsay S T, McSorley J G 1943 Nutritional iron deficiency anaemia in wartime. British Medical Journal 2: 95

Department of Health and Social Security 1987 Promoting better health – the Government's programme for improving primary health care. Secretaries of State for Social Services, Wales, Northern Ireland and Scotland. HMSO, London

Department of Health and Social Security 1989 General practice in the National Health Service: a new contract. Department of Health and the Welsh Office. HMSO, London

Department of Health 1991 The Health of the Nation. HMSO, London

Donaldson R J 1968 Screening procedures and the local authority. Journal of the Royal College of General Practitioners 16 (Suppl 2): 37–41

Donaldson R J, Howell J M 1965 Rotherham multiple screening clinic. British Medical Journal 2: 1034

Engel A 1968 Mass screening for asymptomatic disease as a public health measure. In: Perspectives in health planning. University of London, Athlone Press, London

Evans S M, Wilkes E, Dalrymple-Smith D 1969 Presymptomatic diagnosis. Journal of the Royal College of General Practitioners 17: 237–240

Exton-Smith A N 1952 An investigation of the aged sick in their homes. British Medical Journal 2: 182–186

Ferrer H P 1968 Screening for health. Butterworths, London

Freeling P 1965 Candidates for exfoliative cytology of the cervix. Journal of the College of General Practitioners 10: 261

Gelman A C 1971 Multiphasic health testing systems: reviews and annotations. US Department of Health, Education and Welfare, Rochville

Gershon-Cohen J, Hermel M B, Berger S M 1961 Detection of breast cancer by periodic X-ray examination. Journal of the American Medical Association 176: 1114–1116

Gould G M 1900 A system of personal biologic examination. The condition of adequate medical and scientific conduct of life. Journal of the American Medical Association 35: 134

Gregg I 1966 The recognition of early chronic bronchitis. Journal of the College of General Practitioners 11 (Suppl 2)

Guthrie R 1966a Proceedings of the International Conference on Inborn Errors of Metabolism, 20. US Department of Health, Edcuation and Welfare, Washington DC

Guthrie R 1966b Population screening by the Guthrie Test for phenylketonuria in South-East Scotland. British Medical Journal 1: 764–766

Guttmann D, Naylor G R 1967 Dip-slide: an aid to quantitative urine culture in general practice. British Medical Journal 3: 343

Hart C R (Ed) 1975 Screening in general practice. Churchill Livingstone, London, pp 46–48

Hart J T 1980 Hypertension. Churchill Livingstone, London, p 133

Hodes C 1969 Report of a visit to the United States of America as WHO fellow to study multiphasic screening. BMA Library (cyclostyled copy), London

Holleb A I, Venet L, Day E, Hayt S 1960 Breast cancer detection by routine physical examinations. New York Journal of Medicine 60: 823–827

Hooper P D 1965 Assessment of milestones in general practice. Journal of the Royal College of General Practitioners 51: 89

Hooper P D 1971 Developmental assessment in general practice. The Practitioner 207: 371

Hsieh R K, Gilroy F D, Greberman M 1971 Automated multiphasic health testing: a health services R & D Laboratory. US Department of Health, Education and Welfare, Washington DC

Illingworth D G 1970 The health check in practice. Educare, Hemel Hempstead

Irwin W G, Neill D W 1970 Biochemical screening in general practice. British Medical Journal 4: 56

Jungner G 1965 Chemical health screening. In: Teeling-Smith G (ed) Surveillance and early diagnosis in general practice. Office of Health Economics, London

Jungner G, Jungner I 1968 Chemical health screening. In: Sharp C L, Keen H (eds) Presymptomatic detection and early diagnosis. Pitman, London, pp 67–108

Kaiser R F et al 1960 Journal of the National Cancer Institute 25: 863

Kerr I F 1972 A well women clinic at Ashton-under-Lyne. Journal of the Royal College of General Practitioners 22: 108

Lancet 1989. Editorial: The new GP contract: will patients suffer? Lancet ii: 936–938

Last J M 1963 The clinical iceberg in England and Wales. Lancet ii: 28–31

Lloyd G 1967 Cervical cytology in general practice. Journal of the Royal College of General Practitioners 13: 63

Logan R F 1964 Control of chronic disease in general practice and industry. Journal of the College of General Practitioners 11 (Suppl 1): 94–100

MacDougal I A 1970 Some views on developing the community health team. Health Trends 2: 70–71

Meyrick R 1962 A geriatric survey in general practice. Lancet i: 393–395

Papanicolau G N, Traut H F 1943 Diagnosis of uterine cancer by vaginal smear. Commonwealth Fund, New York

Pearse I H 1970 Periodic overhaul of the uncomplaining. Journal of the Royal College of General Practitioners 20: 146–152

Pearse I H, Crocker L 1943 The Peckham experiment. Allen and Unwin, London

Percy-Robb I W, Cruikshank D, Lamont L, Whitby L G 1971 Biochemical screening in general practice: a clinical follow-up. British Medical Journal 1: 596–599

Pike L A 1972 Screening middle-aged men in a general practice. The Practitioner 209: 690–695

RCGP 1981 Prevention of arterial disease in general practice. Report from general practice no. 19. Royal College of General Practitioners, London

RCGP 1982, 1988 Healthier children — thinking prevention. Report from general practice no. 22. Royal College of General Practitioners, London

RCGP 1984 Combined reports on prevention. Reports from general practice nos. 18–21. Royal College of General Practitioners, London

RCGP, GMSC 1984 Handbook of preventive care for preschool children. Royal College of General Practitioners, General Medical Services Committee, London

RCGP, RCN 1986 Prevention and the primary care team. Report by a joint working party of the Royal College of General Practitioners and the Royal College of Nursing Society of Primary Health Care Nurses. Royal College of General Practitioners, Exeter

RCGP 1987 Preventive care of the elderly. Taylor R C, Buckley E G (eds) Occasional Paper no. 35. Royal College of General Practitioners, London

RCGP, RCOG, RCPath et al 1987 Report of the intercollegiate working party on cervical screening. Royal College of Obstetricians and Gynaecologists, London

RCGP 1988 Members' Reference Book. Royal College of General Practitioners, London

RCGP, BPA, GMSC, HVA, RCN 1989 Health for all children. In: Hall D M (ed) A programme of child health surveillance. Report of a joint working party. Oxford University Press, Oxford

Redhead I H 1960 The incidence of glycosuria and diabetes mellitus in general practice. British Medical Journal 1: 695

Rivett G 1965 Cervical cytology in general practice. British Medical Journal 2: 1531

Rotherham Report 1969 A multiple health screening clinic, Rotherham 1966: a social and economic assessment. Report prepared by the Social Science Research Unit. HMSO, London

Sault J 1973 Diagnoscreen in West Germany. Doctor 3 no. 2

Scott R, Robertson P D 1968 Multiple screening in general practice. British Medical Journal 2: 643–647

Sharp C L 1964 Diabetes survey in Bedford. Proceedings of the Royal Society of Medicine 57: 193–196

Sharp C L 1968 Opportunities and problems presented by screening procedures. In: Sharp C L, Keen H (eds) Presymptomatic detection and early diagnosis. Pitmans, London

Sheps C G 1966 Journal of the Royal College of General Practitioners 11 (Suppl 1): 105–106

Starte G D 1974 Developmental assessment in the young child in general practice. The Practitioner 213: 823

Starte G D 1976 Results from a developmental screening clinic in general practice. The Practitioner 216: 311

Thompson M K 1975 Geriatric screening. In: Hart C R (ed) Screening in general practice. Churchill Livingstone, London

Wilkerson H L, Krall L P 1947 Diabetes in a New England town. Journal of the American Medical Association 135: 209–216

Williamson G S, Pearse I H 1938 Biologists in search of material. Faber and Faber, London

Wilson M 1966 Some principles of early diagnosis and detection. In: Teeling-Smith G (ed) Surveillance and early diagnosis in general practice. Office of Health Economics, London

Winter C J, Clay S, Davis R 1972 Social medical examination in an integrated group practice. Journal of the Royal College of General Practitioners 2: 327

WMA Computer Panel 1973 Report on computers and community health in Japan by Dr Masakazu Kurata. British Medical Journal 3: 292

Wookey B E 1971 A well-woman clinic in general practice. British Medical Journal 1: 396

Wright H B 1971 The implications of automated health screening for the delivery of medical care. Community Health 3: 71–80

Wright J E 1966 The Bedford glaucoma survey. In: Hunt L B (ed) Glaucoma. Churchill Livingstone, London

Yoshisuke I 1973 Recent data and their analysis from the Toshiba multiphasic health screening centre. Medical and Biological Engineering 11: 15–26

2. Theory and its application

Cyril Hart

We have got to elaborate our own theory, suited to screening that is both effective and feasible in the normal conditions in which British general practitioners work.

Julian Tudor Hart 1975

Every specialty has its jargon, which enables workers in the field to define its limits and discuss its relevance to the world outside. Medical screening and surveillance depend for their justification as worthwhile activities on a well established theoretical corpus, but unfortunately little of this is known in detail, and still less is understood, by the average health care professional. Furthermore, its application to British general practice calls for special techniques and resources (especially in the formation of practice data banks), which are still undergoing development and as yet are far from perfect. All too often, an enthusiast will embark upon a screening programme without first defining its objective or its protocols with sufficient rigour. Sometimes insufficient thought is given to its possible repercussions on the community as a whole, and in particular on the individual whose health is under scrutiny. Such a sloppy approach can do more harm than good, and brings the concept of screening into disrepute. It is imperative, therefore, to define the terminology and to consider in some detail the theoretical basis of medical screening and surveillance that underlies the more specialised chapters of this book.

A short definition of medical screening is 'the detection of occult disease or defect by a test'. As long ago as 1957, this was elaborated by the US Commission on Chronic Illness as 'the presumptive identification of unrecognised disease or defect by the application of tests, examinations, or other procedures which can be applied rapidly' (Commission on Chronic Illness 1957). Screening tests sort out apparently well persons who probably have a particular disease or defect from those who probably do not. A further refinement would include, within the definition, the detection of 'a tendency to develop a disease', as well as the detection of diseases that are already established.

In this book the terms 'screening' and 'case-finding' will be used to describe separate and complementary activities. Screening is the application of a test to a symptom-free population, performed on the initiative of a medical professional, while case-finding is the opportunistic application of a test during a routine consultation.

Medical screening may be undertaken for research purposes (actuarial, statistical or epidemiological); to determine eligibility for a particular occupation; with a therapeutic objective, such as the formation of a data bank, or for the prescriptive treatment of disorders that are uncovered by the screen. It is with screening in this last category that we are chiefly concerned here. It may be conveniently divided into *monophasic* screening, in which search is made for a single disease or defect, and *multiphasic* screening, in which search is made for a number of different diseases or defects in the same individual, using a battery of tests, some of which may be automated. Monophasic screening is often limited to those individuals thought to be at risk of developing a particular condition, such as contacts of infectious diseases, e.g. open pulmonary tuberculosis; relatives of cases of familial diseases, e.g. glaucoma; those exposed to environmental or other hazards, e.g. pneumoconiosis in coal miners or blood disorders in radiographers; and vulnerable age/sex groups, e.g. carcinoma of the cervix in sexually active women.

When the feasibility of screening is being considered for a particular disease or defect, one has first to examine its *prevalence* (the percentage of those definitely having the condition) in the population under scrutiny. The prevalence is sometimes called the prior probability in US screening literature. If an ideal test existed, the population being screened would be divisible into two distinct groups — a large group comprising those definitely free from the disease and a smaller group (its relative size being a function of the prevalence) com-

A. Distinct groups

Numbers

Healthy group

Diseased group

Measurement

B. Overlapping groups

Numbers

Healthy group

Diseased group

Equivocal group

Measurement

C. Skew curve

Numbers

Tendency to stay healthy

Tendency to develop disease

Measurement

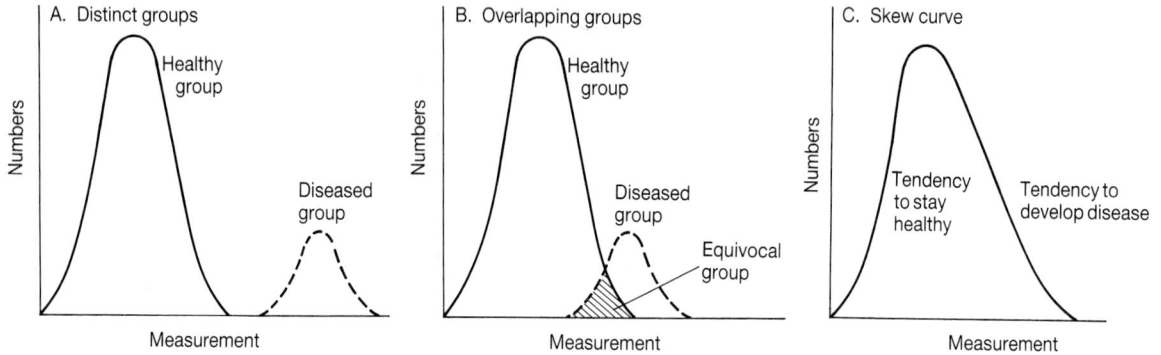

Fig. 2.1 Hypothetical distribution curves of healthy and diseased groups in a population.

prising those who have the disease. The graph of the reaction for each group of individuals to the test would show a normal distribution curve. The peak value for each curve would represent the average figure obtained by the test for that particular group. If the two curves were plotted on the same graph, the result would resemble that of Figure 2.1A. The more perfect the test, or the later the stage of the disease in the average member of the 'diseased' group under test, the further apart, horizontally, the two groups would be on the graph. In the later stages of a disease, of course, the need for screening would not exist, because the signs and symptoms would be so florid as to be self-evident.

Unfortunately, we do not know of any simple test for any condition worthy of consideration for screening, in which the normal and diseased populations (at an early stage in the disease process) can be sorted definitively in this convenient fashion. In practice, our tests are imperfect, so that the 'normal' and 'diseased' groups overlap, as in Figure 2.1B. Those members of each group in the overlapping portion of the graph would yield an equivocal test result and further investigations would then be necessary to sort them into their respective groups. How best to deal with those individuals whose test results lie within this overlapping portion of the graph is considered on page 18.

This is not the end of the problem, however, because as our ability to detect the earliest stages in each disease process becomes more powerful, the two groups will overlap more and more, until they merge completely, producing in most cases a single frequency distribution curve skewed to the right, as in Figure 2.1C. Those with a tendency to develop the disease will then respond to the test with figures that occupy the right-hand side of the graph, while the figures from the healthy section will occupy the left-hand side. A typical example of such a curve is that obtained when a male or female population of a given age group is screened for hypertension, using for the test either the diastolic or the systolic blood pressure (Hart 1980, Figs 4, 5, 7).

THE BORDERLINE BETWEEN HEALTH AND DISEASE

We come now to the problem of defining the borderline between health and disease of the population under test. This depends in the first instance on the selection of an arbitrary figure, the *cut-off point*, which divides the test results into two. Ideally, if the curves of the 'healthy' and 'diseased' groups did not overlap, the cut-off point would lie between them, and produce a perfect division, as with the central line 'A' in Figure 2.2. If the cut-off point were to be set too low (line 'B') this would prove to be too sensitive, and would yield a number of *false positives* from among the 'healthy' group under test. If, on the other hand, the cut-off point were to be set too high (line 'C'), the test would be too specific, and would yield a number of *false negatives* from among the 'diseased' group.

Consider the position when the two curves of the 'healthy' and 'diseased' groups of the population overlap (Fig. 2.3 SP and SE). If the cut-off point is shifted well to the right, there will be a small number of false positives among the 'healthy' group, and a larger number of false negatives among the 'diseased' group: the test will prove to be highly specific. *Specificity* may be defined as the proportion of people without the condition who are correctly identified on being screened. Put in another way, it is the probability that a test result will be negative when the condition is absent.

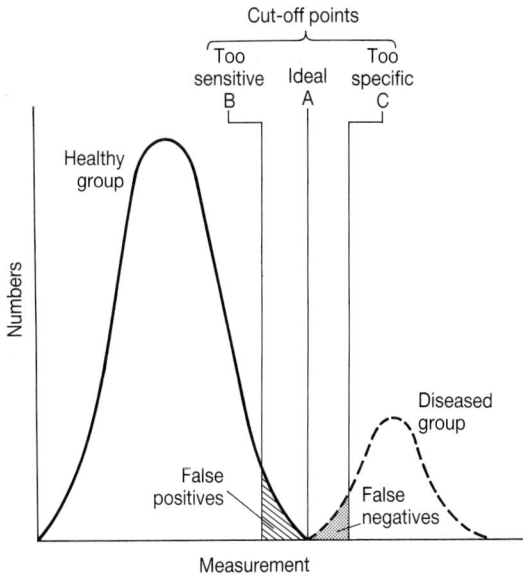

Fig. 2.2 The borderline between health and disease — choosing the cut-off point.

imaginary screening population of 1000, in which it is postulated that 85 persons really have the disease for which the prevalence is being investigated. A highly sensitive test with a high cut-off point, would yield 80 true positives, 15 false positives, and 5 false negatives; conversely, a highly specific test with a low cut-off point would yield only 70 true positives and 5 false positives, with 15 false negatives. The highly sensitive test would have a sensitivity of 94.1% and a specificity of 98.4%; against this the highly specific test would have an unacceptably low sensitivity of only 82.3%, yet its specificity at 99.5% would be a mere 1.1% higher than that obtained for the highly specific test. Either way, the *misclassification rate* in this instance would remain the same, at 2%.

It will be seen that the initial test rarely completes the screening process; the best it can do is to sort out those who may have the disease from those who almost certainly do not have it. Clearly, as the screen has been initiated by the doctor, he/she cannot afford to have any more false negatives than are absolutely unavoidable. The problem of low sensitivity is the ethical one of failing to identify and help those individuals with the disease in its occult stage, for whom the promise of help has been implicit in the invitation to attend for screening (see Chapter 4). The test to aim for must therefore be one that is highly sensitive, in which the net is of fine mesh, so that few people with the disease escape detection (Fig. 2.3 SE). The relatively high number of false positives which may result from this approach will, however, cause unneccesary worry unless these patients are investigated quickly by the application of more precise diagnostic criteria, followed by rapid and powerful reassurance that they do not in fact have the disease.

Conversely, a shift of the cut-off point to the left would result in a highly sensitive test, with a large number of false positives and a relatively small number of false negatives. *Sensitivity* may be defined as the proportion of people with the condition who are correctly identified on being screened. Put in another way, it is the probability that a test result will be positive when the condition is present.

The concepts of sensitivity and specificity are considered mathematically in Table 2.1, using an

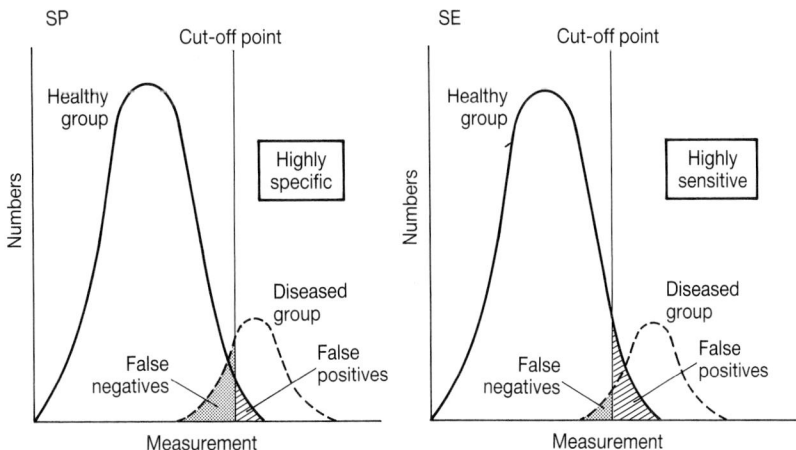

Fig. 2.3 SP and SE Sensitivity, specificity and the cut-off point.

Table 2.1   Mathematical definitions of screening terms (hypothetical figures)

Index		Cut-off point		
		Ideal	Highly sensitive	Highly specific
X = No. of persons screened (= A + B + C + D)		1000	1000	1000
A = No. of true positives (identified correctly)		85	80	70
B = No. of false positives (identified incorrectly)		0	15	5
C = No. of true negatives (rejected correctly)		915	900	910
D = No. of false negatives (rejected incorrectly)		0	5	15
A + D have the disease (= constant)		85	85	85
B + C do not have the disease (= constant)		915	915	915
Prevalence (= constant)	$= \dfrac{A + D}{X}$	8.5%	8.5%	8.5%
Yield	$= \dfrac{A}{X}$	8.5%	8.0%	7.0%
Predictive value	$= \dfrac{A}{A + B}$	100.0%	84.2%	93.3%
Sensitivity	$= \dfrac{A}{A + D}$	100.0%	94.1%	82.3%
Specificity	$= \dfrac{C}{B + C}$	100.0%	98.4%	99.5%
Misclassification rate	$= \dfrac{B + D}{X}$	0	2.0%	2.0%

Bearing this in mind, a convenient way to select the cut-off point is to plot specificity and sensitivity as ordinates against the test figures as abscissa; for a common condition the cut-off should be somewhere near to the point where the two graphs cross. An example of this method was given by Wright and Perini (1987) in their paper on screening for hidden psychiatric illness using the General Health Questionnaire (Fig. 2.4). Please see Chapter 3 for discussion of economic aspects.

YIELD AND PREDICTIVE VALUE

Two other terms that need consideration when examining the effectiveness of a screening test are its *yield* (defined as the number of cases of a condition that are correctly identified by the programme) and its *predictive value* (defined by Last (1988) as the proportion of positive screening results that are correct). Both are explained mathematically in Table 2.1. Yields in excess of 5% are rare in the monophasic screening surveys reported to date; figures of 2–3% are more common (Butler 1989). As might be expected, the higher the yield, the less serious the condition being investigated; nevertheless, some of these trivial conditions, especially in children, can create a high nuisance value for those concerned; plantar warts may be cited as a typical example.

The concept of yield is important in statistical and epidemiological surveys, in which whole populations are screened without prior knowledge of their disease status. It is of considerably less use, however, in the type of prescriptive screening carried out in general practice, because a number of individuals in the practice population will usually already be known to the practice as having the sought-for condition. Our interest when screening in general practice lies in those in whom the condition has been previously unidentified, and is therefore unknown to the practice. Clearly,

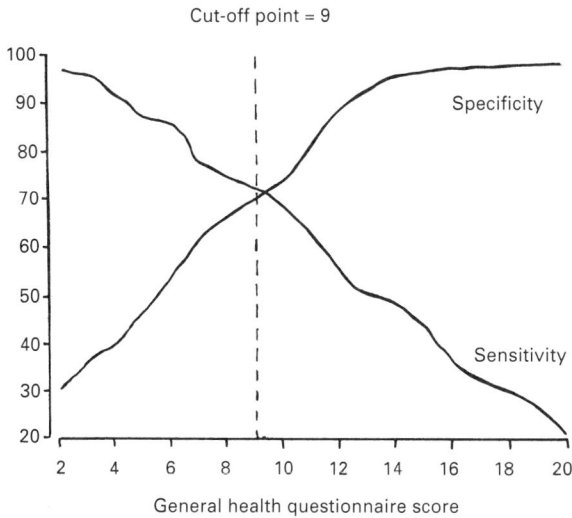

Fig. 2.4   Determining the cut-off point from graphs of sensitivity and specificity (from Wright and Perini 1987).

whenever possible, known cases of a disease should be excluded from a screening programme for that disease; this will have a marked effect on the yield. Moreover, once a continuous programme is under way in a practice population, the yield of fresh cases would be expected to fall progressively in successive screens, according to the law of diminishing returns. The total yield for the whole programme would, however, increase slowly until a plateau is reached. This difference between the yield of epidemiological screening and general practice screening is explored on page 20, under the impact of the time factor on practice screening programmes.

The predictive value is sometimes called the posterior probability in US screening literature. It is related fairly closely to sensitivity. As an indication of efficiency, it is more useful than yield in general practice screening; its importance lies in the fact that when the predictive value is low the programme is faced with the high cost, financially and otherwise, of further investigation of those who are deemed positive on screening but are subsequently found to be normal. Such predictive values for screens as have so far been determined vary widely from around 5% to over 80%, according to the condition being screened. As with yield, however, the predictive value will vary according to whether known cases of the disease are excluded from the screen, and it will also show some variation in successive screens on the same population.

Bayes' theorem, which was described by the eighteenth-century English mathematician, the Reverend Thomas Bayes, states that the predictive value is a function of the

prevalence. The equation is quite complex, not a linear relationship. When the prevalence is high, a positive test is more likely to represent a true positive; conversely, when the prevalence is low, a positive result is more likely to represent a false positive.

Neither yield nor predictive value are easy to calculate from the existing literature reporting most screening programmes because, so far, the true prevalence of the particular condition that is being sought in the population under test seems rarely to have been accurately determined. The process involves identifying unequivocally in the case of each and every individual in the screened population, whether he or she has or has not got the condition being searched for, even in its earliest stages — clearly a most difficult and exacting task. An absolute answer is often impossible; we have to satisfy ourselves with something within reasonable distance of the ideal.

Both these factors — yield and predictive value — are acquiring increasing importance as the planning of screening becomes ever more refined in the relentless search for greater productivity and economy. It is essential, however, to appreciate the difference between epidemiological and prescriptive screening when yield and predictive value are being considered at the planning stage of a programme. Those engaged in academic general practice would do well to note this caveat.

It is possible to apply still more sophisticated statistical analysis to screening programmes, by using the test data to measure the *probability* that a particular individual in the screening population might have the condition sought for. This approach involves an understanding of statistical concepts such as *confidence values* and the application of Bayes' theorem to multivariate analysis. However, the relevance of trying to apply such complicated mathematical techniques to routine prescriptive screening procedures in general practice is questionable, because so many indeterminate factors come into the equation. Those interested are referred to standard textbooks on medical statistics, clinical decision making and epidemiology (Dowie & Elstein 1988, Last 1988).

THE TIME FACTOR

A screening survey result is valid only for the moment which the test is performed. At any one time, a practice population will have within it a healthy group (H), certainly free from the disease under scrutiny, an identified diseased group (I), already known to have the disease before screening starts, an occult diseased group (O), having the disease but as yet unidentified and an equivocal group (E), for whom the screen by

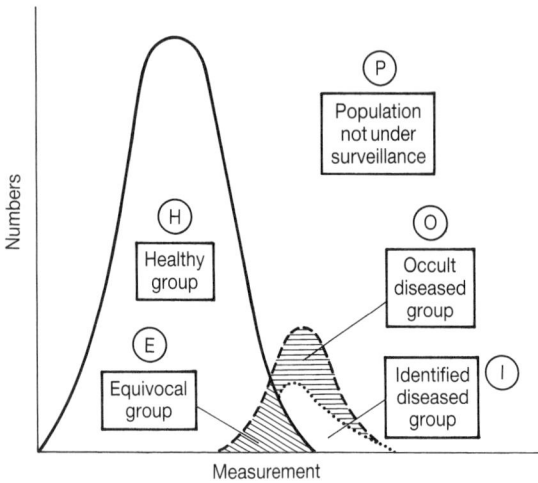

Fig. 2.5   Groups under surveillance.

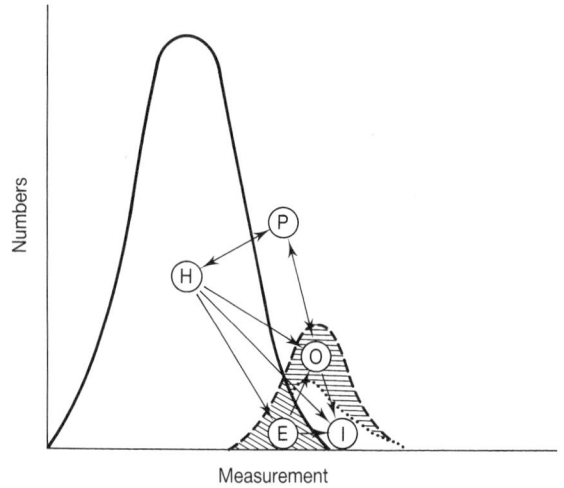

Fig. 2.6   Movement between groups — the time factor.

itself will not yield a definite answer (Fig. 2.5). As time passes, however, some occult disease becomes florid, some individuals cross the border from equivocal to established disease, and some healthy individuals develop occult or florid disease. There is, as a result, a dynamic shift to the right in the graph of our screened population with the passage of time. This is shown in Figure 2.6 by arrows, which indicate the movements between particular groups. The graph is further modified by movement of patients into and out of the population under surveillance. A typical practice population in the UK might well have a 5–8% turnover during the course of a single year. In Figures 2.5 and 2.6, the population *not* under surveillance, i.e. outside the practice, is represented by (P).

Because individuals within each group are forever moving into other groups, it is clearly desirable that *prescriptive screening of the population under scrutiny should be repeated at intervals*. Indeed, many feel that whenever a particular screening activity is started up in a practice, there should be an implicit assumption that the practice has undertaken an on-going commitment to monitor the future prevalence of that condition within the practice population. Such monitoring is an important component of the concept of surveillance. Early detection of disease is one of the distinguishing features of effective primary care.

The frequency of repetition of a particular screening process within a given population will be determined by many factors, which may often be in conflict with each other. Much depends on the natural history of the disease under scrutiny, the rapidity of its development and its disabling or lethal capability. The expense

factor is obviously important and account has also to be taken of the effect of screening on the workload of the practice. A further complicating factor is that it is often convenient and economical to screen for more than one condition at a time. The situation in each practice has to be considered on its merits. It is because of the wide variability of circumstances within different practices that nationwide screening programmes working to a fixed universal protocol are so difficult to establish.

RISK FACTORS AND THE CUT-OFF POINT

Screening parameters are sometimes selected to identify a tendency to develop disease, rather than to detect established disease as such. Such a tendency may depend on one or more risk factors demonstrable in the heredity, environment, metabolism or lifestyle of the individual under scrutiny. For example, hypertension and high blood cholesterol are well known risk factors for ischaemic heart disease and stroke. Most risk factors show a skew curve distribution on screening, and choice of the cut-off level for intervention in the lifestyle of an asymptomatic patient can be very difficult (Fig. 2.7). Julian Tudor Hart, who has perhaps the best understanding of such problems as they affect British general practice today, referred as long ago as 1975 to the dialectical conundrum of 'making rational qualitative decisions from shifting points on continuous distributions of quantity'. Quite apart from the ethical dilemma, strong economic pressures can be brought to bear to keep to a minimum the numbers of asymptomatic patients kept for long

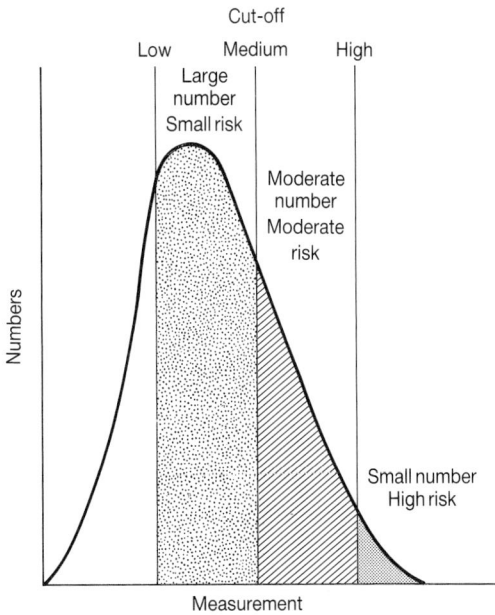

Fig. 2.7   Risk factors and the cut-off.

periods on high-cost drugs and other expensive modifications of lifestyle. Many considerations enter into this equation, not least being the compliance of the patient. For example, most therapists would be reluctant to offer antihypertensive drugs to an obese elderly patient with mild hypertension who found himself unable to give up smoking or to achieve weight reduction. Surveillance in such cases might well start with encouragement to attend the appropriate practice health clinic.

TYPES OF SCREENING ACTIVITY

Screening in British general practice appears to be developing in two different but complementary directions, which may be conveniently labelled as the Swedish and USA models.

The Swedish model (intervention screening)

The Swedish model is based on whole populations, with special emphasis on covering those sections that tend (for whatever reason) to slip through the net. Such activity, by its very nature, usually has to be state-funded in some way, and British general practice is well placed to deal with it. The GP contract, introduced in 1990, exemplifies this approach. It can be monophasic or multiphasic, and it includes, among other areas:

1. antenatal care;
2. paediatric surveillance;
3. geriatric surveillance;
4. screening for cancer of cervix and breast.

The US model (consumer demand-led screening)

The US model is for individuals, and usually it has to be funded privately by individuals or by employers' organisations. Some of this (an increasing amount, whether we like it or not) will take place in general practice. It includes, among other areas:

1. insurance examinations;
2. fitness examinations (for adoption, school, employment, sport, driving, etc.);
3. examinations of individuals for government departments (for Attendance and Mobility Allowances, etc.);
4. health checks, which are usually run by the private health-care market (BUPA, etc.), although limited health checks every 3 years for non-attenders between 16 and 74 are now a feature of GPs' workload (DHWO 1989). A significant difference between these new NHS directives and the programmes of the private health-care market is that the latter usually incorporate sophisticated automated chemical and other tests to buttress physical examination.

Outside these two models are *opportunistic screening* and *case-finding* (see Chapter 9).

SCREENING CRITERIA

What criteria should be adopted when the introduction of a particular screening programme in our own practice is being considered? Clearly there will be many local factors to take into account, which will vary from practice to practice. Before spending time and effort examining these domestic issues, however, it would be as well to look at each proposal from a more detached point of view. In 1965 Dr J Wilson drew up a cautious set of criteria, suggesting that they be applied to all prescriptive monophasic screening (Wilson 1965). These criteria are summarised in Table 2.2. In the USA, modifications were suggested by Dr P S Frame in 1975 and 1986, and these were summarised by Hudson and his colleagues (1988) (Table 2.3). It should be pointed out, however, that while such criteria may have a permanent value, the feasibility of their application in any particular case was not set for all time. What is

Table 2.2   Dr J Wilson's screening criteria (1965)

The disease
  An important problem
  Recognised latent or early symptomatic stage
  Natural history must be understood (including
    development from latent to symptomatic stage)

The screen
  Suitable test or examination (of reasonable sensitivity and
    specificity)
  Test acceptable by population being screened
  Screening must be a continuous process

Follow-up
  Facilities must exist for assessment and treatment
  Accepted form of effective treatment
  Agreed policy on whom to treat

Economy
  Cost must be economically balanced in relation to possible
    expenditure on medical care as a whole

Table 2.3   Recent screening criteria in the USA (Hudson et al 1988)

The problem (the disease)
  Must have a definite effect on length or quality of life
  Must affect substantial numbers of people
  Must have a natural history that is well understood
  Must have an asymptomatic period during which early
    detection and intervention reduce morbidity and/or
    mortality more than with later intervention

The early detection test
  Must be sensitive, specific and predictive (test
    characteristics). Predictive value is probably the most
    important characteristic
  Must be safe. As the test is applied to 'everyone' small
    problems are magnified, and rare, untoward effects
    become significant
  Must be inexpensive. Follow-up costs for further
    evaluation should be considered
  Must be easy to administer. Adequate human and
    equipment resources should be available
  Must be acceptable to health care providers and patients

Early (or primary) intervention
  Must be more effective than late intervention
  Must have benefits that outweigh risks. Small or rare risks
    are magnified, as are small gains
  Resources must be available for follow-up diagnostic or
    therapeutic intervention if required
  Must be acceptable to patients and health care providers

Table 2.4   Suggested additional guidelines for screening in the UK

1. The screening test must be acceptable for the population
    under test
2. It must be applied according to an agreed protocol
3. If the test is clinical, and not recordable in numerical
    terms, then there must be generally recognised and
    strictly applied criteria for distinguishing between the
    healthy and the potentially or established diseased groups
    of the population
4. If the results are recordable in numerical terms then the
    cut-off point must be chosen so that the test is of
    reasonable sensitivity, specificity and predictive value
5. The test result will be communicated quickly and
    humanely to each individual under test
6. When the initial result is equivocal in a particular case,
    further investigations will be undertaken quickly, so that
    the issue is fully resolved
7. Screening must be a continuous process; the frequency of
    repetition must depend primarily on the natural history of
    the disease; recall procedures must be effective
8. Test data for each individual must be preserved and
    passed on to those responsible for subsequent screening
9. Ideally, those responsible for surveillance will be those
    who were responsible for screening
10. There should be an agreed policy on whom to treat
11. The cost of screening and surveillance must be
    economically balanced in relation to possible expenditure
    on medical care as a whole

applicable in the USA might not always be suitable in British general practice. Account must also be taken of medical and economic progress and public expectations, including the increasing risk of litigation. The criteria should therefore be re-examined and their applicability reviewed afresh at the planning stage of each new screening programme. What was desirable, possible and affordable in 1965 differs widely from what is desirable, possible and affordable today. We could do with a new set of basic criteria for British general practice, with greater emphasis on surveillance.

In the case of nationally established programmes, such as that for cervical cancer screening, the major arguments as to desirability and feasibility are unlikely to be of local concern, for they should already have been carried out at national level. But for more modest projects within the practice it may be impossible, or at best very difficult, to obtain reliable statistical and economic information that can safely be applied locally to screening for a particular disorder. The local prevalence of the disorder may be particularly difficult to assess. A search should be made of the literature at one's postgraduate centre library and at the library of the Royal College of General Practitioners. If this fails to provide the necessary information, a pilot study is usually advisable before embarking on a full-blown screening commitment within the practice. Particular care should be taken to monitor screening projects undertaken by trainees within the practice. Trainees are birds of passage, and it is not unknown for a practice to be left with the embarrassing task of winding up a project after its initiator has moved on elsewhere.

When implementing a screening programme it is important to minimise its possible penalties. In addition to the basic criteria mentioned earlier, the guidelines suggested in Table 2.4 may be helpful.

ASSESSMENT AND SURVEILLANCE

The term *assessment* is sometimes used very loosely in screening literature, as if it is just another word for screening. Muddled definitions can sometimes be an indication of muddled thinking in a wider sphere. Thus in *Healthier children — thinking prevention* (RCGP 1982), developmental assessment is defined as 'serially examining children to see if they are growing up normally. It is for healthy children essentially a form of...screening'. Some government publications also use the word in a screening context. Thus in the new GP contract (DHWO 1989), the GP receives an enhanced capitation fee for an annual review of elderly patients, which includes, enthusiastically: 'social assessment; mobility assessment; mental assessment; assessment of the senses (hearing and vision); assessment of continence; and general functional assessment'. Applied to the whole geriatric population, this is an astonishing programme. Full-scale assessment of geriatric problems such as these can be a painstaking and time-consuming task, necessitating the employment of sophisticated and expensive technical procedures by a range of specialised teams. Such detailed assessment, although no doubt desirable, will often be beyond the resources and the competence of the GP; one can only hope (against all experience) that the Government will be able and willing to fund it adequately.

It seems wise, however, to differentiate in this book between *screening* (defined on p. 15), which is usually a function of primary care, and *assessment*, which is essentially a secondary task, concerned with the specialist investigation of a potential or established disorder that has been detected on screening or case finding and referred for consultant advice with a view to establishing a diagnosis and planning the management of the disorder.

Surveillance, like assessment, is a term that needs to be defined closely within the context in which it is being used. It is applied in this book to the on-going supervision of the preventive care of a practice population. Its inclusion in the book's title takes note of the fact that to mount a screening operation in general practice is to incur an obligation to deal with the consequences of the screen. Where the result of the screen is equivocal for a particular individual, we must ensure that the uncertainty is resolved quickly and humanely. Where a new condition is identified, we must ensure that effective treatment and subsequent monitoring of the condition is offered. If there is no effective treatment, then there should be no screen. Screening has to be looked on as a continuous activity, and the interval between repeat screens is crucial. All this is implied in our use of the term 'surveillance'. We would include some health promotion activities within the term, but in practice we have excluded, for the purposes of the book, most health education and all immunisation. Their inclusion would have turned the book into a full-scale but unwieldy treatise on preventive medicine in general practice.

REFERENCES

Butler J R 1989 Child health surveillance in primary case; a critical review. HMSO, London
Commission on Chronic Illness 1957 Prevention of chronic illness. Harvard University Press for the Commonwealth Fund, Cambridge, Massachusetts
Department of Health and Welsh Office 1989 General practice in the National Health Service: a new contract. Department of Health and the Welsh Office, HMSO, London
Dowie J, Elstein A S 1988 Professional judgement: a reader in clinical decision making. Cambridge University Press, New York
Hart J T 1980 Hypertension. Churchill Livingstone, Edinburgh
Hudson T W, Reinhart M A, Rose S D, Stewart G K 1988 Clinical preventive medicine. Little, Brown and Co., Boston
Last J M 1988 A dictionary of epidemiology, 2nd edn. Oxford University Press, New York
RCGP 1982 Healthier children — thinking prevention. Royal College of General Practitioners, London
Wilson J M G 1965 Screening Criteria. In: Teeling-Smith G (ed) Surveillance and early diagnosis in general practice. Office of Health Economics, London
Wright A F and Perini A F 1987 Hidden psychiatric illness; use of the General Health Questionnaire in general practice. Journal of the Royal College of General Practitioners 37: 164–7

FURTHER READING

Frame P S 1986 A critical review of adult health maintenance. Parts 1–4. Journal of Family Practice Vol 22: 341, 417, 511 and Vol 23: 29
Hart J T 1975 Screening in primary care. In: Hart C R (ed) Screening in general practice. Churchill Livingstone, Edinburgh
Wilson J M G and Jungner G 1968 Principles and practice of screening for disease. Public Health Papers No. 34. World Health Organization, Geneva

3. The economics of screening

Calum R Paton

SUMMARY

This chapter outlines some criteria, drawn from economics, that can be used in considering screening and
devising screening programmes. It then considers the key
policy issues confronting screening in Britain. The future
of screening, both generally and in general practice, will
be influenced by the changes in the National Health
Service brought about by the White Paper *Working for
Patients* (Department of Health, 1989a) and the changes
in NHS organization which followed it.

The first question to ask about screening concerns
its purpose and intended benefits, whether conducted
in the public or the private sector. It is then necessary
to set consideration of outcomes and benefits alongside
costs and risks. Naturally, such calculations are not
simple — differing social values and uncertainty are generally prevalent. The qualification of costs and
benefits need not be narrowly construed. Although
economics cannot dictate or change one's values, it
can lead to a clarification of the consequences of a particular value, which may in turn lead to consideration
of how compatible it is with one's other values.

In the context of screening in general practice in the
substantially publicly-funded National Health Service,
a key concept is naturally that of *opportunity cost* — to
what alternative use can the resources used in screening programmes be put (whether to alternative screening programmes or to other programmes altogether)?

Recent trends in UK health policy relevant to the
evolution of screening are discerned and discussed.
Radical proposals for primary care in the UK, generally based on introducing the principles of the market
place into primary care, are now being advocated and,
in some cases, implemented. Likely consequences of
this, based on consideration of economic and other
incentives, are traced.

ECONOMIC CONCEPTS

Economics in itself cannot help us to make choices
between objectives or outcomes. What it can do is provide tools for analysing alternative routes to these
objectives and for comparing the costs and benefits of
so doing.

A *cost-effectiveness* study, for example, tells us either
how to achieve a given objective at the minimum cost
or how to use a fixed pool of resources to maximise an
output. For example, the cost-effectiveness of a family
planning programme could be measured in terms of
the minimum amount of resources that need to be
spent to achieve a given number of averted births, or
alternatively, the maximum number of averted births
achievable from a given sum of resources.

Cost–benefit analysis is used for broader purposes —
namely, to attempt to quantify total costs and total
benefits (perhaps construed very broadly) from rival
activities and to choose how to spend one's resources
accordingly. For example, one might attempt to trace
the costs and benefits of environmental protection as
opposed to road safety. In health care, one might
attempt to compare the costs and benefits of screening
for cervical cancer and of coronary artery bypass graft
operations. Simply to describe this choice shows the
difficulties involved in actually making it.

Cost–benefit analysis in the health arena has been
adapted to *cost–utility analysis* — converting the monetary value into measures of health status. This latter
term is both a measure of outcome from health care
activities and an initial gauge of the challenges that
must be addressed by health care activities. Thus, the
costs of a particular activity may be compared with the
benefits in terms of, for example, life years gained or
quality of life gained. The recently publicized controversial measure known as the Quality Adjusted Life
Year (QALY) is an example of this type of analysis in
practice.

The notion of *opportunity cost* is an important one. The opportunity cost of an activity is the alternative use for the resources: that is the alternative benefits to be derived for a given sum of money. Thus, instead of comparing benefits and costs, one can look at the relative benefits from the expenditure of a given sum of resources. In considering benefits and costs, one should notice that a distinction must be made between the *arithmetical difference* between costs and benefits (if costs outweigh benefits, the idea would be that the project should not proceed) and the *division* of benefits by costs. For example, a project may have benefits only marginally more than costs (producing a benefit–cost ratio of little more than one) yet, because of the large sums of money involved, it may provide *absolutely* more benefit net of cost than a project with a higher benefit–cost *ratio*. In deciding how to allocate resources, the assumption of most economists would be that the aim is to maximise benefit net of cost. (In practice, of course, when comparing like with like, the higher the ratio of benefit to cost, the more likely it is that resources should be invested in that activity.)

However, as one invests more in a particular activity, there may be a *diminishing marginal utility/benefit*. It is a question in practice of paying attention to such factors when 'doing the calculation' concerned to maximise benefit.

APPLICATION TO SCREENING PROGRAMMES

Spending resources on screening programmes is merely one use of the resources generally available in health care, which itself is merely one use of resources generally (whether public or private). Determining the mix between public and private resources is not a question to be decided by economists although, as in other areas, they may have advice as to how to measure relative benefits from the different modes of employing resources. It is then up to society to gauge the importance and salience of different benefits, or indeed the degree to which there is a consensus on what constitutes a benefit and what does not.

If, for example, a society rates the eradication of certain diseases or the equalisation of health status among different social classes above the 'benefits' derived from private consumption, then there may be a case for either wide-scale public ownership of resources or high taxation to provide high government expenditure, or both. At the macro-level, it is naturally a political choice as to which are the more important or 'real' benefits.

In practice, the health care budget is decided in most societies by a political process, rather than by a rational or pseudorational process of comparing alternative uses of resources when distributed to different Ministries. Decisions then have to be made as to how different health care programmes are to receive resources. Thus, before one decides which alternative screening programme can profitably be financed, a more basic question seeks the rationale for spending the money on a screening programme as opposed to another activity altogether. At this level, one is faced with questions such as 'What is the benefit of spending a given resource on prevention or promotion as opposed to cure or care?'

Just as studies have shown that very different sums of money may be spent to 'save one human life' by different Ministries (for example by the Department of Transport as opposed to the Department of Health) (Mooney, 1984), very different sums of money will be spent to save one human life through different screening programmes. This is because such decisions are not made solely by economists using the kind of framework outlined here. Political pressures to institute screening for cervical cancer or breast cancer will usually help to determine the budget for a number of years, perhaps as a result of chance factors spotted by the media highlighting needs in these areas as opposed to others.

The basic criterion for the economist is to work within social preferences. If, for example, these preferences argue that money ought to be spent to maximise the saving of human life, the economist will be able to point to the capacity of different screening programmes to do this, and will therefore be able to advise upon the levels of investment in different programmes to maximise the objective. Given the fact that there are likely to be diminishing marginal rates of return to investment in different activities, then it is likely that a total budget will be allocated amongst different activities, rather than allocated purely to one or two.

Screening may not be worthwhile at all, for example, if the illness being screened for cannot be treated. Even 'productive' screening programmes may reach a limit beyond which investment produces no more benefit to patients. Criteria for screening are discussed below.

Things become more complicated when objectives are multiple. For example, the QALY attempts to incorporate into a measure of outcome not just increases in life (due to increase in length of life lived or to saving of life) but also quality of life. These are two conceptually different things, which cannot be compared unless by making a particular value judgement. For example, 'hard cases' and 'unhappy' conclusions arise from the use of QALYs and these illustrate the difficulty of using the framework on its own to make decisions. Should one save 10 years of one person's life or 1 year of ten peoples' lives, through investing in different health care programmes? Is the quality of life of a mentally handicapped person always judged to be less than that of a 'normal' person? Do QALYs discriminate against the elderly in that the latter will always have less life left, and probably lower quality of life, and therefore do not justify the investment — if rationing is inevitable — of, for example, kidney transplantation or dialysis?

In defining outcomes and benefits, especially in areas dealing with life, death and morbidity within health care, different ethical theories will inform one's initial premises. For example, a utilitarian may be willing to trade off life-years and quality of life. A deontologist may assert that life has a value in itself and that any decision as to where to invest resources that involves 'saving one and condemning another' (in other words playing God) should be done on a non – utilitarian basis — either by lottery or by factors such as mere order of presentation for treatment.

Similar types of value judgements inform the basic premises before economic analysis can be applied to screening programmes. How does one choose, for example, between screening for children's problems, the problems of the elderly, the problems of mid-life women, or for other groups? It may be that benefits can be demonstrated to be greater than costs for all programmes; how, therefore, does one choose? It is a political decision as to how much resource is available for these activities altogether.

One's values may help decide when faced with wide and thorny choices, especially in allocating public resources: for example, whether it is more important to save life through health expenditure, or to improve conditions in prisons and perhaps to preserve life rather than institute capital punishment for certain categories of crime; or, for example, to oppose abortion absolutely (even if one is therefore committing resources, whether public or private, to the protection of severely handicapped children), when resources saved could be used to save lives more generally in the health care system. Alternatively, one may, for example, be 'wholly opposed' on moral grounds to abortion, but see it as a lesser evil in certain circumstances, given a shortage of resources and rationing. In other words, one's values may clash (see also Chapter 4).

Merely alerting the reader to these choices shows that no economist can ever decide on economic principles what the answer is. However, once an adequate degree of consensus has been achieved (a tall order in itself), economists may be able to advise on how to maximise the saving of life through investment — for our purposes here, in different screening programmes.

Private and voluntary screening

It is important to distinguish private screening from voluntary screening. Private screening covers two important categories: first, elective screening for patients in the private sector and, secondly, mandated screening, the successful 'passing' of which is necessary for the individual's receipt of benefit or employment. In this book, voluntary screening is the elective presentation for screening by NHS general practitioners.

In the United States, private health insurance is the norm, and screening prior to acceptance in a health insurance plan is an important area of concern. Such screening has recently become more sophisticated, in an attempt to diminish the problem of 'adverse selection', whereby those enrolled in health insurance plans are already ill or at a higher risk of illness. With the current AIDS pandemic confronting public health, this is an area of drastic importance (Paton, 1989).

It often seems to be assumed that public health screening programmes ought to take account of cost–benefit criteria, but that private screening need not do so — if the patient is willing to pay. This, of course, begs the question as to the justice of the distribution of income that enables such arrangements. If, for example, a controversial 'cost–benefit' decision is made to deny screening programmes through public health care to an individual or group, their ability to pay in the private sector (or the justice of their having to do so) becomes a live political issue.

Another important economic concept arises here. Screening programmes may have as an important function the detection of infectious or other illnesses, which either have implications for the public health or for behaviour in the public realm. That is, whereas cervical cancer affects only the woman in question, on a narrow definition of 'affects', screening for AIDS is geared to the interests of a number of people other than the individual — the individual's current or future sexual partners, potential recipients of the individual's blood and other categories of contact. It is important that any cost–benefit analysis for such screening programmes take into account the full implications.

Economists call these implications *externalities*. Furthermore, screening may be considered to constitute a *public good* in certain circumstances, where it is difficult to discriminate in supplying the good, or a benefit that depends on all receiving it. For example, partial screening, leading only to partial immunisation, can diminish natural immunity in a population and increase risk of disease.

Follow-up

Another consequence of the public/private divide in both screening on the one hand and treatment or caring on the other, concerns follow-up. In other words, what is done as a result of screening? Just as there is no point in instituting a screening programme if problems detected cannot be treated, problems that can be treated but are not because of a lack of resources or poor management in the health service also raise questions about the purpose of screening. One might say that the full cost–benefit implications of a screening programme *with adequate follow-up* should be taken into account.

For example, in their new terms of service GPs are required to offer an annual visit to all their patients over 75 years of age. Whether this is a 'screening programme' that has undergone adequate evaluation is one question. Another question is whether, if the assumption is that the programme is worthwhile, adequate resources will be available to make the exercise worth the costs (including the opportunity cost of a GP's time). It may well be that geriatric and psychogeriatric services, as well as a whole range of support services (such as health visiting and the various local authority social services that would be required to care for the problems unearthed), will simply not be available, whether due to lack of resources or poor management (see also Chapter 25).

The challenge here is to ensure that the full costs and the full benefits of such programmes — with knock-on effects in sectors other than the immediate location of screening — are accounted for.

TYPES OF SCREENING

When considering *prescriptive* screening (i.e. screening undertaken with the deliberate objective of investigating abnormal conditions, as distinct from screening undertaken for actuarial, statistical or research purposes), it is important to distinguish, for economic and epidemiological purposes, between monophasic mass screening on the one hand and multiphasic mass screening on the other. Monophasic screening concerns the application of one or more screening procedures to the detection of an individual disease or defect, e.g. the choice between self-examination, physical examination and mammography in screening for breast cancer. Multiphasic screening concerns accommodation of a battery of tests aimed at the detection of a wide range of diseases or defects, e.g. cervical cytology may be combined with breast cancer screening.

For economic purposes, it is important to distinguish different benefits from, for example, a multiphasic screening programme and then apportion the joint costs as best possible to set against these different benefits, occurring as a result of components of the screening. A simple rule of thumb will sometimes be enough to apportion costs; at other times a more complex economic cost apportionment exercise is required.

Preventive screening is generally thought to be suitable where the disease has serious consequences, where there is a treatment that is more effective when applied after screening than at the symptomatic stage and where the detectable preclinical phase has a high prevalence (otherwise too few cases may be detected to justify the expense of a screening programme). In a context such as this, the opportunity cost of a screening programme may be considered — what can be done with the same resources set to another purpose? One may also, however, consider the opportunity cost of not screening. In other words the resources incurred by a national health service or society as a whole as a result of dealing with preventable disease may also be considered in their alternative uses. Thus, in deriving the benefits of a screening programme, one can look at the benefits for the individuals whose lives benefit and also at averted costs. Against this can be set the cost of the screening programme and the averted benefits of tying up the resources in screening as opposed to another activity. In essence, one is comparing opportunity costs — otherwise known as alternative benefits — for a given expenditure.

The natural history of a disease will tell us the stages at which intervention as a result of screening is possible or worthwhile. A promising innovation in applying economics to the organisation of screening programmes is the development of computer programs that analyse data about the natural history of diseases, populations and available resources for screening to suggest how best to target resources and how often to screen within budget constraints. Thus, while the wider type of cost–benefit questions cannot necessarily be answered by such analysis, cost–effectiveness studies may be considerably furthered. At the simplest level, this may allow us to address policy debates as to whether screening should be opportunistic, generalised

Table 3.1 Identification of costs and benefits in cost-benefit analysis study

Define actual costs and benefits in each alternative

Quantify all costs and benefits in monetary terms

Value all benefits in each alternative

Adjust each alternative for timing and uncertainty

Table 3.2 Costs and benefits of screening for cervical cancer versus not screening

	Costs	Benefits
Screening	Cost of smear	Reduced mortality-life years gained
	Number of smears	Productive capacity gained
	Cost of preventive action, i.e. cone biopsy	Reassurance to patient
	Costs of treating invasive carcinoma	Costs of treatment at symptomatic stage
	Costs of reducing mortality, i.e. pension payments, child allowance Patient costs — attendance for smears and biopsies	'Immeasurables' — peace of mind
Not screening	Cost of treating at symptomatic stage	Saved costs of tests
	Life years lost	Saved pension payments, child allowances and other expenses
	Productive capacity lost	Years of life saved, quality?
	Patient fear of carcinoma	

Table 3.3 A cost-effectiveness study of cervical screening

The Stages	Considerations
The objective	Determine and compare costs/years of life gained
The alternatives	Mass screening; opportunistic screening; targeted screening
The costs	Cost of the smear; call and recall systems; excision of cones; capital costs of equipment; patients' time and own costs Adjust for timing and uncertainty and quality of life

Determine cost/year of
life gained for each alternative

$$\boxed{\text{Total costs} \div \text{Years of life saved}}$$

Decision

Table 3.4 Costs of cervical screening

Cost of taking the smear
1. Fees to GP clerical staff; non-staff costs

Laboratory costs of analysing the smear
1. Consultant and technician time
2. Non-staff costs
3. Capital apportionment

Costs of administering a call and recall service

Consequent costs
1. Further diagnostic tests and treatment arising from a positive smear

The costs to the patient of transport and time

or targeted within a population. However, more precise questions can also be answered.

Cost-effectiveness studies (for example, concerning cervical cytology) may tell us how many smears are necessary and how many excision biopsies are performed for each death averted. Studies may also allow identification of avoidable deaths, i.e. people who die from cervical cancer who could have lived had the programme been more efficiently run. Both *efficiency* and *efficacy* are concepts that are distinguished from *absolute cost*: the relative cost of saving a life may be reduced, although the absolute costs of a screening programme may increase in order to do so.

Tables 3.1–3.4 allow one to think systematically about cost and benefits in particular screening procedures, by way of example.

THE NHS REFORMS

Much has now been written about the theory behind the 1989 White Paper, its likely consequences and the continuing stages of implementation. For the purposes of this chapter it is important to draw attention to the likely effect of budgets held by general practices for selective categories of hospital care, the replacement of planning and the development of market forces to a certain extent in the National Health Service and the introduction of the principle of 'managed health care', whereby patients are not referred wherever the general practitioner wishes but in accordance with preset contracts — whether made specifically by the general practitioner or by the health authority manager acting (one hopes) in cooperation with general practices.

An overall consequence of the reforms may be an emphasis upon quantity rather than quality in the National Health Service. A slogan is now gaining some currency to the effect that 'quantity is now a quality issue'. All health services in future will be delivered by specific contract. A positive side of this is that both doctors and managers will be forced to think more systematically about what, for which specific target groups and for what specific purposes, they can expect to receive for their money — and as a result the concept of programme budgeting will be more firmly established in the National Health Service. However, the entry of market forces on a greater scale than before will lead to the usual problems, and sometimes perverse incentives, that apply in 'competitive' markets. For example, suppliers may be able to collude and establish monopolies or oligopolies whereby prices are increased to the purchaser. There will be vast complexity in monitoring contracts (where, for example, the general practitioner or health service manager is responsible for the budget for patient care but where hospital consultants can affect this budget by tertiary referrals). Furthermore, patients' and doctors' wishes are to be subjugated to managers' wishes when control of budgets may have to be carried out at the expense of patients' wishes.

Despite the title of the White Paper (*Working for patients*), the essence of the Government's proposals is that rationing of health care is done overtly by managers (and to a lesser extent general practitioners), who are the consumers in the new market place, instead of rationing being done ex post and ad hoc by providers. Prior to the White Paper, patients were free to be referred anywhere, although the money did not necessarily follow the patient. General practitioners, of course, often indulged in covert rationing, for example, when they knew that long waiting lists or the inability of particular hospital departments to treat individuals (for example, elderly people requiring access to a urology department), made it simply not worthwhile to refer.

In the new system the money follows the patient, but the patient is not free to go or to be referred anywhere. A specific contract has to be made under which the individual patient's treatment is covered.

The new incentives, in essence geared to relating reward to workload, will have both good and bad effects. A good effect is that there may be a greater incentive 'to do more work' if resources follow the patient. The primary bad effect is likely to be the institutionalisation of rationing in the health service. Previously, there was no assumption that contracts and choices had to be made: patients sought care and somehow the books were balanced at the end of the day, although often with difficulty. (The problem was that authorities often faced silly incentives, e.g. some health authorities confronted with the need to make savings sometimes found that the resource allocation formula made it more rewarding for them to admit patients from outside their boundaries, whereas other authorities found it sensible to put up a ring fence to prevent patients from elsewhere being referred. There was no clarity in incentives to treat patients from outside the district.)

The crucial question here, of course, is the effect the new economic incentives are likely to have upon screening. It has been argued that the US Health Maintenance Organisation (HMO) lies behind the White Paper's reforms (Paton, 1988). The essence of the Health Maintenance Organisation in a US context is that, in contrast with traditional fee-for-service medicine whereby the provider sells health care to the patient and is paid fee-for-service, with an insurer picking up the tab as a third party payer, in a Health Maintenance Organisation the insurer and provider are one and the same. Thus, the perverse incentives of third party payment are removed. Each year the patient/consumer pays a capitation fee to join a Health Maintenance Organisation, which is then responsible out of its global budget for catering for that patient's needs. Some exclusions and deductibles to be paid by the patient may of course be written into the contract. However, the primary economic incentive is certainly not to oversupply care. Doctors who oversupply care while working for Health Maintenance Organisations may not have their contracts renewed because whether the HMO is for-profit or non-profit, it must make a surplus.

It is argued that Health Maintenance Organisations have a specific incentive to keep their enrolled populations well. If they do not, they will incur costs in treating and caring for patients. Thus, it is argued, they have an incentive to evaluate the worth of screening programmes and, where they are economically worthwhile using some of the criteria outlined in the first part of this chapter, they will be implemented. It is true that well-funded Health Maintenance Organisations in the US are often renowned for their screening programmes. One ought, of course, to distinguish between marketing-oriented screening programmes, geared merely to the public relations side of promoting a

Health Maintenance Organisation, and substantive screening programmes geared to detecting disease and preventing it.

In Britain, it is argued that, after the White Paper, District Health Authorities (which have always been a kind of HMO in that they have received money, from the Government in this case, to care for patients within a total global budget) now have a more overt economic incentive to make contracts for the care of their patients and to live within their resources: that is, to evaluate alternative ways of providing care to their patients, whether locally or not, and to contract accordingly.

However, one fundamental difference between the US HMO and the British HMO qua District Health Authority is developing as a result of the White Paper. *Individuals* make contracts with the US HMO, or contracts are made on their behalf by employers or, in some cases, by the Government. In consequence, the individual can expect redress if ill. In Britain, it is *managers* or in some cases *general practitioners* who make contracts for care on *behalf* of their patients. The incentive of the health authority is, of course, to live within its budget, although as a public authority it is not the income of individuals that directly depends on market success, except through bonuses and the like. Patients have contracts made on their behalf.

The British version of the HMO after the White Paper does not, however, have a contract to maintain the health of individuals or to treat them if, for example, due to the lack of screening programmes, the illnesses are not detected. Individuals have to accept the available supply and mix of services provided by health authorities or seek redress in the private sector if the public sector is not willing to pay. In consequence, there is no economic incentive to maintain an individual's health or prevent illness in the same way as in the United States HMO when it works well. That is because a key component of the market-place philosophy — the rights of the consumer protected by law — are absent in Britain. To make the Government's proposals in any way respectable a 'patients' charter' would be needed to accompany them. This fact has been recognized — at least in words — following the implementation of the NHS Reforms (DoH 1991). Such a charter would render the title of the White Paper, *Working for patients*, a little more appropriate. It should be pointed out that such a charter would not be a woolly statement of universal rights of the sort so often derided in the past. It would be a way of backing up the market-oriented responsibilities of health authorities.

The point is that a Health Maintenance Organisation in the United States may incur significant cost through the nature of its contract with an individual, or the individual's representative, if it fails to maintain health or treat the consequences. To reap such advantages in Britain, it would be important to set out specific targets concerning health outcomes for their enrolled populations, for GPs holding practice budgets and for District Health Authorities.

The success of the post-White Paper NHS ought to be judged by the monitoring of specific outcomes by the Department of Health, coupled, of course, with the provision of adequate funds to health authorities to fulfil such outcomes (funding being the original motivation, ironically, of the Prime Minister's Review that led to the White Paper) (Lancet, 1988). Instead, however, the Department of Health is defining the success of the White Paper not in terms of outcome but in terms of process — numbers of hospitals that become self-governing, cost improvements achieved and the like. The Government, in other words, is attempting to have its cake and eat it.

This situation is particularly crucial for screening purposes. Let us consider GPs with a budget for certain types of hospital care. Do they shorten local waiting lists by referring people for elective surgery, spend resources on various types of screening or attempt to 'live within their budget' by avoiding all but the most immediate in terms of health need presenting to the practice? It is not difficult to conceive of a situation whereby the last imperative becomes the most important.

The outlook for screening in general practice has therefore had to be addressed separately, under the aegis of the White Paper's proposals for the future of general practice and the family doctor's contract, by the design of specific norms for screening populations, upon which one component of the GP's income depends (Department of Health, 1989b). We may therefore have the paradox that GPs' salary incentives point in one direction and that budgetary incentives, where they hold a budget for hospital care, point in another.

THE EVOLVING NATURE OF THE GPs' CONTRACT AND ITS EFFECT UPON SCREENING

There was a sea change in the economic incentives offered to GPs by the Government during the 1980s. The assumption that better quality care can be provided by GPs who have fewer patients to cope with on their lists has gradually been replaced by arguments for and incentives towards an increase in the number of patients enrolled with doctors and in practices. It is no longer assumed that high quality is associated with low list sizes.

The Green Paper of 1986 (Secretaries of State, 1986) was the first government document to institutionalise this change and the White Paper has reinforced it. In essence, GPs' income in the future will depend upon the numbers enrolled (i.e. the importance of the capitation factor will increase), upon whether or not they meet norms for screening target populations and, of course, a variety of other factors, including practice allowances.

Broadly speaking, there is a move from reimbursement for individual or opportunistic screening to population-based screening. This may be expected to carry benefits *if* there is adequate flexibility, e.g. to cater for a practice with a low population enrolled in an inner city area where social deprivation, lack of communication and general cultural factors make the achievement of 'normal' targets for screening unattainable.

Competition between practices to attract patients, again promoted by the Green Paper of 1986 and developed further by the White Paper of 1989, may lead to weaker practices — those in inner city, deprived areas or sparsely-populated country areas again being starved of resources when they most need them. Just as 'greater choice' for parents and children in choosing which school to attend may at the end of the day lead to choice of children by schools rather than choice of schools by children (if demand outstrips supply), there is a parallel to be drawn here. Patients may find themselves starved of choice, and tied to practices that can offer them less as they are gradually starved of resources. Weaker consumers in the market place (both economically and sociologically speaking) tend to suffer rather than benefit from the introduction of increased market incentives.

GP budgets generally

It could be argued that the most hopeful means of institutionalising screening in general practice would be to give all budgets for health care to general practices, with appropriate provision for national and regional specialties and other exceptional considerations. Other proposals to establish economic incentives to increase cooperation between the family practitioner services and the hospital community health services have also been tied to the principle of GPs as firms.

For example, Bosanquet has adapted Alain Enthoven's ideas for an internal market amongst District Health Authorities to include primary care (Enthoven, 1985; Bosanquet, 1986). Adapting the idea of the internal market, as proposed by Enthoven,

would allow GPs to bid for district funds in return for providing defined services up to a specified standard. In other words, instead of, or as well as, markets being created *between* health authorities on the Enthoven model, they would be created *within* each district, with GPs as the suppliers. GPs would therefore be encouraged to become active economic agents in the provision of primary care, rather like firms in the wider market, instead of simply responding (as they tend to do now) in a more passive way to the demands made upon them by individual patients. Bosanquet, writing in 1986 and of course prior to the White Paper debate, saw such a proposal in the context of concern about variations in quality (to which attention had been drawn by the 1985 Royal College of General Practitioners Report, *Quality in General Practice*) (RCGP, 1985) as well as variations in efficiency.

In other words, each variable to be addressed — quality, efficiency or cost-effectiveness — could be addressed jointly through more coordinated strategy employing economic incentives.

In the 25 years since the 1965 Family Doctor Charter provided more resources to the family doctor, the employment of resources by different general practices has only recently become a policy issue.

In this context, screening programmes may be a particular focus, but the follow-up that is required to make screening programmes worthwhile may be an even more important focus. A number of services falling somewhere in between primary and secondary care are often not provided at all. Specific examples are preventive care of the elderly, follow-up for people with hypertension, special antismoking clinics and counselling and psychotherapy.

Market-oriented proposals, which allow the GP to contract with districts, might encourage GPs to combine in consortia to offer, for example, services for children, special care for people with long-term illnesses such as diabetes, epilepsy and hypertension, or general services currently provided by hospital and community health services. The argument, presumably, is that if general practices (whether alone or in consortia) could provide such care more cost-effectively, they might be encouraged to do so. Care globally within the NHS would be provided by the component of the NHS best able to do so within a constrained budget.

Thus, the institutional separations that, ironically, were encouraged by the separation in 1982 of Family Practitioner Committees (now called Family Health Services Authorities) from health authority control (although some were reversed by the 1989 White Paper) could be overcome not by yet more institutional tinkering but by direct provision of economic incentives to encourage cooperation and indeed competition between the Hospital and Community Health Services, on the one hand, and Family Practitioner Services, on the other. Overall, concerning the holistic care of the patient, Bosanquet argues that significant problems are caused by a situation where GPs and hospital doctors often treat the same patients yet have very little contact. The post-White Paper role of the Family Health Services Authority, now with increased managerial clout, should provide an institutional framework under which more effective and coordinated management of priorities within primary care can be made (Department of Health, 1989c).

CONCLUSION

This chapter has attempted to tackle two areas. On the one hand it has drawn attention to the basic economic concepts. On the other hand an illustrative, rather than definitive, discussion of how economic incentives can be used to consider general practice, with implications for screening, has been provided.

Much has, inevitably, been left out. For example, specific economic analyses can compare static versus mobile screening projects, and how cost-effectiveness, related to desired outcomes, relates to uptake and other factors (Henderson et al 1988). More generally, it would be useful to outline the epidemiological or 'non-economic' principles of screening and then to apply an economic analysis point by point to such principles. Key principles have been stated, and are listed in Chapter 2, Tables 2.2 and 2.3.

Once the early items of these tables have been 'ticked off', the cost of each stage of instituting the programme and generalising it to the population (if necessary) ought to be evaluated and the different options for screening and numbers of repetitions also costed. Possible 'non-financial' costs at each stage should also be taken into account and given a monetary value, however arbitrary, if a formal cost–benefit analysis is to be done. Benefits at each stage should then be evaluated to produce a total or composite benefit expected from the activity. Benefits and costs can then be compared.

No one prescription for screening policy will be acceptable or independent of individual values. Any screening procedure has to be evaluated as to its effectiveness, acceptability, cost and epidemiological factors, such as sensitivity and specificity. The overall worth of screening as opposed to other activities, such as cure or care of people once they have developed a disease, can also be affected or determined by one's own values. Economics can identify costs but the benefits of, for example, allowing people to develop a disease and then be cured rather than be prevented from having it in the first place are bound to be subjective. Economic concepts can clarify decisions but cannot 'make' them.

REFERENCES

Bosanquet N 1986 GPs as firms. Public Money March 1986
Department of Health 1989a Working for patients. HMSO, London
Department of Health 1989b Working paper 6. HMSO, London
Department of Health 1989c Working paper 8. HMSO, London
Department of Health 1991 The patient's charter. HMSO, London
Enthoven A 1985 Reflections on the management of the National Health Service. Nuffield Provincial Hospitals Trust, London
Henderson J, McKenzie L, Haiart D 1988 Economic evaluations of the Lothian mobile mammography screening project. Health Economics Research Unit, University of Aberdeen, Aberdeen
Lancet 1988 Anonymous editorial: The NHS at 40 –skeletons at the birthday feast. Lancet ii: 79–80
Mooney G 1984 Valuing human life. (Nuffield/York portfolios) Nuffield Provincial Hospitals Trust, London
Paton C 1988 Trouble with the health maintenance organisation. British Medical Journal 297: 934–935
Paton C 1989 Medical testing and health insurance. British Medical Journal 298: 134–135
RCGP 1985 Quality in general practice (policy statement 2). Royal College of General Practitioners, London
Secretaries of State 1986 Primary health care: an agenda for discussion. HMSO, London

4. The ethics of screening

Peter Burke

INTRODUCTION

It will be clear to the reader from the contents of this book that decisions about screening are complex. They are based on considerations of individual and public welfare, on scientific evidence, on economics and on many other factors. Closely linked to all these is the question of medical ethics.

By medical ethics I mean the application of moral philosophy to medical practice, i.e. the critical examination of the arguments and counter-arguments that underlie various moral stances. The use of the term 'moral' does not imply any connection with religious belief. Medical ethics is distinct from the application of the law — the existence of an ethical principle does not imply that there is a corresponding legal sanction.

I will be focussing primarily on screening. Although there are many ethical issues in relation to surveillance in the broader sense, these fall outside the scope of this chapter. So do the more specialised ethical dilemmas, which have been discussed fully elsewhere, in particular antenatal screening for chromosomal disorders (Chapter 10, also Anon 1985, Dunstan 1988), screening for the human immunodeficiency virus (Chapter 36, also Bayer et al 1986), screening in the workplace (Chapter 38, also Bayer 1986, Lappe 1986) and the 'screening' of relatives of those, for example, suffering from Huntington's chorea (Chapter 10). I hope to concentrate on the more general issues, and draw most of my examples from the types of screening likely to be of most immediate relevance to the day-to-day work of general practitioners, such as blood pressure measurement, cervical cytology and screening mammography.

The debate on the ethics of screening has always been highly polarized, the protagonists on each side being described by Sackett & Holland (1975) as 'evangelists and snails'. I hope to be able to steer a middle course between the two, although I would like to make it clear that I am writing from the perspective of a practising GP, rather than that of a philosopher.

In many areas of medical behaviour we are helped by internationally agreed conventions, of which a number originate with the World Medical Association. They include, for example, the Declaration of Geneva on the behaviour of doctors, that of Helsinki on medical research, of Sydney on death, of Tokyo on torture and of Hawaii on the uses of psychiatry. There is no comparable declaration on screening. There are, however, widely-accepted pragmatic codes, in particular the criteria of Wilson & Jungner (1968) (see Chapter 2).

THE DOCTOR–PATIENT CONTRACT

The ethical issues surrounding screening are very different from those relating to routine medical care. The most important difference is in what is being offered, i.e. the nature of the implied contract between doctor and patient (Skrabanek 1988). In the words of Cochrane (1972): 'The "screener" is in an evangelical situation. His cry is "Come unto me, ye faithful, and I will cure your piles." He is definitely advertising and promising a result.' Cochrane and Holland (1971) further point out:

> We believe there is an ethical difference between everyday medical practice and screening. If a patient asks a medical practitioner for help, the doctor does the best he can. He is not responsible for defects in medical knowledge. If, however, the practitioner initiates screening procedures he is in a very different position. He should, in our view, have conclusive evidence that screening can alter the natural history of disease in a significant proportion of those screened.

The ethics of a test or screening programme, therefore, are closely linked to the question of whether it achieves what it purports, in other words they are linked to the programme's efficacy.

In looking at a diagnostic test one needs to consider the test, the patient and the circumstances:

1. To what extent does the test meet the accepted criteria — as described by Wilson and Jungner — of a good screening test? How acceptable, expensive, sensitive and specific is it? What are its predictive value and its yield? (for definitions see Chapter 2). Does the test measure a categorical variable, such as presence or absence of tumour cells, or a continuous variable, such as blood pressure? If the variable is a continuous one, is there a clear concept of where the cut-off point for intervention lies? Has the issue of how borderline findings will be dealt with been considered?
2. To what extent does the patient mandate and understand the test? Is consent implicit, explicit or indeed absent?
3. What undertakings are given by the tester? Is the test done 'opportunistically' at the tester's initiative, or has the patient sought it?

To offer a screening test that does not meet the basic criteria for efficacy, or to offer one that does but in a society where facilities are unavailable to deal with the consequences, is to make a contract that cannot be honoured.

ETHICAL PRINCIPLES

It is useful to look at the four major ethical principles that govern decision-making in medicine. The promotion of individual well-being is known as *beneficience*; the principle of not doing harm is *non-maleficience*; the principle of respect for *autonomy* (literally self-rule) means a respect for the capacity of individuals to think for themselves, make their own decisions and act freely; last but not least is the principle of *justice*.

A given action may involve a conflict between various ethical principles. While it may be argued (the deontological view) that certain duties are absolute and cannot be set aside under any circumstances, the alternative (consequentialist) view is that an action is 'right' when it has a positive benefit/burden ratio, i.e. when its 'benefits' outweigh its 'burdens' (or penalties), and 'wrong' when the reverse applies. In reality, the values to be attached to both benefits and burdens are very often a matter of individual judgement, so that decisions of this nature are far from easy.

Beneficience

A crucial question in any medical intervention is whether the likely benefit to the individual will exceed the likely burdens. A screening procedure is no exception. It will be carried out, first and foremost, in the hope of bringing benefit to the person being screened. I exclude here, of course, procedures with the protection of a third party as their stated purpose, and to which I refer on page 39.

The prime benefit of screening is the detection of treatable disease or abnormality, and for the individual whose life is prolonged or enhanced this is more than enough justification in itself. When a tragedy that could have been prevented by early intervention occurs it is understandable that the finger will sometimes be pointed at the doctor who did nothing. Thus, Hart (1987), who would undoubtedly be regarded as in the 'evangelist' category, states: 'We are surely under a moral if not a legal obligation to record blood pressure at least once in every 5-year span for every registered adult in our practice, if we are to prevent tragedies of this kind'.

The strength of the imperative, if such an imperative exists, depends, of course, to some extent on the test and the population in question. While, as in the case of blood pressure measurement and cervical cytology, it may be difficult to identify the particular individuals who have benefited, it should be possible to assess their number in relation to the number of people tested, i.e. the *yield* of the test. Thus, for example, the yield of cervical cytology, in terms of lives saved, has been estimated at 1 per 40 000 smears (Lancet 1985).

Benefit may come not only to those found positive. One of the hopes of the screener is that by offering a normal result they may: 'give health back to the patient'. Grimes (1988) among others, would argue that a negative smear is valuable because it provides reassurance. It can equally be argued, however, that it provides reassurance about only one relatively uncommon medical condition, of which the majority of patients would be unaware if it were not for the publicity surrounding cervical cytology campaigns.

Non-maleficience

'Primum non nocere' (first do no harm) is one of the oldest aphorisms in medicine. The aphorism is predicated on the belief that harm by commission is in an ethically different category from harm by omission. This belief may be less axiomatic now, at a time when screening features among the British GPs' terms of service. The patient who feels wronged through omission of a screening test may well be more and more ready to seek redress.

It is worth remembering that screening tests themselves have personal and social costs.

Examples of *personal costs* are:

1. The biological effects of the test itself, e.g. the mutagenic potential of mass radiography or even mammography (see Chapter 23). With large numbers of tests, risks that at an individual level are small, can be magnified greatly.

2. The psychological sequelae of having the test. The experience of being tested has been described as a 'memento mori', i.e. it fosters introspection (Skrabanek 1989). That this is more than a theoretical hazard has been demonstrated, for example, by Stoate (1989), who found significant deterioration in General Health Questionnaire scores in patients attending a coronary heart disease screening clinic, compared with controls. This was not attributable to patients who were found to have abnormalities, as these were excluded from the study. As Grimes (1988) put it: 'Promotion of health inevitably results in awareness of sickness'.

3. The very considerable psychological sequelae of being given a positive diagnosis, whether true or false. With a little understatement Marteau (1989) states that: 'a positive result in any screening test is invariably received with negative feelings'. Although Kinlay (1988) describes these as: 'the intangible costs' of screening, they are in fact perceptible, as shown by an increasing number of studies. Haynes et al (1978) drew attention to the increased absenteeism that followed a diagnosis of hypertension and Campion et al (1988) and Wilkinson et al (1990) report a marked increase in anxiety and morbidity among women who had been informed of an abnormal cervical smear result. Britten (1988), describes this response at a deeply personal level. Where the result is a true positive and treatment is available this cost may well be acceptable to the patient. Where, on the other hand, earlier diagnosis prolongs duration of known illness rather than life, it will almost certainly not be. This is the problem of what is sometimes called 'lead time'. There is a further difficulty where continuous, as opposed to categorical, variables are being measured — an example being blood pressure. A look at the blood pressure distribution in the population will show that for every patient with a diastolic pressure above 110 mmHg, there are two in the range 100–110 mmHg and five in the range 90–100 mmHg. Although the latter, in particular, do not require drug treatment and

experience little benefit from having been screened, we face the dilemma of whether to increase their anxiety by putting them on regular follow-up, or whether dishonestly to reassure them. 'Finding an abnormality through screening is a disservice unless effective management follows' (Fowler & Mant 1990). The guidelines in Chapter 2 (Table 2.4) have been drawn up in the hope that they will help mitigate these difficulties.

4. The effects of treatment for a positive test. Such treatments include a lifetime on medication for moderate hypertension — with the prospect of one stroke prevented for every 800 patient-years of treatment (Medical Research Council 1985) — and destructive surgery such as mastectomy and cone biopsy. As Sackett & Holland (1975) point out, screening greatly magnifies the potential for harm arising from unproven remedies.

5. Problems of inaccuracy. No test is 100% sensitive and specific, and it is frequently necessary to make a trade-off between these two characteristics (see Chapter 2). Given limited specificity, there will inevitably be some false positives, and in an uncommon condition these may far outnumber the true positives (90–95% of the positives from once-off mammography will turn out to be false positives). A false positive test will result at least in further investigation and a distressing period of uncertainty, and may indeed lead to inappropriate treatment. Conversely, the consequence of limited sensitivity is the existence of false negatives. Such a result is highly regrettable, as an undertaking has been given to detect the disorder if present, and this undertaking has not been honoured. A sense of false security has been created and in the future symptoms, such as breast lumps, which would otherwise be reported, may be ignored.

6. Misinterpretation of the result. A negative result, e.g. a normal blood pressure or cholesterol level, may be perceived by the patient as a mandate to continue an unhealthy lifestyle, for example to continue smoking. This, of course, would be a misinterpretation of the evidence. A large proportion of deaths due to coronary heart disease occur in individuals with a serum cholesterol — and indeed blood pressure — below the levels normally considered as warranting treatment (see Chapter 20). This problem applies particularly to tests that measure continuous — as opposed to categorical — variables, which are primarily predictive rather than diagnostic.

The costs of screening tests to society are largely economic (see Chapter 3). It must be remembered that such costs include not only the facilities, equipment and personnel to carry out the screening tests, but also those required for secondary assessment and treatment of any individuals found to be positive. They may also include time spent away from work to attend screening examinations. These costs can be considered under the heading of justice.

Some would argue that there is also a more subtle social cost involved in the conversion of 'people' into 'patients'. Illich (1975) describes the medicalization of prevention as a 'major symptom of social iatrogenesis'.

Autonomy

The principle of respect for autonomy is based on the view that mentally competent and mature individuals should make decisions about their own future, subject to the constraints required to ensure social order. The model of the paternalistic doctor who always 'knows best' is giving way to that of partnership between doctor and patient. This trend is no more than a recognition that medical professionals do not have, and have never had, any formal role in regulating their patients' lives.

Autonomy is often invoked by the proponents of screening, who would argue for the 'right' of the individual to know what is going on in his/her own body. The view is sometimes put by consumer groups, in relation to serum cholesterol and cervical cytology, that it is not for the medical profession to ration access to information about what are really personal attributes of the individual. There are screening programmes, particularly in the private sector, which are driven largely or wholly by the pressure of consumer groups based on this belief.

In a world of limited resources, however, questions of social justice must inevitably be weighed against individual autonomy, and we must be aware of the potential cost to others of acceding to requests for annual cervical smears or routine chest X-rays. Experience also shows that the 'inverse care law' (Hart 1971) applies for many screening tests, i.e. those who seek out the test are frequently those who need it least, and therefore a screening programme based largely on consumer demand will achieve a disappointing yield (a possible exception to this is breast cancer, for reasons that may be related in part to its social class distribution). As Hall (1989) puts it: 'In the end, it is not enough to offer tests. Screening without understanding will fail if it does not reach its target populations'.

Furthermore, even if we were to accept the principle of testing on request, the request must be an informed one. Concomitant with the right to be tested is the right to know something about the characteristics of the test, in particular its yield, predictive value and possible adverse effects, and the ability to make a decision based on this information. This is difficult.

To put this another way, in assuming the right to know, it is easy to forget the even more fundamental question of whether there is a wish to know, particularly bearing in mind the possible penalties of such knowledge.

One of the implications of living in a multicultural society is a wide range of perceptions of health and disease. It is easy for us as doctors to become so imbued in the mechanistic/bacteriological model as to deny the possibility of others. Most of us have patients, however, whose philosophy of life — for religious or other cultural reasons — is much more fatalistic than ours (see Chapter 39). To them, immunisation and cervical cytology are at variance with cherished beliefs, and will be unacceptable even after their benefits have been fully explained and understood. Screening programmes come into conflict with the right of autonomy where their introduction assumes that such minority views lack legitimacy. In this context it is worth drawing attention to the distinction between social validity and scientific validity (Atherly et al 1986): a scientifically valid programme may lack social validity because it is applied to a population for which it is unacceptable. 'While an informed consent signed by the patient is required to protect the doctor, no guarantee is signed by the doctor to protect a healthy person who is invited for screening, even though the harm/benefit ratio is much more unfavourable' (Skrabanek 1986).

Screening also becomes problematic where it enters the area of human behaviour. Some of the observations most strongly predictive of long-term outcome relate to lifestyle, e.g. smoking, drinking, diet and sexual habit. 'Screening for lifestyle' is very definitely a feature of the new-look GP contract in the UK, and falls within the ambit of this book. This may be entirely appropriate, leading to the sharing of new information or advice of a morally neutral kind.

Where, however, the end result of screening is apparent condemnation of an individual's lifestyle, there is cause to be reminded of H L Menken's observation:

Hygiene [meaning preventive medicine] is the corruption of medicine by morality. It is impossible to find a hygienist who does not debase his theory of the healthful with a theory of the virtuous. This brings it, at the end, into diametrical conflict with medicine proper. The aim of medicine is surely not to make men virtuous; it is to safeguard and rescue them from the consequences of their vices. The true physician does not preach repentance; he offers absolution. (Menken, Prejudices 1923; quoted in Skrabanek & McCormick 1989).

Decisions about the balance between quantity and quality of life will ultimately be made by the patient. There is a very real conflict between the role of the doctor as an ally, and that of what has been variously termed 'lifestyle police' and 'therapeutic clergy'.

Justice

With recent developments in the health service, dilemmas of distributive justice have very clearly entered the arena of general practice. GPs are increasingly aware that their interventions all carry, in financial terms, an opportunity cost, (see p. 26) i.e. in offering one service I am potentially diverting funds from others, as well, of course, as reducing my availability for routine medical care. Whether decisions about priorities are made by health authorities or by budget-holding practices they are inescapable. The decision may be, for example, whether to spend an extra pound on providing community nursing services, treatment for patients in end-stage renal failure or a breast screening programme. This becomes particularly relevant where the cost of a screening programme competes for funds with the treatment the programme shows is needed. It is ethically unacceptable to spend large sums on, for example, a cervical screening service if the result is that an underfunded colposcopy clinic is overwhelmed with new referrals and there is a backlog of anxious women with untreated dysplasia. It is of course much more difficult to decide at what point — if at all — it becomes mandatory to divert funds from screening to treatment, or vice versa (Doyal 1987).

THIRD PARTY BENEFITS

The question of who is the real beneficiary of screening has been discussed all too rarely (an example includes Berg & Fletcher 1986) but it is crucially important, and not always as obvious as it might seem. Screening is normally offered as bringing benefit to the person screened. However, in some instances the principal beneficiaries of screening are third parties, whether this means society as a whole, an insurance company, an employer or even the screener.

Benefits to society

Benefits to society at large may be of various kinds. Where, for example, routine examination reveals evidence of cardiac arrhythmia in a heavy goods vehicle driver, other road users may be protected, either by appropriate treatment or by well timed career advice. Similar benefits to persons unknown may accrue from the identification of a carrier of the human immunodeficiency virus. In such a case the interests of the individual screened may or may not also be served.

Insurance companies

Many 'routine medicals' are carried out for the purpose of assessing risk for life or permanent health insurance — this is a perfectly reasonable part of every GP's job and raises no ethical problems, providing that doctor and patient are clear about the nature and purpose of the examination. If there are findings carrying an adverse prognosis, this will serve to protect the insurance company and, if all is 'normal', the examination helps to ensure that the patient enjoys a low premium. It must be borne in mind that examination findings may be prognostically significant without carrying any therapeutic message — a single raised blood pressure reading is an example.

Where difficulties arise is in 'routine medicals' that are presented as being in the patient's interests. What happens if I, as a GP, find my patient's blood pressure to be 160/95? I will not normally wish to treat this level of blood pressure. None the less, if, the following week I receive a PMAR (personal medical attendant report) request from the patient's insurance company, I am required, subject to the patient's authorization, to divulge this reading to the company, although I know it will carry as a consequence a higher loading for my patient than would have been the case if he had not been screened. Furthermore, assuming the level of blood pressure is sustained, he will ever after be required to give an indication of this finding in insurance applications. The screening test has, in other words, been of benefit to the insurance company at the expense of my patient. Bearing in mind that blood pressure screening unmasks several borderline readings for every one requiring treatment, should we feel obliged to warn patients of this hazard before we screen them? I do not believe there is an easy answer. It should be added, of course, that consent to the release of such information must be truly informed, and there is good evidence that this is not always the case (Lorge 1989, Noakes 1990).

The employer

Pre-employment examinations raise no problems in themselves, provided again that the role of the doctor is made explicit. However, health status may affect the future of an individual within a company. Suppose an employee is found to have an asymptomatic ischaemic change on a routine electrocardiogram, and is considered the following year for promotion to a post of high responsibility, but asked informally whether he is in good health, what is he to say? Such a finding may, in other words, be prejudicial without there being any breach of confidentiality. What if the screening ECG is carried out as part of a health care package offered as a fringe benefit by the company to its employees? Is such an offer in fact more to the advantage of the individual or the company?

Benefit for the screener

Whatever the benefits to the person screened, the screener is by no means always a financially disinterested party. In many countries, and in the private sector, screening tests are directly reimbursable by the patient or by an insurance scheme, while in the NHS we are now working to targets, at least in relation to cervical cytology. An individual smear may contribute to the achievement of the GP's target — indeed this may be the one patient who can make the difference between achieving and not achieving it, with consequences in terms not only of money but also of kudos. In these circumstances, can doctors be completely certain of their motives when offering patients a smear? As Hart (1988) reflectively puts it: 'For the medical entrepreneurs themselves, the idea of simultaneously assisting the public health and filling their own pockets has been both a powerful spur to enterprise and an effective cure for doubt'.

In these circumstances the doctor's and patient's interests may coincide, but if they do not it would clearly be unethical to use coercion, manipulation or misleading information to achieve the desired objective.

In some projects screening is made possible through the provision of equipment by a third party, commonly one with a vested interest in the detection of abnormalities, e.g. the manufacturer of a lipid-lowering drug. It has been pointed out (Sharp & Rayner 1990) that this may raise difficulties and be in breach of guidelines concerning promotion of drugs issued by the Association of the British Pharmaceutical Industry (ABPI 1988).

There is one additional — and increasingly important — area in which screening may benefit the screener. In societies where litigation has become common, a doctor may well believe that screening tests are needed as a safeguard. Whether this is adequate justification is highly debatable.

SPECIFIC ISSUES

Speculative testing

In carrying out an unsolicited test in an apparently healthy individual, the professional offers an implied undertaking to detect the condition in question if it is present. Many of the procedures being advocated or introduced at present offer little reasonable prospect of this happening. This applies particularly in the area of well person checks among adults. Routine urinalysis as a method of detecting previously undiagnosed diabetics is an example. This test (using a trace on Clinitest as the referent value) may have a sensitivity as low as 34% (Galen & Gambino 1975) and a specificity of 88%, giving it a positive predictive value of only 6% (assuming diabetes is present in 1/50 of the population). A matrix illustrating this point is given in Table 4.1. If a patient is affected, it is thus more likely than not that the condition will be missed, while if the test is positive it is much more likely than not that the person is diabetes-free. Naturally, predictive value is directly related to prevalence (Bayes' theorem; see Chapter 2), so that a test that is of no value as a screening test may still be useful in a high-risk or symptomatic population.

Multiphasic screening

The concept of multiphasic screening (see Chapter 1) arises from the correct perception that the marginal cost of carrying out tests falls as the number of tests increases and therefore, particularly in the private sector, it has become customary to offer a 'package', including, for example, routine haematology, biochemistry, cervical cytology, electrocardiography, etc.

Multiphasic screening, although superficially attractive, carries particular difficulties. The desirable outcomes in screening are normality and unequivocal,

Table 4.1   Urine testing as a test for diabetes. Assume prevalence of diabetes = 2%, referent test is Clinistix (trace), population size = 10000

	Test positive	Test negative	Total
Diabetes	69	131	200
Not diabetes	1146	8654	9800
Total	1215	8785	10000

Sensitivity = 69/200 = 0.35
Specificity = 8653/9800 = 0.88
Positive predictive value = 69/1215 = 0.06
Negative predictive value = 8653/8784 = 0.99

treatable abnormality. A characteristic of multiphasic screening is that with increasing numbers of tests the former outcome becomes progressively less probable, without a necessarily corresponding increase in the latter. To date, despite several valiant efforts (Collen et al 1973, Holland et al 1977), it has proved impossible to demonstrate a clear improvement in health among populations offered multiphasic screening.

Screening and case-finding

So far, discussion has centred primarily on screening, i.e. the testing of populations, initiated by a medical professional. Much preventive medicine, however, is opportunistic, based on contacts initiated by the patient ('case-finding', see Chapter 9).

Sackett & Holland (1975) point out that case-finding is more easily defensible than screening. In screening the implied promise to the patient is that disease, if present, will be detected: 'We suggest that the marketing tactics of screeners imply improved health care just as those of beauty-cream manufacturers imply more youthful complexions; the latter can be punished under consumer and advertising codes if their advertising is misleading or when their products do more harm than good.' The case-finding clinician, on the other hand, offers only the undertaking that he will provide an adequate response to the presenting problem.

Arising from this, Sackett & Holland argue that the burden of proof is different for screening and case-finding. In screening there is a higher value attached to simplicity, acceptability, cost and sensitivity, while in case-finding there is a higher value attached to precision, specificity and predictive value.

On the other hand, there are a variety of special problems associated with case-finding. By its nature, it is not sought by the patient. It therefore represents an unmandated use of consultation time and the imposition of the doctor's agenda (see Chapter 9). The patient, unless unusually determined or vocal, will find it difficult to exercise his/her right not to be tested, or will submit to the test for fear of offending the doctor (this objection may be met, at least in part, if the patient is given the chance to escape, for example, by the offer of a subsequent screening appointment).

TESTING THE TEST

As pointed out by Sackett & Holland (1975), if a screening programme is implemented and later discredited the cost to the credibility of the medical profession is great. Further, the general acceptance of a screening programme, such as cervical cytology, makes effective studies of the validity of the techniques involved very much more difficult, both on practical and on ethical grounds.

A screening programme incapable of achieving certain minimal objectives is meddlesome and ethically suspect. There is, therefore, an imperative to ensure adequate evaluation of a screening programme before its widespread implementation. Although efforts have been made to evaluate many tests by the use of open studies, the only totally valid method is the randomised clinical trial. A trial of this nature entails a potential penalty to those individuals who are assigned to the control group. Proponents of the test may well consider such a study ethically unjustifiable, and argue that the onus is on the person wishing to conduct a trial to demonstrate the deficiencies in current knowledge. The most defensible position is one in which rigorous evaluation occurs at a stage where the test has been shown to have some efficacy, but has not yet come to be regarded as indispensible.

CONCLUSION

This book is written out of a firm commitment to the value of preventive medicine in general, and screening in particular. It does not, however, try to prescribe screening as a universal good. Ultimately decisions about the ethics of screening are dependent upon one's view as to the balance of responsibility for health maintenance between the medical profession and the individual.

Screening examinations can bring substantial benefits to individuals where they seek clearly-defined medical problems for which treatment is possible, available, and of particular benefit during the presymptomatic phase. Such examinations raise no ethical difficulties where these conditions are met and where the individual makes a conscious and informed decision to opt into screening. 'In participating in such services, doctors must be satisfied that the balance of advantage for the potential patient lies in undergoing the test and that some positive action will be taken in the light of the results obtained. In the absence of either of these requirements, it is probably unethical to proceed' (BMA 1988).

The argument that screening is a virtuous activity merely because it increases a person's understanding of his/her own body is problematic. There may be a kernel of truth in the observation that: 'In much wisdom is much grief; and he that increaseth knowledge increaseth sorrow.' (Ecclesiastes i, 18)

REFERENCES

Anon 1985 Geneticists ponder ethical implications of screening. Journal of the American Medical Association 254: 3160

ABPI 1988 Code of practice for the pharmaceutical industry. Association of the British Pharmaceutical Industry, London

Atherley G, Johnson N, Tennassee M 1986 Biomedical surveillance: rights conflict with rights. Journal of Occupational Medicine 28: 958–65

Bayer R, Levine C, Wolf S 1986 HIV antibody screening. Journal of the American Medical Association 256: 1768–74

Bayer R 1986 Biological monitoring in the workplace: ethical issues. Journal of Occupational Medicine 28: 572–577

Berg K, Fletcher J 1986 Ethical and legal aspects of predictive testing. Lancet i: 1043

BMA 1988 Philosophy and practice of medical ethics. British Medical Association, London

Britten N 1988 Personal view. British Medical Journal 296: 1191

Campion M J, Brown J R, McCance D J et al 1988 Psychosexual trauma of an abnormal cervical smear. British Journal of Obstetrics and Gynaecology 95: 175–181

Cochrane A L 1972 Effectiveness and efficiency: random reflections on health services. Nuffield Provincial Hospitals Trust, London

Cochrane A L, Holland W W 1971 Validation of screening procedures. British Medical Bulletin 27: 30

Collen M F, Dales L G, Friedman G D et al 1973 Multiphasic checkup evaluation study 4. Preventive Medicine 2: 236–246

Doyal L 1987 General practice and the ethics of resource allocation. Practitioner 231(1437): 1398–1401

Dunstan G R 1988 Screening for fetal and genetic abnormality: social and ethical issues. Journal of Medical Genetics 25(5): 290–293

Fowler G, Mant D 1990 Health checks for adults. British Medical Journal 300: 1318–1320

Galen R S, Gambino S R 1975 Beyond normality: the predictive value and efficiency of medical diagnoses. Wiley, New York

Grimes D S 1988 Value of a negative cervical smear. British Medical Journal 296: 1363

Hall C 1989 A test of public understanding. The Independent, August 21: p 17

Hart J T 1971 The inverse care law. Lancet i: 405–412.

Hart J T 1987 Hypertension, 2nd edn. Churchill Livingstone, Edinburgh

Hart J T 1988 A new kind of doctor. Merlin, London, pp 304–308

Haynes R B, Sackett D L, Taylor D W, et al 1978 Increased absenteeism from work after detection and labelling of hypertension patients. New England Journal of Medicine 299: 741

Holland W W, Creese A L, D'Souza M F et al 1977 A controlled trial of multiphasic screening in middle age: results of the south-east London screening study. International Journal of Epidemiology 4: 357–363

Illich I 1975 Medical nemesis. Marion Boyars, London, p 48

Kinlay S 1988 High cholesterol levels: is screening the best option? Medical Journal of Australia 148: 635–637

Lancet 1985 Cancer of the cervix - death by incompetence. Editorial. Lancet ii: 363–364

Lappe M A 1986 Ethical concerns in occupational screening programs. Journal of Occupational Medicine 28: 930–934

Lorge R E 1989 How informed is patients' consent to release of medical information to insurance companies? British Medical Journal 298: 1495–1496

Marteau T M 1989 Psychological costs of screening. British Medical Journal 299: 527

Medical Research Council 1985 MRC trial of mild hypertension: principal results. British Medical Journal 291: 97

Noakes J 1990 Double agent. British Journal of General Practice 40: 92–93

Sackett D L, Holland W W 1975 Controversy in the detection of disease. Lancet ii: 357–359

Sharp I, Rayner M 1990 Cholesterol testing with desk-top machines. Lancet 335: 55

Skrabanek P 1986 Preventive medicine and morality. Lancet i: 143–4

Skrabanek P 1988 The physician's responsibility to the patient. Lancet i: 1155–1156

Skrabanek P 1989 Ethics, screening and doctors' paternalism. Medical Monitor 2(47): 33–34

Skrabanek P, McCormick J 1989 Follies and fallacies in medicine. Tarragon, Glasgow

Stoate H 1989 Can health screening damage your health? Journal of the Royal College of General Practitioners 39: 193–195

Wilkinson C, Jones J M, McBride J 1990 Anxiety caused by abnormal result of cervical smear test: a controlled trial. British Medical Journal 300: 440

Wilson J M G, Jungner G 1968 Principles and practice of screening for disease. Public Health Papers No. 34. World Health Organization, Geneva

FURTHER READING

Beauchamp T L, Childress J F 1983 Principles of biomedical ethics, 2nd edn. Oxford University Press, Oxford

Bowman J E 1989 Legal and ethical issues in newborn screening. Pediatrics 83(5 pt 2): 894–896

Dunstan G R 1981 Medical ethics. In: Dunstan AS, Dunstan GR, Welbourn RB (eds) Dictionary of medical ethics, Darton, Longman & Todd, London

Fowler G 1983 Screening. Preventive medicine in general practice. Oxford, p 95

Mant D, Fowler G 1990 Mass screening: theory and ethics. British Medical Journal 300: 916–918

Skarabanek P 1990 Why is preventive medicine exempted from ethical constraints? Journal of Medical Ethics 16: 187–190

Organisation

5. The management of information

Gay Davies

You do not know where you are going
until you know where you are

INTRODUCTION

In order to progress we must learn, and in order to learn we must record, organise, analyse and compare the facts, using the information gained from this for future planning.

Even before the inception of the National Health Service in 1948 it was necessary for doctors to record and manage information regarding their patients. This was required not only for clinical reasons but also to ensure that accounts were submitted and paid. However, practitioners frequently worked singly and it was often impossible to build up a comprehensive medical history for a patient, as he/she did not always consult the same doctor.

The Insurance Act of 1911 eventually led to the birth of the medical record envelope that we use today, still known as 'the Lloyd George envelope'. With the introduction of doctors' 'panels' the need for simple, accurate records became more apparent. Since the commencement of the National Health Service and the setting up of the Central Register of patients (in Southport), each with a unique National Health Service number, it is possible for the medical record to follow the patient anywhere in Britain. This record should contain all the patient's medical history from 'the cradle to the grave'.

THE MEDICAL RECORD

The use of a universal envelope ensures that records can pass from practice to practice easily and that filing systems can be designed to accommodate it. Some years ago it seemed likely that the envelope size would be changed to A4 and although some practices did convert their records this has not materialised on a national

basis (except in Scotland) due, no doubt, to the cost of converting the filing systems of so many surgeries.

The front of the medical record should contain all information necessary to identify the patient, i.e. name, address, date of birth, NHS number, sex and responsible Family Health Services Authority. Simple colour coding, red for male, blue for female, enables the two sexes to be instantly identified. However, the data contained within the medical record are often not so well organised. The contents should be divided into two or more parts; the medical continuation record cards and the correspondence and test results. To maintain maximum efficiency these contents must be constantly reviewed, organised and pruned.

The record cards should be legibly written and arranged in chronological order, preferably secured with a treasury tag.

Correspondence and test results should be arranged in the same way, with the most recent at the top. It is really a matter of preference whether the results are filed with the correspondence or separately. All surplus paper should be trimmed to a minimum and folded carefully to allow insertion in the envelope. Wherever possible, A5 paper should be used (something that District General Hospitals fail to realise).

The abysmal state of record keeping in general practice has been emphasised many times (Heward & Clayton 1980, Fraser & Clayton 1981). There are still a number of practices with no age/sex register (see below) or whose registers are inaccurate. The most dangerous feature of this deficiency is that those children whose names are missing from the register are often those at greatest risk of illness, i.e. children aged under 1 year, those from broken homes, the children of immigrants or from social classes IV and V. No note may have been made of birth history, home background or genetic disorders in the family (Hart 1983).

In our practice at Yaxley, near Peterborough, we have initiated a system whereby all new babies are seen and

IMPORTANT NOTES

....

SIX WEEK CHECK

....

Weight:	Kg. (Cent.)	Head Circ:	cm. (Cent.)
Feeding:	BF/AF	Smile:	Weeks
Motor:		Tone:	
Fixing:			
PHYSICAL:	Chest	Heart	Abdo
	Herniae	Hips	Genit
	Fems	Reflexes	

PKU: ....

T4: ....

OTHER NOTES: ....

....

....

....

....

....

....

....

....

....

This record is the property of the Secretary of State for Social Services

BIRTH DETAILS

DELIVERY:			
WEIGHT:		SCU:YES/NO	
BREAST FED:		DUR^{N}	
GPU	HOSP.	DOM	APGAR:
No. OF SIBS.			
VACCINATION:			

Fig. 5.1 Yaxley group practice 6-week check/birth card.

examined by one of the partners at the age of 6 weeks; the health visitors are also involved in this examination. Full details of the birth are recorded (Fig. 5.1) and a check is made to ensure that the baby has been registered with the practice. At the same time the mother is reminded to make an appointment for her postnatal examination.

There are often many important omissions from the medical records and, at the same time, a great deal of irrelevant information is recorded and retained. Records need to be clear and concise and practitioners should have regard to recent legislation giving patients the right to see their personal medical records. Many practices have started to use problem orientated medical records, where the emphasis is changed from medical diagnosis to stating actual problems (medical or social) and an action plan formulated. 'SOAP' (subjective, objective, assessment and plan) is an excellent method

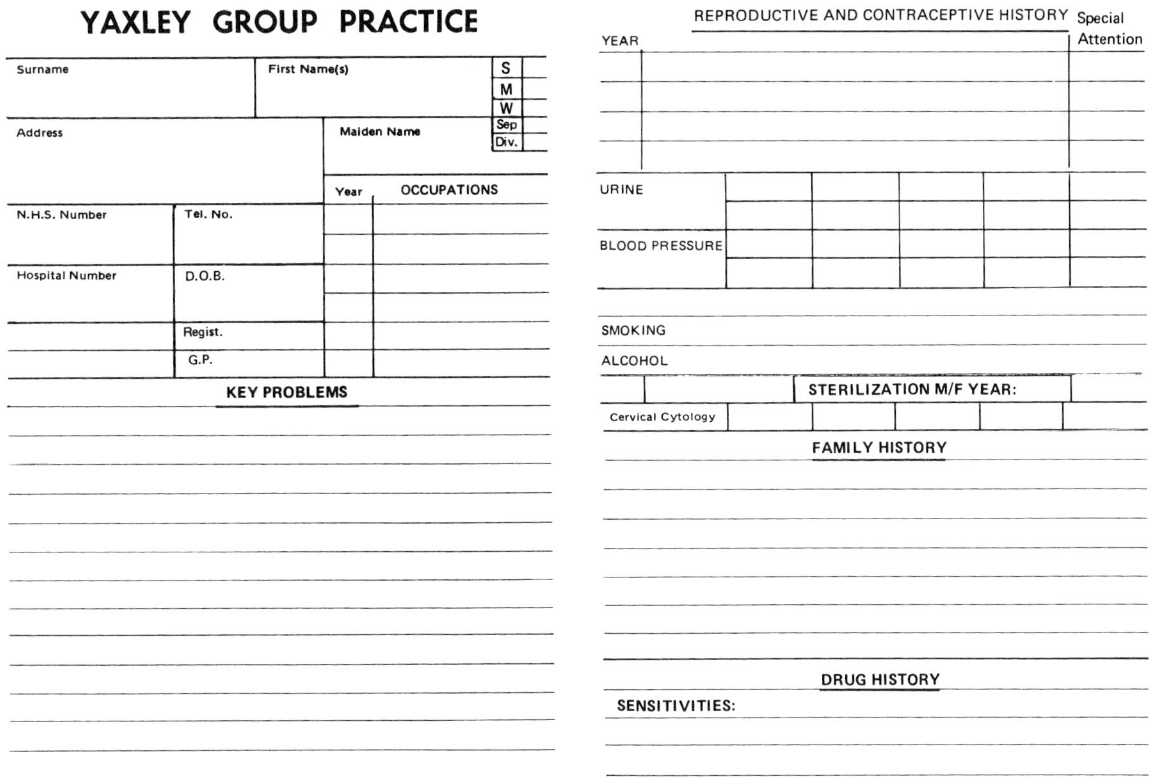

YAXLEY GROUP PRACTICE

Surname	First Name(s)		S
			M
			W
			Sep
Address	Maiden Name		Div.

		Year	OCCUPATIONS
N.H.S. Number	Tel. No.		
Hospital Number	D.O.B.		
	Regist.		
	G.P.		

KEY PROBLEMS

| REPRODUCTIVE AND CONTRACEPTIVE HISTORY | Special |
| YEAR | | Attention |

| URINE | | | | | |
| BLOOD PRESSURE | | | | | |

SMOKING

ALCOHOL

| Cervical Cytology | | STERILIZATION M/F YEAR: | |

FAMILY HISTORY

DRUG HISTORY

SENSITIVITIES:

Fig. 5.2 Summary card used by Yaxley group practice — front and back.

for logical recording of, and dealing with, the patient's presenting problem and, where other doctors continue the follow-up of the patient, it provides a clearer picture of what was intended at the time. Retrospective viewing of existing records in Audit will often demonstrate how difficult it can be to know what was truly happening at the time of consultation.

Whatever system of recording is used, certain features may be 'highlighted', either with boxes, underlining or fluorescent marker pens. Investigations, referrals and receipt of hospital letters may be written (or typed) in different ink, thereby facilitating quick recall of important information. Regardless of the progress of computerisation, the written record will continue to be of permanent importance in general practice.

SUMMARY CARD

The use of a summary card drawing attention to key problems, both social and medical, is essential and many practices devise their own cards rather than use the rather basic card provided by the Family Health Services Authority (Fig. 5.2).

Tait designed several cards (Tait 1978) to cover such aspects as social history. Relevant family histories, including deaths or significant events relating to family members, need to be regularly up-dated for all first-degree relatives to be useful. Hodgkin (1985) describes a graphic method of recording a family structure by means of a Family Gram, a method by which information may be recorded confidentially, and be of inestimable value in the consultation. Whatever method is chosen, an agreement on *what* information is to be recorded and *where* it is to be found is essential. Some practices are keen for all members of the Primary Health Care Team to have access to records and record information for all to share.

Aware of the deficiencies of traditional record systems, a working party of general practitioners from the local medical committees of Devon and Cornwall and the Tamar Faculty of the Royal College of General Practitioners has devised a new preventive care card (Fig. 5.3). This has been piloted in 12 practices, where it received a favourable response.

Training practices now have a set of minimum standards relating to the medical record. These are reg-

PREVENTIVE CARE CARD

Surname	Forenames		D.o.B.	
NHS Number	Blood Group	Height	Male / Female	
Allergies/Risk Factors				

IMMUNISATIONS: Enter date and batch number in each box

	1st	2nd	3rd	Pre-School	15+
Pertussis					
Diphtheria					
Tetanus					
Polio					
Measles		Heaf Test	Date / Result	BCG	
Rubella		Adult Tetanus			
Mumps					

Additional Immunisations: Enter date, vaccine (or test) and batch number in each box

PREVENTION

B.P.	Date					
	Result					
	Date					
	Result					
SMOKING	Date					
	Result					
ALCOHOL	Date					
	Result					
CERVICAL SMEAR	Date					
	Result					
	Date					
	Result					
RUBELLA STATUS	Date					
	Result					
URINALYSIS	Date					
	Result					
WEIGHT	Date					
	Result					
	Date					
	Result					

Additional Information

	Date					
	Result					
	Date					
	Result					
	Date					
	Result					
	Date					
	Result					

Fig. 5.3   Preventive care card (from Grundy and Dwyer 1989).

ularly reviewed at the time of practice visits by the Regional Adviser and local course organisers. These standards include:

1. All medical records and hospital correspondence must be filed in practice notes in date order.
2. Appropriate medical records must contain easily discernible drug therapy lists for patients on long-term therapy.
3. Practices should be starting to create summary problem lists where these do not exist.

THE AGE/SEX REGISTER

Apart from the medical records of individuals, one of the most useful tools in general practice is the age/sex register. This is an integral part of most screening programmes, many of which would be unmanageable without it. It may take one of several forms, from a simple loose-leafed register, through a card index system to a practice computer. As computerisation will be discussed in Chapter 6, the following is addressed to those practices contemplating a manual system.

It is obviously a daunting task for a practice to undertake the establishment of an age/sex register, but with proper organisation this should not be a deterrent. Some Family Health Services Authorities may agree to undertake this task on the doctor's behalf, although it is likely that a charge will be made for this service. More frequently, they are prepared to allow one or more members of the practice ancillary staff to go to their offices to compile the register from the practice nominal index cards. A computer print-out of the register may be provided to the practice on request, although a charge will probably be made. This list can be printed out alphabetically or by date of birth. It must be borne in mind, however, that there will be inaccuracies in the Family Health Services Authority data (Fraser and Clayton, 1981). These could be as much as 20% or more, particularly in urban areas with high patient mobility.

The most usual method is probably to compile the register from the medical records held in the surgery, taking care to ensure that none are missed because they were in use when the register was compiled. This method has several advantages; damaged envelopes can be replaced and all records can be marked to show they have been included in the register. At this stage the opportunity should be taken to return all known 'ghost' records to the Family Health Services Authority.

Whatever method is used, when the task is complete the resultant list should be checked with the list held by the Family Health Services Authority, so that anomalies may be resolved.

It is important to decide at the outset upon the most efficient method of register. The earliest registers were ledgers (Anon 1963) but this form has several inbuilt disadvantages. Although they are portable and initially easy to use, with the passage of time and the number of changes made, ledgers soon become unwieldy and unmanageable. As we now have a fairly mobile population, it is necessary to adopt a flexible system — the answer would appear to be a card index system.

Most practices use the size cards recommended and provided by The Royal College of General Practitioners, which measure 12.7 × 7.6 cm. The sexes are distinguished by colour — males being blue and females pink. Blank cards are used by those practices that prefer to design their own but the structured design developed by the Royal College of General Practitioners is particularly helpful for those practices undertaking screening programmes.

As a considerable amount of work is involved in the initial stages of the compilation of an age/sex register, it may be necessary to employ additional staff or to involve existing staff in overtime. The Family Health Services Authority may, at its discretion, help to fund additional staff hours for this purpose. The summer vacation is an ideal time to employ students for the task. Other possibilities include an additional staff member under the Youth Training Scheme, either to carry out the work personally or to free an existing staff member.

Specially designed filing cabinets are available to house the cards, which can be filed in a number of ways. Usually this is by year of birth, male and female filed separately. It is a matter of practice preference as to whether the patients of individual doctors are filed in different drawers or whether the responsible doctor is merely indicated on the card. Some practices file strictly by date of birth but there are advantages to filing alphabetically within each year.

Once this initial task has been completed the demography of the practice can be defined.

Maintaining the register

It is absolutely essential that the age/sex register is maintained regularly from the moment it is started. It is usually preferable that one member of staff has overall responsibility for this task, although all staff should be familiar with the system. Immediately a patient registers, a card should be initiated. Care should be taken when accepting registrations that all necessary information is obtained. Correct completion of Form FP1 is vital if patients are unable to find their medical card. The patient's National Health Service number should be obtained whenever possible (many patients are unaware that this is usually shown on their birth certificate). Other important items are date of birth and name and address of previous doctor. A little extra time taken at this stage will ensure prompt inclusion of the patient on the doctor's list and speed up receipt of the medical record. Many Family Health Services Authorities ask for the postcode of new registrations and the practice should ensure that these are recorded (the advent of Deprivation Allowances has given an additional incentive for this).

Changes to patients' names and addresses should be entered weekly and it may be beneficial to make a cross-reference when changes of name occur.

It is a good idea to keep new registrations in a separate drawer, enter on them the date the patient is included in the practice list and transfer them to the main index when the record is received. This provides an instant check on awaited medical records or any registrations that might not have been credited.

When a patient leaves the practice the date and the reason for leaving (coded as shown on Form FP22) should be entered and the card removed from the index and filed alphabetically in a 'removed' drawer. This can be extremely useful with patients for whom no record or registration card can be found but who insist they are registered with the practice. It can then be ascertained whether the record has been returned to the Family Health Services Authority, the date of return and the reason for it. Some doctors return the age/sex card with the medical record to the Family Health Services Authority. The card is of no use to the Authority, neither is it likely to be of use to the new doctor. By returning this card a valuable index of past patients is lost.

Use of the age/sex register

The age/sex register has many uses: a check can be kept on the practice list size and of patterns and trends of changes in the list size. This information is essential for the forward-planning of practice policy, including such items as number of partners, premises, attached staff, etc.

For practices in rural areas, a geographical analysis of the practice population may be advantageous, particularly if the possibility of branch surgeries or services is under consideration.

As soon as the register is complete, plans can be made to introduce screening, recall and surveillance. These procedures should include all the practice team and it is important that full discussion and careful planning take place. This applies equally to screening and immunisation, the latter having become a particular focus of attention since the introduction of the new GP contract. Recall systems can be devised for cervical cytology, breast screening, family planning, well-woman and well-man clinics, diabetes and other specific chronic diseases. Once a recall system is under way, it is vital to ensure that all new registrations in the relevant age group are included and that a note is made of patients leaving the practice list. Although it may be decided that a register will be of assistance, the key is the tagging of the age/sex card. There are several types of tags available. Metal ones are very expensive and can sometimes fall off, become affixed to another card or damage the card. The simplest, cheapest and probably most versatile method is coloured tape or tags, which can be used in a variety of combinations.

RESEARCH

Screening programmes may be set up to assist research. One of the first nationwide programmes involving general practice was that organised by the Medical Research Council to screen for mild hypertension (MRC 1985), (see also Chapter 21). The trial involved patients aged between 40 and 65 being invited for screening. Those whose blood pressure readings were within a previously defined range were invited to participate in the trial, the object of which was to determine the effectiveness of the treatment of mild hypertension by various drugs (including a placebo), and whether it proved to be beneficial in the long-term. Screening carried out under the auspices of the practice team usually results in a higher percentage response than that done by an unfamiliar source and has the advantage that, where necessary, treatment not included in the trial can be initiated. In this case, any patients whose blood pressure was found to be higher than the trial levels could be immediately referred to the reception desk to be given an appointment with their own doctor. All costs involved were paid for by the Medical Research Council and an accurate age/sex register was essential for sending out the initial invitation to patients.

Practices may undertake trials of their own, or participate with other practices in local trials, with the aid of the register. Projects involving trainees from one or more practices can also be organised on a local basis.

Audit will play an increasing part in general practitioners' lives, and an up-to-date age/sex register is a minimum requirement. Teaching practices (both for undergraduates and postgraduates) regularly carry out reviews of medical conditions, prescribing and referrals and this will undoubtedly become part of accepted medical practice in the future. Practice reports will be provided for Family Health Services Authorities and contain much basic audit information. Some practices already produce practice reports for their patients (some even have regular newsletters).

Involvement of practice team

Most projects will require the involvement of several members of the practice team: doctors, health visitors, practice nurses, community nurses, secretaries and receptionists. Screening of the elderly, in particular, is likely to be a team effort (see Chapter 25). The number to be screened may be ascertained from the register and, again, the cards could be tagged or marked to indicate whether the patient is regularly visited, and if so, by whom. This project may also include officers from social services, community psychiatric nurses and visitors from voluntary agencies. Coordination will prevent a plethora of professional and voluntary workers dealing with any single individual. Regular meetings should be arranged for the exchange of information and ideas. The limits of confidentiality and access to records should be determined at the outset of each individual screening project.

It is important to ensure that any new patients in the appropriate age group are brought into the programme as soon as possible and an initial visit by the health visitor to assess their needs and to welcome them to the practice may prove useful and be appreciated by the patients.

Many practices have designed their own elderly screening card to complement their programme. The initial offer of a visit is sent to the patient by the health visitor working from the age/sex register.

THE DISEASE INDEX

If practices are to be in a position to review their care of various medical conditions, and indeed to make full use of the data obtained by screening programmes there must be a record of all patients suffering from such conditions; such a record comprises a Disease Index. One of the first such indexes was devised by T S Eimerl in the 1960s (Eimerl & Laidlaw 1969). It is known as the 'E' book and was designed as a diagnostic index for use in general practice. An inexpensive modification of this is the 'E-Box' (Baker & Schilder 1976), in which a box containing loose data sheets for each condition is used instead of a ledger, and only the diseases encountered are indexed. Loose-leaf binders may also be used. Such registers have been established in training practices for some time now.

Various types of diagnostic indexes have evolved from the 'E' book, most of which contain some type of register and are complemented by colour coding of the notes and/or the age/sex card. The Royal College of General Practitioners has devised a colour tagging system for eight important disease groups and this is widely used. The recommended colours are: red, sensitivities; brown, diabetes; yellow, epilepsy; green, tuberculosis (active, arrested or cured); blue, hypertension; white, long-term maintenance therapy, e.g. steroids, thyroid, vitamin B_{12}, antibiotics etc.; black, attempted suicide; black/white check, measles. The College advises as follows:

1. That not more than eight disorders or disease groups be chosen and that these be allotted clear and easily memorised colours.
2. That there be two alternative approved sites for marking records: at the top end of the right edge of the face of the FP5/6 or along the top edge of a projecting insert card or FP7/8.
3. That strip-adhesive plastic tape be the method of choice — 0.5 cm (1/4 inch)-wide tape should be applied in 1.2 cm (1/2 inch) lengths on both the front and back of insert card, envelope or record envelope. If more than one colour code is applicable the next coloured tape should be inserted as close as possible alongside.

These principles are broad enough to cover essentials without the need for an 'interpreter's handbook', whilst leaving enthusiasts free to use striped, hatched, spotted or non-primary colours (placed in non standard sites) for research or their own administrative purposes without confusing the basic system.

By using colours other than those recommended by the Royal College of General Practitioners, or by using combinations of colours, it is possible to include many more diseases than the eight mentioned above. This may prove extremely valuable, both as a teaching aid and for research. As with the age/sex register, establishing a comprehensive disease index within an existing practice is a long and laborious process. For this reason, it is better initially to restrict the index to a small number of important diseases and to build from there. All new records arriving at the practice should be summarised, pruned and included in the register if appropriate. Another method is the analysis of all repeat prescriptions (for diseases requiring medication) issued during a period of, say, 3 months. Many diseases can be identified from the drugs prescribed to patients, e.g. diabetes, hypertension, etc. This method is particularly effective in a dispensing practice, although prescribing practices can adopt this system by keeping a plain carbon copy of each prescription issued.

Another method is for each partner to set aside records for entry in the register during surgery sessions. This method has the disadvantage of involving all the doctors — notoriously unreliable creatures!

Incoming mail from local hospitals can also be used. This needs to be studied before being filed. By this method, for example, it is possible to record all new hysterectomies and to ensure that these patients are not recalled for cervical smears.

There appears to be no quick and easy way to compile the register and users must have regard to the recommendation by the Royal College of General Practitioners, that the use of colour coding is positive, not negative. The presence of a colour tag means that the disorder so coded is, or has been present; the absence of a tag can *never* be taken to imply the absence of such a disorder.

Compilation of the register from existing records can be done alphabetically or in age cohorts. It may be a good idea to commence with the oldest patients, on the premise that these are the most likely candidates for entry in the register, whilst at the same time ensuring any congenital diseases in the newborn are recorded at the outset. Whatever method is chosen, it is imperative that, once established, the register is scrupulously maintained using similar methods.

All outgoing patients should be deleted and all incoming patients included. The register is never complete because it is constantly changing. The changing patterns and distribution of diseases may themselves be important in the research field.

Statistics from such registers enable comparisons with neighbouring and national data practices, but even in the best organised practices they may be notoriously unreliable. As a starting point for a audit project for a student or trainee, however, the register will prove invaluable.

It is by the collection, comparison and analysis of such data that we learn and progress. High numbers of a particular disease or group of diseases in certain areas can be investigated with a view to determining possible causes and solutions. The health implications of such factors as smoking, lead in petrol, aluminium in water supplies and the use of sprays on food products may lead to changes in government policy in our own and other countries. Such statistics are of vital importance in the long-term planning of our health care. Their value outside the practice depends, however, on the uniformity of recording criteria and their efficient application.

NEW PATIENTS

To ensure that new patients are entered in practice registers with the minimum of delay, many practices ask the new patient to complete a health questionnaire upon registration. These may be particularly beneficial while the permanent records are awaited, and in certain cases the receipt of the records can be expedited should this seem desirable. Most Family Health Service Authorities are happy to assist in these matters, although they do not approve of general practitioners making their own arrangements for the transfer of the contents of medical record envelopes, which may result in records becoming fragmented or lost.

When a new patient makes an initial appointment to see the doctor it is helpful if a longer appointment is given, so that his/her medical history can be discussed and assessment and record made of any repeat medication. Indeed, such a health check has now become recognised by the payment of a special fee. At the same time, a check can be made to ensure that the patient's name has been added to any appropriate screening or recall register. A little additional time taken at this stage may prevent problems and confusion later and make for a better doctor–patient relationship.

INFORMATION LEAFLETS

We must never lose sight of the fact that the passing of information is a two-way process. An increasing number of practices produce some form of information leaflet for patients. These should give details of all services provided, surgery times, telephone numbers, out-of-hours arrangements, how to obtain repeat prescriptions, etc. They should also contain the names of *all* the practice team. Again, the information in the leaflet should be regularly reviewed and up-dated. The rules regarding advertising by general practitioners have recently been relaxed and these leaflets may play a key role in attracting patients to a new practice. Practices must also be increasingly aware of the needs and expectations of their patients, so that they maintain their practice lists now that patients have been given the right to change doctor more easily. Frequent changes may lead to fragmented and incomplete records and the loss of continuity of care and, in many cases, will be detrimental to the well-being of the patient.

COMPUTERS

Computers are dealt with in detail in Chapter 6 and they undoubtedly have a major impact on medical records and data management. However, it is a great mistake to believe that a computer can be introduced to a practice and immediately solve the problems of records. Ideally, notes should be improved and accurate registers compiled in *anticipation* of computerisation. The criticism 'rubbish in — rubbish out' is as true as ever when discussing computers in general practice. Despite the greater speed of a computer in certain tasks, a manual system still has a number of advantages. It is completely flexible and can be organised to suit the needs of the individual practice.

Although most computer packages appear to be the answer to our prayers when demonstrated by eager salesmen, in reality it is unlikely that the available software will be tailored exactly as required. Once the system is installed it is not long before its shortcomings are discovered. Manual systems are obviously much cheaper, staff usually find them less daunting and they do not break down when the electricity fails. So far it has not been considered necessary to set up a 'helpline' for practices with manual recall systems!

FUTURE CHANGES

Many changes are occurring in general practice, not least the implementation of the 1990 GP Contract. Greater emphasis will be placed on preventive medicine and screening programmes will need to be the norm for all practices. Technology is developing apace and who knows what new innovations will emerge to help us provide better patient care. However, our first priority should be the correct organisation of medical records and supporting registers. If we build on firm foundations the end product will be worth the effort and we can go forward with confidence.

REFERENCES

Anon 1963 The age/sex register. Records and statistics unit. Journal of the Royal College of General Practitioners 6: 195–197

Baker C, Schilder M 1976 The 'E-box'. Journal of Family Practice 3: 189–191

Eimerl T S, Laidlaw A J 1969 A handbook for research in general practice, 2nd edn. Churchill Livingstone, Edinburgh

Fraser R C, Clayton D G 1981 The accuracy of age-sex registers, practice medical records and family practitioner committee registers. Journal of the Royal College of General Practitioners 31: 410–419

Grundy R, Dwyer D M 1989 Preventive care card for general practice. Journal of the Royal College of General Practitioners 39: 15–16

Hart C J 1983 Child health surveillance in general practice. The Practitioner 227: 256

Heward J, Clayton D 1980 The point accuracy of paediatric population registers. Journal of the Royal College of General Practitioners 30: 412–416

Hodgkin K 1985 Towards earlier diagnosis, 5th edn. Churchill Livingstone, Edinburgh, pp 728–745

MRC Working Party 1985 MRC trial of treatment of mild hypertension: principal results. British Medical Journal 2: 97–104

Tait I G 1978 The clinical record in British general practice. British Medical Journal 2: 683–688

6. Computers in screening and surveillance

Lewis D Ritchie

INTRODUCTION

Good preventive medicine is about the timely and reliable delivery of relevant measures to appropriate subgroups of patients. In turn, this implies the correct and complete identification of these patients, the adequate implementation of chosen activities and the continuous measurement of actual performance set against defined objectives. Targeting, monitoring and evaluating screening activities in general practice therefore demand accurate, flexible and practicable record systems. At one stage, with limited horizons for prevention, good quality paper–based records alone may well have been sufficient. This is no longer the case — the increasing complexity of primary care brings with it information requirements that can be satisfied only by computer assistance.

Computers are, by turns, daunting, challenging and controversial. In the same way that most businesses and professions have recently assimilated microcomputers, general practitioners are embracing the new technology in increasing numbers. Reluctance has slowly given way to acceptance and suspicion has been displaced by a growing familiarity. As attitudes have softened the technology has continued to evolve: computer hardware is becoming more powerful, more reliable and less costly; computer software, or programs, are more accessible — 'user friendly' — and offer increased facilities for the general practitioner and the primary care team. This chapter seeks to address both the potential and the limitations of using computers for screening and surveillance in general practice.

THE CASE FOR COMPUTERS

Information chaos in general practice — the failings of manual records

Structural improvements designed to instil some order into the chaos of traditional manual records have been suggested by numerous workers (Walford 1963 — the practice index, Kuennsberg 1968 — the 'F' book for family morbidity recording, Pinsent 1968 — the age/sex register, Eimerl 1973 – the 'E' book diagnostic/morbidity index), (see also Chapter 5). With the particular exception of the age/sex register, none of these proposals has enjoyed wide-spread implementation by general practitioners. Irrespective of the apparent ingenuity or elegance of suggested manual reforms, the adoption of a novel record improvement is largely made on the grounds of practicability (Ritchie 1986). Arguably, the ultimate shortcoming of the manual record is its passivity — the failure to prompt the user to be aware of some previously recorded important fact or to remind of an investigation, examination or screening procedure that may be outstanding.

Computers — the record continuum

Despite technical advances, the microcomputer will continue to complement rather than replace the manual record for some time to come. Records in general practice can usefully be regarded as a continuum with manual formats (Medical Record Envelope/A4) at one end and the totally computerised record at the other. In between lies the computer-assisted medical record — with varying degrees of assistance, depending on the objectives and priorities of individual practices. This might be represented, at one end of the spectrum, by a practice with a solitary, stand-alone microcomputer based in the office area and running only one or two limited applications, at the other end of the spectrum is a practice with a multiuser system with additional terminals in every consulting room, used for recording details of each patient encounter. Various surveys have attempted to determine the nature of microcomputer used in general practice (Sheldon & Stoddart 1985, NHS Information Technology Branch 1987) and one

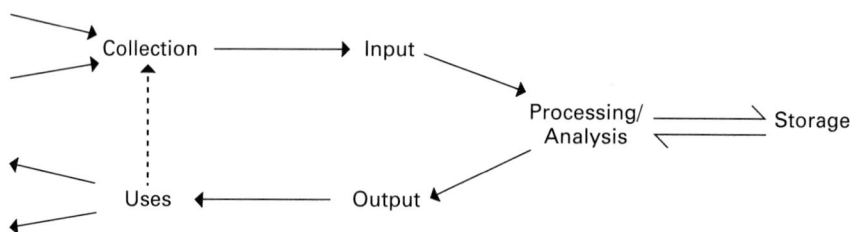

Fig. 6.1   The cycle of data handling in a practice.

study has measured the actual degree of use by general practitioners (Taylor et al 1990). This ongoing 'electronic questionnaire' study of 152 Scottish users of GPASS (General Practice Administration System, Scotland), covering a patient population of 1 052 000, revealed widespread differences in the extent of usage of computer facilities.

WHY COMPUTERS? – PLUSES AND MINUSES

The viability of any professional business is underpinned by the ready availability of accurate, complete and current information about its activities, and general practice is no exception. This requirement for high quality information — and the role of the computer — can be explored by considering the cycle of data handling in a practice (Fig. 6.1).

Data collection — deciding the quantity

Enormous amounts of patient data are generated on a daily basis in general practice. Most of these data hold only transient significance but some are crucial and should be permanently available. To build up a meaningful database, all general practitioners and ancillary staff should have a clear idea of their information requirements, taking into account the needs (and possibly demands) of Family Health Services Authorities/Health Boards. Once these have been established, a core of essential data — the so-called 'minimum dataset' — is collected and updated on a continuous basis. These principles hold equally for manual and computerised record formats. Until recently, pessimism about the likelihood of agreed minimum datasets in primary care may well have been justified. However, several developments are likely to change this outlook, particularly the new GP contract and the NHS reforms (Secretaries of State for Health 1989).

There is now a greater emphasis on screening, surveillance and the achievement of 'targets'. The development of general practice budget-holding is a further powerful force for establishing common datasets.

Data input — improving the quality

Records in traditional manual formats are usually handwritten, with common problems of legibility, accuracy and completeness. The computerised record offers partial solutions for each of these difficulties. Computer data are normally entered using a keyboard; other methods include voice activation, image digitisers, bar codes and optical character recognition, all of which have limited potential for general practice, in the short term.

As data are being entered to a computer, they can be checked for accuracy by means of programs that actively vet their quality. If the data are numeric e.g. weights, heights or blood pressures, the computer could check these against known or anticipated ranges. The check might take the form of query to the operator: 'Value outside expected range: are you sure?' or outright rejection: 'Unacceptable value: check data source'. Similarly, if data are alphabetical, e.g. drugs, diagnoses or procedures, the computer could compare these with internal dictionaries. If no identical entry is found, similar-sounding alternatives might be presented for the operator to consider prior to entry. This facility is commonly found in word processing software with 'spellchecking' capability.

Completeness of entered data is mainly a function of systematic recording, irrespective of format — the limiting factor is the diligence of the user rather than constraints of the record medium. However, the computer can have an advantage over the manual record by preventing the operator from missing or skipping over a particular data field, e.g. when entering individual components of a patient's risk profile at a well-person screening clinic.

Unfortunately, computers are not automatically better than manual formats as far as accuracy and completeness are concerned. Much current general practice software has negligible or rudimentary data-vetting capability. It must also be remembered that any such filter can only reject the impossible and query the implausible. Finally, a computer can only provide information from data that have already been entered on previous occasions.

Data processing — rapid analysis

The superiority of computers for processing and analysing data is indisputable. The retrieval of information from manual records is fraught with problems of legibility, unpredictable or random location of data and obvious time penalties. Although these difficulties can, for example, be offset by the establishment of manual disease registers or diagnostic indices, these instruments are labour intensive, inflexible and usually impose duplication of recording. (By contrast, data need be registered in a computer only once — the benefit of *single data entry*.) The analytical capability of a microcomputer for primary care applications is unlikely to be constrained by the computing power of the hardware, but rather by the limitations of the available software.

Data storage

Quarts into pint pots

Four major aspects should be considered here: efficiency, capacity, security and confidentiality. Computers store information much more efficiently than manual records — a fact best evidenced by the physical space occupied by paper-based records contrasted with the desktop microcomputer. As data storage devices continue to shrink in size and to increase in capacity, previous reservations about limited data capacity no longer apply. In addition to the ubiquitous floppy disk and hard disk magnetic media, data may be stored on optical disk drives, electronic memory chips, magnetic tapes, CD-ROM laser devices and 'smart cards'.

Security

The security of data held on computer is crucial. Vast quantities of data can be irretrievably destroyed by technical failure if no duplicate or back-up copies of the database have been made. Again, technology has moved on, and there is no legitimate excuse for this to happen. Security or 'backup' copies must be made frequently, and they should be carefully stored at some location remote from the site of the computer.

Confidentiality

Confidentiality, the existence of adequate safeguards against misuse of entrusted information, is perhaps the most contentious issue surrounding the use of computers. Legislation, in the form of the 1984 Data Protection Act, with mandatory registration of users who hold identifiable personal data, constitutes a necessary but not sufficient framework for acceptable levels of confidentiality. This can be achieved only by adequate software provisions (limited accessibility and distinct operator passwords), appropriate hardware security (physical and electronic locks) and rigorous operating procedures for all practice staff. In reality, any well maintained in-house practice computer system is likely to be much more secure than manual records and therefore poses less of a risk to confidentiality. This reassurance does not necessarily extend to networks, where computers in different sites are interconnected by telephone lines and may freely exchange data. Such connections may be susceptible to 'hacking' or unauthorised access by a third party. One obvious protection against this — setting aside the doubtful efficacy of proposed UK legislation — is the restriction of information transfer outwith practices to anonymous or deidentified patient data. This will be considered again when looking at the topic of Medical Record Linkage. (p. 61).

Data output: all that glitters

The output from a computer is normally made on a visual display unit (VDU) or by paper printout. A VDU offers the dynamic capability for alerting the operator to key points of information by judicious use of highlighting, flashing display or colour. In addition, tabulated data can be readily transformed into a graphical presentation by suitable software, e.g. serial follow-up measurements of a child's height and weight may be automatically graphed and compared against expected values to demonstrate adequacy of growth.

A permanent paper record may be quickly produced on a printing device with immediate legibility gains over written records. Caution is advocated here, however, because computer printout may be visually impressive and attractive, but is not always error-free — computer output is only as good as the quality of data input.

Data uses

Health professionals tend to be assiduous collectors of patient information but are less adept at making good use of it. The particular capabilities of a computer should result in greater (and more effective) use of data, resulting in improved patient care. The actual and potential uses of microcomputers in screening and surveillance are now considered.

APPLYING COMPUTERS TO SCREENING AND SURVEILLANCE

Identifying patients

Since the inception of the National Health Service, the remuneration of general practitioners in the UK has depended to a lesser or greater degree on capitation fees. This, in turn, led to the practice list or patient population, details of which are held both by general practitioners and by Family Health Services Authorities/ Health Boards. The facility of a readily defined practice population permits complete identification and targeting of subsets of patients for screening and surveillance activities. The availability of a denominator on the one hand allows the calculation of rates, and on the other should draw attention to patients who have failed to attend.

The age/sex register: updated

The manual age/sex register, initially held in ledger form and more recently on individual cards, has undergone a variety of modifications since it was first introduced (Pinsent 1968). Widely adopted by general practitioners, the most basic form contains brief personal (demographic) details, with possible additions of diagnostic, therapeutic, socioeconomic or occupational data. The concept of the age/sex register is an enduring one, although its format is clearly evolutionary.

The age/sex register or, more appropriately, the 'patient database' will continue to form the mainstay of any computer-assisted records system in general practice. Defined lists of patients can be located readily and rapidly on a computer and comprehensive searches of thousands of patients for specified characteristics can be completed successfully within minutes. The actual speed of search will depend on the number of records examined and the computing power of the hardware, in conjunction with the capability of the software.

Inaccurate patient registers — reconciling the differences

The accuracy of computerised patient databases in general practice and of the corresponding population registers held by Family Health Services Authorities (FHSAs) and Health Boards gives much cause for concern. Recognised for some time as a problem in manual age/sex registers (Fraser & Clayton 1981), and also in computerised practices (Difford et al 1985) the problems of missing patients and wrong addresses are serious obstacles to effective targeting of screening invitations in general practice (Bowling & Jacobson

1989). There are various reasons for this universal problem, some of which are patient failures (primarily non-notification of change of address) and others that are the result of poor communications within practices or between practices and FHSAs.

Although efforts to encourage improved self-notification of changes of address by patients are likely to have limited results, there is considerable scope for improvement among health professionals by encouraging a systematic approach to seeking and recording patient movements. Perhaps the most promising avenue here is the automatic comparison or *reconciliation* of data on the same set of patients separately held on general practice and FHSA computers. In the short term this might take the form of a practice sending a copy of its patient database on floppy disks to the FHSA, perhaps on a quarterly basis. The contents of the practice database would then be electronically compared with the FHSA database on a mainframe computer and discrepancies between the two would be printed out, e.g. lists of patients present on one database and not the other, incompatible addresses, dates of birth, etc. Eventually, corresponding records of clinical procedures, such as immunisations and cervical smears could be compared in this way. Practice and FHSA staff could then liaise to reconcile the revealed differences. If this exercise is not performed regularly the contents of general practice and FHSA databases will inexorably diverge over time, leading to administrative chaos, dubious statistics and endless frustrations. The reconciliation of patient registers is particularly important for effective screening and surveillance where a population perspective is essential.

Computers for call and recall

There are two major methods of screening, in the broadest sense, in general practice — true systematic screening and 'opportunistic' screening, or case-finding.

Systematic screening

In systematic screening, letters of invitation are prepared and mailed out to patients requesting them to attend (or to reattend) for a suitable procedure. A computer can facilitate this in several ways. First, the subset of required or at-risk patients can be located rapidly and a complete list of patients complied. Secondly, individually addressed letters can be printed out by linking the selected patient file to a standard or modifiable letter format. This is known as a mail-merge facility and uses the word processor capacity of the computer. Thirdly, most software currently available allows simultaneous production of printed name and address adhesive labels, which are used for the envelopes containing the invitations. Fourthly, some programs contain an appointments facility integrated with a screening clinic schedule — letters of invitation are printed with set appointment times. If the patient is unable to attend at the offered time and notifies the practice in advance, a further appointment can be generated. On the day of the screening activity, a computer printout of expected names and times of attendance is produced for the doctor or nurse responsible for the operation of the clinic. In this way the computer can keep an immediate and accurate record of both attenders and non-attenders.

After the screening, a number of possible results (rather than simply positive or negative) may require distinct letters of explanation, e.g. cervical cytology screening. In turn, result permutations lead to different recall schedules. The computer is well suited to handling complex and recurring tasks — the management of a cervical cytology programme falls into this category.

Computers for opportunistic screening

Opportunistic screening, or case-finding, exploits the opportunity presented by the patient who attends for some other, unrelated reason and is discussed in greater detail in Chapter 9. The method is underpinned by the fact that over 60% of patients see their general practitioner at least once in a 1-year period and that over 95% do so in a 5-year period. There are four basic requirements in opportunistic screening: (i) the screening activity should be worthwhile; (ii) the general practitioner or other team member should be prompted to perform an apparently unrelated activity; (iii) the general practitioner should have the time and inclination to do the screening or to delegate it to an available member of staff; (iv) the patient should be willing.

There are several aspects of this process where a computer can be of assistance. If the practice has a consulting room system, and the patient record is called up on a VDU at each visit, an appropriate reminder could appear on the screen, drawing the doctor's attention to an outstanding procedure. The screening opportunity could be taken by the doctor or be delegated to another colleague. If the prompt was ignored on this occasion the reminder would reappear at the patient's next visit, with a further 'reinforcing message' that one opportunity had already been lost. A basic requirement for this to work is a consensus in each practice, using

available guidelines (or contractual requirements), on what screening or preventive procedures should be performed and how often they should be repeated, e.g. tetanus immunisation boosters and blood pressure recordings at 5-yearly intervals, cervical cytology at 3-yearly intervals, and so on. This opportunistic screening assistance may be further enhanced by specifying margins of latitude on each screening or procedure, e.g. if a blood pressure recording has not been done within the last 7 years (a 2-year margin above the normal 5-year interval) then the individual's record would be flagged by the computer. At regular periods (perhaps weekly) all such flagged patients could be identified and listed by the computer. Letters would then be sent to the individuals concerned offering an appointment to have the outstanding screening or preventive activities performed.

A consulting room computer system is not essential for the facility of opportunistic screening. In practices where a solitary microcomputer is located in the records area, it is possible to produce paper printouts of all patients who have booked consultations. Every doctor would have a printed list of attending patients at each surgery and against each name would appear the overdue relevant screening or preventive procedures. The paper list would then be suitably annotated by the doctor and returned for updating the computer database.

Systematic versus opportunistic screening — either or both?

The merits and demerits of systematic and opportunistic screening have been hotly contested for some time. The former implies considerable investment of effort at the outset, with penalties of letters going to wrong addresses and declined invitations; the latter implies the continuous availability of sufficient resources, time and staff to maximise the opportunities as and when patients consult for other reasons. Both methods may be appropriate. In those procedures where the numbers are small and the time-scale for implementation is critical, e.g. developmental screening or childhood immunisation, a call/recall programme may offer the better solution. Alternatively, where numbers are large and the time-scale is less demanding, e.g. blood pressure screening, the opportunistic method is likely to be more cost effective.

Clearly, both methods are complimentary rather than mutually exclusive and can be greatly facilitated by computer assistance. This has been demonstrated by Difford and colleagues (Difford et al 1987), who found that computer-assisted opportunistic screening for hypertension by itself was insufficient and that numbers were significantly enhanced by sending out addi-

Cervical Cytology Audit
Actual v Target Smears by Age Group

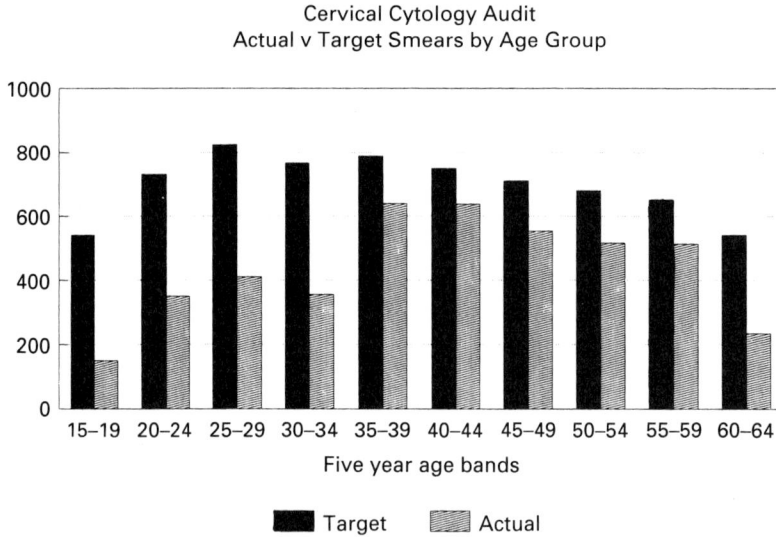

Fig. 6.2 Cervical cytology audit. Actual versus target smears by age group.

tional invitations to attend for blood pressure measurement. Chan and co-workers have described the successful implementation of a computer-based opportunistic health maintenance programme at a general practice teaching clinic in Hong Kong (Chan et al 1988). Benefits reported included a high screening rate, agreement on acceptable standards and improved patient care. Pringle and colleagues have also reported on computer assisted screening within the doctor–patient consultation (Pringle et at 1985). They found that the presence of the computer prompted preventive screening and health education, with a six-fold increase in the number of potentially relevant procedures being mentioned. They also noted that the technology was not found to be stressful by patients. The potential for computer-assisted opportunistic screening of the elderly in Edinburgh has also been reported. (Berrey 1987).

Audit, performance and targets — compliance and default

If a screening procedure is deemed relevant for a particular subset of patients it is essential that the measure is offered to all individuals in the selected group within an acceptable time-scale. In the same way that it is important to measure those who have had a screening or preventive activity performed (compliance) it is even more relevant to identify those who have not had a procedure done (default) — the measurement of omission (Hart 1982). At one stage, audit was a preoccupation of the few and seemed to be irrelevant for

many. Now audit is no longer an optional extra but professional obligation for all and a contractual requirement for most, and NHS targets for cervical cytology and immunisation have now become a fact of life.

In addition to the rapid identification of defaulters and the production of lists of names and addresses with appropriate letters, the graphics capability of the computer can be harnessed to produce an overall view of the selected activity to be audited. Figure 6.2 demonstrates a graphic of cervical cytology performance in a large practice. The figure shows particularly low uptake in the youngest and oldest of the groups (illustrating the potential dilemmas of target setting, e.g. the unknown sexual activities of the youngest group). The graph also demonstrates the results of a practice policy that has emphasised cervical screening in the over 35s at the expense of younger groups. These techniques can be incorporated into the production of an annual practice report, which gives an account of all relevant practice activities, including screening and surveillance, and which can be produced with much greater efficiency and more visual impact than any manual alternative (see also Preece 1989; Shepherd 1989).

Delegation of screening and protocols — opportunities for computer assistance

The recent desire for increased screening and surveillance in primary care has brought with it the requirement for additional consultation time, given that there has been no reduction in the number of patients presenting with established disease. At the same time, questions have been posed as to who should actually be doing most of this additional work. Screening activities in many practices have been delegated to practice nurses who, if properly equipped, trained and supervised, are not only acceptable to patients but may well become more proficient than the delegating doctors themselves. The computer may be exploited not only for dynamic record-keeping in a screening clinic but also for providing guidelines for further investigation and follow-up. In this situation, protocols are decided beforehand by all practice members and the computer is programmed to offer guidance to the nurse in his/her extended role.

A study by Anggard et al (1986) investigated the feasibility of opportunistic screening for cardiovascular risk factors by equipping a specially trained practice nurse with a microcomputer for record-keeping, calculation of a cardiovascular risk score and the management of further follow-up. This 'Life-style Management Model' was initially established in 19 large health centres throughout the UK and it was found to be acceptable to both patients and practice staff. Over 80 000 patients have been screened and long-term assessment of the model is underway. Similarly, in a randomised controlled trial, Robson et al (1989) have demonstrated the effective role of the nurse in preventive activities with computer assisted follow-up.

In the same way that microcomputers can be used to apply protocols to screening and follow-up they have a similar role in the surveillance of chronic disease. This has been investigated by Kenkre et al (1985), who showed that patients with hypertension could be acceptably managed by computer-equipped nurses.

Drug surveillance in primary care

The most commonly used application of computers in general practice is the production and control of repeat prescribing (Taylor et al 1990). The renewed emphasis on rational prescribing, practice formularies, indicative drug budgets and postmarketing surveillance for drug safety provokes demands that can be met only by the monitoring capacity of a computer (Hall et al 1988, Jick et al 1991).

Disease coding — a word on disease classification

The concept of standardised disease coding in surveillance is of immense importance for epidemiological studies and accurate diagnostic labelling in primary care. Screening activities inevitably uncover abnormal-

ities that require accurate classification. Computers can handle numeric data much more efficiently than alphabetical text, and coding systems can be easily implemented. Codes in use include ICD-9, ICHPPC, OXMIS, RCGP and Snomed (Ritchie 1986; Weeks 1989). It is likely, however, that the merits of the Read Clinical Classification/Code will be increasingly recognised and its implementation across the National Health Service in the UK is to be encouraged and welcomed. It now appears that this system will also increasingly be accepted as an international standard. The Read Code is a detailed hierarchical code with the provision of keywords, which are easily recognised and lead to a unique code or rubric. In addition to diagnostic categories (cross-referenced to ICD-9), the Read Code includes occupations, history, symptoms, diagnostic, laboratory and surgical procedures, drugs and preventive activities (Read & Benson 1986).

Technical innovation — the future

Apart from the expected increase in the power and storage capacity of microcomputers, there are other innovations that may well benefit screening and surveillance in general practice. Hand-held portable microcomputers, which can be used in a patient's home for record-keeping are now available. Data are then transferred to a desktop microcomputer — either directly or via a modem and telephone line. These devices are undergoing evaluation by district nurses in the field of community care (Wiseman 1989).

The 'smart card' is another innovation of significant potential. Smart cards are the same size as the ubiquitous credit card. Data may be held on a magnetic strip or the card may contain an integrated circuit or, in the latest versions, the data may be stored optically using a low powered laser etching process. An advantage of the latter is the significantly enhanced storage capacity — allowing enough space for an eventful lifelong medical history. This brings with it the potential and practicability of a patient-held medical record that can be carried by the owner at all times and read at the point of medical care (Jenkinson 1989, Department of Health 1990).

Medical record linkage — computer networks and patient surveillance

Medical record linkage is the gathering together of a patient's medical history, which will have been recorded by different health professionals at different times and usually in different sections of the health service. The reconciliation exercise between general practice and FHSA, referred to above, is one simple example of linkage.

As originally envisaged and subsequently realised in the Oxford Record Linkage Study, the accumulation of successive individual health events facilitated valuable epidemiological research (Baldwin et al 1987). In Scotland, *all* birth, death, hospital in-patient discharge and cancer registration records are held on computer, allowing both epidemiological and health services research (Heasman & Clarke 1979).

In spite of these and similar initiatives, medical record linkage continues to be the exception rather than the rule. This is of particular relevance for screening and surveillance, which are carried out not only by general practitioners and other primary care team members, but by other agencies. Taking the example of cervical cytology screening, a smear may be taken in general practice, at a Health Authority family planning clinic, at an out-patient clinic, on a hospital ward or by an occupational health service. Each of these continues to generate distinct records, points of care and communication of relevant findings between them, by letter, is frequently unsatisfactory. As a result, cytology results may go unrecorded or unrecognised by the general practitioner, possibly leading to the repetition of smears with unnecessary distress and inconvenience for patients and duplication of laboratory workload. It is unrealistic to expect that such difficulties will be automatically resolved with the advent of computerised records systems. Nevertheless, the gradual evolution of computer networks with connections between practice, FHSA, hospitals, out-patient clinics and laboratories will hopefully lead to much enhanced communications and, as a result, improved uptake and monitoring of screening activities.

Computers in perspective

Despite technological advances, it will be some time before computers supplant manual notes, which continue to be the normal format for recording patient encounters. Although most experience has been gained by using microcomputers located in the practice reception or office areas, increasing numbers of consulting room systems are being deployed. In the former, data are usually entered by administrative staff, rather than doctors, and therefore the information recorded is usually selective and incomplete. In the latter, doctors can enter data directly to a computer-based record during a consultation, and at the same time be prompted by the computer to perform some extra activity or to enter additional data. As such, the true potential of the computer as an essential adjunct for screening and surveillance will be realised only when it becomes part of the standard patient encounter.

Like any innovation, computers incur costs as well as yielding benefits. The downside is, however, limited and the potential is impressive. Computers are, after all, only tools — albeit powerful tools. Properly used they are likely to make a significant contribution to patient care in general and to screening and surveillance in particular.

REFERENCES

Anggard E E, Land J M, Lenihan C J et al 1986 Prevention of cardiovascular disease in general practice: a proposed model. British Medical Journal 293: 177–180

Baldwin J A, Acheson E D, Graham W J, 1987 Textbook of medical record linkage. Oxford University Press, Oxford

Berrey P N E 1987 A computerised case-finding system: the Stockbridge Project. In: Taylor R C, Buckley E G (eds) Preventive care of the elderly: a review of current developments. Occasional Paper 35. Royal College of General Practitioners. London

Bowling A, Jacobson B 1989 Screening: the inadequacy of population registers. British Medical Journal 298: 545–546

Chan D H, Chan N F, Chan C et al 1988 Journal of the Royal College of General Practitioners 38: 360–362

Department of Health: NHS Management Executive 1990. The care card: evaluation of the Exmouth project, HMSO, London

Difford F, Hook P M, Sledge M 1985 Maintaining the accuracy of a computer practice register: household index. British Medical Journal 290: 519–521

Difford F, Telling J P, Davies K R et al 1987 Continuous opportunistic and systematic screening for hypertension with computer help: analysis of non-responders. British Medical Journal 294: 1130–1132

Eimerl T S 1973 The E book system for record keeping in general practice. Medical Care xi (Suppl): 138–144

Fraser R C, Clayton D G 1981 The accuracy of age/sex registers, practice medical records and family practitioner committee registers. Journal of the Royal College of General Practitioners 31: 410–419

Hall G C, Luscombe D K, Walker S R 1988 Post marketing surveillance using a computerised general practice database. Pharmaceutical Medicine 2: 345–351

Hart J Tudor 1982 Measurement of omission. British Medical Journal 284: 1686–1689

Heasman M A, Clarke J A 1979 Medical record linkage in Scotland. Heath Bulletin (Edinburgh) 37: 97–104

Jenkinson S 1989 Medical credit cards. British Medical Journal 299: 472

Jick H, Jick S S, Derby L E 1991 Validation of information recorded on general practitioner based computerised data resource in the United Kingdom. British Medical Journal 302: 766–768

Kenkre J, Drury V W M, Lancashire R J 1985 Nurse

management of hypertension in general practice assisted by computer. Family Practice 2: 17–22

Kuennsberg E V 1968 A new record system for general practice. Report from Research Committee, Scottish Council of the Royal College of General Practitioners. British Medical Journal 2: 420–423

NHS Information Technology Branch 1987 Survey of computerised general practices. Department of Health and Social Security, London

Pinsent R J F H 1968 The evolving age-sex register. Journal of the Royal College of General Practitioners 16: 127–134

Preece J 1989 Electronic communicator and monitor. Practice Computing. May: 3–4

Pringle M, Robins S, Brown G 1985 Computer assisted screening: effect on the patient and his consultation. British Medical Journal 290: 1709 – 1712

Read J, Benson T J R 1986 Comprehensive coding. British Journal of Healthcare Computing 3: 8–11

Ritchie L D 1986 Computers in primary care, 2nd edn. Heinemann, London

Robson J, Boomla K, Fitzpatrick S et al 1989. Using nurses for preventive activities with computer assisted follow up: a randomised controlled trial. British Medical Journal 298: 433–436

Secretaries of State for Health, Wales, Northern Ireland, Scotland 1989 Working for patients, Cmnd 555. HMSO, London

Sheldon M, Stoddart N (eds) 1985 Trends in general practice computing. Royal College of General Practitioners, London

Shepherd S 1989 Audit for all — but how? Practitioner 233: 433–436

Taylor M J, Ritchie L D, Taylor R J et al 1990 General practice computing in Scotland. British Medical Journal 300: 170–172

Walford P A 1963 The practice index. Journal of the College of General Practitioners 6: 225–232

Weeks R 1989 Coding colds. British Journal of Healthcare Computing 6: 9–10

Wiseman J 1989 A portable answer to the Griffiths challenge. British Journal of Healthcare Computing 6: 24–26

FURTHER READING

Johnson N, Mant D, Jones L et al 1991 Use of computerised general practice data for population surveillance: comparative study of influenza data. British Medical Journal 302: 763–765

Lawrence M, Coulter A, Jones L 1990 A total audit of preventive procedures in 45 practices caring for 430 000 patients. British Medical Journal 300: 1501–1503

Ritchie L D, Watt A, Taylor M W 1991 Large computer data-bases in general practice. British Medical Journal 302: 1081

Weed L L 1969 Medical records, medical education and patient care. Case Western Reserve Press, Cleveland

Willis A, Stewart T 1989 Computers: a guide to choosing and using. Oxford University Press, Oxford

7. Health teams: the preventive interface

John Robson   Nicki Spiegal

HEALTH TEAMS: THE PREVENTIVE INTERFACE

The preventive agenda gets longer and longer. Coronary heart disease has hardly begun to be tackled in a systematic way and major new items such as screening for breast cancer or cystic fibrosis have, or are about to, appear on the list of outstanding tasks. Although adaptation by primary health teams to the work of prevention is often slow, haphazard and contentious, the emergence of a new orientation in the aims and organisation of primary services is clearly apparent. This chapter summarises some of the main developments, obstacles and requirements for teams delivering effective anticipatory care.

THE DISCRIMINATION OF RISK

Over the last 20 years there has been a marked change in general practice to encompass the anticipation of risks, as well as responses to demand. The reorientation of primary care is characterised by a shift in medical perception to include not only the clinical definition and treatment of disease but also the discrimination and modification of risks. Pickering, who helped make continuous risk medically acceptable, captured elements of these changes when he quoted from *The epidemiology of country practice* by William Pickles. Pickles wrote in his introduction:

And as I watched the evening train creeping up the valley with its pauses at our three stations, a quaint thought came into my head and it was that there was hardly a man, woman or child in all those villages of whom I did not know the Christian name and with whom I was not on intimate terms of friendship. My wife and I say that we knew most of the dogs and indeed some of the cats (Pickering 1987).

Pickering contrasted this with a passage from Tudor Hart's book on hypertension, written almost 50 years later. The changing medical gaze was perceptible when

Hart wrote:

For the past 18 years I have given day to day care to and lived most of my life among a stable community of 1400 men and women of 20 years and over, for every one of whom I have known the mean of at least two or more casual pressures. From this I have learned that there is no outward feature of personality or physique or other outward sign that gives any clue to the pressures found on measurement (Pickering 1987).

Weed has argued that the creation of a context for the discrimination of risk is a central task for health services (Weed 1977) and Van den Dool coined the term *anticipatory care* for this process in primary care (Van den Dool 1973). Epidemiology, with its population profiles, risk ascertainment and measurable outcomes is increasingly the lingua franca of primary care (Hart 1974, Hart 1984, Mant & Anderson 1985, Tuomilehto & Puska 1987) and, as the evidence accumulates, so do public expectations and the necessary tasks of providers.

But ascertainment of risk is only a first step. An early trial, which relied on screening alone, failed to yield demonstrable benefit and the authors concluded: 'that the use of general practice multiphasic screening in middle age can no longer be advocated' (South East London Screening Study Group 1977). Other screening programmes also had less than optimum results. The failure has been primarily one of delivery — a failure to reach the entire population rather than low risk attenders and a failure to change risks once identified (Hart 1982, Heath 1984, Stott & Pill 1988).

The process of informing, educating and sustaining treatment over a lifetime for individuals who are frequently constrained by social and financial limits has received low priority. Advice is often unplanned, perfunctory and prescriptive, frequently contradictory or simply wrong. In our own practice, measles immunisation rates improved from 60 to 90% over 3 years, largely as a result of giving common and consistent advice, a message reinforced by the Peckham report on immunisation (Peckham et al 1989). Similar problems of professional performance have arisen for lipid-lowering diets, cervical cytology, diabetes and asthma. The problem has been compounded by the absence of clear national or district strategies or the development of local consensus among primary care staff. Maintaining an appropriate programme of advice, with targets monitored by staff and understood by patients, is a skilled and labour intensive task (Kranshein et at 1988). Where organisation is rudimentary, at least half the population have not had their risks identified, half those found to be at risk are lost to follow-up and even where care is sustained, control is frequently poor. The problems of compliance apply equally to professionals and patients.

THE DELIVERY GAP

No practice can hope to deal with all these needs, although there are now few who have not made a start. If surveillance were to be achieved simply by increasing the number of visits to the doctor, consultation rates would have to be increased by 50% for surveillance of blood pressure alone — a solution unlikely to be welcomed by patients or their doctors (Robson 1986). The distribution of risks for coronary heart disease illustrates the magnitude of the problem. About 70% of the adult male population has at least one major risk factor for ischaemic heart disease and 20% have two or more major risk factors. There are few practices that can claim to be systematically tackling the top quintile. This delivery gap has stimulated change both in the content of patient contacts and in the division of work within the practice. People in their communities do not readily fit into the single disease categories that characterise hospital outpatients. Their multiple risks are personal attributes and change is constrained by personal priorities and social pressures. General practitioners have been concerned to build on existing patient contacts where possible and the 'health check' and opportunistic use of existing consultations have both been utilised (Marsh & Chew 1984). At the same time the clinical and administrative work has been divided amongst an expanding team. The institutional model for disease treatment based on hierarchy has begun to give way to devolved responsibility for the tasks of sustained modification of multiple risks.

OBSTACLES TO TEAMWORK

The obstacles to change are formidable, not least the structural issues of finance, premises and registers. The 1966 package gave the financial impetus for the division of work to include nursing and administrative staff. Twenty-four years later, finance and premises remain major obstacles to the employment of staff, particularly in urban areas (Bosanquet & Leese 1988). If general practitioners had made full use of their entitlement to employ staff, an additional 27 000 nurses or administrative staff could have been added to available resources for prevention (Hart 1985).

In 1972, the Briggs Report on nursing hoped the profession would pay more attention: 'to teamwork (which includes leadership of the right kind) instead of formal hierarchy, and to function instead of status' (Briggs Report 1972). But enthusiasm for teams was often received with suspicion by doctors and nurses alike. The division of labour often became synonmous with the delegation of boring tasks without responsibility for care or any means to assess outcome (Bowling 1981). Bruce (1980) outlined three forms of cooperation between staff:

1. *Nominal cooperation*, in which there are no structural links and communication is largely a matter of obligation — a feature of much social work contact.
2. *Convenient cooperation*, which is often a one-way referral or delegation — a feature of many staff attachments where meeting is largely a matter of chance.
3. *Committed cooperation*, where staff work for agreed and common goals with an awareness of their mutual interdependence, is most likely to result in success and satisfaction.

In 1981 a survey of 366 general practitioners in Manchester found that although 82% had attached staff, one-third felt they did not have a team and less than one-quarter had regular meetings (Whitehouse 1986). 'It is naive' wrote Rubin 'to bring together a highly diverse group of people and expect that by calling them a team they will behave like a team' (Rubin & Beckhard 1971).

The absence of agreed goals exacerbates interpersonal differences, which are frequently characterised on the basis of gender, culture and authority (Dingwall 1980, Bowling 1983, McClure 1984, Colliere 1986, Cartilidge et al 1987). The resulting conflict in roles and responsibility may make effective cooperation difficult (Hannay 1980). In the USA, failure to develop cooperative methods of working, coupled with the changing medical market, is leading to the demise of the nurse practitioner. In 1974 Spitzer demonstrated the capabilities of nurses with appropriate training; 10 years later he described their declining fortunes (Spitzer et al 1974, Spitzer 1984).

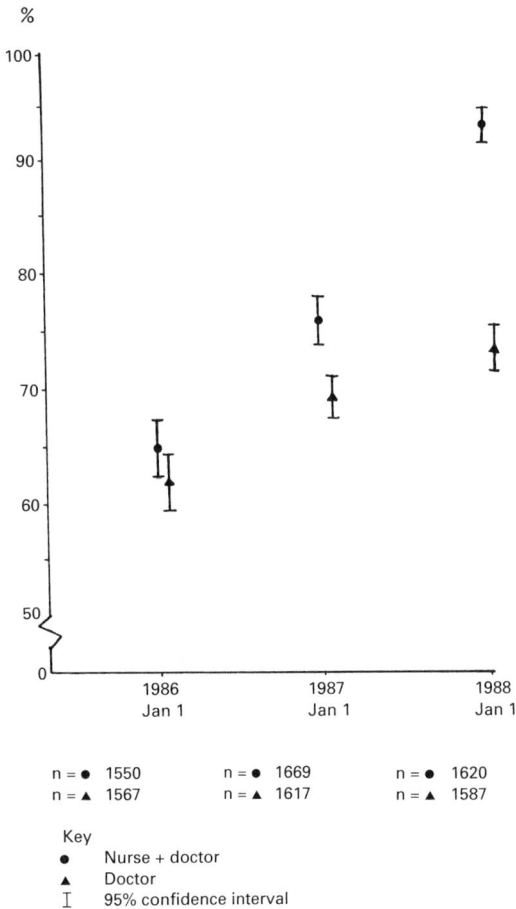

Fig. 7.1 Randomised trial comparing an organized programme with a doctor working without a programme (Robson et al 1989). Percentage of people with blood pressure recorded within 5 years.

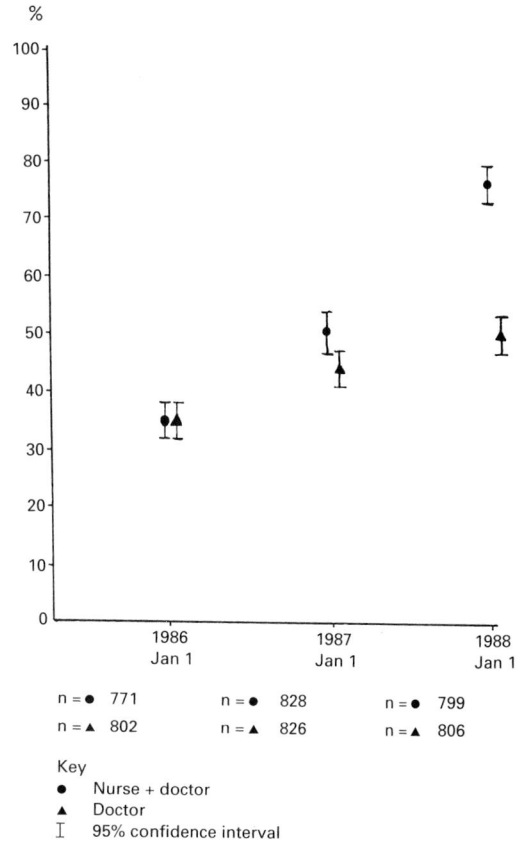

Fig. 7.2 Percentage of women with a cervical smear recorded within 3 years.

NURSES

Despite the problems, local initiatives have continued to challenge inertia at the centre (Brown et al 1986). Although contentious, the Cumberlege Report (Jarman & Cumberlege 1987) acknowledged the issues and the Edwards Report (1987) envisaged far reaching changes in Wales, not least the development of common geographical strategies.

While the work of maternity care and child health are shared with midwives and health visitors, there are no similar staff or structures for prevention among adults. Where successful preventive programmes for adults have been initiated, nurses have been a key component. Practice nurses have been used in Oxford, health visitors in Glasgow and nurses in East London

have been jointly funded from general practice and the District Health Authority (Goodhearted Glasgow 1987, Fullard et al 1987). Nurses have proved effective and acceptable (Drury et al 1988, Robson et al 1989). Figures 7.1 and 7.2 show the improved performance in adults aged 30–64 in an organised prevention programme, which included nurses, compared to usual care by the general practitioner. Both groups had access to computer-assisted follow-up.

Nurses are increasingly involved in preventive care. Of 300 practice nurses surveyed, 90% were measuring blood pressure, 70% were taking cervical smears and around one-half were performing lung function and breast examination. Lack of further training was the most frequently cited obstacle to further development of their role (Greenfield et al 1987). Training was often rudimentary and failure to provide written contracts, and anomalies in pay and conditions, exacerbated the difficulties faced (Reedy 1980).

THE PRIMARY CARE FACILITATOR

The role of a 'facilitator' in an organisation is not new. 'Advisor', 'consultant' or 'coordinator' could be substituted for the term, although facilitator is quite descriptive, from the Latin to 'make easy or easier'. Facilitators are well known in industrial management, where they act as catalysts for change and development. Margerison defines a facilitator as someone who had developed a role beyond that of the traditional personnel officer. He states: 'We have the *technical* knowledge and skills to solve problems, but it is difficult to get *people* to change' (Margerison 1978).

Facilitators within the health service are a more recent development. Following the Acheson Report on inner city care (London Health Planning Consortium 1981), Arnold Elliot, a general practitioner, was appointed as one of the first facilitators to work in primary health care (Elliott 1984). His function was to help general practitioners and other workers in primary care to upgrade their organisation of services — to improve clinical care by improving clerical care. Dr Elliott visited all practices in Islington to discuss their organisational needs and succeeded in improving premises through advice on grants and staffing opportunities.

In a more recent development of facilitation, Elaine Fullard was appointed to a study organised between general practice and community medicine (Fullard et al 1984). The brief was to explore the contribution of a facilitator to the organisation of screening for cardiovascular risk factors. The post developed to include direct help, with regular audits of medical records, recruitment and training of practice staff and advising on protocols for screening and life style counselling. She has pointed out her importance as a 'cross-pollinator' of good ideas between practices and the importance of coordinating the resources of community medicine, the Family Health Services Authority and the primary care team in developing effective prevention. A preliminary evaluation of the scheme has been undertaken in three Oxford practices and has shown a significant increase in recording after 2 years compared with control practices who had no access to facilitators (Fullard et al 1987).

Although the majority of facilitators focus mainly on screening for coronary risk factors, there are those who operate in areas such as alcohol abuse, AIDS and the management of chronic disorders in general practice. The success of this initiative is reflected in the growing numbers of facilitators throughout the UK (over 100 at the time of writing), with their own training programme and national coordinator.

THE ORGANISATION OF PREVENTIVE CARE

The size and complexity of the preventive task are daunting, but substantial progress can be made even in areas of high workload. 'The key to the process is an acceptance of measurable objectives with regular audit of the extent to which they are being achieved. Authority must be based on evidence rather than status' (Hart 1987). The achievement of these goals within a practice requires both educational and administrative change. Above all, it depends upon involving, informing and securing the active cooperation of all the relevant staff, whether they are receptionists, doctors, clerks or nurses. Doubtful partners and cautious nurses require time to express their reservations with the sympathetic accommodation of dissent.

When planning a preventive programme, key information includes an assessment of the practice's readiness to change. Industrial experience suggests that innovation is most likely to be successful in organisations that display certain characteristics (Rogers 1982). These include the availability of 'slack resources'. Resources such as time, money, personnel and space are stretched to the limit in most general practices and innovation may be possible only if new resources can be found or existing ones reallocated. For example, the introduction of a nurse-coordinated diabetic clinic will depend on the nurse being given 'protected' time in which to run the clinic. If available time is already fully committed, an innovation such as this will depend on generating more nurse sessions or restructuring existing commitments. Innovations fail when enthusiasm denies the existence of such practical constraints.

It is also important to reflect upon who has the power to make decisions within the organisation. If this power is concentrated in one person, an innovation may be introduced without overt opposition. However, the cost of such coercion may be the limited success of the innovation in the longer term. Without adequate consultation the innovator forfeits the constructive contribution of the other team members and their potential for enthusiastic support. Conversely, where decision-making is distributed more evenly among all members of the team, negotiating agreement may be much more difficult and time-consuming. However, if it is well done, the potential for sustaining success in the long term is much greater. In both these cases, recognising how decisions are made in a particular practice is an important first step.

The next step is to identify all those people who may be affected by the proposed change, or who may be in a position to obstruct or promote it within the practice. For example, doctors could invest considerable time introducing a computer into the practice, but if reception staff have a computer imposed upon them without effective discussion, their reluctance to cooperate may lead to an inaccurate and poorly functioning system. Success of an innovation depends upon effective discussion and negotiation with all interested parties and involvement at an early stage.

Having listed all these individuals with a 'stake' in the innovation, it is helpful to consult with them and assemble their current involvement in the organisation, the potential benefit and cost to them of the new project and their power to achieve or obstruct its success.

Consensus can be formulated around aims and administration over a series of meetings. While a maximum programme may not be achieved, a set of minimum goals can usually be agreed in a way that informs and educates those involved, secures their commitment and clearly demarcates their roles and responsibilities.

Meetings of this kind are notoriously difficult. People with bright ideas are keen to get others to support them. They approach colleagues, stress the benefits and play down difficult aspects. Gaining support for an innovation can become linked with the innovator's own personal sense of worth, so that criticism of the innovation is seen as criticism of the innovator. The response of team members to proposals may be linked to their status within the organisation. Where individuals have limited power in relation to the innovator, they may feel that they are unable to express criticism, and that whatever their opinions the change will be imposed. Little meaningful discussion can take place unless this sense of impotence can be contradicted. Alternatively, individuals whose power is comparable to the innovator's may use negative criticism to undermine the innovator. The challenge of these meetings is to set them up in such a way that they are positive opportunities for constructive discussion. A useful structure is to start by briefly presenting your idea and eliciting in turn the benefits and cost of the innovation as perceived by each team member. The success of this discussion depends upon creating a sense of collaboration rather than confrontation. It is important that everyone feels they not only have their say, but are actually listened to. Techniques that have been found helpful in creating such an atmosphere include:

1. Being explicit about why you think it's important to involve this person. For example, if a computerised appointment system were being considered, the subject might be introduced to the receptionists by referring to their expertise and central role in coordinating appointments. Stressing the cre-

dentials of the individual helps empower them to think constructively and act responsibly.

2. Behaving as if you trust your colleagues with your idea and expect them to be able to look at it objectively. Entering discussions in a defensive or aggressive frame of mind is likely to generate the negative response you wish to avoid.

3. Being receptive to positive and negative responses to your ideas, and being seen to value each stakeholder's opinion, even if it contradicts your own. In particular, encouraging colleagues to expand on negative feelings can convince them that you are not simply trying to manipulate them. It is more powerful to arrive at agreement when negative reactions have been explored than to obtain premature agreement by evading areas of potential conflict. In the short term this can be tedious and threatening, but in the longer term may be crucial for the sustained success of the project.

4. Where potential benefits are identified, it is important that these should be seen as realistic and attainable. Where costs to individuals are identified, these must be addressed, however trivial they may seem. Strategies for minimising these costs can then be explored. People often need this opportunity to express and deal with the fear that may accompany proposals for change. Having carried out discussions with key individuals, the feasibility of the proposed preventive service can be re-evaluated. As well as generating strategic information, these discussions will have given an opportunity to refine the original proposal. Trusting colleagues with your thinking and giving them an opportunity to contribute to its development also encourages a sense of ownership at this crucial early stage.

Having decided to introduce a preventive service into the practice, the next step is to define the main objectives of the new service. It may be useful to divide the meeting into small groups to discuss 'What do you think it is important for the service to achieve?' It may help to have a structure for these groups such that each individual has the same opportunity to speak and be listened to, allowing ideas to be refined in relative safety. The principal points can be fed back to the main meeting and listed on a blackboard, where they can be discussed.

Once objectives have been agreed upon, the next step is to consider the range of options to realise them. The preliminary meetings may well have identified a number of alternative ways of implementing the innovation. These can be listed and discussed and other alternatives encouraged before going on to discuss which option is best. Having chosen one or more of these options, the implications for relevant individuals within the practice need to be outlined. All the tasks that need to be undertaken to implement the innovation can be listed and agreement on whose responsibility it is to carry each one out can be reached. In particular, it is helpful to choose someone for a central coordinating role to oversee progress as a whole.

Where individual responsibilities have been agreed, the resources and skills needed to fulfil them can be identified. Some of these may already be available in the practice, and where there are gaps in skills or resources, strategies can be planned for filling them. A nurse may need to improve her clinical knowledge of diabetes on a course, or extra clerical time may be needed to administer the diabetic register. Common criteria for measurement may need to be adopted. Manuals exist for the measurement of most common conditions and these provide an invaluable starting point for discussion.

The provision of a planned programme of advice to patients needs to be addressed and the leaflets, checklists of issues covered and other resources for patient education should be discussed and agreed. The development of counselling strategies that take account of patients' priorities and constraints may prove a rich and continuing source of education and more complex educational programmes involving individuals, groups and families may continue to evolve.

There are four administrative tasks for which members of staff need to take clear responsibility.

1. A coordinator is required to ensure overall cohesion of the programme.
2. Maintenance and validation of the register.
3. Administration of call, recall and follow-up, including procedures for non-respondents.
4. Provision of continuing audit.

Much of the preceding discussion can now begin to be summarised in a concise working document outlining the agreed aims and administration of the project. Procedures can often be complex, particularly for new staff, and the document can serve as a basis for training. The document also serves as an aide-memoire to cut-off points, grades of risk and action to be taken, as well as to complex administrative procedures. It serves as a starting point for discussion in the event of dispute and a source of amendment where procedures fail to produce the desired result. The document summarises the practice consensus and, as such, it evolves over time.

Having agreed objectives, chosen the best option for meeting these and identified the personnel, skills and resources necessary to carry them through, it is realistic to agree a timetable for implementation. How long will training take and how long will it take to validate the register? Who will be the first people to be called or recalled? When does it all start? And when it does start, will there be additional time to allow staff to highlight weaknesses and generate ideas for improvement? Frequent meetings in the early days of the new project provide a forum for continuing support and improvement.

THE REGISTER

It must be rare for an entire new programme to start all at once. The component parts may be prepared at different times and a schedule of what becomes operational and when is a useful spur to action. The register is one of the most complex and key elements. An accurate register is a prerequisite for whole population ascertainment. Fifteen to fifty per cent of the practice population may not be at the address stated (Stott & Pill 1988, Bowling & Jacobson 1989). With meticulous documentation at practice level, clear procedures for the notification of entry and exit and simple and continuing validation of the register, inflation can be maintained below 10–15% in most inner urban areas. Areas with many hostel dwellers or other highly transient groups may experience particular difficulties.

Fraser has devised simple cross-checks between the practice record, the practice register and the Family Health Services Authority register that identifies most current patients (Fraser & Clayton 1981). Where doubt remains, home visits or a letter may quickly clarify that the patient is no longer resident. Computerisation allows fairly rapid validation of data. Checks may be built into the software, e.g. date today may not be allowed as a date of birth, or printed lists of new registrations can be manually checked once a month for completeness and accuracy.

DOCUMENTATION AND NON-RESPONDENTS

Display of the date of next test due on the front of the notes is the simplest plan for action. By itself this will identify only those who turn up to see the doctor. More complex registers, both manual and computerised, may provide lists for call, recall and audit. Cross-checks between the recall register and the patient record will reveal that tests are undertaken but not reported on the recall register, a source of irritation both for the patients and for those who have contacted them unnecessarily.

The follow up of non-respondents is as much concerned with eradicating those who have in fact left the practice from the register, as it is with the location of patients who have not replied. How many reminders will be sent? Who will do it and how will records be flagged so that the offer may be repeated should the opportunity arise during a routine consultation? The follow-up of non-respondents provides continuing validation of the register.

AUDIT

Sustaining enthusiasm and commitment to what is often repetitive work with marginal gains is a continuing task. Regular meetings of staff allow the organisation to be examined and improved, and concerns about either patients or the administration discussed.

Audit criteria might include measures such as patient attendance, procedures performed per consultation, staff or patient satisfaction, percentage of those with or without a test result and the percentages overdue. Data sheets need to be designed to collect this information prospectively and a member of staff designated to collate the information and check that it is entered by staff in a standard fashion. Alternatively, a random sample of the notes might be selected, although the variability inherent in too small a sample may make comparisons difficult.

Progress reports from team members lend colour to these figures and the changes required where there are weaknesses. It is important that evaluation should be used to enhance learning and performance rather than to pillory the shortcomings of the past. Celebration is an important element of the review, and even where there have been difficulties there are usually some areas where there has been progress and success can be credited.

Clinical review of patients is best carried out with adequate protected time. One thorough review and explanation may be more useful than frequent hurried and incomplete contacts. Content and periodicity of clinical review need to be decided, and strategies devised for improving control where this is poor. Review is as much for the patient as for the provider and a report of progress with revision of priorities, strategy and aims may improve progress towards targets.

The results of audit meetings may be summarised in the annual report. This permits review by peers and public and also enables a comparison of practices. It also helps formulate the goals for the coming year for all members of staff and the proposed changes to improve performance. Lawrence has published guidelines for peer review through team visiting (Lawrence 1989).

Without organisation, neither doctors nor nurses do very well at prevention. The size and complexity of the task make it impossible simply to delegate the responsibility to someone else or hope that computerisation will solve the problem. At best such a strategy will reduplicate the current sins of omission and commission. At worst, the defunct computer on the shelf or the failed diabetic clinic that the nurse was told to set up can be bruising experiences for all concerned. There will inevitably be false starts and blind alleys, but providing these have been fully discussed and were entered into by informed, involved and committed staff, the problems that arise can usually be surmounted without too much damaging recrimination. It has taken our practice in Chrisp Street, London, 10 years of patient, painstaking and at times frustrating meetings to achieve consensus on a programme of effective action around smoking, blood pressure, cervical cytology, heart disease risk factors and immunisation. The process has certainly changed the perceptions of the practice team and hopefully enabled patients to deal more effectively with the risks they face.

REFERENCES

Bosanquet N, Leese B 1988 Family doctors and innovation in general practice. British Medical Journal 296: 1576–1580

Bowling A 1981 Delegation to nurses in general practice. Journal of the Royal College of General Practitioners 31: 485–490

Bowling A 1983 Teamwork in primary health care. Nursing Times November: 56–58

Bowling A, Jacobson B 1989 Screening. The inadequacy of population registers. British Medical Journal 298: 545–546

Brown A M, Jachuck S J, Walters F, van Zwanenberg T D 1986 The future of general practice in Newcastle upon Tyne. Lancet i: 370–371

Briggs Report 1972 Report of the Committee on Nursing, Cmnd 5115. HMSO, London

Bruce N 1980 Teamwork for preventive care. Research Studies Press, Chichester

Cartilidge A, Bond J, Green B 1987 Interprofessional collaboration in primary health care. Nursing Times 83: 45–48

Colliere M F 1986 Invisible care and invisible women as health care providers. International Journal of Nursing Studies 23: 95–112

Dingwall 1980 Problems of teamwork in primary care. In: Lonsdale S, Webb A, Briggs T (eds) Teamwork in the personal social services and health care. Croom Helm, London

Drury M, Greenfield S, Stillwell B, Hull F M 1988 A nurse practitioner in general practice. Patient perceptions and expectations. Journal of the Royal College of General Practitioners 38: 503–505

Edwards Report 1987 Review of community nursing in Wales. Nursing in the community — a team approach for Wales. Welsh Office, Cardiff

Elliott A 1984 General practice facilitator — a personal view. Health Trends 16: 74–79

Fraser R C, Clayton D G 1981 The accuracy of age/sex registers, practice medical records and family practitioner committee registers. Journal of the Royal College of General Practitioners 31: 410–419

Fullard E, Fowler G, Gray M 1984 Facilitating prevention in primary care. British Medical Journal 289: 1585–1587

Fullard E, Fowler G, Gray M 1987 Promoting prevention in primary care: controlled trial of low technology, low cost approach. British Medical Journal 294: 1080–1082

Goodhearted Glasgow 1987 Goodhearted Glasgow: the first year. Greater Glasgow Health Board, Glasgow

Greenfield S, Stillwell B, Drury M 1987 Practice nurses. Social and occupational characteristics. Journal of the Royal College of General Practitioners 37: 341–345

Hannay D R 1980 Problems of team work. In: Barber J H, Kratz C R (eds) Towards team care. Churchill Livingstone, London

Hart J T 1974 The marriage of primary care and epidemiology. Journal of the Royal College of Physicians London 8: 299–314

Hart J T 1981 A new kind of doctor. Journal of the Royal Society of Medicine 74: 871–883

Hart J T 1982 The measurement of ommission. British Medical Journal 284: 1686–1689

Hart J T 1984 Community general practitioners. British Medical Journal 288: 1670–1673

Hart J T 1985 Practice nurses: an underused resource. British Medical Journal 290: 1162–1163

Hart J T 1987 Hypertension: community control of high blood pressure. Churchill Livingstone, London, p 122

Heath M C D 1984 Failure of the cervical cytology screening programme . British Medical Journal 289: 1223–1224

Jarman B, Cumberlege J 1987 Developing primary health care. British Medical Journal 294: 1005–1008

Kranshein P, Jorgen V, Mulhauser I et al 1988 Evaluation of a structured treatment and teaching programme on non-insulin dependent diabetes. Lancet 2: 1407–1411

Lawrence M 1989 Practice team visiting. Anticipatory care teams working party, Department of Community Medicine Radcliffe Infirmary, Oxford

London Health Planning Consortium 1981 Primary care in inner London. Primary care study group, Department of Health and Social Security, London

Mant D, Anderson P 1985 Community general practitioner. Lancet ii: 1114–1117

McClure L M 1984 Teamwork myth or reality. Community nurses' experience with general practice attachment. Journal of Epidemiology and Community Health 38: 66–74

Margerison C 1978 Influencing organisational change: The role of the personnel specialist. Lonsdale University Printing, USA

Marsh G N, Chew C 1984 Well man clinic in general practice. British Medical Journal 288: 200–201

Peckham C, Bredford H, Senturia Y, Ades A 1989 The Peckham Report. National immunisation study: factors influencing immunisation uptake in childhood. Department of Paediatric Epidemiology, Institute of Child Health, London

Pickering G 1987 Foreword to the first edition. In: Hart J T Hypertension: community control of high blood pressure. Churchill Livingstone, London

Reedy B L E C, Metcalfe A V, de Roumanie M, Newell D J 1980 The social and occupational characteristics of attached and employed nurses in general practice. Journal of the Royal College of General Practitioners 30: 477–482

Reith W 1985 Should nurses practice prevention? British Medical Journal 291: 1349

Robson J 1986 Bridging the expectation delivery gap. In: Pereira Gray D J (ed) The Medical Annual. John Wright, Bristol

Robson J, Boomla K, Fitzpatrick S et al 1989 Using nurses for preventive activities with computer assisted follow-up: a randomised controlled trial. British Medical Journal 298: 433–436

Rogers E 1982 Diffusion of innovations. New York Free Press, New York

Rubin I M, Beckhard M 1971 Factors influencing the effectiveness of health teams. MIT working paper 561–71. Massachusetts Institute of Technology, Cambridge, Ma

South East London Screening Study Group 1977 A controlled trial of multiphasic screening in middle age. Results of the South East London screening study. International Journal of Epidemiology 6: 357–363

Spitzer W O, Sackett D L, Sibley J C et al 1974 Burlington randomized trial of the nurse practitioner. New England Journal of Medicine 290: 251–256

Spitzer W O 1984 The nurse practitioner revisited. Slow death of a good idea. New England Journal of Medicine 310: 1049–1052

Stott N C H, Pill R M 1988 Health checks in general practice. Why some people attend and others do not. Department of General Practice, University of Wales College of Medicine, Cardiff

Tuomilehto J, Puska P 1987 The changing role and legitimate boundaries of epidemiology. Community based intervention programmes. Social Science and Medicine 25: 589–597

Weed L 1977 The expectation delivery gap. Oklahoma State Medical School Journal 70: 12–15

Whitehouse C R 1986 Conflict and cooperation between doctors and nurses in primary health care. Nursing Practice 1: 242–245

Van den Dool 1973 From multiple screening to anticipatory medicine. Allgemein medizin International 3: 100–101

8. Questionnaires

Alastair F Wright

INTRODUCTION

When information has to be gathered in a systematic and reliable way, the best method is usually to use a questionnaire. All of us are, of course, familiar with marketing surveys and opinion polls, which use specially constructed questionnaires. A simple use for a questionnaire in general practice would be for recording registration details of new patients, with perhaps details of immunisations, date of last cervical smear and some past medical history. Other uses might be in geriatric surveillance, or screening to uncover hidden psychiatric illness.

Successful screening, surveillance or research depends on the quality of the information on which action can be based or conclusions drawn. The quality of the information in turn depends on the quality of the questionnaire used to obtain it. Clinical audit (performance review) requires appropriate information to be gathered accurately and systematically before any conclusions may be drawn on the quality of care.

Definition

A questionnaire is a *prepared* set of written questions used to gather or compare information. It is not just a form to be filled in but is a scientific tool for measuring and collecting specific types of data. This data can then be used to classify or categorise events, behaviour, attitudes or performance.

Questionnaires are thus used to solve many different types of clinical problem. They can be used to build up a database of clinical information on new patients so that case summaries can be more easily prepared. They can be used in performance review to compare a doctor's care of diabetic patients with standards established for good practice. The work need not stop at collecting or comparing routine data but can go on to become a proper research project, which discovers new facts about disease or about the organisation of care

and leads to the development of better forms of treatment.

Sheldon (1982a) describes the use of a questionnaire in his practice to collect background information for individual patient summaries. This background information on all patients in the practice is routinely collected by patient-filled questionnaires and subsequently checked by the general practitioner at the next consultation. The information is compared with the medical record when it arrives and summary forms are completed by the practice secretary. A computer print-out of the medical summary is prepared and filed in the patient's records. A duplicate summary is then checked by the general practitioner and amended if necessary.

As Sheldon points out (1982b): "...the consultation between the doctor and the patient is stressful for patients and makes them forget, exaggerate or minimise important information. Most of this stress can be removed using a questionnaire technique... and more accurate answers, especially to personal questions or areas of anxiety to the patient, can be obtained." The main disadvantage of such questionnaire systems is that not all patients will fill them in.

Patient questionnaires have also been found to be of value at hospital out-patient clinics (Short 1986). In Short's study, the patient-completed questionnaire mentioned more symptoms than the referral letter, gave more detailed family history and more accurate information about therapy. There is evidence that even in consultant clinics the history is of more value than either the physical examination or the investigations and a questionnaire completed while the patient is waiting improves the quality of the subsequent consultation. The author points out that the idea of using a questionnaire may be less acceptable to doctors than to patients, who often welcome the questionnaire as evidence of the doctor's special interest in their problem.

Specially prepared research questionnaires (Goldberg 1972) can also be used with advantage in a practice, for example in uncovering hidden psychiatric illness in attending patients (Wright & Perini 1987).

BASIC CONSIDERATIONS

Gathering facts can be intriguing and exciting and the questionnaire seems to make this simple. Take care: good questionnaires are more difficult to design and construct than you might think. Beware of collecting worthless data that cannot be analysed or understood.

Constructing a questionnaire does not have to be complicated but some basic principles should be observed. The first step must always be to define the problem to be tackled and hence to decide on what questions to ask. It is always tempting to try to cover too much ground, to enquire about everything that might turn out to be useful or interesting. This leads to long boring questionnaires, which yield little worthwhile information and are very difficult to analyse. Certain questions are obviously important and include themselves. It is necessary to ask classification questions such as name, sex, date of birth and perhaps employment to identify patients and be able to classify answers. Try to exclude any questions that are not strictly relevant to the objectives you set for the survey.

The patient or respondent has information we need and we must aim to get it from him/her with a minimum of distortion. It is important for designers of questionnaires to remember that people often do not have clear or consistent ideas of what they want, like or expect; and there is a danger that neat precoded questionnaires give the impression that they do. The first idea that comes to mind does not reflect a considered opinion.

Answers are affected by wishful thinking, a desire to please the doctor and the wish to put oneself in a good light. In addition, most people forget details with the passage of time.

There is no point in asking people's opinion about something they do not understand. Neither is it safe to assume that patients will voluntarily admit ignorance. So even when asking for factual information, make sure that the person asked is in a good position to give it and don't expect infallible memory. Consider providing a 'don't know' option. Although patients are willing to complete the questionnaire, there is no certainty that the answers will be accurate if the questions are on a delicate subject about which people are reluctant to talk. Many people might tend to understate their age and how much alcohol they drink and to exaggerate their education.

Some people will answer questions on 'how often' or 'when' or 'what is the average' in terms of what they think they usually do or aim to do rather than what they actually do. Similarly, some people, when asked to choose a numerical estimate, will choose a figure near the middle of a series. This can be partially avoided by choosing an even number of possible answers so that the middle answer is not possible.

Avoid ambiguity and jargon

Good questionnaires should avoid ambiguity and jargon so that all patients understand and interpret the questions in the same way. Likewise, good questionnaires should be valid and reliable. That is to say they should measure closely what you aim to measure and must give consistent results over time and with different respondents. It is pointless to ask a patient 'Are you bothered with sickness or diarrhoea?' First, it is a double question. What should be the answer of the patient who has loose stools and who feels well? Does 'sickness' mean malaise or vomiting? Does 'bothered' mean having symptoms or being upset by them? Is the questioner asking about symptoms today or over the last month? Not all patients will know what is generally meant by diarrhoea, just as some may believe that 'having the bowels open' means vomiting.

Meaningful questions

If questions are too broadly based they will generate answers that are difficult to classify and summarise. It is crucial to ask meaningful questions, which will receive truthful reactions. Direct questions about smoking, drinking and sex-life have personal and intimate overtones and may not be answered truthfully, especially when asked face to face. In this instance, written and computer-based questionnaires tend to give more accurate responses. Frequently, patients may not answer or may furnish the answer they think is expected of them. Intimate questions must be handled very tactfully and are best answered anonymously or put by someone who has the patient's complete confidence. It seems doubtful whether the badly asked questions on present-day insurance proposals about sexual lifestyle and HIV risk will produce scientifically reliable answers.

Reliability and validity

A reliable questionnaire is one that obtains consistent results from different respondents and at different times. A valid questionnaire is one that accurately measures the factor under investigation. However, if a questionnaire gives inconsistent results it cannot be expected to produce valid answers.

It may be possible to compare the results of a questionnaire with an independent measure of the same variable, often called a criterion. Several questionnaires are available to measure whether or not patients are psychiatric 'cases' and could be regarded as suffering from psychiatric illness. This measure of 'caseness' can be compared with the opinions of consultant psychiatrists or the questionnaire can be shown to distinguish between 'normal' individuals and patients under treatment in a mental hospital. Another way of approaching validation of a questionnaire is to compare the results obtained with the results of other studies.

A descriptive study

This type of investigation is descriptive or enumerative; in other words its purpose is to count. It often uses a representative sample and makes inferences about the whole group. It estimates *how many* have the characteristic in question or *how often* an event occurs. It is not designed to explain anything or show relationships. However, using a questionnaire before and after a screening exercise can provide a measure of the effectiveness of the programme.

A comparative study

Another type of investigation is the analytical/relational survey. The aim is to look at associations and to find explanations for differences between groups of patients. This type of survey is often set up to test specific hypotheses.

Opinion and attitude surveys

Opinion and attitude surveys are a special type of enquiry. They also use questionnaires to gather the data but have special problems of bias that make the interpretation of the results particularly tricky. Studying attitudes and behaviour is very complex. Difficulty with criteria is the main problem in trying to assess the validity of questions on attitudes. Opinion polls, say on voting intentions, may attempt simply to estimate what proportion of the survey population say they will vote for a particular political party.

Research questionnaires

These follow the same rules as any other questionnaire, although the rules must be more stringently followed and more attention must be paid to the reliability and validity of the questionnaire. The answers are likely to be subjected to statistical analysis.

DESIGN

Designing the questionnaire is by no means the first step. By this stage you should be clear about the aims of the project, what information you need and from which group of patients the information is to be collected. You should consider confidentiality as well as any sampling technique to be used. It would be wise to have looked over publications on the same subject and at the questionnaires used by other workers. You should think about how the questionnaire is to be used: would there be problems with illiterates or ethnic minorities in the practice and how would these be overcome? Would the omission of these patients matter to the research aims?

Once the data are collected how are they to be processed and analysed? If the questionnaire is to be used in a research project have you formulated a hypothesis and considered the testing of your data for statistical significance?

Specific design questions that need to be considered include:

1. Will the questionnaire be completed by an interviewer, who may be the doctor, nurse or receptionist or a worker specially trained for the purpose?
2. If the questionnaire is to be self-completed, will it be a mail questionnaire or filled in by the patient at the surgery, where additional explanation can be given if necessary? A mail questionnaire will need a letter of introduction from the doctor and may require more elaborate written instructions.
3. Are the questions to be open or closed or a mixture of both?
4. What is to be the order of the questions? 'Funnnel' questions start by being broad and general and later concentrate on specific points. 'Filter' questions can be used to exclude the respondent from a subset of questions that are irrelevant to him or her. The order of the questions must be logical for these devices to be effective. Forms used for clinical interview should follow the natural order of the consultation from retrieval of information to patient assessment.

Interview versus self-administered

The questionnaire-based interview has much in common with the traditional consultation but the information is acquired and written down in a predetermined and structured way. In research on mental illness, psychiatrists often use structured interviews based on prepared questionnaires (Goldberg et al 1970) so that they can write down their findings in a way that is more easy to compare.

The interview questionnaire is more sensitive and spontaneous than the self-completed questionnaire and is also more flexible. However, it is much more expensive, uses a lot of doctor or interviewer time and there is the danger that the interviewer may unwittingly influence the patient to give the desired answer (interview bias). An interesting variant, common in the USA, is the interview by telephone. This method may be particularly suitable for enquiries on sensitive subjects such as sexual behaviour. A computer-assisted telephone interviewing system has recently been used to study AIDS-related knowledge, attitudes and sexual practice (University of Edinburgh 1989).

Self-report questionnaires are inexpensive and simple to administer, and interview bias is eliminated. Not all patients will complete the form and some will complete it incorrectly. There is an advantage for patients in that they are spared the stress of an interview and are thus less likely to forget, exaggerate or minimise important information. Self-administered questionnaires can be used in the waiting room before the patient sees the doctor. This ensures a high response rate and accurate sampling of attending patients with no interview bias. The receptionist may provide any necessary explanations (but may not interpret the questions or suggest answers) and provide the advantage of a measure of personal contact. The doctor may then make an interviewer assessment during the consultation.

Self-report questionnaires are often used for postal surveys accompanied by a letter of introduction and more detailed instructions. Mail surveys are cheap, do not need trained staff but postage must be allowed for. Data processing and analysis are also simpler and cheaper, as the forms can be precoded. This allows the researcher to have a larger sample at small cost and the sampling can be very accurate because the envelope is addressed to a particular individual (although it is occasionally not completed by that person). As there is no interviewer, the questionnaire must be relatively simple because little explanation is possible and there is a limited possibility for comments from the patient. When investigating sensitive areas such as sexual behaviour or illicit drug taking, an anonymous mail questionnaire will often produce more (socially unacceptable) true responses than an interview.

The main disadvantage of this type of questionnaire is the possibility of low response rates, so there should be a plan for follow-up of non-respondents. Non-response does not occur randomly, it varies from study to study and can be reduced by careful planning. A personal letter from the doctor to the patient, bearing the patient's name and signed individually by the doctor, can greatly improve the response rate.

Open or closed questions

The questions on a questionnaire can be open or closed. Open questions give much more freedom to the respondent but replies are difficult to classify and code for analysis. Both types of questions have their advantages and disadvantages.

If the question is closed the respondent does not need to write an answer but simply marks with a tick, underlines or circles his/her choice from a list of possibilities. A modern example of closed questions is the multiple choice questionnaire, now much used in medical examinations to test factual knowledge. Closed questions are less flexible but coding and analysis is simpler. It is particularly important that the questions are direct and easily understood and that the permitted answers are relevant. This is ensured by careful pilot work. The GHQ-28 (Goldberg 1972) is a questionnaire that uses closed questions.

Open questions allow the respondent to reply in his or her own words. Very loquacious patients can be restrained by limiting the space available for answers. The main advantages with open questions are the freedom they give to the respondent and the sensitivity of the answers. This type of question is easy to ask, difficult to answer and much more difficult to analyse. Coding of open questions requires skill and takes time and, unless the researcher means to do all his/her own work, trained staff are expensive. Open questions call for more thought in replying and have lower yield than a simple prompt list.

Question wording

Poorly worded, ambiguous questions produce unmanageable ambiguous answers that cannot be compared. Vague questions receive vague answers and leading questions produce biased answers.

Even simple words can be misunderstood. A week may mean seven days in some contexts but can also be taken to be the five working days. Shift workers can have working 'weeks' of differing lengths, so it is best to be precise. Similarly, using 'forename' and 'family name' rather than 'Christian name' and 'surname' covers different ethnic and religious groups. Leading questions and loaded words are not neutral. Try to avoid loaded phrases like 'doctors say that', 'as you know' or 'research has shown'.

Vocabulary that is common in medical texts may be quite unfamiliar to those who are completing the questionnaire. Words like 'hypothetical', 'initiate' or 'consider' may be familiar to the doctor but are uncommon in everyday conversation. Use 'help' rather than 'assist', 'say' rather than 'state' and 'think' rather than 'consider'. 'Live' is better than 'reside', 'want' is better than 'require' and 'end' or 'stop' is better than 'terminate'.

Even simple words can cause problems if not used carefully. For example, 'about', 'any' or 'few' must be used (and understood) with precision or answers may be unreliable. All patients ought to interpret the question in the same manner. Adjustment of question wording or in the order of words may significantly affect the answers.

Answers to opinion questions are more sensitive to changes in wording, emphasis, sequence and so on than those to factual questions. Consider changes carefully and remember to retest. One should avoid giving the impression that respondents would be stupid if they did not know the answer.

Apparently factual questions can also present unexpected problems, especially if they deal with drinking, smoking or carbohydrate consumption. Answers may be a mixture of fact, uncertain memory, a desire to please or plain wishful thinking. It can help a patient's memory to link questions to a memorable event such as Christmas or the local summer holidays. A number of simple tests can often be used to check the reliability of factual questions. For example, one can cross-check with other sources of data, e.g. medical record cards or a list of voters.

The same problems may occur with tactlessly worded questions on employment, financial status or sex-life. Embarrassing questions must be handled with sensitivity, preferably by someone who has the patient's complete confidence. It may help to lead in to the target topic indirectly, with subsequent questions becoming more specific. Additionally, one can guarantee that the questionnaire is anonymous and create a permissive atmosphere by the wording and sequence of the questions.

Classification questions

Classification questions are factual questions on age, sex, marital status, social class or family size to enable patients to be placed in groups. It is polite to explain the reason for such questions, which may seem to pry, e.g. 'To help classify and compare your answers with those of other patients, I need to ask about yourself and your family.' It is often best to leave classification questions to the end, to prevent packing the beginning of the questionnaire with personal questions that may distract from the main purpose.

Format of the questionnaire sheet

Forms should be planned to aid accurate recording and easy transfer to a computer for analysis. A well structured form makes analysis and summarisation much simpler and mistakes less likely. The layout should follow a natural order if possible. It may be helpful to use boxes for answers and these should be aligned both vertically and horizontally.

Pilot run

It is tempting with a new questionnaire to start using it as soon as the ink is dry. This would be foolish. Designing questionnaires depends as much on experience and following hunches as it does on scientific rules and every questionnaire must be tested before it can be used reliably. The pilot survey shows defects in wording and structure and points out questions that have been misunderstood by the respondents. The pilot run is a 'health check' for the questionnaire.

Apart from pinpointing sources of misunderstanding and bad questions, the pilot run can suggest how to turn free answer questions into multiple choices, which are much easier to analyse. The pilot helps one think ahead to the analysis. It is very frustrating to realise at the time of analysis that important questions have been missed or that the wrong questions have been asked. Also, at the pilot stage, the method of approaching patients can be reviewed and the letter of introduction can be perfected. It is advisable to allow enough time between pilot and main study to allow lessons learnt from the pilot to be incorporated in the main study.

ANALYSIS

If the earlier stages have been well handled, analysing the results should present few problems but it is very important to be systematic and to label each sheet of figures very carefully. A simple analysis can be done by ticking columns in an arithmetic exercise book. Another simple method is to use edge-punched cards. The computer system offers the most flexible means of storing data, analysing them quickly and producing reports. Data are best stored in their basic form when possible, i.e. date of birth, date of onset of illness rather than age or how long the illness has been present. In this way, calculations are left to the computer and errors of mental arithmetic avoided.

At the design stage, provision will have been made for coding the answers, i.e. converting them into numbers that can be analysed mathematically. The coding can be devised by the researcher, e.g. 0 = no symptoms,

1 = mild symptoms, 2 = moderate symptoms, 3 = severe symptoms. When coding, for example, occupations or diagnoses, nationally recognised lists are available and this helps when making comparisons with other studies. The Royal College of General Practitioners publishes a list, *Classification and analysis of general practice data* (RCGP 1986), as does the World Organisation of National Colleges, Academies and Academic Associations of General Practitioners/ Family Physicians (WONCA) — *International classification for primary care* (WONCA 1987). More exhaustive lists are prepared for international comparisons but these can be too bulky and complex for easy desktop use unless a computer is available.

Precoded and most closed questions are easily represented numerically but open questions are more difficult to process. Individual answers to each question have to be collected together and tabulated in a form that seems to make sense. The data are converted into numerical form by classifying the answers strictly and fairly. This is possible only if the aims of the study and the questions asked have been defined accurately at the planning stage and if these are strictly followed at the time of analysis. Converting free form answers to numerical form inevitably means rejecting information. There are no hard and fast rules and the process calls for some judgement and experience. For simple projects in general practice it is probably wise to use as many closed questions as possible.

Statistical analysis

The purpose of statistical analysis is to draw conclusions about a general population based on data collected from a sample of that population.

A doctor might need to know how many women patients had recently had a cervical smear done in hospital or well-woman clinic to estimate the need for a practice screening programme. Asking every adult woman would be impracticable, so the doctor sends a questionnaire to a sample of women *representative* of all adult women on the practice list and, from this, can estimate, within known limits of error, the staff time required for the practice screening programme.

For simple projects, it may be sufficient simply to tabulate the results of the questionnaire. If statistical analysis is contemplated, or comparisons are to be drawn, it is essential to consult a statistician at a very early stage. Even the best statistician cannot make presentable data that have been collected in a haphazard way or that are badly biased and are not representative of the group of patients being studied. Statisticians may be found in most health districts and at universities. The local university Department of General Practice is a valuable source of advice, as is the local faculty of the RCGP.

Using punch cards

For very small projects, or to test out ideas, edge-punched cards provide a simple cheap method of analysis. The only equipment required is a hand punch, or pair of scissors, and a few knitting needles of an appropriate diameter. Standard multipurpose cards are easily obtained (e.g. Cope-chat cards, from the Copeland Chatterson Company, Seymour House, 17 Waterloo Place, London SW1Y 4AR) but cards can be prepared for specific projects. It is possible to use the card as the questionnaire on which the patient's answers can be directly marked by the investigator.

For any one answer, the cards can be separated out by inserting a single needle into the appropriate hole. Those cards that have the hole punched out simply drop down and are easily counted. Several needles can be used at once to identify patients who have several characteristics in common. It is often best for the investigator to handle the cards, because the size of the various piles of cards gives a good 'feel' of the numbers involved and helps in the understanding of the results in a simple way. When many different categories are required, or when there are more than a couple of hundred patients, cards become unwieldy unless they are to be handled by a machine, and in this case it is better to use a microcomputer.

Simple microcomputer methods

The arrival of microcomputers in practices has simplified many of the processes involved in surveys and surveillance. The power of even a simple microcomputer to organise information, count numbers, perform statistical calculations and print out the results is awesome. Instead of filling in a questionnaire form, practice patients can even sit at a computer screen, be presented with a series of multiple choice questions and pass their answers directly to the computer memory (Wright 1990). In this way several stages of an investigation can be combined and transcription errors minimised.

The main disadvantage of computers with great processing power is that it is possible to summarise and analyse large volumes of data, some of which may be of questionable quality. Researchers can collect too much data and find it too complex to provide a satisfactory analysis. Comparisons of hundreds of different items collected from a few dozen patients do not make convincing reading.

While good statistical advice is as vital as ever, it is no longer necessary for data to be processed and statistical tests done on a university mainframe computer, unless the project is very large indeed. If the doctor wishes to become involved in computer analysis of the data, and can handle a keyboard, there are good commercial computer programs available to manipulate and analyse data and print out results (see also Chapter 6).

PRACTICAL TIPS

1. I have found it useful to start my thinking with open questions and then try to close them. There is always a loss of information when questions are converted to the closed type but this need not be important if more questions are answered satisfactorily and the analysis is more manageable.
2. A long questionnaire can intimidate both the doctor or interviewer and the respondent. Over-long, boring questionnaires lead to higher refusal rates and affect the quality of the data.
3. Think of the office staff as well as the doctor and the patient. Clear layout and printing are fundamental if coding and checking of answers are to proceed smoothly.
4. Make clear which questions are to be answered by whom. Using capital letters to emphasise important words makes instructions easier to follow. Tell patients that accuracy is most important and that a negative answer is as good as a positive one.
5. Staff may explain the nature of the enquiry and encourage patients to complete the form but should not have to explain the questions themselves or the patient's answers will be biased. If a question has to be explained it may mean that you are asking the wrong question. Try to rephrase it or split it into two separate questions.
6. A personalised letter of explanation from the patient's own doctor is a very effective way of ensuring that patients participate in the enquiry.
7. Printed instructions are needed for self-report and mail questionnaires. Capital letters are widely used to emphasise particular words and instructions. The main purpose of instructions is to compensate for the absence of an interviewer, so they must be clear and in simple language.
8. Above all don't try to do too much at the first attempt. Keep it simple.

REFERENCES

Goldberg D P 1972 The detection of psychiatric illness by questionnaire. Oxford University Press, London
Goldberg D P, Cooper B, Eastwood M R 1970 A standardised psychiatric interview for use in community surveys. British Journal of Preventive Medicine 24: 18–23
Royal College of General Practitioners 1986 Classification and analysis of general practice data. Occasional paper 26. RCGP, London
Sheldon M G 1982a Giving patients a copy of their computer medical record. Journal of the Royal College of General Practitioners 32: 80–86
Sheldon M 1982b The use of patient questionnaires in practice. Medicine in Practice 13: 320–323
Short D 1986 Why don't we use questionnaires in the medical out-patient clinic? Health Bulletin, Edinburgh 44: 228–233

University of Edinburgh, Research Unit in Health and Behavioural Change 1989 AIDS-related knowledge attitudes and practices provisional data. University of Edinburgh, Edinburgh
WONCA 1987 International classification for primary care. Oxford University Press, Oxford
Wright A F, Perini A F 1987 Hidden psychiatric illness: use of the general health questionnaire in general practice. Journal of the Royal College of General Practitioners 37: 164–167.
Wright A F 1990 A study of the presentation of somatic symptoms in general practice by patients with psychiatric disturbance. British Journal of General Practice 40: 459–463.

9. Opportunistic screening

Colin P Bradley

There is a tide in the affairs of men, which, if taken at the flood, leads on to fortune... (Shakespeare, *Julius Caesar* IV iii)

SCREENING, SURVEILLANCE AND CASE-FINDING

Before beginning to discuss what is meant by opportunistic screening, it is important to clear up some of the semantic confusion that exists in the use of terms related to screening. Screening has been rather narrowly defined as the 'seeking out of people with no overt symptoms and asking them to undergo examination to see whether the condition to be identified is present' (HMSO 1977). This distinguishes it from the related activities of surveillance and case-finding. Surveillance, in its narrowest sense, is the close observation or supervision of people to identify health problems at an early, and possibly more easily treated, stage of their development. The term 'case-finding' has been used by some authors (Fowler & Gray 1983) to describe an approach to screening that involves the detection of disease or risk factors at consultations for unrelated health problems. This may also be described by the terms 'opportunistic screening' or 'opportunistic case-finding', depending whether it is asymptomatic or symptomatic conditions that are being sought. The first medical use of the term 'screening' was to describe the detection of asymptomatic or predisease states (Wilson 1966). Its use is now sometimes extended to describe health promotion or the detection of risk factors for disease, such as smoking. In this context the word is being used in a sense closer to its colloquial meaning of simply testing for the presence or absence of a quality (Sykes 1982).

OPPORTUNISTIC SCREENING

Opportunistic screening is only one approach to the screening of a population. It aims to exploit the fact that general practitioners see many of their practice

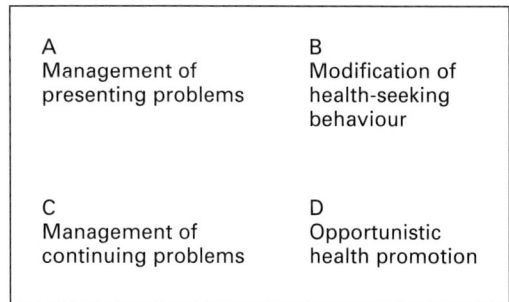

A Management of presenting problems	B Modification of health-seeking behaviour
C Management of continuing problems	D Opportunistic health promotion

Fig. 9.1 The exceptional potential in each primary care consultation (after Stott & Davis 1979).

population over a relatively short period of time. It has been estimated that over two-thirds of the patients on a general practitioner's list will visit in any given year and 90% will have been seen within a 5-year period (Fowler & Gray 1983). In opportunistic screening, the opportunity presented by the patient consulting his or her GP is capitalised upon to carry out any number of screening or surveillance activities. The concept was popularised by Stott & Davis (1979) in their seminal paper on the exceptional potential of the general practice consultation. In this paper they argued that the occasion of the patient consulting his or her doctor provides opportunities for much more than a reactive response to the condition presented. In the paper they identified four broad areas of activity that could widen the scope of ordinary general practice consultations and exploit their full potential. These areas are shown in Figure 9.1. This diagram was presented by them as an aide memoire to help doctors become more proactive in their care of patients. One of the opportunities they saw presented was for the doctor to promote health in whatever way seemed appropriate at the time. This could include a screening test, such as the measurement of blood pressure, or simply a discussion of potential risk factors of future disease. This gave birth to the notion of opportunistic screening in the very broadest sense of the term.

ALTERNATIVE METHODS OF SCREENING

There are, however, a number of other possible approaches to screening and each has its proponents. The value of the opportunistic approach can be gauged by comparing it to these other methods. Each method has strengths and weaknesses and the opportunistic approach can be seen as combining some of the strengths of other methods, although it may inherit some of the weaknesses too. When the idea of screening for disease at an early or presymptomatic stage was first mooted it was greeted with great enthusiasm and there was a vogue for mass screening campaigns of various sorts. A classic example was the mass radiographic screening for tuberculosis in the UK. This was a rather unsystematised mass screening endeavour but was not unsuccessful for all that. It was soon appreciated, however, that one of the features of screening and other preventive activities was that they address the needs of populations rather than those of individuals. In this case, the degree of 'population cover' achieved becomes an issue. In some instances, such as the case of immunisation for infectious diseases, a definable level of population coverage is essential to make the preventive endeavour worthwhile at all. The same principle applies, to a certain degree, to screening, although the levels of coverage needed to justify the effort have never been so clearly defined. This appreciation did lead to more systematic mass screening campaigns and efforts were then made to identify the target population at the outset. If target populations were recruited to be screened for one disease it was soon advocated that they be screened simultaneously for several. Hence the popularity of so-called 'multiphasic screening' grew. A variant of this same approach may be seen in some well-woman and well-man clinics in general practice. A further approach to screening is exemplified by the screening of neonates for various metabolic disease. This screening for several diseases in a systematically identified and sought out population is organised on a continuous basis rather than as an occasional screening drive.

PROBLEMS WITH OTHER SCREENING METHODS

Mass screening drives, even if unsystematised (as in the mass X-ray campaign), can be successful. Their success, however, depends on the benefits of the procedure being very readily apparent to the members of the target population and the absence of 'consumer resistance'. Population coverage in an unsystematised campaign is rather haphazard. Where there is a need to employ some high technology or only intermittently available staff or facilities, a 'once-off' type of campaign is useful. But a once-off campaign also requires that the condition being screened for can be readily treated over a wide time span in its natural history and that, once treated, little or no further monitoring is likely to be required. If such conditions are not met a recurrent campaign will be needed. Initial enthusiasm will usefully carry along more systematic attempts at mass screening for a time. Such enthusiasm is often easy to muster and so such campaigns are fairly easy to launch. The administrative system needed may also be quite simple to set up, although, outside general practice, there are real difficulties in identifying the population to be screened. Even within general practice, where there are registered patient populations, there are difficulties (Bowling & Jacobson 1989). As it is a new activity, the administrative protocol needs only limited integration into existing health care systems. By employing the multiphasic approach maximum benefit is achieved from the recruitment effort. Such a screening campaign usually involves the creation of a special 'clinic'. This facilitates a timing that suits the occasional availability of the particular staff or facilities that may be required. However, a major drawback of this approach to screening is that enthusiasm runs out. Furthermore, it tends to flag at the point when efforts are being made to recruit those who missed the first run. Evidence suggests it is just such non-attenders who are most likely to need the health surveillance being offered (Pill et al 1988). This may well account for the apparent failure of the various attempts at multiphasic screening to alter mortality or morbidity patterns. And if there is a need for repeated campaigns, the energy found for the first campaign may not be so readily forthcoming for subsequent ones.

The more continuous approach avoids these problems with flagging enthusiasm by being established as part and parcel of day-to-day practice, although *becoming* so established is not easy. It is a low key approach to screening and, as such, it is easily forgotten unless well established. It requires substantial change in ways of working. Experience teaches us that long-term behavioural change is always difficult to achieve. The continuous screening approach requires very tight administrative systems to ensure that patients do not slip through the net. These systems must be well integrated with existing administrative arrangements and such a degree of integration may not be so readily achieved. This approach works well for neonatal screening because of the comprehensive nature of birth registrations and it has also been successfully employed in general practice for cervical cytology screening (Standing & Mercer 1984), although its success was dependent on a very reliable age/sex register. Bowling & Jacobson (1989) have recently pointed out how inaccurate age/sex registers generated from Family Health Services Authorities may be. It can probably be regarded as a prerequisite of any on-going screening programme that it is accompanied by diligent maintenance of any administrative tools needed. Being continuous may also preclude the use of high technology or staff who are only occasionally available.

ADVANTAGES OF THE OPPORTUNISTIC APPROACH

The opportunistic approach to screening suffers from no difficulties in indentifying and recruiting the target population and it avoids the problems of non-attendance. As pointed out above, most people consult their GP at least once every 5 years. Furthermore, those who do attend are de facto the more ill members of the population and, in certain circumstances, are at greatest risk of the conditions being screened for. This is the very segment of the population unlikely to attend specifically for preventive procedures (Townsend & Davidson 1980). Attendance at the surgery is also associated with a higher than usual level of health concern and hence greater motivation to follow health advice (Russell 1971, Stott 1976, Stott & Davis 1979). Conversely, there is evidence that non-attenders are likely to be healthy and unlikely to benefit from screening (Thompson 1990). Relatively simple administrative procedures will usually ensure that prompts are provided to the doctor regarding screening to be done and duplication of effort is avoided. The opportunistic method has all the advantages of the continuous approach to screening described for neonates and it avoids the problems of flagging enthusiasm associated with once-off efforts.

There has been some debate over two alternative preventive strategies. Many doctors advocate that screening be directed at 'high risk' subgroups of the population. This assumes that such high risk groups can easily be identified without the need for an initial screening measure. In such individuals the pay-off of intervention is usually greater (providing the disease is treatable), although the impact on the population is less. The less selective mass screening strategy suffers from what Rose (1981) has described as the 'preventive paradox'. This is the observation that 'a measure

that brings a large degree of benefit to the community offers little to each individual'. This makes it difficult for doctors and their patients, both of whom expect that any treatment or intervention arising from the screening effort will be rewarded with benefit that they will readily appreciate. This is not the case. If, say, the treatment of blood pressure will save one person for every 50 treated, then 49 individuals have to take the treatment at no personal benefit. Even the one saved from the stroke will not be able to tell that he/she has been saved by the treatment. Waine (1989) has argued that the high risk versus the unselective approach is a false antithesis. He can say this from the perspective of general practice where both approaches can easily coexist. Such simultaneous, population-wide and selective strategies are particularly feasible when an opportunistic approach to screening is adopted. One can opportunistically provide a low-key minimal intervention approach on a whole population basis and at the same time have a more active interventionist approach to high risk subjects who are identified as and when they appear.

DRAWBACKS OF OPPORTUNISTIC SCREENING

The opportunistic approach does, however, require a substantial change in doctor behaviour during the consultation. It also requires a fundamental change in the doctor's perception of the task of general practice – it requires a knowledge of and an appreciation of the perspective of population medicine. There are real difficulties in establishing and maintaining new habits and ways of working. Another major drawback reported is that opportunistic screening takes up time, and that time is not abundant in general practice consultations. It is possible to make consultations longer and there is, fortunately, encouraging evidence that a change to a longer time does lead to more opportunistic preventive activity (Wilson 1989). As more and more screening activities are investigated and found to be worthwhile, however, the pressure on time in the consultation will increase and there is the danger of not being able to fit all the useful screening procedures into the standard consultation time, even if this is increased (Pringle 1985). Also, if screening is to take place in ordinary consultations, then tests requiring special facilities are clearly not feasible.

All screening activities pose ethical difficulties (Mant & Fowler 1990, see also Chapter 4) but there are particular ethical difficulties involved in the opportunistic approach. If one is to exploit the opportunity provided by the patient's consulting it is mandatory that one has fully dealt with all matters on the patient's agenda before moving on to the doctor's agenda (Middleton 1989, and see also Fig. 9.1, above). Furthermore, an explicit mandate must be sought when moving on from the reasons for the consultation to preventive matters — one cannot rely on the implied mandate given by the patient's consulting. To deal with these ethical issues properly requires the learning of extra communication skills and greater sensitivity to the patient's view.

COMPARATIVE STUDIES

There have been few studies to compare the relative merits of the opportunistic and more traditional approaches. Houston et al (1990) and Houston & Davis (1985) have compared opportunistic child health surveillance and the more usual method of child health clinics. Their results did not point to any substantial difference in the two approaches in either pickup rate of abnormalities or in population coverage. However, they did point out that more of the children judged to be more 'at risk' were seen by the general practitioner for routine consultations than were seen at baby clinics by the health visitor. Burton (see Chapter 21) has similarly compared opportunistic and systematic approaches to screening adults for hypertension. He found the opportunistic approach detected more cases of more elevated blood pressure than did a systematic approach. Hall (1985) has also described how the application of an opportunistic philosophy alone led to an 80% recording rate for blood pressure, which was difficult to improve upon. Pierce et al (1989) compared the uptake of cervical cytology testing in women invited for smears as part of a systematic campaign and those invited by their general practitioners opportunistically while attending for other matters. They found no significant difference in the two methods. They did, however, find that both groups were significantly more likely to have a smear test than a control population who were offered smears opportunistically but with whom there was no system for cuing the doctor to the need to offer the test. The lesson from this study is that either method is adequate if systematically applied and not just left to chance. There have been many studies into the health needs of the elderly, which have indicated the existence of unmet needs, and have led to calls for some form of systematic health screening. Freer (1987) has shown how this can be done opportunistically in the surgery using a flow chart (see also Chapter 25). It is clear from all these studies that opportunistic screening is feasible for all ages and groups of the population. It does, however, require systematic application and some form of regular review to ensure it is being done. One of the major difficulties that even the enthusiasts for opportunistic screening encounter is the gap that can grow between what one thinks one is doing and what one is actually doing. Audit is the key to closing this gap.

OPPORTUNISTIC RECRUITMENT

In the early 1980s the Royal College of General Practitioners published a series of papers on prevention in general practice (RCGP 1981a, b). These papers advocated slightly different approaches to prevention for different problems, but in the case of coronary heart disease and stroke they came down firmly in favour of the opportunistic approach. Fullard et al (1984), in Oxford, used this as the starting point for a study to test the feasibility of applying existing knowledge about coronary heart disease and stroke to its prevention in general practice. They set out to use an opportunistic approach, but came up with a new approach to screening that can be said to combine the best of two worlds. The key to their success can be encapsulated in the term 'opportunistic recruitment'. In this method, the opportunity presented by the patient's consulting for another reason is exploited, not to carry out a range of screening tests, but to recruit the patient to an ongoing and systematic screening and health promotion programme. This exploits the patient's motivation and likely health concern and yet avoids the problems of lack of time. Indeed, further time can be set aside if, at some future date, more screening procedures prove worthwhile. As the screening visit is explicitly for that purpose, it is easier and more permissible to follow a predetermined protocol. Important health promotion opportunities are less likely to be missed and the ethical difficulties of misappropriating the patient's time and agenda at patient-initiated consultations are circumvented. The patient's captivity in the consulting room is not so ruthlessly exploited. An offer is made and may be refused. Even if the pressure of the doctor's presence forces patients to agree unwillingly, they can always miss the appointment for screening, although experience suggests that few do. For the doctor, opportunistic recruitment requires a much less fundamental shift in the conduct of consultations. Indeed, the experience in Oxford suggests that the enthusiastic participation in the recruitment drive by the practice reception staff can virtually obviate the need for the doctor to do anything very new. By tagging of the notes and priming the patient to ask the doctor about the screening procedure, the doctor is provided with sufficient cues to ensure that he/she recruits the patient into the programme. The actual screening may be done by practice nurses, and some would argue that this is a task more suited to their skills and training. Nurses are also seen by patients as appropriate professionals to be involved in health promotion. The involvement of the whole practice team shares the burden of extra work and helps motivation. If extra high technology facilities are needed, these, too, could be made available at the time of the screening visit. For instance, opportunities presented by attendance could and, in my view, should be used to encourage women in the relevant age group to attend for mammography in the current breast screening campaign.

Fullard et al (1987) report that this method of implementing a screening programme is highly successful, with 92% of the practice target population attending for health checks. It must be said that this success has not been universal. One practice adopting the Oxford model was disappointed at the lack of uptake (Waller et at 1990). It seems the success of such a screening programme may be extremely sensitive to the type of practice population, to the exact method of recruitment and to the effect of enthusiasm waning with the passage of time, although it is still more successful than the unsystematised opportunistic approach previously being used in some practices. There are also some encouraging trends now being observed in the mortality data from Oxfordshire, which suggest that the county-wide enthusiasm for opportunistic screening of cardiovascular risk factors may be paying off in reductions in cardiovascular mortality (E M Fullard, personal communication).

In the Oxford study, the move to opportunistic recruitment was stimulated by the presence of a 'nurse facilitator' (see Chapter 7) and the initial study of the method was in a relatively affluent area of the country. This raises questions of whether the same model would work elsewhere and how central the role of the 'nurse facilitator' is to the succes of such endeavours. Robson et al (1989) have shown that an active approach and an on-going health promotion and screening clinic can work even in a deprived inner city area. However, they recruited both systematically and opportunistically and this belt-and-braces approach to patient recruitment may be what is needed in some areas. They also emphasise the key role of the nurse, who was employed by the practice rather than coming as a facilitator from outside. Marsh and Channing (1988) have also shown how a practice can, on its own initiative, start up an opportunistic campaign to promote health in even a very deprived population. They too found that opportunistic recruitment raised the uptake of a whole range

of preventive services by a deprived population who had previously been shown to be poor partakers of these services. In their study they included all ages and showed that the principle of opportunistic recruitment can improve immunisation rates in children and cervical cytology rates in women, as well as adult health screening. All these studies emphasise the key role of the nurse. It seems probable that, in the future, health promotion nurses will become as important a part of primary health care teams as they are an integral part of successful opportunistic recruitment and screening programmes.

THE NATIONAL HEALTH SERVICE REFORMS

The recent changes in the National Health Service, as first described in the White Paper, *Working for Patients* (HMSO 1989) and the 1990 Contract for NHS General Practitioners (Health Departments of Great Britain 1989) seem on first reading to reject the importance of opportunistic screening. The contract advocates the setting up of special clinics as the way forward for screening and health promotion, and offers financial incentives accordingly. Some Family Health Service Authorities (FHSAs) have taken a rather broader interpretation of the regulations relating to these clinics and have chosen to recognise opportunistic screening endeavours as being acceptable in lieu of formally set up clinics, although, at the time of writing, it is uncertain whether this can be sustained. Even where this is not the case, one may take the opportunistic recruitment approach to ensure a good attendance at the screening sessions, for which a fee will be payable. Indeed, the Oxford experience suggests that this would be an inexpensive way of ensuring that the contractual obligation to see patients every 3 years is fulfilled.

It must also be said that the use of the opportunistic screening approach does not preclude the use of other methods. Indeed, under the terms of the new contract it is understood that doctors will send for those patients not attending the practice and offer them a health check, although the actual clinical benefit of this has been questioned (Thompson 1990).

SUMMARY

The opportunistic approach to screening, as most broadly defined, aims to exploit the high probability of patients being seen by a general practitioner. Other approaches to screening find it more difficult to achieve similar population coverage, although they may allow more systematic screening for a wider range of conditions, especially where special technology is required. Opportunistic screening reaches the most at-risk members of the population and is administratively simple to implement. It does require substantial changes of habit for the doctor and more time in the consultation. It also demands a high level of communication skill to avoid ethical pitfalls. Comparative studies suggest it is at least as good as other systematic approaches to screening and it is applicable to all ages and patient groups. Opportunistic recruitment tries to achieve the best of both worlds by exploiting the opportunity of a consultation to recruit to a systematic screening programme. Experience suggests this is highly successful and applicable in many practice settings and to a variety of preventive health measures. The new health service reforms do not, as might first appear, discourage opportunistic screening, although they do encourage its advance on the lines of the opportunistic recruitment model.

REFERENCES

Bowling A, Jacobson B 1989 Screening: the inadequacies of population registers. British Medical Journal 298: 545–546

Fowler G, Gray M 1983 Opportunities for prevention in general practice. In: Gray M, Fowler G H (eds) Preventive medicine in general practice. Oxford University Press, Oxford

Freer C B 1987 Consultation-based screening of the elderly in general practice: a pilot study. Journal of the Royal College of General Practitioners 37: 455–456

Fullard E M, Fowler G H, Gray J A M 1984 Facilitating prevention in primary care. British Medical Journal 289: 1585–1587

Fullard E M, Fowler G H, Gray J A M 1987 Promoting prevention in primary care: a controlled trial of low technology, low cost approach. British Medical Journal 294: 1080–1082

Hall J A 1985 Audit of screening for hypertension in general practice. Journal of the Royal College of General Practitioners 35: 243

Health Departments of Great Britain 1989 General practice in the National Health Service: the 1990 contract. HMSO, London

HMSO 1977 Prevention and Health Cmnd 7047. HMSO, London

HMSO 1989 Working for Patients CM 555. HMSO, London

Houston H L A, Davis R H 1985 Opportunistic surveillance of child development in primary care: is it feasible? Journal of the Royal College of General Practitioners 35: 77–79

Houston H L A, Santos K, Davis R H 1990 Opportunistic development surveillance in general practice. British Journal of General Practice 40: 230–232

Mant D, Fowler G 1990 Mass screening: theory and ethics. British Medical Journal 300: 916–918

Marsh G N, Channing D M 1988 Narrowing the gap between a deprived and an endowed community. British Medical Journal 296: 173–176

Middleton J F 1989 The exceptional potential of the consultation revisited. Journal of the Royal College of General Practitioners 39: 383–386

Pierce M, Lundy S, Palanisamy A, et al 1989 Prospective randomised controlled trial of methods of call and recall for cervical cytology screening. British Medical Journal 299: 160–162

Pill R, French J, Harding K, Stott N 1988 Invitation to attend a health check in a general practice setting: comparison of attenders and non-attenders. Journal of the Royal College of General Practitioners 38: 53–56

Pringle M 1985 Computer assisted screening: effect on the patient and his consultation. British Medical Journal 290: 1709–1712

Robson J, Boomla K, Fitzpatrick S, et al 1989 Using nurses for preventive activities with computer assisted follow up: a randomised controlled trial. British Medical Journal 298: 433–436

Rose G 1981 Strategies of prevention: lessons from cardio-vascular disease. British Medical Journal 282: 1847–1851

Royal College of General Practitioners 1981a Health and prevention in primary care. Royal College of General Practitioners, London.

Royal College of General Practitioners 1981b Prevention of arterial disease in general practice. Royal College of General Practitioners, London

Russell M A H 1971 Cigarette dependence: doctor's role in management. British Medical Journal 2: 393–395

Standing P, Mercer S 1984 Quinquennial cervical smears: every woman's right and every GP's responsibility. British Medical Journal 289: 883–886

Stott H H 1976 The Valley Trust sociomedical project for the promotion of health in a less developed rural area. M D Thesis University of Edinburgh, Edinburgh

Stott N C, Davis R H 1979 The exceptional potential in each primary care consultation. Journal of the Royal College of General Practitioners 29: 201–205

Sykes J B 1982 The Concise Oxford Dictionary of Current English. Oxford University Press, Oxford.

Thompson N F 1990 Inviting infrequent attenders to attend for a health check: costs and benefits. British Journal of General Practice 40: 16–18

Townsend P, Davidson N 1980 Inequalities of health: the Black Report. Penguin, London

Waine C 1989 Everyone's business — everyone's responsibility. Journal of the Royal College of General Practitioners 39: 5–10

Waller D, Agass M, Mant D et al 1990 Health checks in general practice: another example of inverse care? British Medical Journal 300: 1115–1118

Wilson J M G 1966 Some principles of early diagnosis and detection. In: Teeling Smith G (ed) Surveillance and early diagnosis in general practice (Proceedings of Colloquium held at Magdalen College, Oxford, 7 July 1965). Office of Health Economics, London

Wilson A 1989 Extending appointment length — the effect in one practice. Journal of the Royal College of General Practitioners 39: 24–25

Antenatal and preconceptional care

10. Genetic risks and their management

Nicholas R Dennis

INTRODUCTION

It is estimated that 1% of newborn infants have a medically significant single gene disorder, 1% have a microscopically visible chromosome abnormality and 1–2% have a congenital malformation whose cause is at least partly genetic (Weatherall 1985, Jacobs 1990). Most of the common diseases affecting children and adults arise from a combination of genetic predisposition and environmental factors. The statement 'It can't be genetic — nothing like it has ever happened before in our family' is often heard in genetic clinics, but genetic disease usually strikes unheralded. A proportion of cases, resulting from recent damage to, or rearrangement of, genetic material, will remain, for the forseeable future, unpredictable. But recent scientific advances have increased the proportion of at-risk and affected pregnancies that can be identified.

This chapter will focus on those situations where a genetic risk is less than obvious, but can be identified by screening and surveillance tactics. Risks to unborn children are most readily identified in the nuclear family when a previous affected child has been born with, or one parent suffers from, a well defined single gene disorder. Most doctors now recognise the need for genetic counselling in these situations, which are not addressed by this chapter. They are well covered, together with relevant genetic principles, in some good introductory texts, e.g. Harper (1988), Connor & Ferguson-Smith (1987), Thompson & Thompson (1985).

The tactics that may be used to cast the net wider, and ascertain more pregnancies at risk, include:

1. Investigating family relationships not normally investigated — it is sometimes important to consider the extended rather than just the nuclear family.
2. Making genetic diagnoses that might have escaped being made.
3. Population screening to identify at-risk individuals or couples.

This chapter looks at the methods, the costs (emotional as well as financial) and the benefits in a number of genetic disorders.

A brief discussion of the benefits of genetic counselling is necessary here. To identify couples or pregnancies at increased risk of serious disorders will usually lead to a reduction in the number of affected births, by means of the avoidance of conception or by prenatal diagnosis and selective abortion. Many people think that a reduction in disease frequency in the population is the first aim of genetic counselling. It is, rightly, the main reason why governments and health authorities allocate money to genetic services. But for the clinical geneticist advising a family, the preventive role must be secondary to the aim of helping that family to choose what is, for it, the best outcome. Experienced genetic counsellors have almost without exception decided that they must be non-directive (Wertz & Fletcher 1988); families who make an informed decision to risk or to have an affected child do not represent a failure of genetic counselling. To think otherwise is either to believe that one knows more about other people's lives than they do themselves, or to embrace a form of eugenics that our society has rejected. Affected births will be prevented as a by-product of informing people of their risks and options, and in numbers sufficient to cover the cost of genetic screening, counselling and testing several times over, but it is not for us to seek specific outcomes in individual cases.

Most medical screening is a method of ascertaining people with an undiagnosed disease who will benefit from early treatment. Genetic screening is a way of identifying a potential patient either before conception, when various options for avoidance of an affected birth may exist, or during pregnancy, when the options are fewer. To screen for established disease may be a form of genetic screening if it indicates a risk to further pregnancies, as for example in the case of newborn screening for phenylketonuria or X-linked muscular dystrophy.

The early diagnosis of many paediatric and some adult disorders is important because of their genetic implications. The approach to these conditions is surveillance rather than screening, denoting an alertness to the diagnosis followed by willingness to manage the question of risk in the family.

PRECONCEPTIONAL SCREENING

Two forms of genetic screening are applicable to a young healthy couple without obvious risk factors. The first is a careful review of the family history — unsuspected risks may come to light and even when risks are known to the family they are often ignored until pregnancy has been achieved. The second is to enquire whether the couple is at risk of one of the autosomal recessive disorders that have reached a high frequency in particular ethnic groups and for which heterozygote (carrier) screening is available. Until recently this has meant the haemoglobinopathies and Tay–Sachs' disease. At the time of writing, carrier tests for cystic fibrosis are being developed, which will carry far reaching medical and social implications in the UK and other countries with populations of European origin.

Taking a family history

Taking and recording a family history is one of the basic techniques of clinical genetics and is necessary for sorting out many of the problems discussed in this chapter. Not surprisingly, given the special sense of guilt and responsibility surrounding genetic disorders, a person's true concerns may take some time to emerge.

It is useful to record the family history as a pedigree diagram, with information such as name, date of birth, occupation and clinical status either written next to each individual or recorded below using a key. A representative pedigree with a key to the standard notation is given in Figure 10.1. Consanguinity (parents who are blood relatives) increases the chance that a child will suffer from a recessively inherited disorder and parents should be asked about any chronic undiagnosed condition.

Couples who are cousins sometimes ask prospectively about risks to their children. In the case of first cousins with no relevant family history (of definite or possible autosomal recessive conditions), the population risk of early death or serious handicap is approximately doubled, from 3 to 6% (Magnus et al 1985), the excess being accounted for by autosomal recessive disorders, which include cystic fibrosis and many causes of mental retardation, deafness, blindness and neuromuscular problems. If the couple have an affected child, it is important to establish the correct diagnosis, because an autosomal recessive disorder will have a 25% recurrence risk, but cousin parents are not immune to conditions with a low recurrence risk.

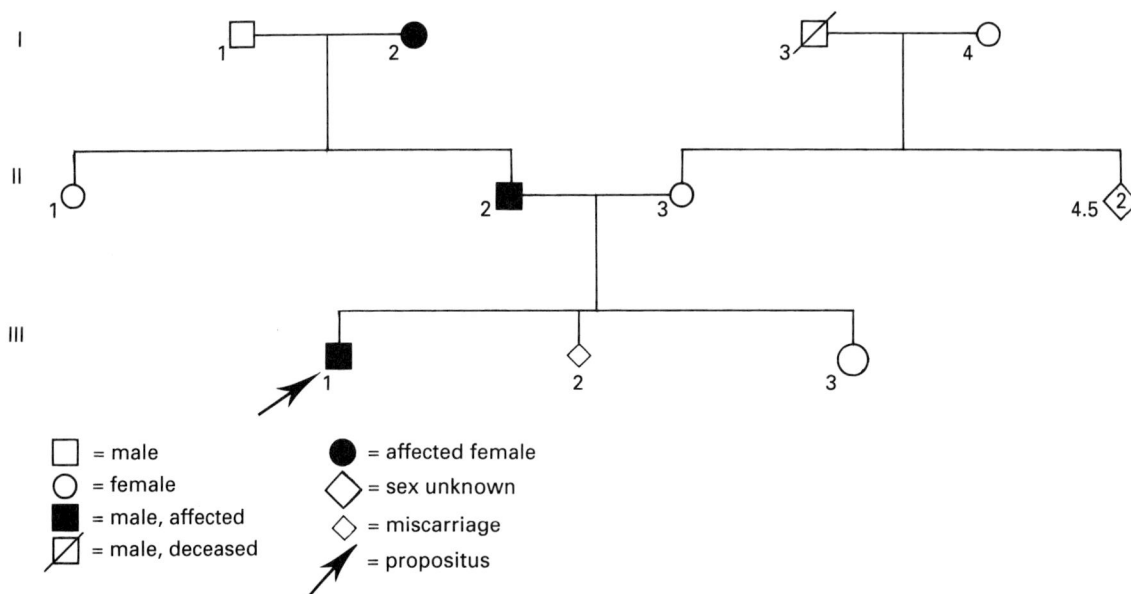

Fig. 10.1 Pedigree diagram showing conventional notation.

Table 10.1 Some clinical features of possible genetic significance, which may be elicited by a routine family history

Presentation	Possible genetic diagnostic	Genetics
Recurrent (3 or more) miscarriages	Balanced chromosome anomaly in one partner (check couple's chromosomes)	May be familial
Presenile dementia or 'nervous breakdown'	Huntington's disease or Alzheimer's disease; schizophrenia or manic depressive illness	Huntingdon's — AD* Alzheimer's — sometimes AD Schizophrenia and manic depression — familial but risks usually less than AD
Renal failure or hypertension in early to mid-adult life	'Adult' type polycystic kidney disease	AD
Brown patches, skin lumps, 'tumours'	Neurofibromatosis	AD
Early onset coronary heart disease	Familial hypercholesterolaemia or other hyperlipidaemia	AD
Multiple rodent ulcers or skin cancers	Gorlin (basal cell naevus) syndrome	AD
Renal or brain tumours	von Hippel–Lindau disease	AD
Epilepsy and skin abnormalities	Tuberose sclerosis	AD
Early onset (under 60) colon carcinoma	Polyposis coli	AD
Muscle weakness and wasting, intellectual deterioration, cataracts	Myotonic dystrophy	AD
Muscular dystrophy in males	Duchenne and Becker muscular dystrophy	XLR†
Mental retardation in a male	Fragile X syndrome or other type of X-linked mental retardation	XLR

* AD, autosomal dominant; † XLR, X-linked recessive

Consanguinity elsewhere in the pedigree, other than between the parents themselves, is irrelevant.

It is particularly important for consanguineous couples to be offered heterozygote screening for any autosomal recessive disorders that are known to be common in their ethnic group (see below).

When recording the pedigree it is preferable to ask about pregnancies rather than children, so that miscarriages, stillbirths and infant deaths are included. If each relative is recorded individually and his or her state of health or cause of death enquired about, more comes to light than is elicited by questions such as 'Any illness running in the family?'

Table 10.1 lists some of the clinical presentations that may alert a doctor to a genetic risk when taking a routine family history. Most of these conditions are dealt with in more detail below.

Preconceptional carrier screening for autosomal recessive disorders

Autosomal recessive disorders arise when both parents pass on a defective allele of the same gene to a child; such mutant alleles are harmless in single dose, paired with a normal allele, as in heterozygous carriers. Nearly all affected births have parents who are both carriers (the contribution of fresh mutations to this group of conditions is very small), so theoretically, given a test for carriers, nearly all affected births could be foreseen.

Most of the 600 or so recognised autosomal recessive disorders are rare, and the labour of carrier screening for all but the most common, even when tests are available, will probably never be justified. A few autosomal recessive disorders have become common in certain populations, and these are the ones yielding the clearest benefits from carrier screening.

Cystic fibrosis is the most common autosomal recessive in populations originating from northern Europe, with carrier frequencies of up to 1 in 20. It is now known that in the UK around 75% of the cystic fibrosis alleles are of one type, the delta F 508 mutation, which deletes one phenylalanine from the protein product of the gene. This mutation can readily be detected by techniques that are adaptable for population screening. The remaining 25% of mutations may be diverse and individually rare. Screening for only the delta F 508 mutation can detect just over $\frac{1}{2}$ ($[\frac{3}{4}]^2$) of couples at risk, so that in about 1 in 800 couples screened, both will be shown to be carriers. At the time of writing, pilot studies to assess the feasibility of population screening for cystic fibrosis carriers are being carried out in the UK.

Couples from outside northern Europe should be offered screening for haemoglobinopathies (mainly sickle-cell anaemia and the thalassaemias), and Ashkenazi Jewish couples should also be offered screening for Tay–Sachs' disease. Genetic screening of ethnic minorities is covered in more detail by Modell and Modell (1990) and elsewhere in this book (Chapter 39).

In offering testing the following points should be made:

1. Being a carrier is in itself of no serious medical importance.
2. The aim of screening is not to reduce the frequency of carriers in the population.
3. Each couple is free to decide how to proceed if they both turn out to be carriers. The options are:
   (i)   do not reproduce;
   (ii) go ahead and take the 1 in 4 risk of an affected child;
   (iii) request prenatal diagnosis with the option of aborting affected fetuses;
   (iv) (possibly available in future) request in vitro fertilisation with preimplantation testing, replacing only unaffected embryos;
   (v)   attempt a pregnancy using donor sperm or egg to ensure that one (genetic) parent is not a carrier.

The concept of population carrier screening is not widely understood. Many people find it threatening, probably because they think that it has eugenic overtones, and that people will be encouraged to abort affected fetuses. Any carrier screening programme needs to provide adequate education to the target population, plus pre- and post-test counselling. So far, programmes in the UK, limited to ethnic minorities, have not had the resources to provide this type of back-up. With the imminence of cystic fibrosis carrier screening, health authorities should ensure that all genetic screening services are integrated and provided with resources adequate to cover health education, counselling, quality control and audit. See the Report on Prenatal Diagnosis and Genetic Screening from the Royal College of Physicians (1989) for a full discussion of these issues.

The best stage of life at which to offer carrier screening is unclear and may depend on local social customs. Although the testing of schoolchildren has been advocated, this could offend against current notions of informed consent. Experience suggests that few adults

will seek testing until they have a pregnancy in view. Testing pregnant women was an economical option as long as prenatal testing of the fetus was confined to the middle trimester. If a woman was negative there was no need to test the male partner. The use of first trimester diagnosis gives too little time for this approach; in any case, once pregnancy has begun, some of the options listed above are excluded. Once a carrier has been found, screening the rest of the family is an efficient way of detecting more carriers.

It thus seems likely that the most acceptable option for carrier screening will be 'walk in' preconception clinics designed for adults, either as individuals or as couples, at which counsellors are available. Ideally, all disorders for which screening is available should be dealt with in the same clinic, and these clinics could also deal with general enquiries about genetic risks and tests in pregnancy. The more complicated problems would be referred on to the medical genetics or obstetric service.

The arrangements for haemoglobinopathy testing in the UK, including a list of centres and details of record cards and leaflets, are available from the Department of Health (DHSS 1988)(see also Chapter 39).

If blood or other samples are being obtained from a large number of couples to test for their particular 'ethnic' recessive disorder, it may be possible to perform tests for other recessive disorders, as long as these are reasonably common (say 1 in 10 000 or more, giving a carrier frequency of 1 in 50 or more) and, if direct DNA analysis is being used, as long as only one or a few well characterised mutations are responsible for the condition. In the UK at present, this approach could be used to detect couples at risk of severe alpha-1 antitrypsin deficiency (PiZZ) and some cases of phenylketonuria and congenital adrenal hyperplasia. In all three conditions, however, a majority of people would probably not welcome screening because of variable severity or treatability. It remains to be seen whether the addition of extra conditions to screening programmes will be desirable or cost effective.

SCREENING IN PREGNANCY

The main techniques available for screening in pregnancy are mid-trimester amniocentesis, chorion villus sampling, maternal serum measurements and ultrasound scanning.

Chromosomes

The use of maternal age as a screening test for chromosome anomalies is relatively inefficient. If all women aged 35 or over at the due date opted for

Table 10.2 Risks of chromosome abnormality in relation to maternal age (adapted from Gardner and Sutherland (1989) and based on data from Ferguson-Smith and Yates (1984) and Hook (1983). Risks are given as the denominator x in the expression '1 in x'

Maternal Age (years)	Live birth		Amniocentesis	
	Down syndrome	All unbalanced chromosome abnormalities	Down syndrome	All unbalanced chromosome abnormalities
35	380	240	260	110
36	290	185	200	95
37	230	161	160	80
38	180	115	120	65
39	140	105	100	55
40	110	75	75	45
41	80	56	60	34
42	65	46	45	27
43	50	36	35	22
44	40	30	30	19
45	30	24	20	15

Differences between rates for Down syndrome and for any unbalanced chromosome abnormality are accounted for by:

1. Abnormalities of the sex chromosomes (mainly 47, XXX, 47, XXY, 47, XYY and 45, X), which are less severe than Down syndrome and which do not usually cause problems in early childhood.
2. Abnormalities as severe as or more severe than Down syndrome — mainly trisomies 18 and 13 — and unbalanced structural rearrangements of the autosomes.

Overall rates of abnormality at chorion villus sampling are 1.5–2 times higher than those at amniocentesis across most of this maternal age range (35 years and over), the difference being attributable to the detection of severe and lethal abnormalities destined to miscarry (Hook et al 1988).

amniocentesis, 40% of all cases of Down syndrome (formerly referred to as Down's syndrome) would be detected by testing 8% of the pregnant population (Ewings et al 1991: these figures will vary with the age distribution of pregnant women). The risks of Down syndrome and of other unbalanced chromosome abnormalities at various maternal ages are given in Table 10.2.

Most of the other numerical chromosome abnormalities show a maternal age effect (47, XYY and 45, X do not, being wholly (47, XYY) or most commonly (45, X) paternal in origin). The standard notation for a person's chromosome constitution gives the chromosome number, followed by a comma, then the sex chromosome constitution, (normally XX in females and XY in males), then, if applicable, extra chromosomes and other abnormalities are listed.

Wald et al (1988), using a function of maternal serum alphafetoprotein (AFP), chorionic gonadotrophin, oestriol and maternal age, identified a group comprising 5% of pregnant women who were carrying 60% of all Down syndrome fetuses. Despite the attraction of this approach in limiting the number of unnecessary amniocenteses, it has not yet been widely adopted.

Maternal serum screening cannot yet be used in conjunction with first trimester prenatal diagnosis by chorion villus sampling. Yet there is no doubt that many women are prepared to accept an increased miscarriage rate in return for an earlier result, and sometimes the experience of amniocentesis, with or without a mid-trimester termination, seems to act as a strong disincentive to repeat this form of testing. The delay of 3 weeks in obtaining a chromosome result from amniotic fluid cells is one of the main drawbacks, and reduction of the delay to 1–2 weeks with chorion villus sampling is perceived as a great advantage.

The risk of fetal loss attributable to chorion villus sampling in experienced hands is 2–3% (Canadian Clinical Trial Group 1989, Rhoads et al 1989, Jackson 1990, MRC working party 1991), on top of a spontaneous miscarriage rate of 2–5% for sonographically normal pregnancies at 10 weeks (Wilson 1984). This compares with a fetal loss rate attributable to amniocentesis of about 1 in 200 (National Institute of Child Health and Human Development (NICHD) Registry 1976, Simpson et al 1976, MRC Working Party 1978, Tabor et al 1986).

Couples who request fetal karyotyping should be aware that abnormalities other than Down syndrome may be detected. Sex chromosome anomalies, of which the most common are 47, XXY, 47, XYY, 47, XXX and 45, X are an important group. Together, these are roughly as common as Down syndrome, but their effects are far milder. Apart from short stature in 45, X and infertility in 45, X and 47, XXY, there are no consistent clinical features in these conditions. Although, as a group, children with sex chromosome anomalies show significant impairment in learning ability, which is most severe in 47, XXX girls and least so in 45, X girls, most of them still fall within the normal range (Ratcliffe & Paul 1986). The decision facing a couple on diagnosis of a fetal sex chromosome anomaly may be the most difficult they will ever have to make. Information on the prognosis of these conditions, which has been accumulating from the various newborn follow-up studies, has shown that they are generally milder than the perception of 10–15 years ago; however, the children ascertained at birth in these studies have not yet been followed into adult life, so the picture remains incomplete.

Another situation where the fetal chromosome result carries an uncertain prognosis is when a structural abnormality, such as a translocation or an inversion, or a small extra 'marker' chromosome is found. The next step is always to check the parents' chromosomes. If one of them has the same abnormality as the fetus, it is almost certainly balanced and harmless (later pregnancies may, however, be at increased risk of chromosome imbalance and the wider family will need to be studied).

When the parental chromosomes are normal and the fetal chromosome abnormality has arisen de novo, the prognosis is uncertain. Empirically, structural abnormalities that look balanced, and very small extra 'marker' chromosomes, are usually associated with a normal outcome, but are sometimes associated with mental retardation. Specific staining reactions or DNA studies may clarify the situation. These uncommon complications of prenatal diagnosis should be dealt with by a clinical geneticist in close collaboration with the laboratory and the obstetrician.

Neural tube defects

The use of maternal serum alphafetoprotein (AFP) levels as a screening test for neural tube defects has not been adopted in every district, despite the fact that, when carried out with due care, it is demonstrably effective (Thom et al 1985). The high false positive rate of the test will inevitably cause anxiety in some parents of what turn out to be normal pregnancies; however, high quality ultrasound, with or without amniotic fluid AFP and acetyl cholinesterase assays, will usually resolve the positives into neural tube defects, other malformations associated with raised AFP levels, e.g. abdominal wall defects, compromised pregnancies with fetomaternal bleeds, and normals.

Some authors have suggested that maternal serum AFP screening for neural tube defects should be superseded by the offer of a detailed fetal anomaly scan in every pregnancy (Nicolaides & Campbell 1987). In one study (Richards et al 1988) this technique had a sensitivity of 100% for anencephaly and 81% for open spine defects, with no false positives. While the use of fetal scanning as a screening test for fetal anomalies will undoubtedly continue to increase, in most districts the use of maternal serum AFP will remain a useful screening test for neural tube defects for some time to come. The development of serum AFP screening for Down syndrome (see above) is an extra incentive to provide this form of screening.

Ultrasound scanning

Ultrasound scanning, originally used to date pregnancies, monitor fetal growth and facilitate

Table 10.3 Fetal structural abnormalities that may be diagnosable by middle trimester ultrasound scanning

System	Diagnosable abnormalities
Central nervous system	Hydrocephalus Microcephaly Anencephaly Spina bifida
Skeleton	Symmetrical shortening of limb bones (includes bone dysplasias) Bowing of long bones Focal abnormalities (absence defects) Polydactyly Positional deformities, e.g. talipes
Renal tract	Pelviureteric junction obstruction with hydronephrosis Dilated ureters Dilated bladder Renal agenesis Cystic kidneys (various types)
Gastrointestinal tract	Diaphragmatic hernia Abdominal wall defects (exomphalos and gastroschisis) Atresias
Cardiovascular system	Congenital heart defects (some) Rhythm disorders
General	Nuchal cysts (including cystic hygroma) Hydrops Tumours

invasive manoeuvres, such as amniocentesis, has gradually been refined to a point where a high proportion of fetal anomalies can be detected during the middle trimester. Since most of these occur in pregnancies with no prior risk factors, and a full fetal anomaly scan calls for considerable time and expertise, this form of screening is not uniformly available. However, regardless of whether there is a stated intention to scan every pregnancy for fetal anomalies, increasing numbers of anomalies are picked up by ultrasonographers performing routine dating scans, and the result may be a de facto screening programme with profound implications for the pregnant population but for which no consent is sought. The main categories of congenital abnormality likely to be noticed on scanning are listed in Table 10.3.

Prognosis for some of these findings is difficult because the normal range is still ill-defined, there is a lack of information about the natural history of the condition, or survival involves an operation with significant mortality. One source of uncertainty should be minimised: if a decision to continue the pregnancy is being considered, a search should be made for other abnormalities that may be associated with the presenting one, and this may include checking the fetal chromosomes. Several of the structural anomalies detected by ultrasound scanning occur as features of chromosome syndromes (Nicolaides et al 1986), especially diaphragmatic hernia, cleft lip, exomphalos, heart defects and neural tube defects. An exception is gastroschisis, which is rarely associated with other abnormalities. The presence of severe intrauterine growth retardation is also suggestive of a chromosome anomaly, especially trisomy 18. In such circumstances there may not be time to wait for an amniocentesis result and urgent fetal karyotyping via fetal blood sampling or late chorion villus biopsy may be necessary, usually requiring referral to a fetal medicine centre.

There are also single gene-determined syndromes, which include major structural anomalies such as CNS malformations, hydrops fetalis and limb shortening. A precise prenatal diagnosis in these cases will often be impossible for the first case in the family, but clinical geneticists who see dysmorphic infants after birth should be consulted about the possible significance of unusual combinations of fetal ultrasound findings.

The management of a pregnancy in which a malformation is detected is difficult and demanding. A decision on the continuation of the pregnancy must be made in a limited time, and may need information from specialists, such as the paediatric surgeon, paediatric cardiologist or geneticist. The couple, who must make a decision based on complex and sometimes uncertain data, are usually emotionally devastated.

In some centres, all prenatal diagnoses are reviewed by a regional multidisciplinary group, and this seems desirable as a way of gaining experience and setting standards in a complex and developing field. If the couple decide to terminate the pregnancy, they will need follow-up, with support from the community medical services and a review of the medical details, including pathology of the fetus, by the obstetrician, who may at that stage wish to refer the couple to a genetic counselling clinic. All prenatal diagnoses should be confirmed by tests on the child after birth or on the aborted fetus. Clayton-Smith et al (1990) showed that a high proportion of ultrasound diagnoses were inaccurate or incomplete.

The Royal College of Physicians' report *Prenatal diagnosis and genetic screening* (Royal College of Physcians 1989) discusses in detail the delivery of prenatal diagnosis services. Its recommendations are likely to influence both planners and clinicians over the next few years. One of its suggestions is that each health district should have prenatal diagnosis counsellors available to guide couples through the procedures, liaise between the departments, and provide some supportive counselling. The Report also draws attention to the need for more public education, so that couples are able to clarify their attitudes to the various screening tests before embarking on a pregnancy. This will apply particularly if first trimester testing is required. At present, few women are seen by obstetricians during the first trimester

NEONATAL SCREENING

The screening of neonates for phenylketonuria and hypothyroidism is justified by the treatability of those conditions. The diagnosis of phenylketonuria (but not usually of hypothyroidism) also identifies a high genetic risk to further children of the couple. So far, few couples have chosen to avoid this risk by prenatal diagnosis, although highly reliable DNA markers allowing first trimester diagnosis are available. The condition is generally regarded by parents as being too mild, given early diagnosis and treatment, to justify abortion. These conditions are discussed in greater detail in Chapter 15.

Newborn screening has also been advocated, and shown to be technically feasible, for cystic fibrosis, congenital adrenal hyperplasia, galactosaemia and Duchenne muscular dystrophy. None has yet gained widespread acceptance; the relevant arguments are considered by Sardharwalla and Wraith (1989).

CLINICAL PRESENTATIONS IN THE PAEDIATRIC AGE GROUP

Genetic disease may present with mundane symptoms. Failure to make a correct diagnosis may result in the neglect of genetic risks in the family as well as inappropriate management of the patient. Genetic disorders are comparatively rare, however, and we all, rightly, learn not to jump to the small print before considering the common. A sense of proportion is therefore important in discussing the presentation of genetic disorders in general practice. Those conditions that produce an unusual clinical picture, such as multiple malformations, will not be considered here.

Metabolic defects

Inherited metabolic defects may cause sudden deterioration in the newborn period, or occasionally later in infancy, when they may be a cause of sudden, unexpected death in a previously apparently healthy baby. A history of a previous child behaving similarly is an important clue in some families, as is parental consanguinity, as most of the relevant disorders are autosomal recessive.

The diagnosis and management of this group of conditions is reviewed by Saudubray et al (1989). It is a specialised area of paediatrics, but any doctor who is first on the scene should be aware of the diagnostic importance of blood and urine samples collected during the acute phase of the illness.

Neonatal liver disease, which may cause prolonged jaundice or bleeding, may be the first sign of alpha-1 antitrypsin deficiency in a family. About one-tenth of infants homozygous for the Z allele (ZZ) develop liver disease during early infancy (Sveger 1978). Some of these recover but others progress to cirrhosis. The other important effect of the ZZ genotype is to predispose to emphysema in adult life. Around 1 in 4000 infants born in Northern Europe has this genotype, with about 1 in 30 carrying the Z allele in single dose. Families who have had a child with serious liver disease will often opt for prenatal diagnosis in further pregnancies, which can be carried out by first trimester DNA analysis. The families of clinically affected index patients should be offered testing to detect carriers of the Z allele. Usually both parents of a ZZ child will be heterozygous (MZ), with a 1 in 4 risk of another ZZ, but occasionally one of the parents will also be ZZ. An MZ x ZZ mating will have a 1 in 2 risk of another ZZ child, and the ZZ parent may need advice on avoiding smoking because of the increased risk of emphysema.

Glucose-6-phosphate dehydrogenase deficiency is a cause of neonatal jaundice whose distribution largely coincides with that of the haemoglobinopathies (see Chapter 39). It is X-linked, so most sufferers are male. Families should be offered testing, as the diagnosis also has pharmacological and dietary implications.

Developmental delay and mental retardation

Developmental delay and mental retardation (see also Chapter 17) are common diagnostic and management problems for the paediatrician and for the general practitioner, especially if carrying out routine development checks, and they are common reasons for referral to genetic counselling clinics. One responsibility of the general practitioner to the families of mentally handicapped people is to ensure that concerns about recurrence risks are aired and dealt with, preferably before pregnancy. The key to recurrence risk is an accurate diagnosis in the index patient. It is not possible to review here the genetic causes of mental handicap, but one, the fragile X syndrome, should be mentioned because it is the most common cause of familial mental handicap. For further details see Davies (1989).

The fragile X syndrome is caused by a mutant gene near the end of the long arm of the X chromosome, which causes mental handicap in at least 80% of the males who inherit it and (usually more mildly) in about 30% of carrier females. Very unusually for a single gene defect, the mutant allele is associated with a visible change in the chromosome at or near the site of the gene, the so-called fragile site, but this is never seen in all cells examined; typically it occurs in 5–50% of cells, and this proportion varies with the cytogenetic methods used.

Although the clinical features are not highly distinctive, males with the fragile X syndrome have large heads, long faces, large projecting ears and large testes. These features, and/or a family history of mental handicap, should prompt chromosome analysis.

When the diagnosis is made, the family should be referred to the regional genetics service. Carrier females, who are at risk of having affected children, can be identified using cytogenetic and DNA analysis and offered prenatal diagnosis. Unlike X-linked disorders generally, this condition can be transmitted by clinically unaffected males, whose daughters may be carriers.

Another type of familial mental handicap, less common than the fragile X syndrome but important because those at risk can easily be identified within affected families, is that resulting from a parental balanced[*] structural chromosome anomaly. Such anomalies were found in 1 in 500 births in newborn screening studies (Jacobs et al 1974), but more modern methods of analysis with higher resolution give frequencies of about 1 in 150 (Jacobs 1990). Most consist of translocations, where material is exchanged between two non-homologous chromosomes, or inversions, where a segment of chromosome has acquired reverse orientation, i.e. ABEDCFG instead of ABCDEFG. These rearrangements are usually entirely harmless to carriers, but may confer a high risk of chromosomally unbalanced gametes that lack, or have extra doses of, certain chromosomal regions. The result, depending on the rearrangement, may be infertility, miscarriages, or children with mental handicap, often associated with physical abnormalities.

---

[*]The term 'balanced' means in this context that there is no deficiency or duplication of important genetic material, so the person concerned is clinically normal.

Families carrying structural abnormalities may be detected incidentally, usually in prenatal diagnosis, or as a result of investigation for multiple miscarriages (see p. 99) or the birth of a child with developmental abnormalities. The risk of an abnormal birth is usually low or negligible in the first two categories, but it is accepted practice to offer fetal chromosome analysis to any carrier of a balanced structural rearrangement, with the possible exception of a paracentric inversion, because the occurrence of an unbalanced but still viable offspring cannot be excluded. In the case of a balanced translocation, which has been ascertained through an unbalanced offspring, the recurrence risk may be as high as 10–15% (Gardner & Sutherland 1989).

Family follow-up should be carried out when a balanced structural rearrangement is found. All available relatives who are at risk of carrying the rearrangement should be offered testing and counselling. It is usually necessary to reassure those found to be carriers, as the risks are often overestimated.

Where parents are asking about the recurrence risk of mental retardation after one affected child, possible high risk situations include:

1. An autosomal recessive disorder (25% risk).
2. The presence of an autosomal dominant disorder in one of the parents (50% risk of transmitting the gene, prognosis often variable).
3. An X-linked disorder — the affected child will usually be male, but some X-linked disorders, including the fragile X syndrome, affect females (risk depends on careful analysis of pedigree and other data).
4. An unbalanced chromosome anomaly in the child, resulting from a balanced chromosome rearrangement in one parent (risk variable, see Gardner & Sutherland, 1989).
5. A maternal metabolic disorder producing intrauterine damage — most can be excluded by checking maternal blood amino acids.
6. Maternal medication producing a teratogenic effect.

If a precise diagnosis cannot be made in the affected child, an empirical risk figure can be quoted. For example, the recurrence risk of severe undiagnosed mental retardation in sibs is 3–4% but it may be as high as 11% for brothers of retarded males (Herbst & Baird 1982). Recurrence risks of undiagnosed mild mental retardation may be higher (Bundey et al 1989).

When someone with a mentally retarded sibling seeks advice on risks to his or her children the high risk possibilities are more limited. The most worrying is a woman with a mentally handicapped brother. In this case, every effort should be made to exclude an X-linked disorder in the brother, which will usually call for a careful clinical assessment and chromosome analysis for the fragile X syndrome. In other situations it is usually enough to check the mentally handicapped brother's or sister's chromosomes to exclude a structural abnormality that could be transmitted in balanced form through unaffected relatives.

Cystic fibrosis

The potential role of preconceptional heterozygote screening and newborn screening for affected infants is mentioned above, but for some time to come cystic fibrosis will be met most often as a clinical diagnosis in an affected child. The classic picture of an infant or toddler with recurrent chest infections, failure to thrive and steatorrhoea is well known. Sometimes, early symptoms are milder and the diagnosis may be made later in childhood or even in the teens.

Prenatal diagnosis for cystic fibrosis in families where both parents are known to be carriers (either because they have already had an affected child or because of carrier testing) is almost always possible by chorion villus sampling and is highly reliable (the rare exceptions are where the mutations cannot be defined and one parent is homozygous for all the linked DNA markers, but as more becomes known about the cystic fibrosis gene these will become vanishingly rare). Use of the polymerase chain reaction means that the fetal DNA analysis will be very rapid (1–2 days) and should be adaptable to preimplantation embryos in due course.

When cystic fibrosis is diagnosed in a family, many people are identified as potential carriers. Although most of them are at low risk of having affected children (as long as they do not mate with a cousin or another person with a family history of cystic fibrosis), an offer to the extended family to test for carrier status is worthwhile. When a carrier is identified, his or her partner must be tested. Normality on current tests, which detect about three-quarters of cystic fibrosis alleles, for a person with no family history of cystic fibrosis, reduces his or her carrier risk from 1 in 20 to about 1 in 80. When 90% of mutations are detectable, the risk will fall to 1 in 200, and so on. Prenatal diagnosis will be appropriate only when both partners are shown to carry a cystic fibrosis mutation.

Deafness

Between 1 and 2 children per 1000 suffer from severe sensorineural deafness, and a definite cause such as prenatal rubella infection can be identified in only a small minority. Autosomal recessive inheritance is responsible for a high proportion of cases (Fraser 1976). Severe deafness of unknown cause in an otherwise healthy child of hearing parents is quite likely to be an autosomal recessive, with an empirical recurrence risk in the region of 1 in 6. If two or more deaf children have already been born, or the parents are consanguineous, autosomal recessive inheritance is virtually certain (if both children are male, X-linked severe deafness, although rare, is a possibility). The positive side to this unpalatable information is that the risk of deafness in the next generation is correspondingly low. If the deaf proband marries another deaf person, an estimate of the recurrence risk can be made from a careful assessment of the pedigree and clinical features. In such a family, however, deaf children will often be acceptable to the parents (see also Chapter 18).

CLINICAL PRESENTATION IN THE ADULT AGE GROUP

Many genetic disorders of late onset are autosomal dominant. These conditions tend to have only a small effect on reproductive fitness and are maintained in the population more by transmission from affected parents than by fresh mutation. It follows that a high proportion of at-risk pregnancies can be foreseen by identifying cases in the preceding generation, with corresponding opportunities for prevention of affected births by genetic counselling and prenatal diagnosis. The late onset and sometimes relatively benign nature of these conditions, however, often lead families to question the relevance of genetic counselling and testing.

Huntington's chorea

About 1 person in 4000 carries the gene for this important genetic disorder and between 1 in 1000 and 1 in 500 of the population are affected, presymptomatic, at risk or married to someone in one of these categories.

For various reasons, many of the at-risk group are not aware of their risk. The family may in the past have been given an incorrect diagnosis, or the genetic implications of the diagnosis may not have been explained. Many people were separated from their affected parent in childhood. The condition is often a taboo subject within families, particularly between parents and children. It is therefore common for clinical geneticists to be asked to see adults who have just become aware of their at-risk status. A common reac-tion is to request immediate testing for the Huntington gene. Presymptomatic testing is, however, possible for only a minority of at-risk people, mainly because the use of linked markers requires the elucidation of the linkage phase, i.e. which markers are linked to the Huntington gene in that particular family, by examining DNA samples from relatives who are known to be affected or to have escaped (Harper & Sarfarzi 1985).

It is necessary to store DNA, which can easily be extracted from blood samples, from the potentially informative members of families: affected people, their spouses, and unaffected people who have reached an age (say 70) which makes it very unlikely that they have inherited the condition. Blood should not be taken from at-risk people except as part of an explicit presymptomatic testing procedure with a clearly defined protocol.

Protocols currently in use by genetic units offering presymptomatic testing call for detailed clinical and psychological assessments and at least two counselling sessions specifically to address the issues of predictive testing before the test is administered. This should take place over a period of not less than 2–3 months. The use of linked markers, with its need to investigate the family, often imposes such a time lag, but when the gene is identified, 'free standing' testing may become possible. It will then be important to ensure that adequate pretest counselling and post-test support, are maintained (International Huntington Association and World Federation of Neurology 1990).

Crauford et al (1989) found that 15% of an unselected series of at-risk people elected to enter a predictive testing protocol. Experience suggests that a proportion of these will withdraw during the pretest period, when the issues are discussed and they are required to think through their responses to the possible outcomes.

Most regional genetic services in the UK now maintain a computerised register of affected and at-risk people from Huntington's chorea (HC) families, so that they can offer information and testing to those at risk and identify informative relatives from whom DNA should be stored to help in the interpretation of future tests. These contacts should, whenever possible, be made and maintained via the general practitioner.

Adult polycystic kidney disease

This highly variable autosomal dominant disorder (Watson et al 1990) is present in about 1 per 1000 births. It occasionally causes renal enlargement from birth, more typically causes symptoms in middle age, and may remain clinically silent until old age. Cerebral berry aneurysms are an occasional feature of the condition.

Presymptomatic relatives can be offered ultrasound scanning, which detects renal cysts in about 90% of affected adults. In most affected families, the faulty gene is on chromosome 16 and DNA analysis will usually be informative. Because of the variable and often benign prognosis there has so far been little demand for prenatal diagnosis.

Neurofibromatosis (von Recklinghausen disease)

Brown skin patches are always present in neurofibromatosis and there are usually also subcutaneous neurofibromata. The other features are far more variable, but many of them are serious. Of all the people who carry the gene for neurofibromatosis (1 in 4000 of the population), one-half to two-thirds go through life without any serious problems resulting from it (Huson et al 1989a,b). Many families are aware of the skin signs but consider them trivial. It is debatable whether one should disturb their peace of mind, but most parents of seriously affected children would probably say they wish they had been informed of the possibilities beforehand. Thus, when the diagnosis is made, genetic counselling should be offered to all at-risk relatives, but one should be prepared for a low uptake rate.

Relatives who, on careful examination of the skin, show no sign of being affected (conventionally, six or more cafe au lait patches measuring 1.5 cm or more in diameter) can be reassured that they and their children are not at risk.

There has so far been little demand for prenatal diagnosis by DNA testing using linked markers on chromosome 17. This approach is hardly necessary for presymptomatic diagnosis, as affected children are clinically diagnosable by 5 years of age.

Myotonic dystrophy

Asymptomatic relatives of a person affected by myotonic dystrophy may be shown to be affected by careful clinical examination, electromyography and slit lamp examination of the lenses for cataracts. The wide variation in severity that can occur within a family makes genetic counselling difficult, but it is important to recognise the risk of severe congenital symptoms in the offspring of affected females.

DNA testing with markers on chromosome 19 can be used for diagnosis, and may be helpful when the clinical tests mentioned above are confusing. Testing can also be carried out prenatally.

The condition is well reviewed by Harper (1989).

Marfan syndrome

This condition is also very variable, so that 'classic' Marfan patients are outnumbered, when families are systematically examined, by more mildly affected relatives. Sometimes an obligatory gene carrier, e.g. a person with an affected child and sibling, shows no abnormality on any of the tests in current use.

Families may request investigation and genetic counselling after the diagnosis of a relative. The association with sudden death and cardiac defects usually adds greatly to the anxiety surrounding this procedure. Careful clinical examination, with measurement of skeletal proportions (upper/lower segment ratio, arm span/height ratio), and joint laxity, plus echocardiography and expert eye examination are the best diagnostic tests. Apparently unaffected but at-risk children should be offered follow-up by echocardiography every 2–3 years.

The location of the gene or genes causing Marfan syndrome and the precise nature of the protein defect are still unknown.

Spontaneous abortion and infertility

Although about half of all first trimester miscarriages are caused by fetal chromosome abnormalities, the great majority of these are sporadic and have no significance for further pregnancies. Couples who have had three or more spontaneous abortions should have their chromosomes checked, because in about 1 in 30 such couples one of the pair will be found to carry a balanced chromosome rearrangement, such as an inversion or translocation (Gardner & Sutherland 1989).

When a chromosome rearrangement is discovered, the family should be offered testing to identify other carriers. If ascertainment was coincidental or via miscarriages, the risk of a surviving abnormal child is likely to be low, but prenatal diagnosis should be offered to all carriers.

Infertility is sometimes caused by balanced chromosome rearrangements, some of which may interfere with meiosis. Other chromosome findings relevant to infertility include males with 47, XXY (Klinefelter syndrome) or 46, XX ('XX males'), and females with 45, X (Turner syndrome), a structural abnormality of one X chromosome, or 46, XY (usually testicular feminisation or XY gonadal dysgenesis).

Table 10.4   Some autosomal dominant conditions with a high risk of cancer

Condition	Genetics	Type of malignancy	Appropriate test in at-risk relatives	Age of maximum risk (years)
Polyposis of colon	AD* chr 5†	Adenocarcinoma of colon—usually multiple	Colonoscopy, eye examination for hypertrophy of retinal pigment epithelium	15–40
Retinoblastoma	AD chr 13	Retinoblastoma (osteosarcoma)	Retinoscopy	0–5
Multiple endocrine neoplasia type II	AD chr 10	Medullary thyroid carcinoma Phaeochromocytoma	Calcitonin levels with pentagastrin stimulation Urinary catecholamine levels	9–35
von Hippel–Lindau syndrome	AD chr 3	Renal carcinoma, Cerebellar haemangioblastoma Phaeochromocytoma	CT–cranium and abdomen Retinoscopy Urinary catecholamine levels	5–50

*AD, autosomal dominant; †chr, chromosome

Cancer

While cancer is a genetic disease of cells, most cancers do not show strong family clustering. There is, however, a small but important group where susceptibility to specific types of malignancy is conferred by a single gene defect showing autosomal dominant inheritance. These conditions are summarised in Table 10.4 and the management of risk in the affected families is reviewed by Littler and Harper (1989). In most cases, surveillance by means of periodic examinations during the at-risk period will greatly improve the prognosis, making the recognition of these conditions important. The type of tumour or clinical presentation in the index patient is generally enough to prompt consideration of the diagnosis in this group.

Familial aggregation of more common cancers has also been reported, and in these cases it is the family history that is suggestive (although individual patients may present unusually early or with multiple primary tumours). The tumours most commonly involved in this so-called 'cancer family syndrome' are of the colon, rectum, stomach, ovary, uterus and breast. Although the genes responsible have not been identified and empirical risk data are still imprecise, families can be helped by advice on risks and screening procedures. Often, the risk estimates will be lower than feared. Genetic counseling services should be able to deal with these families, or to refer them on to the (so far few) genetic counselling clinics specialising in cancer.

The questions of genetic risk in cancer, and the importance of genetic studies are reviewed by Ponder (1987) and by Parry et al (1987).

Coronary heart disease

Genetic risks may be important in coronary heart disease, particularly in families showing unusually early onset. The topic is covered in Chapter 21.

THE ORGANISATION OF MEDICAL GENETICS SERVICES

Following the suggestions of the Clinical Genetics Society, clinical and laboratory genetics services in the UK have been organised along regional lines. The benefits of such organisation include a clear definition of responsibility for geographic areas, a large and epidemiologically meaningful population base, and the ability to plan what is increasingly a preventive medicine service.

Most regional clinical genetics centres hold satellite genetic counselling clinics at their main district general hospitals. There is an increasing use of specialist genetic nurses or other non-medical associates, who are able to gather information before the clinic and provide continuity in follow up. These associates may provide, or at least register the need for, supportive counselling and monitor the understanding of information given in the clinic.

Self-help groups devoted to specific disorders or groups of disorders are now playing an important part in stimulating and financing research, supporting affected people and families, and disseminating information to the public and professionals. For families coping with a rare disorder, contact with the national group may be a lifeline. Recently, most of the lay groups concerned with genetic disorders in the UK have combined into an 'umbrella' organisation — the Genetic Interest Group.

Most clinical genetics services now hold computerised registers of individuals at risk of genetic disorders for which testing is available, and which are sufficiently severe to justify some form of outreach into the community. Conditions for which this approach is generally agreed to be appropriate are Huntington's chorea, Duchenne and Becker muscular dystrophies, X-linked mental retardation, colonic polyposis and the other dominantly inherited cancer syndromes, and balanced translocations known to have produced an unbalanced but viable segregant. Conditions for which the benefits of a genetic register approach are less clear include neurofibromatosis, adult polcystic kidney disease, myotonic dystrophy and haemophilia.

Familial hypercholesterolaemia and other major gene effects on coronary disease risk also call for a register approach, but will need a joint effort by cardiologists and geneticists, which has not so far been widely developed.

CONCLUSIONS

The scope of genetic screening and testing is expanding rapidly. Clinical genetics is beginning to have far-reaching implications for the planning of community medical services. The more genetic markers of disease susceptibility are identified, the more testing, counselling and perhaps treatment will need to be offered to the relatives of the presenting patient. General practitioners provide an essential link between the regional genetic services and the community. They can disseminate information about the availability and implications of screening tests. Their help is essential in contacting relatives for family studies or offering risk information and they are ideally placed to provide support for their patients who are coming to terms with genetic risks.

The supplanting of prenatal diagnosis by the correction of genetic defects is not, for most conditions, just around the corner. In the enthusiasm for ever more elegant ways of testing for genetic disorders we must remember that abortion of an affected fetus is an option that will never be chosen by a significant minority of our society and, for most of those who do choose it, the process will, for a long time afterwards, seem a loss rather than a gain. These are some of the reasons for approaching genetic counselling non-directively. General practitioners will find increasing numbers of their patients facing such issues and should not be inhibited from offering help by the fear that the genetics are too complicated. It is the job of the genetic counsellor to present the options and their possible consequences clearly to the family and to the referring doctor.

REFERENCES

Bundey S, Thake A, Todd J 1989 The recurrence risks for mild idiopathic mental retardation. Journal of Medical Genetics 26: 260–266

Canadian Collaborative CVS-Amniocentesis Clinical Trial Group 1989 Multicentre randomised clinical trial of chorion villus sampling and amniocentesis. Lancet i: 1–6

Clayton-Smith J, Farndon P A, McKeown C, Donnai D 1990 Examination of fetuses after induced abortion for fetal abnormality. British Medical Journal 300: 295 297

Connor J M, Ferguson-Smith M A 1987 Essential medical genetics. Blackwell Scientific Publications, Oxford

Crauford D, Dodge A, Kerzin-Storrar L, Harris R 1989 Uptake of presymptomatic testing for Huntington's disease. Lancet 2: 603–605

Davies K E (ed) 1989 The fragile X syndrome. Oxford University Press, Oxford

DHSS April 1988 Letter on haemoglobinopathy cards. DHSS, London. Obtainable from Central Stores, No. 2 site, Manchester Road, Heywood, Lancashire, OL10 2PZ, UK

Ewings S, Gregson N, Jacobs P A 1991 The efficacy of maternal age screening for Down's syndrome in Wessex. Prenatal Diagnosis: in press

Ferguson-Smith M A, Yates J 1984 Maternal age specific rates for chromosome aberrations and factors influencing them: report of a collaborative European study on 52 965 amniocenteses. Prenatal Diagnosis 4: 5–44

Fraser G R 1976 The causes of profound deafness in childhood. Bailliere Tindall, London

Gardner R J M, Sutherland G R 1989 Chromosome abnormalities and genetic counselling. Oxford University Press, Oxford

Harper P S 1988 Practical genetic counselling, 3rd edn. Wright, Bristol

Harper P S 1989 Myotonic dystrophy, 2nd edn. Saunders, Philadelphia

Harper P S, Sarfarazi M 1985 Genetic prediction and family structure in Huntington's chorea. British Medical Journal 290: 1929–1931

Herbst D S, Baird P A 1982 Sib risks for non specific mental retardation in British Columbia. American Journal of Medical Genetics 13: 197–208

Hook E B 1983 Chromosome abnormalities and spontaneous fetal death following amniocentesis: further data and associations with maternal age. American Journal of Human Genetics 35: 110–116

Hook E B, Cross P K, Jackson L et al 1988 Maternal age-specific rates of 47, +21 and other cytogenetic abnormalities diagnosed in the first trimester of pregnancy in chorionic villus biopsy specimens: comparison with rates expected from observations at amniocentesis. American Journal of Human Genetics 42: 797–807

Huson S M, Compston D A S, Clark P, Harper P S 1989a A

genetic study of von Recklinghausen neurofibromatosis in South East Wales. I Prevalence, fitness, mutation rate and effect of parental transmission on severity. Journal of Medical Genetics 26: 704–711

Huson S M, Compston D A S, Harper P S 1989b A genetic study of von Recklinghausen neurofibromatosis in South East Wales. II Guidelines for genetic counselling. Journal of Medical Genetics 27: 712–721

International Huntington Association and World Federation of Neurology 1990 Ethical issues policy statement on Huntington's disease molecular genetics predictive test. Journal of Medical Genetics 27: 34–38

Jackson L G 1990 CVS newsletter No. 29. Jefferson Medical College, Philadelphia

Jacobs P A 1990 The role of chromosome abnormalities in reproduction failure. Reproduction, Nutrition, Development Suppl 1, 63–74

Jacobs P A, Melville M, Ratcliff S et al 1974 A cytogenetic study of 11 680 newborn infants. Annals of Human Genetics 37: 359–376

Littler M, Harper P S 1989 A regional register for inherited cancers. British Medical Journal 298: 1689–1691

Magnus P, Berg K, Bjerkedal T 1985 Association of parental consanguinity with decreased birthweight, and increased rate of early death and congenital malformations. Clinical Genetics 28: 335–342

Modell M, Modell B 1990 Genetic screening for ethnic minorities. British Medical Journal 300: 1702–1704

MRC working party on amniocentesis 1978 An assessment of the hazards of amniocentesis. British Journal of Obstetrics and Gynaecology 85 Suppl 2, 1–41

MRC working party on the evaluation of chorionic villus sampling 1991 Medical Research Council European Trial of chorionic villus sampling. Lancet 337: 1491–1499

NICHD Registry, national registry for amniocentsis study group 1976 Midtrimester amniocentesis for prenatal diagnosis, safety and accuracy. Journal of the American Medical Association 236: 1471–1476

Nicolaides K H, Campbell S 1987 Diagnosis and management of fetal malformations. In: Rodeck C H (ed) Fetal diagnosis of genetic defects. Bailliere Tindall, London

Nicolaides K H, Rodeck C H, Gosden C 1986 Rapid karyotyping in non lethal fetal malformations. Lancet 1: 284–286

Parry D M, Berg K, Mulvihill J J et al 1987 Strategies for controlling cancer through genetics: report of a workshop. American Journal of Human Genetics 41: 63–69

Ponder B A J 1987 Familial cancer: opportunities for clinical practice and research. European Journal of Surgical Oncology 13: 463–473

Ratcliffe S G, Paul N 1986 Prospective studies on children with sex chromosome aneuploidy. Birth Defects Original Article Series 22(3) AR Liss New York

Rhoads G G, Jackson L G, Schlesselman S E et al 1989 The safety and efficacy of chorionic villus sampling for early prenatal diagnosis of cytogenetic abnormalities. New England Journal of Medicine 320: 609–617

Richards D S, Seeds J W, Katz V L et al 1988 Elevated maternal serum alphafetoprotein with normal ultrasound: is amniocentesis always appropriate? Obstetrics and Gynaecology 71: 203–207

Royal College of Physicians 1989 Prenatal diagnosis and genetic screening. Community and service implications. Royal College of Physicians of London, London

Sardharwalla I B, Wraith J E 1989 A clinician's view of the mass screening of the newborn for inherited diseases: current practice and future considerations. Journal of Inherited Metabolic Disease 12 (Suppl 1): 55–63

Saudubray J M, Ogier H, Bonnefont J P et al 1989 Clinical approach to inherited metabolic diseases in the neonatal period: a 20 year survey. Journal of Inherited Metabolic Disease 12 (Suppl 1): 25–41

Simpson N E, Dallaire L, Miller J R et al 1976 Prenatal diagnosis of genetic disease in Canada: report of a collaborative study. Canadian Medical Association Journal 115: 739–748

Sveger J 1978 Alpha-1 antitrypsin deficiency in early childhood. Pediatrics 62: 22–25

Tabor A, Philip J, Madsen M, et al 1986 Randomised controlled trial of genetic amniocentesis in 4606 low risk women. Lancet i: 1287–1293

Thom H, Campbell A G, Farr V et al 1985 The impact of maternal serum alphafetoprotein screening on open neural tube defect births in north-east Scotland. Prenatal Diagnosis 5: 15–19

Thompson J S, Thompson MW 1985 Genetics in medicine. W B Saunders, Philadelphia

Wald N J, Cuckle H J, Densem J W et al 1988 Maternal serum screening for Down's syndrome in early pregnancy. British Medical Journal 297: 883–887

Watson M L, Macnicol A M, Wright A F 1990 Adult polycystic kidney disease. British Medical Journal 300: 62–63

Weatherall D J 1991 The new genetics and clinical practice. Oxford University Press, Oxford

Wertz D C, Fletcher J C 1988 Attitudes of genetic counsellors: a multinational study. American Journal of Human Genetics 42: 592–600

11. Antenatal and postnatal care

David Jewell

INTRODUCTION

Antenatal care has been an established part of general practice for many years. In any discussion of prevention it is held up as an example of effective prevention at work, sharing with better intrapartum care the responsibility for the steady improvement in maternal and perinatal health in the last 50 years. Ten years ago the Short Committee, reporting on the maternity services stated: 'We unhesitatingly accept the often reiterated claim of antenatal care as a means of reducing perinatal and neonatal mortality' (House of Commons Social Services Committee 1980). Such attitudes, sincerely held and fostered by the medical establishment, have until recently been neither questioned nor rigorously tested. The established tradition of antenatal care, together with the improvement in maternal and perinatal mortality, have largely insulated antenatal care from the scrutiny to which screening tests would now be subjected before introduction into general clinical practice. However, as this chapter will show, there are grounds for challenging the accepted beliefs.

History

Despite its established presence in modern obstetric practice, antenatal care has a comparatively short pedigree. Oakley (1982) has charted the development of antenatal care from the opening of the first outpatient clinic in Edinburgh in 1915, through clinics run under the auspices of Local Authorities between the wars, to the present day practice of antenatal care largely conducted by general practitioners and midwives in general practice premises. The impetus for this development was a series of government reports, starting in 1929 and continuing through the 1930s, which concluded that many maternal deaths would have been preventable by better care. Development was haphazard until a further report recommended a

pattern of attendances and procedures based on a consensus of the current practice in local authority clinics. This pattern has remained largely unchanged to the present time, and practice has only been altered by the addition of more technically based tests.

This illustrates the now familiar fallacy of identifying a problem and prescribing a solution, without taking the trouble to ascertain the strength of the causal link, if any, between them.

Evaluating antenatal care

The evaluation of antenatal care poses a number of methodological problems, some shared with other screening programmes but others arising from the particular problems of pregnancy.

Content

In a complete programme of antenatal care there is a mix of activities. At the simplest level there are three components: education, treatment of medical problems occurring in pregnancy and preventive care. However, even the preventive component consists of activities that differ from each other in their nature and intent. For instance, women's heights are measured, in theory, to assess the risk of cephalopelvic disproportion during labour. Like social class and previous obstetric history, height is a fixed component of an individual's risk. Testing for protein in the urine, on the other hand, is aimed at identifying a risk that might, again in theory, be altered by medical intervention. The problem is further complicated by procedures that are repeated during each pregnancy, but whose functions alter as pregnancy progresses. For instance, repeated palpation of the abdomen at first has the function of verifying dates and checking for twin pregnancy; it is subsequently used for screening for growth retardation; and its final function is to identify malpresentation or pelvic obstruction sufficient to cause disproportion. Some conditions may affect mother and fetus so that, for instance, screening for severe pre-eclampsia is intended to protect mothers from eclamptic fits and fetuses from growth retardation and increased mortality.

Predictive value

Antenatal screening shares with other programmes the problems inherent in the relationship between the prevalence of a condition and the predictive value of a test intended to identify it (Grant & Mohide 1982; see also Chapter 2). First, there is the possibility that screening tests, which have been developed on high-risk populations under ideal conditions, are applied to a normal population under normal working conditions, where the predictive value will be lower. Second, circumstances in pregnancy may change rapidly with time. A test that gives reliable information about fetal well-being at and after delivery, may be much less accurate if used some time before labour. For instance, analyses of records in research studies on antepartum cardiotocography have mostly been restricted to records taken within 7 days of birth. However, a clinician doing a cardiotocograph on a patient has to interpret the results without knowing whether the patient is within a week of giving birth. Once again the conclusions of research would tend to overestimate the predictive value of the test. Third, one aim of antenatal care has always been to reduce maternal and perinatal mortality, and the various components of the programme have been thought to predict these, either directly or indirectly. In fact, the screening tests now applied were not properly evaluated in the past. Ideally they would have been evaluated, found to be accurate and then incorporated into the antenatal care programme. Maternal and perinatal mortality rates have now fallen considerably, so the predictive value of previously accurate tests would be expected to have fallen.

Screening tests and gold standards

Knowing the sensitivity, specificity and predictive values of a screening test implies the existence of a gold standard against which the test is measured. For a complete programme there may be a need for a diagnostic test, whose properties are closer to the gold standard and on which some action can be taken. As will be shown, some components of antenatal care include all of these components. For instance, serum alphafetoprotein (AFP) factors is the screening test for

the detection of anencephaly and neural tube abnormality. The test properties can be calculated, using the final diagnosis of abnormality after birth, as the gold standard. The intermediate diagnostic test was, until recently, the amniotic fluid alphafetoprotein level. The same applies to genetic amniocentesis for detection of Down syndrome, except that in this case the screening test also functions as a diagnostic test. As Wilson and Jungner (1968) pointed out in their classic monograph on screening, diagnostic tests differ from screening tests primarily in the necessity to demonstrate greater accuracy.

However, for other components of antenatal care the position is more complex. Given the low perinatal mortality rate it is difficult, and not helpful, to use perinatal or neonatal death as the gold standard for tests of fetal well-being, and attempts have been made to identify alternatives. The problem begins with defining what is meant by poor outcome. Diagnoses of fetal distress could be validated by comparison with Apgar scores, but the relationship between Apgar scores and long-term morbidity is not at all clear. The incidence of early neonatal convulsions has been proposed as a measure of good obstetric care (Dennis & Chalmers 1982). This is fortunately also a rare occurrence, and a recent report of a long-term follow-up from a study of electronic fetal monitoring in labour has cast doubt on its ability to predict long-term morbidity (Grant et al 1989b). In the absence of an agreed and easily used gold standard, studies to identify screening tests are forced to use substitutes whose own relationship to usually unstated gold standards is speculative.

The same point is illustrated by the detection of intrauterine growth retardation. In research studies the results of screening tests can be compared with the actual weight measured after birth. In practice a suspicion of growth retardation leads to further tests, such as non-stress cardiotocography and ultrasound scanning, which when used as screening tests themselves have low predictive values.

Finally, the success of any screening programme depends on the ability to intervene effectively to improve outcome. As will be seen, the assumption of effective intervention to improve obstetric outcomes has increasingly become impossible to sustain. Even electronic fetal monitoring during labour has failed to demonstrate any benefits. In two large and well-controlled trials, electronic fetal monitoring increased the rate of caesarean section without benefits to the babies both immediately after birth (MacDonald et al 1985, Leveno et al 1986), and at 4 years of age (Grant et al 1989b). In a third trial in women in preterm labour, electronic fetal monitoring appeared to increase the rate of cerebral palsy measured at 18 months of age (Shy et al 1990).

In the remainder of this chapter the various components in the antenatal care screening programme will be considered in more detail and the evidence to support their use will be discussed. Any activity that is undertaken to improve overall outcome has been included, excluding only the general provision of health promotion and education, and the care and treatment of the common symptomatic problems of pregnancy.

SCREENING FOR MATERNAL CONDITIONS

Screening in early pregnancy

Initial risk assessment

The first step in antenatal care is an attempt to assess risk based on the sociodemographic status, medical and obstetric history of pregnant women. Perinatal mortality rate is known to be closely associated with social class (Knox et al 1980, Chalmers 1985), and also with the extremes of maternal age. Ethnic background influences both perinatal mortality rate and birthweight, with Asian and Afro-Caribbean groups having higher perinatal mortality rates than Europeans. It is not clear whether this effect is genetic or related to diet, although there is some evidence that it is related to the environment during the early years of the mother's life.

The likelihood of recurrence of adverse events in previous pregnancies depends on the nature of the previous problem. For instance, the likelihood of recurrence of genetic abnormalities may follow classic Mendelian inheritance patterns; other congenital abnormalities may confer little or no risk of recurrence. Preterm delivery is more frequent in those women with a previous history, although again the risk may be less when the previous preterm delivery can be ascribed to a non-recurrent cause, such as twin delivery. Caesarean section is also more likely after one, or more strongly still, two, previous caesarean sections, although this may owe as much to clinicians' attitudes as to the intrinsic problem. If pelvimetry indicates a major degree of cephalopelvic disproportion then a decision will usually be made to plan an elective caesarean section.

There may be a complex relationship between pregnancy and medical disorders. Medical problems can cause problems in pregnancy, and pregnancy itself may exacerbate certain medical conditions. Hypertension does not seem to cause an increase in risk in itself, but does cause an increase in the rate of pre-eclampsia. Diabetes mellitus causes the problems of large babies and late intrauterine death, and pregnancy usually makes diabetic control more difficult. In epilepsy the frequency of fits may be altered in either direction, or remain unchanged. Provided the condition remains reasonably controlled there does not seem to be any increased risk to the fetus. One of the problems in managing medical conditions in pregnancy is balancing the need for good pharmacological management of the maternal problem with the potential risk the drugs may cause to the fetus. The problems associated with other medical disorders have been reviewed by James (1988).

The theoretical reason for assessing risk in early pregnancy is to plan appropriate care for the pregnancy. When a larger proportion of births was under the care of general practitioners, either at home or in general practitioner units, then it was possible to use the information gained to book for delivery in the most appropriate setting. However, such a decision now has to be made only rarely (Jewell & Smith 1990), and conventional risk assessment does not seem to be a good predictor of obstetric outcome (Lilford & Chard 1983, Reynolds et al 1988). Nor, as will be shown, is there much that intensive antenatal or intrapartum care has to offer as a means of improving outcome in those at increased risk. It would be absurd to argue that carers should neither take an obstetric history nor try to make an initial assessment of risk. However, the limitations of such an exercise must be recognised.

Screening for lifestyle factors

Diet. At times of severe famine the birth rate falls, such as happened in The Netherlands at the end of the Second World War. However, at lesser degrees of maternal malnutrition the fetus is well protected, becoming thinner but not stunted in growth (Hytten 1980). Controlled trials of both calorie and protein supplements to undernourished women in New York (Rush et al 1980) and a nutritionally vulnerable area of East Java (Kardjati et al 1988) have failed to show any overall effect on birthweight, although the latter study did show some benefit to those in greatest need.

More specific attention has been directed to diet in early pregnancy following the studies on the effect of folate supplementation in preventing neural tube defects (Smithells et al 1980, 1983), although there were methodological problems with this work. More recent studies have seemed to confirm (Milunsky et al 1989) and refute (Mills et al 1989) the early claims of the beneficial effects of folate and vitamin supplement. The recently reported MRC study (MRC Vitamin Study Research Group 1991) showed a recurrence rate of neural tube defects of 1% among 600 women given folic acid, compared with 3.5% among controls.

Department of Health guidelines now support the use of folic acid for the prevention of neural tube defects in patients with a relevant past history.

There is therefore no indication for any general advice to be given to pregnant women concerning their diet. As with some other areas, discussing diet may provide an opportunity for exploring patients' beliefs about diet in pregnancy. In particular, women who tend to be overweight can be reassured that controlling their food intake to keep the weight gain in pregnancy to a minimum is unlikely to do their babies any harm.

Smoking. Smoking in pregnancy is associated with a reduction in mean birthweight, an increase in perinatal mortality rate (Butler et al 1972) and a higher rate of preterm delivery (Fedrick & Anderson 1976). The effect appears to operate on placental function (Meyer et al 1976); after correcting for social class smoking has no effect on the rates of congenital abnormality (Golding & Butler 1983; Hemminki et al 1983).

Stopping smoking before 16 weeks' gestation largely removes its deleterious effects (MacArthur & Knox 1988). Women are well enough informed to choose to give up spontaneously: in a study of women attending antenatal clinics in Nottingham 31% smoked during pregnancy, 36% had never smoked, 26% had stopped before becoming pregnant and 7% on hearing that they were pregnant (Madeley et al 1989). Advice and encouragement can increase the numbers of women stopping smoking. In one controlled study using a variety of strategies for giving up, 43% in the treatment group had given up by 8 months' gestation, compared with 20% of the control group (Sexton & Hebel 1984). Such advice is not always offered by professionals involved in antenatal care (McKnight & Merrett 1986).

The conclusion is therefore that smoking does increase risk to the fetus and that encouragement from doctors and midwives may help women already motivated to give up. However, a cautious approach needs to be taken. The actual increase in risk is not enormous, so that the average reduction in birthweights of babies born to smokers is only 170 g (MacArthur & Knox 1988). On the other hand, smoking may be of benefit to some women. Graham (1976) found that smoking helped women cope with other family responsibilities, broke up the daily routine and delineated a time for relaxation. Too much attention to 'bad habits' that women find impossible to give up may only make them feel guilty.

Alcohol. The fetal alcohol syndrome of growth retardation both prenatally and postnatally, microcephaly, short palpebral fissures, maxillary hypoplasia and cardiac abnormalities, was first described in 1973 (Jones & Smith 1973; Jones et al 1973). Persistent mental retardation has been found at the ages of 1 year (Olegard et al 1979) and 7 years (Jones et al 1974). At lower levels of consumption alcohol has been associated with reduced birthweight (Lumley et al 1985). The effect is seen only in those women consistently drinking at least 2–3 units of alcohol daily; alcohol consumption below this level, which is the amount consumed by most women in pregnancy, does not confer any increased risk on the fetus (Mills & Graubard 1987).

Work. Early research on the effects of work suggested a reduction in birthweight of babies born to women who worked in pregnancy, and it was suggested that this might account for the effect of class on birthweight. More recent evidence has arrived at the opposite view, with women working late in pregnancy having lower rates of both preterm delivery and low birthweight babies in both the United Kingdom and France (Murphy et al 1984; Saurel & Kaminski 1983). The effect on low birthweight disappeared, however, when allowance was made for those with an adverse medical or obstetric history. This suggests a 'healthy worker effect', in which employment selects a group of healthy individuals. By contrast, a study of women in Addis Ababa found that there was a reduction of birthweight of babies born to women who had physically demanding tasks to perform both inside and outside their homes (Tafari et al 1980).

This illustrates the difficulty of generalising about work and pregnancy. What 'work' means in terms of physical effort, reward and social contact will vary with the occupation. Paid employment is also, for most women, only part of their work, as they usually have the responsibility for housework. Garcia and Elbourne (1984) have concluded that there is no overall risk that work confers on pregnancy, but that this advice needs to be tailored for individual women.

Certain occupations do confer specific risks. There is an increase in miscarriage rate for women exposed to anaesthetic gases, most probably nitrous oxide (Vessey & Nunn 1980), an increase in perinatal mortality rate for women working in the chemical and laundry/dry cleaning industries and an increase in congenital abnormalities for those working in the glass and pottery industries (Peters et al 1984). A recent review concluded that there was no risk to women working at video display terminals, not least because the level of radiation from the screens is very low (Blackwell & Chang 1988).

Exercise. Neither regular exercise (Hauth et al 1982) nor the level of fitness measured on a bicycle ergometer (Pommerance et al 1974) have any effect on the health of the fetus, although fitness was associated with shorter labours in multiparous women. Increasing the fitness of women during pregnancy by graded exercises had no effect on obstetric outcomes when compared with a control group (Collings et al 1983).

Screening for infection

Bacteriuria. The rational basis for screening for bacteriuria in pregnancy is the finding that 2–7% of pregnant women can be found to have symptomless bacteriuria, and approximately 30% of these will develop acute pyelonephritis if untreated (Cunningham 1987). Evidence for an association with preterm delivery is much less definite (Whalley, 1967), although one study suggested a link between infection with group B steptococci and both preterm labour and primary rupture of membranes (Thomsen et al 1987). A meta-analysis of eight controlled trials shows that treatment of asymptomatic bacteriuria in early pregnancy significantly reduces the risk of subsequent pyelonephritis (Wang & Smaill 1989). However, a programme of a single urine culture early on in pregnancy will not eradicate pyelonephritis, as this condition can occur in some women without bacteriuria on screening (Gilstrap et al 1981) and in others treated for bacteriuria following screening (Chng and Hall 1982, Campbell-Brown et al 1987, Foley et al 1987). At a prevalence for asymptomatic bacteriuria of 5%, a test specificity of 90% gives a single culture a positive predictive value of only 30% (Wang & Smaill 1989). (For definitions see Chapter 2.) Therefore a rational policy is for all pregnant women to have a screening urine culture; for those found to be positive to have a second test and be treated if that too is positive; and for those who have been treated to have further cultures done at intervals in the remainder of the pregnancy. Even this will not prevent all episodes of pyelonephritis (Gilstrap et al 1981), and similar policies have been questioned, on the grounds both of effectiveness (Chng & Hall 1982) and of cost (Campbell-Brown et al 1987).

Rubella. Rubella in pregnant women is a well known source of congenital infection. The risk of a fetus being infected is 80% if the mother is infected in the first 12 weeks. After this the risk falls to approximately 25% at the end of the second trimester but rises towards 100% at term (Miller et al 1982). Previous infection or immunisation results in high levels of maternal immunity; one study showed 2.6% of nulliparous women and 1.1% of multiparous women to be susceptible to rubella early in pregnancy (Miller et al 1987). However rubella was confirmed in some women reported as previously immune or immunised, and a minority of them gave birth to infants with features of congenital infection. The study concluded that congenital rubella would be prevented only by improved herd immunity. It remains to be seen whether the introduction of rubella immunisation at the age of 1 year, with the MMR vaccine, will achieve this goal.

Multiparous women are more likely to contract rubella in pregnancy than nulliparous women. Two-thirds of women affected by rubella in pregnancy are multiparous, presumably because they contract the infection from their own children (Miller et al 1982). This provides a justification for continuing to test the rubella immunity of pregnant women, and offering immunisation postpartum for the non-immune.

Syphilis. The incidence of congenital syphilis is now very low and the value of continuing to screen for syphilis in pregnant women has been questioned (Clay 1989). However, congenital syphilis does still occur (Mascola 1984) and from 1986 to 1988 in New York the incidence increased, and was associated with use of cocaine (Morbidity and Mortality Weekly Report 1989). Infection of the fetus is believed to occur only after 20 weeks' gestation, and treatment of infected mothers prevents fetal infection (Sequeira & Tobin 1984). Therefore serological testing of mothers early in pregnancy creates a latent stage in which the disease (congenital syphilis) can be prevented. A cost–benefit analysis, comparing the costs of screening and treatment with the lifetime costs of supporting the small number of children affected with congenital syphilis showed that substantial benefits are to be achieved from continuing to screen in pregnancy (Stray-Pedersen 1983) (see also Chapter 36).

Other infections. Other organisms that can infect fetuses include toxoplasma, human immunodeficiency virus (HIV), cytomegalovirus (CMV), herpes simplex virus, and *Listeria monocytogenes*. Unfortunately, the natural history of all of these infections, together with the limited opportunities for treatment, preclude the development of effective screening programmes.

There is a screening programme for toxoplasmosis in France, where the infection is much more common. Women are tested early and late in pregnancy and a rise in antibodies is taken as evidence of maternal infection (Sequeira & Tobin 1984). Only a minority of fetuses in women who seroconvert become infected, and a minority of these subsequently develop cerebral complications. Screening might nevertheless be indicated, but the available treatment is not wholly effective at eradicating fetal infection (Desmonts & Couvreur 1974).

HIV affects approximately one-third of infants born to affected mothers (Bradbeer 1989). The route of transmission is not clear (Italian Multicentre Trial 1988), treatment is not currently an option in pregnancy and there are considerable ethical problems. For these reasons screening in pregnancy is not considered appropriate. This condition is discussed further in Chapter 36.

CMV infection of fetuses can cause microcephaly and other neurological problems. The only method of treatment would be termination of affected pregnancies, but this has not been introduced since only 15% of maternal infections result in congenital infection of fetuses (Hanshaw et al 1985).

Herpes simplex virus is thought to be acquired by fetuses during labour by direct contact with lesions in the birth canal (Hanshaw et al 1985). The consensus is that, in the presence of active viral infection, fetal infection can be prevented by casearean section. In this case the screening test is a visual inspection of the mother's cervix at the onset of labour.

Listeria monocytogenes is a rare cause of second trimester miscarriage or pneumonia and meningitis if contracted later in pregnancy (Spencer 1987). The non-specific nature of the maternal illness makes it difficult to distinguish from other flu-like illnesses, and the latent period between maternal and fetal infection is believed to be as short as 1 or 2 days (Fleming et al 1985; Khong et al 1986). This rules out the possibility of screening for this condition.

Screening for cervical cancer

Pregnant women constitute a population of sexually active women available for cervical smear examinations when they attend antenatal clinics. The Department of Health has recommended examination of cervical smears every 5 years for women between the age of 20 and 64, and each health district has been given the responsibility of organising call and recall systems to ensure maximum coverage. A specific recommendation to take cervical smears in pregnant women would be justified only if pregnancy itself increased the risk of invasive cervical cancer, but there is no evidence of such an effect.

Anxiety has been expressed about the rising rate of abnormal smears in young women (Wolfendale et al 1983). However, death rates from cervical cancer in the younger age cohorts, while they have been rising since 1971, remain much lower than those in the older age groups (Peto 1986). There is no evidence of a higher incidence of rapidly progressive cervical cancer affecting younger women (Silcocks & Moss 1988) and the prognosis of cervical cancer is the same for women above and below the age of 35 (Smales et al 1987).

There is no argument, therefore, to recommend cervical smears in pregnancy except in those women whose last cervical smear was examined more than 5 years previously, and those over the age of 20 who have never had a cervical smear examined. Even then the difficulties in interpreting smears taken in pregnancy (Coleman & Evans 1988), together with the practical problems of responding to abnormal smears taken from pregnant women, may dictate deferring the smear until the postnatal examination or later. General practitioners are in a position to check that a smear is not required and to inform specialist colleagues that this is the case (see also Chapter 24).

Screening during pregnancy

Anaemia

Accepted practice has now moved away from recommending iron supplementation for all pregnant women. However, it remains routine to measure the haemoglobin concentration at least twice in each pregnancy. The problems of this approach have been reviewed by Mahomed and Hytten (1989). Anaemia in pregnancy is difficult to define. Haemoglobin concentration depends on the ratio of two variables, red cell mass and plasma volume, and both of these change during pregnancy so that changes in haemoglobin concentration may result from changes in either. Increases in plasma volume, and therefore lower haemoglobin measurements, are associated with increases in birthweight; conversely, high haemoglobin measurement is associated with lower birthweight, fetal death and pre-eclampsia (Koller et al 1980). It it suggested that increases in haemoglobin lead to larger cells and greater blood viscosity, which may be harmful in pregnancy.

Ferritin is thought to be a better guide to iron deficiency. Without supplementation the serum ferritin level falls in early pregnancy, reaching a steady level at about 28 weeks' gestation, then rises after birth. However, even at 6 months postpartum the level may not have recovered to the level found at 12 weeks gestation (Taylor et al 1982). Supplementation with oral iron has been shown in controlled trials to reduce or even reverse the early second trimester fall in ferritin; after delivery the level may fall, but the results postpartum are then unlikely to be below the earliest measurements, as they were for the control groups (Taylor et al 1982, Wallenburg & Van Eijk 1984).

Such studies do not, however, give any information about pregnancy outcome. In one US study the graph of pregnancy outcomes compared with haemoglobin showed a U-shaped curve, with problems occurring more frequently at high and low extremes of haemoglobin. The optimum haemoglobin concentration was 11–12 g/dl for white women, but only 10–11 g/dl for black women (Garn et al 1981).

The available evidence does not support widespread iron supplementation in pregnancy, but neither does it offer useful guidelines for a more selective policy. It is probably prudent to offer iron supplements to women whose ferritin levels are considerably depressed at the start of pregnancy. Otherwise changes in both haemoglobin and ferritin concentrations in pregnancy appear to be physiological and it is impossible to say with any confidence that supplementation will do more good than harm.

Rhesus isoimmunisation

Strictly speaking, the screening programme for rhesus isoimmunisation belongs both in antenatal and in postnatal care. However, it is convenient to discuss the different components of the programme under antenatal care: testing begins before birth and testing and treatment can be regarded as preventive care for future pregnancies.

The theoretical possibility of preventing rhesus isoimmunisation appeared with the demonstration that sensitisation could be avoided by injection with rhesus antibodies half an hour after transfusion with rhesus positive blood (Clarke et al 1963). Controlled trials provided overwhelming evidence of the actual benefits when administered to rhesus negative women after delivery (Ascari et al 1968, Chown et al 1969, Robertson & Holmes 1969). A meta-analysis of nine such controlled trials revealed that out of 2972 women receiving anti-D gammaglobulin, six became sensitised, compared with 186 out of 2488 controls (Gravenhorst 1989). It is now standard practice to give prophylactic anti-D to rhesus negative women after events likely to cause sensitisation other than transplacental haemorrhage at delivery, such as miscarriage and amniocentesis (Hill et al 1980). Despite such measures, or because of their incomplete application, some rhesus isoimmunisation still occurs. Screening for rhesus antibodies, with monitoring of affected fetuses and intrauterine transfusion in severe cases, remains an important component of antenatal care (Larkin et al 1982). Bowman (1984) has assessed the benefits of the complete programme in Manitoba: in 1963 rhesus isoimmunisation had an incidence of

10.6 per 1000 pregnancies, with a perinatal mortality rate of 151 per 1000 in affected babies. The comparable figures were 1.6 per 1000 (1980) and 18 per 1000 (1974–79), respectively.

Pre-eclampsia and hypertension

The risks of severe pre-eclampsia are well known: placental abruption, thrombocytopenia and intravascular coagulation, renal failure and fits in mothers, and stillbirths and neonatal deaths in fetuses (MacGillivray 1985; Sibai et al 1985). The risks of mild pre-eclampsia or hypertension preceding pregnancy are, in themselves, much less; only proteinuria or diastolic blood pressure greater than 110 mm Hg increases perinatal mortality rate compared with the normotensive group (De Swiet 1984). MacGillivray (1985) quotes one study in which the perinatal mortality rate for women with late hypertension and no proteinuria was lower than for those with normal blood pressure. The major risk of diastolic blood pressure between 90 and 100 mm Hg is of progression to severe pre-eclampsia (De Swiet 1984, Sibai & Anderson 1986). Women subsequently developing pre-eclampsia have consistently higher blood pressures from an early stage of pregnancy than non-affected women (Moutquin et al 1985). Similarly, the use of diastolic blood pressures above 90 mm Hg as the cut-off point for pre-eclampsia is of much less value in predicting risk for mothers and babies than using an increase in diastolic pressure of 25 mm Hg or more (Redman & Jefferies 1988).

Results of trials of hypotensive and anticonvulsive therapy show, on the whole, few benefits of drug treatment. In controlled trials in mild or moderate pre-eclampsia, diuretics have been shown to reduce blood pressure, but to have no influence on progression to severe pre-eclampsia or perinatal death (Collins et al 1985). The use of bed rest and drugs to prolong pregnancy in severe pre-eclampsia, compared with earlier termination of pregnancy, i.e. delivery, increased the risk to mothers, with meagre benefits, if any at all, to fetuses (Sibai et al 1985). Intensive drug therapy in severe hypertension detected early in pregnancy reduced maternal morbidity without influencing the incidence of pre-eclampsia (Sibai & Anderson 1986).

Results from recent studies have suggested that aspirin treatment, with or without dipyridamole, can reduce the incidence of pre-eclampsia, intrauterine growth retardation and perinatal death (Beaufils et al 1985, Wallenburg et al 1986). Another study suggested that aspirin and dipyridamole reduced the incidence of fetal growth retardation in a high-risk group of mothers (Wallenburg & Rotmans 1987). A larger study to test these findings is currently in progress.

Severe pre-eclampsia is still a problem, with significant morbidity that can be treated by termination of pregnancy. Hypertension and mild pre-eclampsia are risk factors for severe pre-eclampsia. Blood pressure and proteinuria are simple measurements to take and continued screening for this condition can be recommended.

Gestational diabetes

The consequences of maternal diabetes mellitus on fetal outcome (late intrauterine death and macrosomia) and the beneficial effects of tight diabetic control are well known. However, the purpose of screening is to identify women with gestational diabetes, defined as glucose tolerance that is abnormal during pregnancy but normal both before and after it. Gestational diabetes has been reported to cause an increase in macrosomia and fetal loss (O'Sullivan 1975), an increase in the incidence of large for gestational age babies from 22 to 33%, an increase in the rate of caesarean sections from 11 to 18% (Philipson et al 1985, Spellacy et al 1985), an increase in the rate of congenital abnormalities (Widness et al 1985) and an increase in perinatal morbidity, chiefly feeding difficulties (Nordlander et al 1989).

Screening is usually by testing for glucose in the urine. If frequent testing is done, then up to 50% of women will have positive tests for glycosuria; blood glucose testing at 28 weeks has been recommended for screening rather than diagnostic purposes (Lind 1984). Several studies have shown the benefits of insulin treatment to women with gestational diabetes mellitus. These benefits include reduction in the rates of macrosomia (O'Sullivan 1975, Coustan & Imarah 1984), operative delivery and birth trauma (Coustan & Imarah 1984) and in the perinatal mortality rate (Roversi et al 1980). However, all these studies had non-random allocation to study and control groups or relied on historical controls. Controlled studies have shown little benefit from treatment and have concluded that routine treatment with insulin is unnecessary in gestational diabetes (Persson et al 1985, Widness et al 1985, Nordlander et al 1989).

Hunter and Keirse (1989), reviewing the evidence, have pointed out that the risks of gestational diabetes are linked to conditions, such as stillbirth, which are indications for the glucose tolerance test. Similarly, macrosomia is more common in those with gestational diabetes, but both occur more commonly in heavier mothers and glucose intolerance may be no more than a marker for other risks. Nevertheless, they conclude that gestational diabetes is associated with an increase in macrosomia and operative delivery, and that these risks can be reduced by treatment with insulin. However, a policy of screening and active treatment will result in unnecessary treatment of many women with gestational diabetes who would otherwise deliver normal birthweight babies, and will cause only a small reduction in the overall proportion of babies born with macrosomia, most of whom are born to women who have not developed gestational diabetes. It is therefore impossible to say at this time whether the benefits of screening outweigh the disadvantages. Under the circumstances any practical suggestions must be tentative: screening for gestational diabetes is probably still indicated; for affected women treatment with diet is unlikely to do harm; and insulin is recommended only when blood sugar remains persistently raised despite such dietary measures.

SCREENING FOR FETAL CONDITIONS

Assessment of fetal growth

Measurement of fetal growth occupies a large part of antenatal care. However, even with an apparently clear subject such as this, problems of definition and semantics abound, and these have been reviewed by Altman and Hytten (1989). First, it is important to distinguish between size and growth. Intrauterine growth retardation is not the same as small for gestational age, although the two terms are often used synonymously. The distinction can be illustrated by pointing out how different the response would be to a fetus growing steadily just below the 10th centile, compared with one whose growth had fallen from the 90th to the 30th centile (assuming that such detailed information about growth were available). Second, there is the problem inherent in all biological systems of having to decide arbitrary cut-off points to define abnormality, in this case usually the 10th centile. Such a strategy applied to fetal weights seems particularly inappropriate because it defines as problems an unchanging proportion of developing fetuses, despite any general improvement in perinatal health or overall increase in birthweights for the whole population.

Construction of fetal growth charts poses particular problems. There is the problem of using charts derived from cross-sectional data to draw inferences about a longitudinal process. Centile charts for birthweight have been derived from the birthweights of babies born at different gestational ages and these are not necessarily the same as the weights of fetuses remaining in utero at the same gestational age. Secker et al (1987) found that the birthweights of babies born at 32 and 37 weeks gestation were lower than those of the babies remaining in utero, estimated by ultrasound. The discrepancy was greater at 32 weeks gestation, so that for those born at 32 weeks the 10th centile corresponded to the 4th centile for fetuses still in utero. Even in the group of babies born preterm, those delivered electively were shown in one study to have lower birthweights than those born by spontaneous labour. This may distort the norms in a regional centre with many high-risk pregnancies (Yudkin et al 1987).

Finally, there is the importance of ensuring that the growth charts are based on, and applied to, similar populations. Fundal height charts have been constructed using measurements only of those infants with birthweights between 10th and 90th centiles, but which then show 10th and 90th centile lines derived from this selected population (Calvert et al 1982, Persson et al 1986). Such norms will tend to increase the numbers of fetuses falsely identified as being small for gestational age.

Clinical methods of assessing fetal growth

By tradition, women have been weighed regularly during pregnancy to assess fetal growth. Abrams and Laros (1986) have confirmed that maternal weight gain correlates with birthweight, although the relationship did not apply to women with the highest body mass indices. However, maternal weight gain, even when it is combined with abdominal palpation in the traditional way, is a poor predictor of small for gestational age babies. Rosenberg et al (1982), in a retrospective analysis of the records of 226 babies with birthweights below the 10th centile, found that 50% were unsuspected antenatally. Forty one per cent of those with birthweights below the 5th centile were unsuspected. Even this result is misleading because it takes no account of those suspected of being small for gestational age and subsequently having normal birthweights.

The poor performance of traditional methods led to the development of fundal height measurement as a better predictor of small for gestational age infants. Studies on populations including a high proportion of high-risk women have reported positive predictive values of 60–70% for a test with sensitivity of 73% and

specificity of 77% (Quaranta et al 1981, Mathai et al 1987). Studies of unselected populations have found lower positive predictive values of 18–29% (Calvert et al 1982, Persson et al 1986).

Ultrasound assessment

Ultrasound scanning can provide detailed measurements of fetal size. Scanning early in pregnancy is known to be the most accurate method of dating pregnancies and is a better predictor of delivery dates than the date of the last menstrual period. Neilson et al (1980) used a scan at 12–14 weeks for dating and a second one at 34–36 weeks to identify small for gestational age fetuses. The most accurate index, crown–rump length multiplied by trunk area, gave a sensitivity of 94%, but with a positive predictive value of only 39.5%. Pearce and Campbell (1987), in a similar study comparing abdominal circumference on ultrasound scanning and symphysis–fundal heights, found ultrasound to have a higher sensitivity (83% compared with 76%), but with a positive predictive value of 39% (compared with 36%). Geirsson et al (1985) studied a group of women referred at 36 weeks gestation because of obstetric complications, and who delivered infants with a mean birthweight on the 31st centile for the reference population. Fetal abdominal area had a sensitivity value of 72%, and a positive predictive value of 68%. As was shown above, the drawback of this approach is that the initial clinical identification of the high-risk group probably fails to identify half of those delivering small for gestational age babies.

The critical test, here as elsewhere, is whether the knowledge gained from screening makes any difference to clinical practice. In one study of women with uncomplicated pregnancies ultrasound scans were done between 34 and 36 weeks gestation. In half the cases the results were reported to the obstetricians; there were no differences between the two groups in obstetric management or fetal outcome, measured by rates of antenatal admission, induction of labour, operative delivery and Apgar scores (Neilson et al 1984).

Risks of ultrasound scanning. No risks to the health of fetuses have ever been ascribed to ultrasound scans. Two case-control studies found no evidence to link ultrasound scanning in pregnancy with childhood cancer or leukaemia (Kinnier et al 1984, Cartwright et al 1984). There may be gains for the patients. A series of studies has compared the effect of showing and discussing with women the image of the baby on the screen with giving little or no immediate information. 'High feedback' has been shown to reduce anxiety more than 'low feedback' (Cox et al 1987), and made women more likely to give up smoking and drinking (Reading et al 1982). Such benefits depend not only on the amount of feedback but also the circumstances of the patients. For instance, the difference between high and low feedback was greater in low-risk women; high-risk women gained considerable psychological benefit from even a minimal amount of feedback (Cox et al 1987). A study in Manchester, based in two hospitals with different scanning policies, found that women in the hospital where scanning was selective were less likely to think they would find a scan reassuring than those where scanning was routine. While there was a possibility that scans done insensitively might do psychological damage, there was no support for the view that they tended to medicalise pregnancy (Hyde 1986).

Conclusions

The advantages of symphysis–fundal heights over traditional clinical methods in assessing fetal growth justify the use of this practice, although it should not be relied on as an accurate measure.

Despite the enormous technical advances in ultrasound scanning the evidence does not support a policy of routine scanning in late pregnancy for all pregnant women. It remains to be seen whether cheaper scanners, allowing repeated scanning throughout pregnancy (albeit by less skilled operators) will allow longitudinal growth to be plotted for individuals with the degree of accuracy that would identify true intrauterine growth retardation, as opposed to small for gestational age fetuses. At present ultrasound can be recommended only for evaluation of a group identified clinically as being high risk, knowing that this strategy will fail to identify approximately half of those with birthweights below the tenth centile.

Assessment of fetal well-being

Fetal movement counting

The observation that some stillbirths were preceded by a reported decrease in fetal movement led to the development of formal methods of fetal movement counting. It has proved difficult to devise a standard method of counting. The Cardiff system records the time taken to count ten fetal movements and can lead to some women counting until the evening. In comparison the method of counting for fixed periods can leave some women with very low counts. Grant & Hepburn (1984) attempted to solve this problem by devising guidelines based on individuals' own experience, using the average number of movements felt by each individual in 1 hour. Nevertheless, approximately one-quarter of the women in this study experienced no consistent pattern of fetal movement. A further problem with fetal movement counting is defining cut-off points for diagnostic testing and what to apply as a diagnostic test. A reported abnormality is often followed by further tests, such as cardiotocography which, as will be shown, is itself not accurate enough to be an effective screening test, let alone a sound diagnostic test.

The difference in value when applying a test to high-risk or low-risk populations is again apparent. One study of 264 women with problems identified during pregnancy tested the ability of fetal movement counting to predict stillbirth and low Apgar scores. In this high-risk group the sensitivity was 86%, specificity 91%, and the positive predictive value 46% (Leader et al 1981). In comparison, a similar study of 1515 unselected women found sensitivities of only 16–38% (Valentin et al 1986).

In a randomised controlled trial of 2250 unselected women attending a hospital in Denmark, half were asked to count fetal movements for 2 hours and to contact the hospital if no movements were felt. Eight deaths in infants with birthweights greater than 1.5 kg occurred in the control group, and none in the counting group (Neldam 1980). In contrast, a study in the UK compared 6597 women attending a maternity unit using Cardiff count-to-ten charts with 13 705 attending a unit not using fetal movement charts. The rate of apparently preventable stillbirths was similar in the two groups, and this applied in infants with birthweights above and below 1.5 kg (Lobb et al 1985). A further randomised, multicentre trial of 68 654 women showed no difference at all in the number of late antepartum deaths in counting and control groups (Grant et al 1989a).

Acceptability of fetal movement counting. Studies have found variable levels of acceptability. In one study, 90% of women found it easy to count, and 70% were fully compliant; 66.5% found it more convenient to count in the evening than in the morning (Valentin et al 1984). The multicentre trial referred to above, probably a better indicator of how the test would work in routine practice, found only 58.9% completion of charts in the counting group (Grant et al 1989a). Draper et al (1986) questioned 132 women about their use of fetal movement charts 6 weeks postpartum. Eighty seven per cent were aware of the reason for keeping charts, but few seemed to have any clear idea what they should do if they felt no movement. Fifty five per cent were reassured by filling in the chart and 23% were worried, either by variability or diminution of movement. Unfavourable comments were made by 16%: busy or active women found them difficult to complete, some lost count or forgot, and some complained that the doctors did not pay attention to their charts.

Cardiotocography

Measurement of fetal heart rate in pregnancy is an extension of monitoring in labour. Initially, oxytocin was used to induce uterine contractions; this is now omitted, and the procedure is known as antepartum non-stress cardiotocography. If it is combined with ultrasound examination to assess fetal breathing movements, fetal tone, gross body movements and amniotic fluid volume, it is know as a biophysical profile.

The biophysical profile has been shown to be better at predicting perinatal death, intrauterine growth retardation, low Apgar scores, or fetal distress in labour, with positive predictive values of 56.5–87.5%, compared with 13.1–33.3% for the non-stress test in a group of high-risk patients (Manning et al 1984, Platt et al 1985). However, it is expensive and time-consuming and cannot be considered as a valid screening test (Mohide & Keirse 1989). The dangers of measuring the value of these tests against fetal distress or low Apgar scores have been discussed above (see p. 000).

Several trials have assessed the value of antepartum non-stress cardiotocography in high-risk patients. Lumley et al (1983) randomized patients admitted with antenatal problems to having or not having cardiotocography. There were no differences between the two groups in terms of rate of instrumental delivery, period of gestation at birth, Apgar scores, birthweights and admission rates to special care units in the babies. Analysis of the subgroup found to have abnormal heart readings on cardiotocography showed them to have fewer spontaneous labours, a higher rate of caesarean section, more small for gestational age infants and more perinatal deaths. The authors reported the 'totally unexpected finding' that the trial group had a non-significant excess of stillbirths. They also noted that the perinatal mortality rate for the study groups taken together was lower than that for the whole hospital, and that this was partly a result of excluding babies born preterm, who constitute the group at highest risk. Two trials where all women

entered had cardiotocography, but where half in each case were randomly assigned to have the results communicated to clinicians, both reported similar results. In both studies there were no differences between the groups in incidence of operative delivery, or in indices of fetal well-being at delivery. Both reported a non-significant increase in perinatal deaths in the 'revealed' group (Brown et al 1982, Kidd et al 1985).

Conclusions

Fetal movement counting is intended to prevent antepartum late fetal deaths, a group that has diminished less than other categories. Grant & Elbourne (1989) point out that only 50–60% of such deaths may be preventable, that in practice it is not clear when they will occur and therefore when counting should begin, and that there are problems in recording when there is considerable variation in fetal activity, both within and between observers. Despite early enthusiasm, this technique does not seem to offer any benefit to pregnant women, beyond reassurance to some. It certainly does not justify the use of resources, in terms of midwives' time, and resulting cardiotocography and hospital admissions, that would be entailed in its application to the entire pregnant population.

Studies of antepartum non-stress cardiotocography have failed to show any benefit when applied to a group of high-risk women. The technique of Doppler scanning of fetal vessels may be a sensitive predictor of fetal hypoxaemia and perinatal asphyxia, but will need more careful study before its value is established, and it is unlikely to be widely applied as a screening test (James 1990).

Screening for fetal abnormalities

While traditonal antenatal care has remained largely unchanged for the 60–70 years of its existence, the explosive development of new techniques to detect specific fetal abnormalities, and their rapid introduction into routine care, have radically improved the prospects for healthy infants in certain groups of high-risk families. The range of techniques offered is likely to continue expanding in the foreseeable future.

Screening by amniocentesis for neural tube defects and chromosomal abnormalities, such as Down syndrome, has been available for several years (Harris 1980, Murday & Slack 1985, Richards et al 1988). Fetal blood sampling allows prenatal diagnosis of haemoglobinopathies (Weatherall et al 1985). With the advent of chorionic villus sampling (CVS) and

Table 11.1 Minimum programme of effective antenatal care

Gestation	Screening test	Purpose
During first trimester	Interview	Discussion of lifestyle factors Review past obstetric history Identify risk factors in medical/social history
	Measure height, weight and blood pressure	Identification of risk factors: low height or weight, existing hypertension
	Urine culture	Screening for bacteriuria
	Blood test	Screening for major iron deficiency Screening for rubella and syphilis
16-18 weeks	Abdominal examination Ultrasound scan (optional)	Screen for multiple pregnancy Verify dates Screen for multiple pregnancy Screen for neural tube defect and other abnormalities
	Blood test	AFP as screen for neural tube defect and Down syndrome
Approx 32 weeks	Blood pressure	Identification of women with, or at risk of developing pre-eclampsia
	Urine test	Screen for proteinuria Screen for gestational diabetes
Approx 36 weeks	Abdominal examination Repeat blood pressure and urine tests	Identify fetal presentation As at 32 weeks
40–42 weeks	Interview	Discuss action in the event of pregnancy continuing beyond 42 weeks' gestation

recombinant DNA synthesising techniques, numerous other genetic disorders, such as muscular dystrophy (Forrest et al 1987), are coming within the reach of prenatal diagnosis. These techniques are discussed in greater detail in Chapter 10.

THE ORGANISATION OF ANTENATAL CARE

The organisation of antenatal care can be analysed under four headings: what procedures should be done, how frequently women should be seen, where they should be seen, and who should see them.

Content of antenatal care

Given the evidence reviewed above, it is difficult to give clear guidelines as to what modern antenatal care should contain. The procedures that can be unequivocally recommended are shown in Table 11.1. This is clearly a substantial reduction from current common practice and poses a problem for practitioners. For instance, the evidence suggests that regularly measuring fundal heights and weighing all pregnant women are of little value. However deciding to abandon the practice is difficult, as it would entail seeing women for an antenatal consultation without doing an abdominal examination and thereby giving up any pretence at identifying fetuses affected by intrauterine growth retardation.

Frequency of visits

It is similarly difficult to give a clear recommendation concerning the number of antenatal visits that should be made. Hall et al (1980) questioned the conventional wisdom in an analysis of visits to antenatal clinics that showed how rarely abnormalities were detected. They concluded that antenatal care was a very inefficient form of care. In a subsequent, non-controlled experiment, a revised programme achieved a reduction in the number of visits and a shift from hospital- to community-based clinics. Women's responses suggested not only that they found general practice antenatal care a more pleasant experience than hospital antenatal care, but also that they gained more benefit from general practice care (Hall et al 1985). Marsh (1985) has reported a similar programme of reduced visits in his own practice.

The most frequently voiced criticisms of antenatal clinics are those of the consumers: some years ago there were numerous reports of women's negative feelings towards the organisation of the clinics, that they were kept waiting too long and treated as if they were on a conveyor belt. One benefit of reducing the number of visits should be a more relaxed and personal atmosphere in antenatal clinics.

Site and staffing of antenatal clinics

Experiments to determine the best setting for antenatal care have mostly been driven by a desire to respond to negative feelings about hospital clinics, and to make antenatal care more accessible. In two programmes of care in Edinburgh and Cambridge, antenatal care was moved entirely into general practice, with an experienced obstetrician working alongside general practitioners. In the Sighthill clinic, Edinburgh, an enormous reduction in perinatal mortality rate has been claimed in a deprived area of the city (Sighthill Maternity Team 1982). In the Cambridge project, the benefits were measured by increased satisfaction and ease of access (Draper et al 1984).

The Cambridge project also identified one unexpected major problem that accompanied the changes introduced. While high levels of satisfaction were recorded by the obstetricians and general practitioners who participated in the experiment, midwives felt uncertain about their role and excluded from antenatal care. This was supported by a survey of midwives, which found that they were frequently not given independent responsibility for some of the tasks of antenatal care, such as abdominal palpation, when working alongside general practitioners (Robinson 1985). Midwives' ability to manage antenatal care without help or supervision has been shown by the 'Know Your Midwife' experiment (Flint & Poulengeris 1985). This was an attempt to evaluate the benefits of continuity of care provided by midwives through pregnancy and labour. The authors predictably found benefits to mothers in continuity of care provided by midwives. They also concluded that there were advantages in care provided by general practitioners, but that when the general practitioners were not involved in intrapartum care the advantages were not sustained in labour. The only difficulty in accepting the conclusions of the 'Know Your Midwife' report is in accepting the authors' definition of continuity. Not surprisingly, they measure it only through pregnancy, whereas for general practitioners it extends both before and after. Indeed, some general practitioners not involved in intrapartum care have stated informally that the only purpose of participating in antenatal care is to get to know their patients as preparation for their future role caring for mothers and children.

SURVEILLANCE IN POSTNATAL CARE

Postnatal care is a similar mixture of treatment of medical problems, education and preventive care. Strictly, the preventive care component for the mother is small and is limited to administration of anti-D antibodies and rubella immunisation where indicated, and a discussion about contraception.

There is, however, some evidence that a strategy for prevention of postnatal depression may be appropriate. Study of this subject has been bedevilled by disagreements over definition: the distinction between prolonged postnatal depression and transient 'blues'; the length of time during which depression should be considered to be postnatal; whether postnatal depression exists as a unique entity or is depression that happens to coincide with the postnatal period; and whether it should be regarded as a medical problem at all (Romito 1989). The 'blues' can be defined as transient mood disturbance in the first few days after birth. It is both common and distinct from later depression (Kumar & Robson 1984). Seventy four per cent of women reported weeping, not for joy, in the first week after birth, and 33% thought they had had the blues when interviewed at 3 months (Kumar & Robson 1984). Such feelings might be helped by different practice in labour or pregnancy. In a separate study, 40% of women reported feelings of indifference towards their newborn babies at birth, although by 1 week only 4 out of 120 still felt indifferent. Initial feelings of indifference were associated with a recall of pain being worse than had been expected (Robson & Kumar 1980).

Romito (1989) points out that the prevalence and duration of postnatal depression reported in studies depends on the time at which the study was carried out. The maximum prevalence of postnatal depression has been reported as 16% (Kumar & Robson 1984). Zajicek (1981) and Paykel et al (1980) have reported higher figures of 20–35%, but these both included groups in whom postnatal depression seemed to be a continuation of depression before and during pregnancy. Using a method of repeated interviews, Kumar and Robson (1984) showed the prevalence of postnatal depression increasing to a maximum at 3 months after delivery, and falling thereafter.

Paykel et al (1980) found that women with postnatal depression reported more life events, with a particular excess of undesirable life events. Kumar and Robson (1984) found an association with marital conflict, infrequent sexual intercourse, negative feeling for babies, subfertility, thoughts about abortion and problems with women's own mothers. Postnatal depression is therefore similar to other forms of depression in being caused by social events (Brown & Harris 1978), and distinguished only by the events specific to the postnatal period.

Accepting a theory of social causation of postnatal depression provides an opportunity for prevention. Entwisle and Doering (1981) found that practical help from husbands beyond the end of the first week after delivery had some protective effect. Of more use to health professionals is the study of regular visiting to women identified as being depressed at 6 weeks after delivery, by health visitors trained in simple counselling techniques. This programme reduced the subsequent prevalence from 62 to 31%, and the discrepancy was not explained by differences in antidepressant prescription (Holden et al 1989). Those women reporting positive personal feelings towards postnatal groups are presumably using the same mechanisms, although the objective success of such groups has not been established. The issue of postnatal depression is discussed further in Chapter 37.

CONCLUSIONS

The combination of falling risk, probably a result of general improvements in health, and increasingly critical scrutiny has meant that it is difficult to justify continuing antenatal care as it has been practised for many years. The key has to be thorough application of screening tests whose effectiveness is well established. Thus, screening for bacteriuria, rubella and syphilis in early pregnancy is still capable of preventing avoidable morbidity. Encouraging women to give up smoking and to drink less than two to three measures of alcohol daily is one of the few measures known to be able to improve the outcome for developing fetuses, however small the gains. Modern techniques, such as the prevention of rhesus isoimmunisation and the

detection of genetic abnormalities, have been shown to be highly effective, and it is likely to be in such areas that new developments will have the most impact.

These measures must, however, be distinguished from the universal application of high technology techniques, of doubtful value, to all pregnant women in the quest for perfect outcomes. Both professionals and patients will surely benefit from a more honest statement from the obstetric establishment about what it can and cannot achieve (Lancet 1989). Antenatal care may then follow postnatal care in becoming more concerned with the emotional and psychological well-being of pregnant women, and not seeing them merely as passive receptacles for developing fetuses (Pollitt 1990).

It is likely that, at least in terms of their physical needs, pregnant women could safely attend antenatal clinics much less frequently than at present. At the current level of knowledge the most appropriate model is for most women to receive care from midwives working in general practice premises.

This conclusion is, however, based on evidence that has tested each component of antenatal care separately, and that ignores two important questions. First, what are the benefits to women of regular attendance at antenatal clinics in terms of their sense of emotional and psychological well-being? Second, what are the consequences to the confidence of doctors and midwives of reducing the frequency of antenatal visits, in terms both of their knowledge of each patient and their confidence in their clinical skills? Loss of confidence in personal skills may lead to increased reliance on technology, more willingness to refer to specialists and hence more intervention and avoidable morbidity. Until such questions have been answered, traditional patterns of antenatal care, of doubtful effectiveness, will continue to be applied for a combination of contractual motives and uncertainty on the part of the professionals applying them.

REFERENCES

Abrams B F, Laros R K 1986 Prepregnancy weight, weight gain, and birth weight. American Journal of Obstetrics and Gynecology 154: 503–509

Altman D G, Hytten F E 1989 Assessment of fetal size and fetal growth. In: Chalmers I, Enkin M, Keirse MJNC (eds) Effective care in pregnancy and childbirth. Oxford University Press, Oxford, pp 441–418

Ascari W Q, Allen A E, Baker W J, Pollack W 1968 Rh$_0$(D) immune globulin (human). Journal of the American Medical Association 205: 71–74

Beaufils M, Uzan S, Donsimoni R, Colau J C 1985 Prevention of pre-eclampsia by early antiplatelet therapy. Lancet 1: 840–842

Blackwell R, Chang A 1988 Video display terminals and pregnancy. A review. British Journal of Obstetrics and Gynaecology 95: 446–453

Bowman J M 1984 Rhesus haemolytic disease. In Wald N J (ed) Antenatal and neonatal screening. Oxford University Press, Oxford, pp 314–344

Bradbeer C S 1989. Mothers with HIV. Risks to baby need to be balanced against benefits of breast feeding. British Medical Journal 299: 806–807

Brown B, Harris T 1978. Social origins of depression. Tavistock Press, London

Brown V A, Sawers R S, Parsons R J, et al 1982 The value of antenatal cardiotocography in the management of high-risk pregnancy: a randomized trial. British Journal of Obstetrics and Gynaecology 89: 716–722

Butler N R, Goldstein H, Ross E M 1972 Cigarette smoking in pregnancy: its influence on birthweight and perinatal mortality. British Medical Journal 2: 127–130

Calvert J P, Crean E E, Newcombe R G, Pearson J F 1982 Antenatal screening by measurement of symphysis-fundus height. British Medical Journal 285: 846–849

Campbell-Brown M, McFadyen I R, Seal D V, Stephenson M L 1987 Is screening for bacteriuria in pregnancy worth while? British Medical Journal 294: 1579–1582

Cartwright R A, McKinney P A, Hopton P A, et al 1984 Ultrasound examinations in pregnancy and childhood cancer. Lancet 2: 999–1000

Chalmers I 1985 Short, Black, Baird, Himsworth and social class differences in fetal and neonatal mortality rates. British Medical Journal 291: 231–233

Chng P K, Hall M H 1982. Antenatal prediction of urinary tract infection in pregnancy. British Journal of Obstetrics and Gynaecology 89: 8–11

Chown B, Duff A M, James J et al 1969 Prevention of Rh immunization: first report of the Western Canadian trial, 1966–1968. Canadian Medical Association Journal 100: 1021–1024

Clarke C A, Donohoe W T A, McConnell R B, et al 1963 Further experimental studies in the prevention of Rh haemolytic disease. British Medical Journal 1: 979–984

Clay J C 1989. Antenatal screening for syphilis. Must continue. British Medical Journal 299: 409–410

Coleman D V, Evans D M D 1988 Biopsy, pathology and cytology of the cervix. Chapman & Hall, London

Collings C A, Curet L B, Mullin J P 1983 Maternal and fetal responses to a maternal aerobic exercise program. American Journal of Obstetrics and Gynecology 145: 702–707

Collins R, Yusuf S, Peto R 1985 Overview of randomised trials of diuretics in pregnancy. British Medical Journal 290: 17–23

Coustan D R, Imarah J 1984 Prophylactic insulin treatment of gestational diabetes reduces the incidence of macrosomia, operative delivery, and birth trauma. American Journal of Obstetrics and Gynecology 150: 836–842

Cox D N, Wittmann B K, Hess M et al 1987 The psychological impact of diagnostic ultrasound. Obstetrics and Gynecology 70: 673–676

Cunningham F G 1987 Urinary tract infections complicating pregnancy. Bailliere's Clinical Obstetrics and Gynaecology 1: 891–908

De Swiet M 1984 Hypertension. In Wald NJ (ed) Antenatal and neonatal screening. Oxford University Press, Oxford, pp 396–408

Dennis J, Chalmers I 1982. Very early neonatal seizure rate: a possible epidemiological indicator of the quality of perinatal care. British Journal of Obstetrics and Gynaecology 89: 418–426

Desmonts G, Couvreur J 1974 Toxoplasmosis in pregnancy and its transmission to the fetus. Bulletin of the New York Academy of Medicine 50: 146–159

Draper J, Field S, Thomas H 1984 The early parenthood project. An evaluation of a community antenatal clinic. Hughes Hall, Cambridge

Draper J, Field S, Thomas H, Hare M J 1986 Womens' views

on keeping fetal movement charts. British Journal of Obstetrics and Gynaecology 93: 334–338

Entwisle D R, Doering S G 1988 The first birth. A family turning point. Johns Hopkins University, Baltimore

Fedrick J, Anderson A B M 1976 Factors associated with spontaneous preterm birth. British Journal of Obstetrics and Gynaecology 83: 342–350

Fleming D W, Cochi S L, MacDonald K L et al 1985 Pasteurized milk as a vehicle of infection in an outbreak of Listeriosis. New England Journal of Medicine 312: 404–407

Flint C, Poulengeris P 1985 The 'Know Your Midwife' report. KYM report, London

Foley M E, Farquharson R, Stronge J M 1987 Is screening for bacteriuria worth while? British Medical Journal 295: 270

Forrest S M, Smith T J, Cross G S, et al 1987 Effective strategy for prenatal prediction of Duchenne and Becker muscular dystrophy. Lancet 2: 1294–1297

Garcia J, Elbourne D 1984 Future research on work in pregnancy. In: Chamberlain G (ed). Pregnant women at work. Royal Society of Medicine, London, pp 273–287

Garn S M, Keating K T, Falkner F 1981 Hematological status and pregnancy outcomes. American Journal of Clinical Nutrition 34: 115–117

Geirsson R T, Patel N B, Christie A D 1985 Intrauterine volume, fetal abdominal area and biparietal diameter measurements with ultrasound in the prediction of small-for-dates babies in a high-risk obstetric population. British Journal of Obstetrics and Gynaecology 92: 936–940

Gilstrap L, Cunningham F C, Whalley P 1981. Acute pyelonephritis in pregnancy: an anterospective study. Obstetrics and Gynecology 57: 409–413

Golding J, Butler N R 1983 Maternal smoking and anencephaly. British Medical Journal 287: 553–554

Graham H 1976 Smoking in pregnancy: the attitudes of expectant mothers. Social Science & Medicine 10: 399–405

Grant A, Elbourne D 1989 Fetal movement counting to assess fetal well-being. In: Chalmers I, Enkin M, Keirse M J N C (eds) Effective care in pregnancy and childbirth. Oxford University Press, Oxford, pp 440–454

Grant A, Hepburn M 1984 Merits of an individualised approach to fetal movement counting compared with fixed-time and fixed-number methods. British Journal of Obstetrics and Gynaecology 91: 1087–1090

Grant A, Mohide P 1982 Screening and diagnostic tests in antenatal care. In: Enkin M, Chalmers I (eds) Effectiveness and satisfaction in antenatal care. Heinemann Medical Books, London, pp 22–59

Grant A, Elbourne D, Valentin L, Alexander S 1989a Routine formal fetal movement counting and risk of antepartum late death in normally formed singletons. Lancet 2: 345–349

Grant A, O'Brien N, Joy M-T et al 1989b Cerebral palsy among children born during the Dublin randomised trial of intrapartum monitoring. Lancet 2: 1233–1235

Gravenhorst J B 1989 Rhesus isoimmunisation. In: Chalmers I, Enkin M, Keirse M J N C (eds) Effective care in pregnancy and childbirth. Oxford University Press, Oxford, pp 565–577

Hall M H, Chng P K, MacGillivray I 1980 Is routine antenatal care worthwhile? Lancet 2: 78–80

Hall M, MacIntyre S, Porter S 1985. Antenatal care assessed.

A case study of an innovation in Aberdeen. Aberdeen University Press, Aberdeen

Hanshaw J B, Dudgeon J A, Marshall W C 1985 Viral diseases of the fetus and newborn. Philadelphia Saunders Company, W B

Harris R 1980 Maternal serum alphafetoprotein in pregnancy and the prevention of birth defect. British Medical Journal 1: 1199–1202

Hauth J C, Gilstrap L C, Widmer K 1982 Fetal heart rate reactivity before and after maternal jogging during the third trimester. American Journal of Obstetrics and Gynecology 142: 545–547

Hemminki K, Mutanen P, Saloniemi I 1983. Smoking and the occurrence of congenital malformations and spontaneous abortions: multivariate analysis. American Journal of Obstetrics and Gynecology 145: 61–66

Hill L M, Platt L D, Kellogg B 1980 Rh sensitization after genetic amniocentesis. Obstetrics and Gynecology 56: 459–461

Holden J M, Sagovsky R, Cox J L 1989 Counselling in a general practice setting: controlled study of health visitor intervention in treatment of postneonatal depression. British Medical Journal 298: 223–226

House of Commons Social Services Committee 1980 Report on perinatal and neonatal mortality (Chairman R. Short). HMSO, London

Hunter D J S, Keirse M J N C 1989 Gestational diabetes. In: Chalmers I, Enkin M, Keirse M J N C (eds) Effective care in pregnancy and childbirth. Oxford University Press, Oxford, pp 403–410

Hyde B 1986 An interview study of pregnant women's attitudes to ultrasound scanning. Social Science & Medicine 22: 587–592

Hytten F E 1980 Nutritional aspects of human pregnancy. In: Aebi H & Whitehead R (eds) Maternal nutrition during pregnancy and lactation. Hans Huber, Bern, pp 27–38

Italian Multicentre Study 1988 Epidemiology, clinical features and prognostic factors of paediatric HIV infection. Lancet 2: 1043–1045

James D K 1988 Risk at the booking visit. In: James D K, Stirrat G M (eds) Pregnancy and risk: the basis for rational management. John Wiley, Chichester, pp 45–80

James D 1990 Diagnosis and management of fetal growth retardation. Archives of Disease in Childhood 65: 390–394

Jewell D, Smith L 1990 Is there a future for general practitioner obstetrics In: Royal College of General Practitioners. Members' handbook. Royal College of General Practitioners, London, pp 229–232

Jones K L, Smith D W 1973 Recognition of the fetal alcoholic syndrome in early infancy. Lancet 2: 999–1001

Jones K L, Smith D W, Ulleland C N, Streissguth A P 1973 Pattern of malformation in offspring of chronic alcoholic mothers. Lancet 1: 1267–1271

Jones K L, Smith D W, Streissguth A P, Myrianthopoulos N C 1974 Outcome in offspring of chronic alcoholic women. Lancet 1: 1076–1078

Kardjati S, Kusin J A, De With C 1988 Energy supplementation in the last trimester of pregnancy in East Java: I Effect on birthweight. British Journal of Obstetrics and Gynaecology 95: 783–794

Khong T Y, Frappell J M, Steel H M, et al 1986 Perinatal listeriosis. A report of six cases. British Journal of Obstetrics and Gynaecology 93: 1083–1087

Kidd L C, Patel N B, Smith R 1985 Non-stress antenatal cardiotocography — a prospective randomized clinical trial. British Journal of Obstetrics and Gynaecology 92: 1156–1159

Kinnier Wilson L M, Waterhouse J A H 1984 Obstetric ultrasound and childhood malignancies. Lancet 2: 997–999

Knox E G, Marshall T, Kane S et al 1980 Social and health care determinants of area variations in perinatal mortality. Community Medicine 2: 282–290

Koller O, Sandvei R, Sagen N 1980 High hemoglobin levels during pregnancy and fetal risk. International Journal of Gynaecology and Obstetrics 18: 53–56

Kumar R, Robson K M 1984 A prospective study of emotional disorders in childbearing women. British Journal of Psychiatry 144: 35–47

Lancet (leading article) 1989 Cerebral palsy, intrapartum care, and a shot in the foot. Lancet 2: 1251–1252

Larkin R M, Knochel T Q, Lee T G 1982 Intrauterine transfusions: new techniques and results. Clinical Obstetrics and Gynecology 25: 303–312

Leader L R, Baillie P, Van Schalkwyk D J 1981 Fetal movements and fetal outcome: a prospective study. Obstetrics and Gynecology 57: 431–436

Leveno K J, Cunningham P G, Nelson S et al 1986 A prospective comparison of selective and universal electronic fetal monitoring in 34,995 pregnancies. New England Journal of Medicine 315: 615–619

Lilford R J, Chard T 1983 Problems and pitfalls of risk assessment in antenatal care. British Journal of Obstetrics and Gynaecology 90: 507–510

Lind T 1984 Antenatal screening for diabetes mellitus. British Journal of Obstetrics and Gynaecology 91: 833–834

Lobb M O, Beazley J M, Haddad N G 1985 A controlled study of daily fetal movement counts in the prevention of stillbirths. Journal of Obstetrics and Gynaecology 6: 87–91

Lumley J, Lester A, Anderson I et al 1983 A randomized trial of weekly cardiotocography in high-risk obstetric patients. British Journal of Obstetrics and Gynaecology 90: 1018–1026

Lumley J, Correy J F, Newman N M, Curran J T 1985 Cigarette smoking, alcohol consumption and fetal outcome in Tasmania 1981–2. Australia and New Zealand Journal of Obstetrics and Gynaecology 25: 33–38

MacArthur C, Knox E G 1988 Smoking in pregnancy: effects of stopping at different stages. British Journal of Obstetrics and Gynaecology 95: 551–555

MacDonald D, Grant A, Sheridan-Pereira M et al 1985 The Dublin randomized trial of intrapartum fetal heart rate monitoring. American Journal of Obstetrics and Gynecology 152: 524–539

MacGillivray I 1985 Pre-eclampsia. The hypertensive disease of pregnancy. WB Saunders, London

McKnight A, Merrett J D 1986 Smoking in pregnancy — a health education problem. Journal of the Royal College of General Practitioners 36: 161–164

Madeley R J, Gillies P A, Power F L, Symonds E M 1989 Nottingham mothers stop smoking project — baseline survey of smoking in pregnancy. Community Medicine 11: 124–130

Mahomed K, Hytten F 1989 Iron and folate supplementation in pregnancy. In: Chalmers I, Enkin M, Keirse M J N C (eds) Effective care in pregnancy and childbirth. Oxford University Press, Oxford, pp 301–317

Manning F A, Lange I R, Morrison I, Harman C R 1984

Fetal biophysical profile score and the nonstress test: a comparative trial. Obstetrics and Gynecology 64: 326–331

Marsh G N 1985 New programme of antenatal care in general practice. British Medical Journal 291: 646–648

Mascola L, Pelosi R, Blount J H et al 1984 Congenital syphilis. Why is it still occurring? Journal of the American Medical Association 252: 1719–1722

Mathai M, Jairaj P, Muthurathnam S 1987 Screening for light-for-gestational age infants: a comparison of three simple measurements. British Journal of Obstetrics and Gynaecology 94: 217–221

Meyer M B, Jonas B S, Tonascia J A 1976 Perinatal events associated with maternal smoking during pregnancy. American Journal of Epidemiology 103: 466–476

Miller C L, Miller E, Waight P A 1987 Rubella susceptibility and the continuing risk of infection in pregnancy. British Medical Journal 294: 1277–1278

Miller E, Cradock-Watson J E, Pollock T M 1982 Consequences of confirmed maternal rubella at successive stages of pregnancy. Lancet 2: 781–784

Mills J L, Graubard B I 1987 Is moderate drinking associated with an increased risk for malformation? Pediatrics 80: 309–314

Mills J L, Rhoads G G, Simpson J L et al 1989 The absence of a relation between the periconceptual use of vitamins and neural-tube defects. New England Journal of Medicine 321: 430–435

Milunsky A, Jick H, Jick S S et al 1989 Multivitamin/Folic Acid supplementation in early pregnancy reduces the prevalence of neural tube defects. Journal of the American Medical Association 262: 2847–2852

Mohide P, Keirse M J N C 1989 Biophysical assessment of fetal well-being. In: Chalmers I, Enkin M, Keirse M J N C (eds) Effective care in pregnancy and childbirth. Oxford University Press, Oxford, pp 477–492

Morbidity and Mortality Weekly Report 1989 Congenital syphilis — New York City, 1986–1988 Morbidity and Mortality Weekly Report 38: 825–829

Moutquin J M, Rainville C, Giroux L et al 1985 A prospective study of blood pressure in pregnancy: prediction of pre-eclampsia. American Journal of Obstetrics and Gynecology 151: 191–196

MRC Vitamin Study Research Group 1991 Prevention of neural tube defects: results of the Medical Research Council Vitamin Study. Lancet 338: 131–137

Murday V, Slack J 1985 Screening for Down's syndrome in the North East Thames Region. British Medical Journal 291: 1315–1318

Murphy J F, Dauncey M, Newcombe R et al 1984 Employment in pregnancy: prevalence, maternal characteristics, perinatal outcome. Lancet 1: 1163–1166

Neilson J P, Whitfield C R, Aitchison T C 1980 Screening for the small for dates fetus: a two-stage ultrasonic examination schedule. British Medical Journal 1: 1203–1206

Neilson J P, Munjanja S P, Whitfield C R 1984 Screening for small for dates fetuses: a controlled trial. British Medical Journal 289: 1179–1182

Neldam S 1980 Fetal movements as an indicator of fetal wellbeing. Lancet 1: 1222–1224

Nordlander E, Hanson U, Persson B 1989 Factors influencing neonatal morbidity in gestational diabetic pregnancy. British Journal of Obstetrics and Gynaecology 96: 671–678

Oakley A 1982 The origins and development of antenatal care. In: Enkin M, Chalmers I (eds) Effectiveness and satisfaction in antenatal care. Heinemann Medical Books, London, pp 1–29

Olegård R, Sabel K-G, Aronsson M et al 1979 Effects on the child of alcohol during pregnancy. Acta Paediatrica Scandinavica Supplement 275: 112–121

O'Sullivan J B 1975 Prospective study of gestational diabetes and its treatment. In: Sutherland H W, Stowers J M (eds) Carbohydrate metabolism in pregnancy and the newborn. Churchill Livingstone, Edinburgh, pp 195–204

Paykel E S, Emms E M, Fletcher J, Rassaby E S 1980 Life events and social support in puerperal depression. British Journal of Psychiatry 136: 339–346

Pearce J M, Campbell S 1987 A comparison of symphysis-fundal height and ultrasound as screening tests for light-for-gestational age infants. British Journal of Obstetrics and Gynaecology 94: 100–104

Persson B, Stangenberg M, Hansson U, Nordlander E 1985 Gestational diabetes mellitus. Comparative evaluation of two treatment regimes, diet versus insulin and diet. Diabetes 34 (Suppl 2): 101–105

Persson B, Stangenberg M, Lunell N O, et al 1986 Prediction of size of infants at birth by measurement of symphysis fundus height. British Journal of Obstetrics and Gynaecology 93: 206–211

Peters T J, Adelstein P, Golding J, Butler N R 1984 The effects of work in pregnancy: short- and long-term associations. In: Chamberlain G (ed). Pregnant women at work. Royal Society of Medicine, London, pp 87–104

Peto R 1986 Geographic patterns and trends. In: Peto R, Zur Hausen H (eds) Viral etiology of cervical cancer. Cold Spring Harbor Laboratory, New York, pp 3–15

Philipson E H, Kalhan S C, Rosen M G et al 1985 Gestational diabetes mellitus. Is further improvement necessary? Diabetes 34, (Suppl 2): 55–60

Platt L D, Walla C A, Paul R H, et al 1985 A prospective trial of the fetal biophysical profile versus the nonstress test in the management of high-risk pregnancies. American Journal of Obstetrics and Gynecology 153: 624–633

Pollitt K 1990 Tyranny of the foetus. New Statesman & Society 3 (94): 28–30

Pommerance J J, Gluck L, Lynch V A 1974 Physical fitness in pregnancy: its effect on pregnancy outcome. American Journal of Obstetrics and Gynecology: 119: 867–876

Quaranta P, Currell R, Redman C W G, Robinson J S 1981 Prediction of small-for-dates infants by measurement of symphysial-fundal height. British Journal of Obstetrics and Gynaecology 88: 115–119

Reading A E, Campbell S, Cox D N, Sledmere C 1982 Health beliefs and health care behaviour in pregnancy. Psychological Medicine 12: 379–383

Redman C W G, Jefferies M 1988 Revised definition of pre-eclampsia Lancet 1: 809–812

Reynolds J L, Yudkin P L, Bull M J V 1988 General practitioner obstetrics: does risk prediction work? Journal of the Royal College of General Practitioners 38: 307–310

Richards D S, Seeds J W, Katz V L, et al 1988 Elevated maternal serum alphaprotein with normal ultrasound: is amniocentesis always appropriate? Obstetrics and Gynecology 71: 203–207

Robertson J G, Holmes C M 1969 A clinical trial of anti-$Rh_0(D)$ immunoglobulin in the prevention of $Rh_0(D)$ immunization. Journal of Obstetrics and Gynaecology of the British Commonwealth 76: 252–259

Robinson S 1985 Maternity care: a duplication of resources. Journal of the Royal College of General Practitioners 35: 346–347

Robson K M, Kumar R 1980 Delayed onset of maternal affection after childbirth. British Journal of Psychiatry 136: 347–353

Romito P 1989 Unhappiness after childbirth. In: Chalmers I, Enkin M, Keirse M J N C (eds) Effective care in pregnancy and childbirth. Oxford University Press, Oxford, pp 1433–1446

Rosenberg K, Grant J M, Hepburn M 1982 Antenatal detection of growth retardation: actual practice in a large maternity hospital. British Journal of Obstetrics and Gynaecology 89: 12–15

Roversi G D, Gargiulo M, Nicolini U et al 1980 Maximal tolerated insulin therapy in gestational diabetes. Diabetes Care 3: 489–494

Rush D, Stein Z, Susser M 1980 A randomized trial of prenatal nutritional supplementation in New York City. Pediatrics 65: 683–697

Saurel M J, Kaminski M 1983 Pregnant women at work. Lancet 1: 475

Secker N J, Kern Hansen P, Lykke Thomsen B, Keiding N 1987 Growth retardation in preterm infants. British Journal of Obstetrics and Gynaecology 94: 115–120

Sequeira P J L, Tobin J O'H 1984 Intrauterine infections: syphilis, viral diseases, toxoplasmosis, and chlamydial infections. In: Wald N J (ed) Antenatal and neonatal screening. Oxford University Press, Oxford, pp 358–381

Sexton M, Hebel J R 1984 A clinical trial of change of maternal smoking and its effect on birth weight. Journal of the American Medical Association 251: 911–915

Shy K K, Luthy D A, Whitfield M et al 1990 Effects of electronic fetal-heart-rate monitoring, as compared with periodic auscultation, on the neurologic development of premature infants. New England Journal of Medicine 322: 588–593

Sibai B H, Anderson G D 1986 Pregnancy outcome of intensive therapy in severe hypertension in first trimester. Obstetrics and Gynecology 67: 517–522

Sibai B H, Taslimi M, Abdella T N et al 1985 Maternal and perinatal outcome of conservative management of severe pre-eclampsia in midtrimester. American Journal of Obstetrics and Gynecology 152: 32–37

Sighthill Maternity Team 1982 Community antenatal care — the way forward. Scottish Medicine 2: 5–7

Silcocks P B S, Moss S M 1988 Rapidly progressive cervical cancer: is it a problem? British Journal of Obstetrics and Gynaecology 95: 1111–1116

Smales E, Perry C M, Ashby M A, Baker J W 1987 The influence of age on prognosis in carcinoma of the cervix. British Journal of Obstetrics and Gynaecology 94: 784–787

Smithells R W, Sheppard S, Schorah C J et al 1980 Possible prevention of neural-tube defects by periconceptual vitamin supplementation. Lancet 1: 339–340

Smithells R W, Nevin N C, Seller M J et al 1983 Further evidence of vitamin supplementation for prevention of neural tube defect recurrences. Lancet 1: 1027–1031

Spellacy W N, Miller S, Winegar A, Peterson P Q 1985 Macrosomia — maternal characteristics and infant complications. Obstetrics and Gynecology 66: 158–161

Spencer J A D 1987 Perinatal listeriosis. British Medical Journal 295: 349

Stray-Pedersen B 1983 Economic evaluation of maternal screening to prevent congenital syphilis. Sexually Transmitted Diseases 10: 167–172

Tabor A, Philip J, Madsen M et al 1986 Randomised controlled trial of genetic amniocentesis in 4606 low-risk women. Lancet 2: 1287–1293

Tafari N, Naeye R L, Gobezie A 1980 Effects of maternal undernutrition and heavy physical work during pregnancy on birth weight. British Journal of Obstetrics and Gynaecology 87: 222–226

Taylor D J, Mallen C, McDougall N, Lind T 1982 Effect of iron suplementation on serum ferritin levels during and after pregnancy. British Journal of Obstetrics and Gynaecology 89: 1011–1017.

Thomsen A C, Mrup L, Brogaard Hansen K 1987 Antibiotic elimination of Group-B streptococci in urine in prevention of preterm labour. Lancet i: 591–593

Valentin L, Lofgren O, Marsal K, Gullberg B 1984 Subjective recording of fetal movements. I Limits and acceptability in normal pregnancies. Acta Obstetrica et Gynecologica Scandinavica 63: 223–228

Valentin L, Marsal K, Wahlgren L 1986 Subjective recording of fetal movements. III Screening of a pregnant population; the clinical significance of decreased fetal movement counts. Acta Obstetrica et Gynecological Scandinavica 65: 753–758

Vessey M P, Nunn J F 1980 Occupational hazards of anaesthesia. British Medical Journal 281: 696–698

Wallenburg H C S, Rotmans N 1987 Prevention of recurrent idiopathic fetal growth retardation by low-dose aspirin and dipyridamole. American Journal of Obstetrics and Gynecology 157: 1230–1235

Wallenburg H C S, Van Eijk H G 1984 Effect of oral iron supplementation during pregnancy on maternal and fetal iron status. Journal of Perinatal Medicine 12: 7–12

Wallenburg H C S, Dekker G A, Makovits J W, Rotmans P 1986 Low-dose aspirin prevents pregnancy-induced hypertension and pre-eclampsia in angiotensin-sensitive primigravidae.Lancet 1: 1–3

Wang E, Smaill F 1989 Infection in pregnancy. In: Chalmers I, Enkin M, Keirse M J N C (eds) Effective care in pregnancy and childbirth. Oxford University Press, Oxford pp 534–564

Weatherall D J, Old J M, Thein S L, et al 1985 Prenatal diagnosis of the common haemoglobin disorders. Journal of Medical Genetics 22: 422–430

Widness J A, Cowett R M, Coustan D R, 1985 Neonatal morbidities in infants of mothers with glucose intolerance in pregnancy. Diabetes 34, (Suppl 2): 61–65

Whalley P 1967 Bacteriuria of pregnancy. American Journal of Obsterics and Gynecology 97: 723–738

Wilson J M G, Jungner G 1968 Principles and practice of screening for disease. World Health Organization, Geneva

Wolfendale MR, King S, Usherwood M Mc D 1983 Abnormal cervical smears: are we in for an epidemic? British Medical Journal 287: 526–628

Yudkin P L, Aboualfa M, Eyre J A, et al 1987 Influence of elective preterm delivery on birthweight and head circumference standards. Archives of Disease in Childhood 62: 24–29

Zajicek E 1981 Psychiatric problems during pregnancy. In: Wolkind S, Zajicek E (eds) Pregnancy: a psychological and social study. Academic Press, London pp 57–73

Children

12. Paediatric surveillance

John Wilmot

Surveillance, in the sense of 'watchful observation', is a term now frequently applied to the preventive health care of children, especially in the years before school entry. General practitioners continue to disagree about how far surveillance is useful in principle, or how much it is an appropriate task for them. Some of the controversy arises from vague, unclear, or undefined terms. As Butler (1989) points out, the term 'surveillance' is variously used in the limited sense of the detection of remediable diseases or defects, as in the *Handbook of preventive care for preschool children* (General Medical Services Committee and Royal College of General Practitioners 1984 and 1988), or applied to the whole range of screening, immunisation, treatment, advice and referrals of children outside hospital, as in the Court Report (Committee on Child Health Services 1976).

DEFINITIONS

From the foregoing it is clear that definitions are important. Child health surveillance can be simply described as 'the serial unsolicited professional observation of the health and development of the child, and of the well-being of the family as a whole' (DHSS unpublished 1972, cited by Rogers 1980). In the sense to be used here, a fuller definition of the term would include a range of activities: the oversight of the physical, social and emotional health and development of all children; measurement and recording of physical growth; monitoring developmental progress; offering and arranging intervention where necessary and prevention of disease, especially by immunisation and health education (Hall, 1989) (Fig. 12.1).

Developmental examination is a term applied to procedures, including a history of development, observation of behaviour and various specific tests, that define the stage of the child's development and detect deviations from the normal pattern. *Developmental screening* involves the performance of developmental examinations at specified key ages in populations of children to detect hitherto unrecognised abnormalities. *Developmental assessment* is, by contrast, the detailed, expert, and usually multidisciplinary, appraisal of suspected or overt abnormality in development. This is a definitive and problem-solving (rather than screening) exercise (Hall 1989).

HISTORICAL ASPECTS

The principle of attention to children when they are overtly healthy to detect remediable problems has a long history, with roots reaching back to the time of the Enlightenment.

The Court Report (Committee on Child Health Services 1976) was probably the seminal British influence on present-day professional views. This government-appointed committee made numerous recommendations, including the provision of surveillance for all children by a new group of general practitioner paediatricians, working closely with somewhat differently trained health visitors in primary care teams.

This degree of specialisation was unpalatable to general practice and, in the event, few of the Court recommendations were implemented, for reasons including the consequent professional rivalries and the cost to the Exchequer (Butler, 1989).

Healthier children — thinking prevention was the title of a report of a working party of the Royal College of General Practitioners in 1982 (RCGP 1982). This again recommended that surveillance should be offered to all children, and performed by family doctors and their practice teams. Many disagreed with the report, on both practical and philosophical grounds; but there was sufficient support from the academic and political wings of general practice for a new working party to be

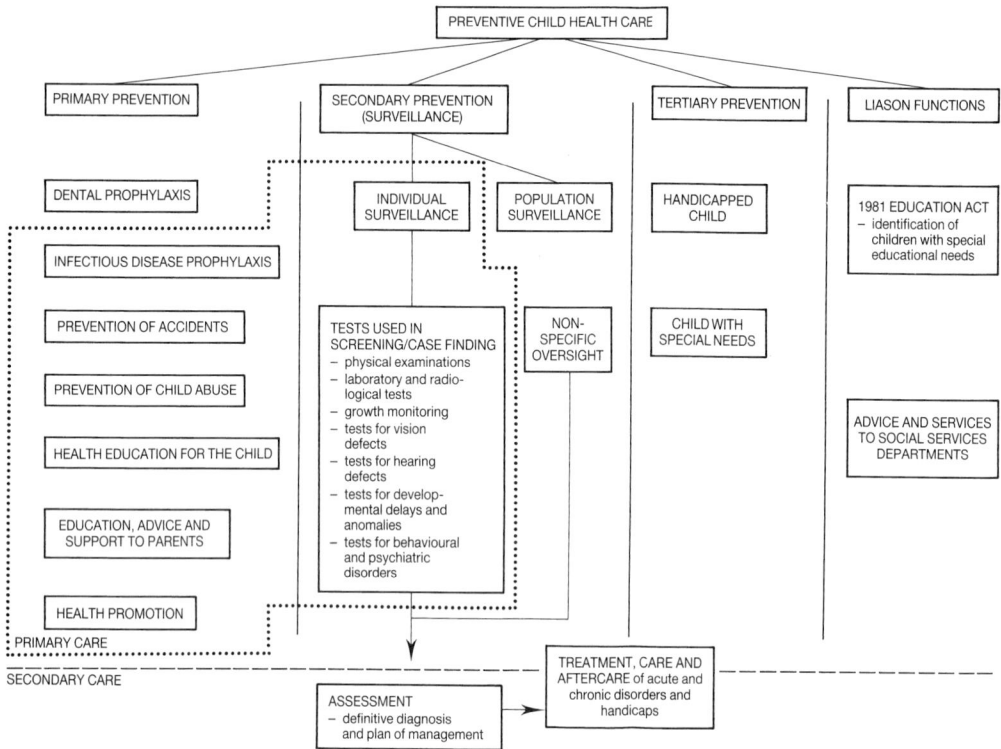

Fig. 12.1 The preventive health care of pre-school children: a definitional framework. The dotted line represents the author's view of surveillance in primary care (from Butler 1989).

formed from the College and the General Medical Services Committee of the British Medical Association. This group produced two editions of the *Handbook of preventive care for preschool children*, detailing surveillance examinations at different stages (General Medical Services Committee and Royal College of General Practitioners 1984 and 1988).

While general practitioners were moving towards a degree of consensus, other professional groups (health visitors, community medical officers, hospital paediatricians and public health doctors) often took a radically different stance, especially as regards the division of labour in child health work.

A Joint Working Party was formed by the British Paediatric Association, with members from all the relevant professional bodies, and produced a report, *Health for all children* (the Hall Report) (Hall 1989), incorporating agreed recommendations for health surveillance of children. The professional response was muted, but the report appeared to receive a welcome from the government (See the foreword to the Hall report (Hall 1989, Department of Health 1989).

A recent monograph by the health services researcher, Professor John Butler, reviews the evidence for surveillance and provides a perceptive discussion of the history of recent proposals for child surveillance within primary care (Butler 1989). Health visitors have misgivings about how far family doctors are motivated or trained for surveillance (Marsh et al 1989b). Likewise, clinical medical officers have understandably been concerned that much of their long-standing raison d'etre would be usurped by the more numerous and powerfully represented general practitioners.

ARGUMENTS FOR AND AGAINST CHILD SURVEILLANCE

As reviewed by Butler (1989), the case made out for surveillance is that it is effective, cost-effective, helpful to parents, good for doctors and provides useful support to families. The counter-arguments are that its effectiveness is unproven, that it is unduly costly, that it medicalises healthy individuals, and that it distracts attention from the pervasive effects of poverty and inequality on the health of children.

As noted above, surveillance programmes for young children are widely advocated because of the several advantages they are believed to confer (Hall, 1989). First, contact with health professionals separated from the pressing needs of acute illness can result in a relationship with greater potential for support and the promotion of positive health. There are also likely to be specific preventive effects, such as a reduction in childhood accidents, and improved immunisation uptake rates (as demonstrated by practices offering comprehensive surveillance; Curtis Jenkins et al 1978, Wilmot et al 1984). Thirdly, professionals can offer guidance relating to child development, behavioural problems and appropriate use of services. Finally, surveillance work can foster a helpful increase in knowledge about child health among parents and professionals.

The disadvantages of surveillance need to be recognised, and include the direct and opportunity costs for families, practices and health services generally. Secondly, the identification of a suspected problem in a screening programme results in much anxiety and stress in the period before resolution or definitive diagnosis. Thirdly, the preventive efforts of professionals must not distract attention from the wider social and economic causes of ill health in children, such as poverty, inappropriate nutrition, environmental hazards and marital strife and breakdown.

EVIDENCE ABOUT SURVEILLANCE

There are several large-scale research studies that, unfortunately, do not provide definitive answers regarding the benefits of surveillance. Studies in Dundee (Drillien & Drummond 1983, Drillien et al 1988) show that three-quarters of the total defects identified in children up to school age were found through screening, but many were only minor. Children with these problems had greater difficulty in their first 2 years at school, suggesting that screening may be useful more in the identification than prevention of disabilities. A controlled prospective study in Canada also showed that educational problems in the first school year could be predicted by performance on the Denver Development Screening Test or screening for vision and hearing defects (Cadman et al 1988). Conversely, a similar study in Sweden showed few differences between screened and unscreened children.

Such findings led Butler to conclude that '...surveillance may not be particularly useful in

reducing the subsequent prevalence of handicapping or disabling conditions'. He went on to say that interpretation was difficult, because as many defects were found in other ways as were detected through screening. There might be more benefit in encouraging parents and teachers to spot potential problems than in increasing professional involvement. Interested readers are recommended to consult Butler's monograph for a detailed discussion of the evidence.

In considering similar evidence, Bain (1989) concluded that the benefits of screening of preschool children were slight. The Hall Committee considered that, while formal screening of all children for *developmental impairments* did not meet the recognised criteria for screening programmes (see Chapter 2), a number of other tests offered to children did do so (Hall, 1989).

The different components of a surveillance programme will be considered more fully. Much of the detail is closely based on *Health for all children* (Hall 1989), with special emphasis on reports from general practice when these are available.

IMMUNISATION

The prevention of infectious diseases, mainly through immunisation, must be one of the key preventive services offered to children. In their different ways the virtual eradication of measles and whooping cough in North America and the continuing reduction of premature mortality in developing countries, show what can be done.

The World Health Organization set regional targets for immunisation levels for Europe. These stated that 90% of children should have completed courses of injections against diptheria, pertussis, poliomyelitis, tetanus and measles. This target has now been incorporated in the system of remuneration of British general practitioners. In October 1988, the United Kingdom followed the USA and other countries in adopting the MMR (measles, mumps and rubella) vaccine, which is now given early in the second year, shortly after the completion of the course of triple antigen (Badenoch 1988). For the time being, this vaccine is also to be given to children reaching school age and girls aged 10–14 years will still require rubella vaccination.

A detailed consideration of immunisation is beyond the scope of this book, and useful advice can be found in the *British National Formulary*, in practical handbooks on immunisation (Joint Committee on Vaccination and Immunisation 1990, Sefi and Macfarlane 1989) and in flow charts designed to help professionals in decision-making (Nicoll and Jenkinson 1988).

Any practice team considering a surveillance programme must consider how best to achieve high levels of immunisation. Protection against major infections is one of the more attractive aspects of the preventive package that can be offered to parents, even given some recent misgivings among the British public. The pros and cons for the individual child can be discussed at scheduled surveillance examinations, most importantly at 6 weeks.

Deprived groups will find it much less easy to attend prearranged appointments, so ad hoc and opportunistic action will be the key to improving uptake among such children. Enthusiastic groups have thus been able to report immunisation rates exceeding 90% even in the inner cities (Rossdale et al 1986). The children of travellers and some others may be best covered by a peripatetic nurse (employed by Health Authorities or perhaps by practices) who can be very effective without direct medical supervision (Sefi and Macfarlane 1989).

Computerisation can remove much of the drudgery involved in sending appointments, mailing reminders and providing information on coverage levels. The computer schemes developed by individual Health Authorities will shortly be replaced by the National Child Health Computer system. It will be much easier for practices to monitor immunisation uptake levels given the information feedback elements to the new arrangements.

MONITORING GROWTH

The weighing of babies is, like immunisation, a frequent activity in preventive child health care in many countries, but is it worth doing? The Hall report critically assessed the evidence and found much of it wanting (Hall 1989).

The ceremony of weighing a baby is valued by parents, who may use it as the focus for a clinic visit, with its potential for social contact with other young families and discussion of various factors affecting child health and development. There is, however, the potential for harm in inexpert measurement or erroneous interpretation of recordings or points on centile charts (Hall 1989).

Measurements of weight and height need to be considered in the same light as any screening test, in that children whose growth pattern appears less than optimal need more careful appraisal. Only a minority of such children, however, are likely to be suffering any serious disorder. The Hall report commented, in particular, that weight may fluctuate by several hundred grams, that static weight or even weight loss

for a week or two is common and that infants gaining weight slowly or crossing percentile lines are likely to be following a genetically programmed growth trajectory. There are likely to be other symptoms or reasons for concern accompanying organic diseases or the form of child abuse known as 'non-organic failure to thrive' (Hall 1989).

Among the important childhood disorders that affect height gain are growth hormone deficiency (incidence 1 in 3000–5000), hypothyroidism (1 in 3000) and Turner syndrome (1 in 2500 females) (Hall 1989). Other diseases, such as inflammatory bowel disease, chronic renal failure and bone dysplasia may present with short stature, often without other symptoms. Measurement of height may permit the early detection of these conditions, leading to corrective treatment and, at least in some instances, genetic counselling.

The measurement of height is thus an important part of the routine surveillance of those children with a known or suspected growth disorder, e.g. small for dates at birth, suspected failure to thrive, or dysmorphic syndromes. The Hall committee recognised the problems in accurately measuring height in infants and toddlers and so argued that universal height measurement as a screening procedure should be performed at about 3 years of age.

PHYSICAL EXAMINATION

Physical examination developed in medical practice as a method that could confirm or refute diseases or defects suggested by other cues. At the same time the 'laying on of hands' can demonstrate concern and provide reassurance. The use of a general examination for screening purposes is recent and calls for careful critical appraisal. For neonates especially, however, the examination acts as a multiple screening tool whose yield is high (Hall 1989). The conditions that are particularly likely to be detected in this way include eye defects, congenital heart disease, congenital dislocation of the hip and abnormalities of the genitalia.

DEVELOPMENTAL EXAMINATION

One of the most striking conclusions of the Hall report was that not all children should be subjected to formal developmental testing, largely because such examinations did not satisfy the criteria for screening tests. The important developmental impairments were identified in other ways, often around the time of birth or because of parents' concern about a child's progress.

The most important disorders and their incidence rates are as follows: cerebral palsy, 1.5–3 cases per 1000 births; Duchenne muscular dystrophy, 3 per 10 000 male births; severe learning difficulties, 3.7 cases per 1000; autism, 3 cases per 10 000; specific language difficulties, probably more common than the above. The conditions are thus uncommon and, while rarely medically treatable, their early detection prevents some avoidable suffering and may reduce secondary handicaps (genetic counselling and antenatal diagnosis also being relevant to muscular dystrophy). The diagnosis of these conditions is difficult in infancy and many mistakes occur, often because of the inappropriate reassurance of professionals in response to the concerns of parents.

The Hall committee, therefore, recommended that universal developmental screening should be replaced by an approach to developmental surveillance that makes more explicit use of the views and observations of parents. Professionals (health visitors and doctors) could satisfy themselves that most children were developing within normal limits through the developmental history and by general observation of the child. In doubtful cases, the established developmental schedules could then be used for detailed developmental testing, to clarify whether closer observation or referral was necessary.

Of the methods that can be used for this more detailed testing of selected children, the most familiar in the United Kingdom will be the Sheridan scales (Sheridan 1975), which were updated and slightly modified in the Woodside system (Barber et al 1976, Barber 1981) and the schedule of growing skills (Bellman and Cash, 1987). The Denver Developmental Screening Tests or DDST, developed in the United States and used in many countries, are favoured by some British professionals (Frankenburg et al 1975). The choice of a system will depend on the experience of the individual professional, training in a specific method and local arrangements. The application of the different schedules will be considered in detail in Chapter 17, and either the relevant practical manuals or detailed texts, such as Illingworth (1983), can be consulted.

LABORATORY TESTS AND X-RAYS IN CHILDHOOD SURVEILLANCE

As childhood metabolic disorders are to be considered elsewhere in this book (Chapter 15), it will be sufficient merely to note that screening programmes are now established for the detection of phenylketonuria and hypothyroidism using a capillary blood sample obtained by heel-prick a few days after birth (Hall 1989). It has been suggested that the same sample should be used to screen for cystic fibrosis and Duchenne muscular dystrophy. Early treatment might benefit cystic fibrosis, and trials of enzyme assays are underway for neonatal screening of this condition.

Genetic counselling is all that can be offered when muscular dystrophy is diagnosed after birth. An alternative strategy with this condition would be to check the serum creatine kinase of boys who first walk later than 18 months. See Chapter 11 for a discussion of the prenatal diagnosis of these conditions.

Haemoglobinopathies

Abnormal types of haemoglobin are a cause of childhood ill-health among certain ethnic minorities (representing about 3.3% of the total United Kingdom population (Hall 1989) (See also Chapter 39).

There are thought to be 4000–5000 sufferers from sickle cell disease in the UK with about 70 babies born each year. The incidence is one in 80 among West Africans and one in 200 among those of Jamaican origin. The disease causes impaired immunity, with painful splenic crises and fulminating pneumoccal infection, resulting in high morbidity and mortality up to 3 years of age. Penicillin prophylaxis is safe and effective and pneumococcal vaccine is of some benefit (Lancet 1987).

Thalassaemia is less dramatic in its presentation, resulting in anaemia and failure to thrive; treatment is by blood transfusion and iron chelation therapy.

Neonatal screening for both types of disorder is feasible, using the same sample that is tested for phenylketonuria, at a cost of about 33p. A screening programme in Birmingham managed, over eight years, to increase sensitivity from 66% to nearly 100%, through technical changes and improved interpretation (Griffiths et al 1988).

Screening for haemoglobinopathies, and more particularly their longer-term management, really calls for a team approach involving haematologists, geneticists, paediatricians and counsellors. Present provision is generally patchy (Franklin 1988). Population screening is probably worthwhile in industrial cities, with a more selective approach to testing in other areas (Griffiths et al 1988).

Iron deficiency anaemia

Iron deficiency is common in preschool children, occuring in about 5–10% with a peak at 3 years. The condition is more prevalent among the poor and in ethnic minorities, where the responsible dietary factors probably include insufficient iron-rich food, fresh cow's milk and tea drinking (as this chelates iron) (Hall 1989).

Iron deficiency anaemia is associated with behavioural problems, developmental defects and increased liability to infection. The condition is simply treated by a 2 month course of oral iron, although the dietary and health education aspects need to be considered and warrant further research.

General recommendations are that health professionals conducting surveillance should be aware of the prevalence of iron deficiency and should consider blood testing and consequent treatment, especially among the toddler age group (Hall 1989). A surveillance scheme in an inner city general practice has incorporated screening for haemoglobinopathies and iron deficiency, combined with treatment and dietary education (James et al 1989).

Atlantoaxial instability

Atlantoaxial instability occurs in Down syndrome, especially in girls, but the interpretation of X-rays is difficult in relation to this condition. Most cases develop insidiously following road accidents and whiplash injuries, with effects on the tendon reflexes. The most appropriate preventive manoeuvre is, therefore, the use of head restraints during car journeys (Hall 1989) (See also Chapter 16).

HEALTH EDUCATION

Health education is defined by the Hall report as 'any activity which provides health-related learning, i.e. some relatively permanent change in an individual's capabilities or dispositions' (Hall 1989). It is one of the principal methods of health promotion, namely the process of enabling people to increase control over and improve their health.

It follows from the above definition that health education is not simply a matter of health professionals instructing members of the public in a straightforward set of rules for healthy living. The modern view would emphasise the mutuality of the learning process, with professionals imparting their scientific knowledge (and how often have our certainties been unwarranted?) and parents sharing their day-to-day experience of their children's behaviour and aptitudes. Recent research suggests that doctors and health visitors should relate their detailed advice to the values and beliefs of the families they deal with.

The complexity of the processes involved in health education makes evaluation difficult. Where a clear end-point is possible, there is good evidence that general practitioners can influence smoking (Russell et al 1979) and excessive drinking (Wallace et al 1988) among adult patients.

There are clear needs for educational efforts in relation to breast feeding, smoking by parents, immunisation, children's safety in home and car, and dental care. Advice about nutrition is a long-standing role of the health visitor and in high-risk populations this can include advice about rickets. Doctors and health visitors can advise on appropriate responses to acute illness, including self-care for minor illness and when to seek urgent medical help.

Anticipatory or developmental guidance

Anticipatory or developmental guidance involves explanations of what developmental milestones to expect, how to encourage learning and how to recognise problems. This again tends to be an important activity of health visitors.

Many of the children at risk of child abuse can be recognised around the time of birth, through risk factors that include the parents' age, parents' childhood experiences, separation of mother and infant and a lack of nurturing behaviour (Lynch and Roberts 1977, Ounsted and Roberts 1982). Child abuse may be reduced through special support by the practice team, which includes education in children's capabilities, practical help and facilitating a support network (Aylett 1979). There are encouraging suggestions that primary care teams delivering a comprehensive surveillance programme may be able to reduce child abuse among the populations they serve (Hardy et al 1979, Wilmot et al 1984).

SURVEILLANCE FOR EMOTIONAL DISORDERS

Emotional and social difficulties are common in childhood and include problems with sleeping, eating and growth impairment, conduct disorder, behaviour problems and, in older children and adolescents, anorexia nervosa and drug abuse. While there was insufficient evidence for the Hall committee to recommend specific screening, it is clearly appropriate to make enquiry about difficulties with children's behaviour and management.

Postnatal depression, occurring in about 12–15% of mothers, has adverse effects on several aspects of children's development. Both the general practitioner and health visitor must be on the alert for evidence of depression. A small randomised trial has shown significant benefits from brief counselling provided by specially trained health visitors (Holden et at 1989).

SPEECH AND LANGUAGE PROBLEMS

Normal children (especially boys) learn to talk at a very variable rate. There is thus great difficulty in distinguishing between 'late normal' children and those with marked articulatory problems or the rare childhood dysphasias and related conditions, at least below the age of 3 years (Hall 1989). Many 4 year-olds who are poor talkers later 'catch up', and the ability to tell a story from pictures seems the best predictor (Bishop and Edmundson 1987).

SPECIAL EDUCATIONAL NEEDS

One of the aims of preschool surveillance is to identify children who need special help, either from health professionals or during their schooling. Up to 20% of children may need some special teaching at some time but there are perhaps 2% with complex or severe problems who will need comprehensive, multidisciplinary assessment (Taylor 1989). In recent years, Child Development or Assessment Centres, usually jointly funded by health and education authorities, have met the latter need. They are staffed by paediatricians, specialist teachers, psychologists, physiotherapists, speech therapists and other professionals.

The 1981 Education Act has formalised the principle that children with all but the most severe impairments should be educated in ordinary schools. If parents, teachers or health professionals consider it appropriate, a Statement of Special Education Needs is prepared. This is a lengthy and time-consuming process and unfortunately resource shortages have often led to compromises in the decisions made (Taylor 1989).

IMPAIRMENT AND HANDICAP

Children may be born with, or may acquire, *impairments*, which cause *disability* in the activities of daily living; they are *handicapped* by the attitudes or behaviour of others, as well as the physical barriers found in the environment (see Chapter 17 for detailed definitions of these terms).

The process of attempting to meet the multiple needs of children with severe impairments, such as cerebral palsy, can lead to fragmentation of care, with the accompanying risk that the primary care team will lose touch with the child. The Court Report recommended that each district should appoint a consultant community paediatrician, leading a district handicap team, to coordinate provision (Committee on Child Services 1976). The creation of these posts in more recent times, albeit in a slow and patchy fashion, may be instrumental in improving care in many areas (Bain 1989). The 1989 Children Act lays new responsibility on local authorities to ensure the welfare of children 'in need', i.e. with actual or potential impairments. Resulting benefits for children remain to be seen, especially considering present constraints on local authority resources.

ORGANISATION OF SURVEILLANCE

Teamwork

The 'core' or 'functional' team that provides surveillance is the health visitor, doctor (general practitioner and/or clinical medical officer), nurse (usually a practice-employed treatment room nurse) and the reception and clerical staff.

The health visitor

Ideally, the health visitor should have adequate space and other facilities within the practice building, either privately owned or a publicly financed health centre, to facilitate ready communication. It is obviously desirable for the different members of the team to meet regularly to discuss the overall practice strategy for child health, as well as discussing individual patients. The health visitors are, or have hitherto been, far more constrained by district health authority policies and their own management structure than general practitioners. A recent survey of general practitioners and health visitors in the north of England (Marsh et al 1989a, b) revealed that only 25% of 407 health visitors considered they had office space for their sole use (while 52% of 210 doctors considered that they did). The professionals did agree that they met to discuss patients, about 70% meeting at least weekly. Formal policy meetings were much less common, 17% of the health visitors and 29% of the doctors reporting that these occurred. Many health visitors commented that doctors only poorly understood their role and training, while the fact that 47% had been in their practices for 3 years or less presents another obstacle to smooth collaboration. Clearly there is considerable room for improvement in the teamwork in our practices.

Should health visitors actually perform all surveillance screening examinations? One-third of health visitors in the Northern region survey considered they should (Marsh et al 1989b). The logic of the Hall committee proposals would be that a doctor should perform the physical examinations recommended for infants neonatally, at 6 weeks and around 9 months, with health visitors performing the later checks. This indeed is the pattern to be adopted in the author's health district. Some enthusiasts for developmental surveillance have argued against the fragmentation likely to result from the doctor doing some checks and the health visitor testing hearing and vision (Curtis Jenkins et al 1978). On the other hand, Bain (1977) has shown that general practitioners adequately perform physical examinations, but at the expense of adequate testing of hearing and vision. Certainly, health visitors have carried out these tests in the author's practice and district, with rates for the detection of abnormality very similar to Curtis Jenkins and his colleagues (Wilmot et al 1984).

Other team members

The nurse

The nurse's main direct involvement in preventive care is likely to be immunisation. Nursing training should thus include instruction in techniques of immunisation, contraindications and how to respond to the very infrequent anaphylactic episode. Appropriately trained nurses seem to be very competent in dealing with this rare emergency (Sefi and Macfarlane 1989), although it has been argued that ideally a doctor should be within a few minutes' call, which would normally mean in the practice building.

The clinical medical officer

Clinical medical officers have considerable experience and skills in child health and are active members of some practice teams offering comprehensive surveillance (Curtis Jenkins et al 1978, Wilmot et al 1984). Most Northern region practices (Marsh et al 1989a) had very infrequent contact with clinical medical officers, but close collaboration could enhance the care that primary care teams offer their child patients. It would seem desirable for practice principals to plan meetings with health visitors, perhaps inviting clinical medical officers, if they are not already involved, to decide policies for preventive child health care. Practice nurses and relevant reception or clerical staff should participate, because of the educational benefits, to give them a sense of worthwhile involvement, and to ensure smooth implementation.

Is there a need for special sessions?

This question was considered in *Healthier children — thinking prevention* (Royal College of General Practitioners 1982). The advantages of the health visitor, doctor and practice nurse being present together, the particular needs of fit young children and the requirement for at least some special equipment, point towards a scheduled clinic session, although this is not always suitable for groups such as the urban deprived or rural populations with poor transport services. Surveillance examinations during ordinary consulting hours thus have a place, if only as a supplement to special sessions (Williams 1985). Some have argued that 'opportunistic surveillance', during consultations for other matters, can be relied upon as the sole approach (Houston and Davis 1985) (See also Chapter 9). Only a little under half of practices surveyed in the North of England, or nationally, had specific sessions for paediatric screening (Marsh et al 1989a, Burke and Bain 1986, respectively).

Time and space

The number of appointments needed for surveillance can be simply calculated. For instance, the scheme in the author's practice and district requires two examinations by a doctor in the first year. Our practice of 11 700 persons produces about 140 births each year. In addition to the 280 appointments thus needed, at least an extra 25% should be allowed for extra appointments (including problems suggested by the health visitor checks, children considered to be 'at risk' — developmentally or otherwise — and those moving into the area who may have higher rates of abnormality; Curtis Jenkins et al 1978). Thus 350 appointment slots have to be provided over 44 weeks (to allow for holidays, study leave, etc.) in a five doctor practice, or eight per week — say 2 hours of a doctor's time. The health visitor examinations are in addition to this and, while checks of toddlers can usefully be performed at home, the distraction test of hearing at 8 months needs a quiet room (and would be performed 175 times each year on the above calculations). The space required includes a child-friendly waiting area, a room for the doctor, and perhaps one also for the health visitor.

Records

There are a variety of records that are used for child surveillance. The standard health visitor record is the white quarto NM+CW46 envelope. This has been variously adapted, and other records include the similar-sized card in the Woodside system (Barber et al 1976), the A4-size self-copying sheets in the Schedule of Growing Skills (Bellman and Cash, 1987) and the smaller cards produced specifically for general practitioners (General Medical Services Committee and Royal College of General Practitioners 1984 and 1988). The last-named are designed to fit in the FP5 or FP6 'Lloyd George' medical record envelopes.

These various records are likely to be rendered partly obsolete by two factors. One, of course, is the introduction of computers. A national child health computer scheme is being introduced (Rigby 1987) and will replace earlier local systems. The software provides for a computer in the district health authority to send appointments for immunisations and surveillance examinations, to produce an updated record sheet for the professional concerned and to produce data regarding coverage rates and abnormalities detected.

The second development is parent-held records. This accords with the philosophy that parents are active participants in their children's developmental progress and are partners in their health care. Such records, well established in maternity care, are welcomed by parents (who do not lose them!) (O'Flaherty et al 1987).

Within the next few years, we are likely to see parent-held records becoming more widespread, with computers used in parallel to support an information system that incorporates feedback to professionals and the material needed for audit.

AUDIT

Several forms of audit were suggested in *Healthier children — thinking prevention* (Royal College of General Practitioners 1982), including attendance rates, rates of coverage for surveillance examinations and immunisation and the frequency of detection of abnormality. These can be applied by practices (Wilmot et al 1984), but are time-consuming. Computer systems can greatly reduce the drudgery and provide prompt feedback for practice teams. Arrangements in Northumberland provide for the feedback to practices of rates of surgery for congenital hip dislocation, cataract extraction and orchidopexy, as

well as data on mean age of diagnosis for major handicapping conditions (Colver and Steiner 1986).

EDUCATION AND TRAINING

It is difficult to make firm recommendations for the training that general practitioners require for child health surveillance. A starting point would be agreement on the educational needs. Two developmental paediatricians have suggested that the following should be the objectives of any training given: a *knowledge* of child development and its variability, of immunisation, of sensory screening, of local resources and treatment for handicapping conditions; *skills* in the examination of children, in communication and counselling; and an insight into one's own *attitudes* towards the views and beliefs of parents, to children themselves and to minority groups (Bellman and Cash 1987).

A consideration of the competencies needed for the community care of children suggests a reordering of priorities for undergraduate education, which only exceptionally enlightened medical schools have so far taken into account (Waterston 1987).

Those responsible for organising vocational training for general practice have assumed that a 6 month hospital post in paediatrics is desirable. Recent surveys of trainees and younger principals suggest that 70–75% of doctors entering general practice in the past 15 years have occupied such a post (Ronalds et al 1981, Wilmot 1984, Polnay and Pringle 1989, Marsh et al 1989a). All such doctors now obtain a certificate from the Joint Committee for Postgraduate Training in General Practice, whose own records on 8326 doctors between 1984 and 1987 show that 57% had occupied paediatric posts (Styles 1989). Of course, such posts tend mostly to provide experience of ill children, but about 30% of recent trainees report experience of child health clinics and handicap services (Wilmot 1984, Polnay and Pringle 1989).

A national survey of training practices revealed that 54% were holding developmental screening sessions, as against 34% of non-training practices (Burke and Bain 1986). Only one-third of trainees in the West Midlands region felt sufficiently confident to conduct the surveillance of preschool children (Wilmot 1984, Cyna and Pryslo 1987); the proportion was 44% in the Trent region (Polnay and Pringle 1989). Such findings have prompted the Joint Committee on Postgraduate Training in General Practice to recommend that all practices provide teaching on, and experience in, paediatric surveillance.

Established general practitioners are likely to need specific courses related to surveillance. Again, there is little agreement on appropriate content and duration, but Bellman and Cash (1987) have suggested the following for a 1-week (10 half-day) course: training in developmental screening, updating on immunisations, sensory testing, speech and language problems, emotional disorders, chronic handicaps, nutrition, minority needs, the 1981 Education Act, local community services, professional attitudes and counselling. Doctors need practical hands-on experience of examining children, either during such courses or in additional sessions in surveillance clinics.

In 1989, an ad hoc working party of the British Paediatric Association and the Royal College of General Practitioners (RCGP/BPA 1989) produced recommendations for entry to the child health surveillance lists being established by Family Health Services Authorities. These comprise: attendance at a theoretical course covering the areas outlined above, but lasting normally for three full days and a minimum of two full days, and a series of supervised practical sessions (normally six), either in health authority child health clinics, appropriate practice premises or at specially arranged sessions. These recommendations seem to have been adopted fairly widely, but once again in a patchy fashion in different parts of the country. Subsequently, the Royal College of General Practitioners has undertaken to modify the MRCGP examination to the extent that the possession of this qualification would be sufficient evidence of competence.

As others have already predicted, the situation regarding child health care in general practice is undergoing rapid change, especially since the Hall Report and the 1990 Contract changes. (Burke and Bain 1986, Marsh et al 1989a, b).

SURVEILLANCE IN DIFFERENT AGE GROUPS

The doctor, nurse or health visitor needs to understand the appropriate content of surveillance checks at different ages, which will be outlined in this section, based on the recommendations of the Joint Working Party (Hall 1989).

The relevant body systems are covered in greater detail in separate chapters in this book, but the essentials are summarised in Table 12.1.

Neonatal examination

Examination soon after birth is the longest-established childhood screening test. Immediately after delivery, the infant can be scanned for the grosser defects of skull, palate, trunk or limbs, but full normal examination is generally performed on the next day. The usual sequence is roughly 'top to toe', first palpating the skull and palate for defects. The eyes should be carefully inspected, and use of the ophthalmoscope at 20–30 cm (using a +3D lens) should reveal the red reflex; a cataract may manifest as an absent reflex or as a silhouette. A family history of serious visual disorder, e.g. congenital cataract, glaucoma or retinoblastoma, calls for very careful examination, perhaps by an ophthalmologist. Auscultation of the heart and lungs may reveal cardiac murmurs which may be accompanied by cyanosis, tachypnoea, or palpable thrills.

The genitalia should be examined. One or both testes are undescended at birth in 6% of boys, the rate being much higher in preterm infants. Three-quarters have resolved by 3 months, but spontaneous descent is unlikely after this age. Surgical referral should be made before 18 months because of the risks of infertility and malignancy. After gentle manipulation into the lowest position, without traction, the centre of the testis should be more than 4 cm below the pubic tubercle (2.5 cm in infants under 2.5 kg). The femoral pulses need palpation to exclude aortic coarctation, while the hips require examination because congenital dislocation is much more treatable if detected early. Barlow's and Ortolani's manoeuvres should be performed and the hips should be re-examined at later surveillance checks until the child is walking normally (see Chapter 16).

The issue of screening for hearing impairment in the neonatal period is difficult. Significant sensorineural hearing loss occurs in between one and two births per thousand. Children who require intensive care or exchange transfusion, who have congenital infection or dysmorphic syndromes, or who have a family history of hearing loss, are at increased risk. Some maternity units perform universal screening, for instance using the auditory response cradle (ARC); in many localities it will be necessary to consider referral of high-risk infants for this test, or for brain stem-evoked response audiometry (BSER) (See also Chapter 18).

Examination at 6–8 weeks

Parents should be asked for their concerns, or indeed observations about their baby's behaviour. Particular enquiry should be made regarding vision and hearing. Physical examination should be performed, including eye inspection, examination of the hips and palpation of the testes. Weight and head circumference should be

Table 12.1 Outline of surveillance scheme (based on Hall Committee recommendations (Hall 1989))

Screening/examination	Health Education and developmental guidance (including safety topics*)
Neonatal	
Family and perinatal history	
Full physical including weight, head circumference	
CDH and testes	
Eyes (red reflex)	
ARC or BSER if high risk of hearing loss	
PKN and thyroid	
6 weeks	
History and concerns	Feeding
Physical examination	Family relationships
Weight and head circumference	Contraception
CDH	
Inspect eyes	Immunisation
Refer if high risk of hearing loss	Safety in home and car
8 (7–9) months	
Parental concerns (especially vision and hearing)	Parents' relationships
Weight, if requested or indicated	Stairs
CDH	Fire and cooker guards
Testes	Glass
Distraction test of hearing	Scald risks
Visual behaviour and observe for squint	Car seats
	MMR vaccine
1¹/₂–2 years	
Concerns (especially behaviour, vision and hearing)	Car seats
Walking with normal gait?	Medicines and chemicals
Few words	Electric plugs
Understanding speech?	Water outside
(Iron deficiency anaemia)	Behaviour problems (e.g. tantrums)
3–3¹/₂ years	
Vision, squint, hearing, behaviour and development	Separation from parents
Height (plot on chart)	Playgroups
Testes (if not examined since 8 months)	Dentist
Hearing test if indicated	Road dangers
Special educational needs?	
School entry (4-5 years)	
Concerns by parents and teachers	Schooling
Physical examination (including heart)	Immunisation
Height (plot on chart)	Roads and bicycles
Vision (Snellen chart)	Strangers
Hearing by sweep audiometry	
School years	
Visual acuity 8, 11 and 14 years	
Colour vision at 11	
Height measurement when indicated	

*from Colver and Steiner 1986
ARC, auditory response cradle; BSER, brain stem evoked response; CDH, congenital dislocation of the hip; MMR, measles, mumps, rubella; PKN, phenylketonuria

measured. Immunisation and risks to infants in cars or from falling, can be discussed with parents. Check-lists can be given regarding hearing problems.

Examination at 8–9 months

Again, parents should be asked about their concerns regarding health and development, especially regarding vision and hearing. Weight should be checked. Physical examination should particularly include the testes and hips. A distraction test should be performed to check hearing by two suitably trained individuals (perhaps the health visitor and an assistant).

Surveillance check at 1½–2 years

After enquiry for parental concerns, the health professional needs to confirm that the child is walking with a normal gait (the possible disorders relevant here including congenital hip dislocation and Duchenne muscular dystrophy), is beginning to say words and understands when spoken to.

Surveillance check at 3–3½ years

Enquiry should be made about vision, squint, hearing, behaviour and development. The question of any possible educational problems or needs should be discussed with parents. Further action will be needed if there appear to be potential problems. Height should be measured and plotted on a chart. Testicular descent should be confirmed in boys and a hearing test should be performed if indicated.

School entry

Examination should be preceded by review of preschool records and enquiry about the concerns of parents or teachers. Physical examination can include auscultation of the heart. Height should be measured, vision tested using a Snellen-type chart and hearing checked using sweep audiometry.

School age

Visual acuity can be tested at ages eight, eleven and fourteen. Colour vision should be tested by Ishihara plates at age 11 (in boys) and height checked if indicated. Otherwise medical attention can be based on problems reported by child, parents or teachers.

CONCLUSIONS: THE ROLE FOR PAEDIATRIC SURVEILLANCE IN GENERAL PRACTICE

The involvement of general practitioners in the preventive care of children can be roughly at three levels: first, the traditional responsibility for symptomatic illness, perhaps also offering immunisations. Secondly, an intermediate level of establishing a well-infant or well-child clinic, or performing some of the surveillance examinations. The third level represents a move towards comprehensive care, almost certainly in close concert with the health visitor as well as the practice nurse and clerical or secretarial staff.

The first level, or traditional approach, is likely to become increasingly less viable over the next few years. While the medical profession may object to the prescriptive nature of the tasks set out in the new GP contract (Department of Health 1989), this document has given firm official recognition to modern concepts of family medicine, embracing prevention and responsibility for populations as well as high-quality care in acute and chronic illness.

REFERENCES

Aylett M 1979 Preventing child abuse: the primary health care team. Update: 537–540
Badenoch J 1988 Big bang for vaccination. British Medical Journal 297: 750–751
Bain D J G 1977 Methods used by general practitioners in developmental screening of pre-school children. British Medical Journal 2: 363–365
Bain J 1989 Developmental screening for pre-school children: is it worthwhile? Journal of the Royal College of General Practitioners 39: 133–137

Barber J H 1981 Pre-school developmental screening — the results of a four year period. Health Bulletin (Edinburgh) 40: 170–178
Barber J H, Boothman R, Stanfield J P 1976 A new visual chart for pre-school developmental screening. Health Bulletin (Edinburgh) 34: 80–91
Bellman M Cash J 1987 The schedule of growing skills in practice. NFER — Nelson, Windsor
Bishop D V M, Edmundson A 1987 Language impairment in four year olds: distinguishing transient from permanent

impairments. Journal of Speech and Hearing Disorders 52: 156–173

Burke P, Bain J 1986 Paediatric developmental screening: a survey of general practitioners. Journal of the Royal College of General Practitioners 36: 302–306

Butler J R 1989 Child health surveillance in primary care: a critical review. HMSO, London

Cadman D, Walter S D Chambers L W et al 1988 Predicting problems in school performance from pre-school health developmental and behavioural assessments. Canadian Medical Association Journal 139: 31–36

Colver A F, Steiner H 1986 Health surveillance of pre-school children. British Medial Journal 293: 258–260

Committee on Child Health Services 1976 Fit for the future (Court Report) Cmnd 6680 HMSO, London

Curtis Jenkins, Collins G H , Andrews C 1978 British Medical Journal 1: 1537–1540

Cyna A M, Pryslo F R 1987 Are the recommendations being met in the general practice year of vocational training? Trainees' view in the West Midlands Region. British Medical Journal 294: 416–418

Departments of Health 1989 General practice in the National Health Service: the 1990 contract. Department of Health, London

Department of Health and Social Security 1972 unpublished, cited in Rogers 1980

Drillien C M, Drummond M B 1983 Development screening and the child with special needs. Spastics International Medical Publications/Heinemann, London

Drillien C M, Pickering R M, Drummond M B 1988 Predictive screening for different areas of development. Developmental Medicine and Child Neurology 30: 294–305

Franklin I M 1988 Services for sickle cell disease: unified approach needed. British Medical Journal 296: 592

Frankenburg W, Dodds J B, Fandal A W 1975 Denver Developmental Screening Test Reference Manual, revised edn. Ladoca, Denver, Colorado

General Medical Services Committee and Royal College of General Practitioners 1984 (2nd edn. 1988) Handbook of preventive care for pre-school children. Royal College of General Practitioners, London

Griffiths P D, Mann J R, Darbyshire P J, Green A I 1988 Evaluation of eight and a half years of neonatal screening for haemoglobinopathies in Birmingham. British Medical Journal 296: 1583–1585

Hall D M B (ed) 1989 Health for all children: report of joint working party on child health surveillance. Oxford University Press, Oxford

Hardy M, McElroy E, Patchett D R 1979 Prevention of baby battering. Practitioner 222: 243–247

Houston H L A, Davis R M 1985 Opportunistic surveillance of child development in primary care: is it feasible? Journal of the Royal College of General Practitioners 35: 77–79

Holden J M, Sagovsky R, Cox J L 1989 Counselling in a general practice setting: controlled study of health visitor intervention in treatment of postnatal depression. British Medical Journal 298: 223–226

Illingworth R 1983 Development of the infant and young child, 8th edn. Churchill Livingstone, Edinburgh

James J, Lawson P, Male P, Oakhill A 1989 Preventing iron

deficiency in pre-school children by implementing an educational and screening programme in an inner city practice. British Medical Journal 299: 838–840

Joint Committee on Vaccination and Immunisation. Vaccination against infectious disease 2nd edn. HMSO, London.

Lancet 1987 Iron deficiency — time for a community campaign (editorial): Lancet 1: 142

Lynch M A, Roberts J 1977 Predicting child abuse in the maternity hospital. British Medical Journal 1: 624–626

Marsh G N, Russell D, Russell I T 1989a Is paediatrics safe in general practitioners hands? A study in the North of England. Journal of the Royal College of General Practitioners 39: 138–141

Marsh G N, Russell D, Russell I T 1989b What do health visitors contribute to the care of children? A study in the North of England. Journal of the Royal College of General Practitioners 39: 201–205

Nicoll A, Jenkinson D 1988 Decision making for routine measles/MMR and whooping cough vaccination. British Medical Journal 297: 405–407

O'Flaherty S, Jandera E, Llewellyn J, Wall M 1987 Personal health records: an evaluation. Archives of disease in childhood 62: 1152–1155

Ounsted C, Roberts J C 1982 Fourth goal of perinatal medicine. British Medical Journal 1: 879–82

Polnay L, Pringle M 1989 General practitioner training in paediatrics in the Trent region. British Medical Journal 298 1434–1436

Rigby M J 1987 The national child health computer system. In: Macfarlane J A (ed) Progress in child health, vol 3. Churchill Livingstone, Edinburgh.

Rogers M G H 1980 Preventive aspects of child health practice. In: Mitchell R G (ed) Child health in the community, 2nd edn. Churchill Livingstone, Edinburgh

Ronalds C, Douglas A, Gray D J P, Selley P 1981 Fourth national trainee conference. Occasional Paper No.18 Royal College of General Practitioners, London

Rossdale M, Clark C, James J 1986 Improved health care delivery in an inner city well-baby clinic run by general practitioners. Journal of Royal College of General Practitioners 36: 512–513

Royal College of General Practitioners 1982 Healthier children — thinking prevention. Report from general practice No. 22. RCGP, London

Royal College of General Practitioners and British Paediatric Association 1989 Recommendations on the training and accreditation of general practitioners performing child health surveillance. Royal College of General Practitioners, London

Russell M A H, Wilson C, Tayler C, Baker C D 1979 Effect of general practitioners advice against smoking. British Medical Journal 2: 231–235

Sefi S, Macfarlane A 1989 Immunising children. Oxford University Press, Oxford

Sheridan M D 1975 From birth to five years: children's developmental progress, 2nd ed. NFER-Nelson, Windsor

Styles W McN 1989 Analysis of the hospital experience completed by general practitioner trainees in 1984–1987. Journal of the Royal College of General Practitioners 39: 96–97

Sunderlin C, Mellbin T, Vuille J C 1982 From four to ten: an overall evaluation of the general health screening of four-year olds. In: Anastivov N J, Frankenburg W S, Fandal A N (eds) Identifying the developmentally delayed child. University Park Press, Baltimore, Maryland

Taylor B 1989 Educating children and young people with special needs. British Medical Journal 298: 905–906

Wallace P, Cutler S, Haines A 1988 Randomised controlled trial of general practitioner intervention in patients with excessive alcohol consumption. British Medical Journal 297: 663–668

Waterston T 1987 Medical education in child health. In:

Macfarlane J A (ed.) Progress in child health, vol 3. Churchill Livingstone, Edinburgh

Williams P R 1985 Opportunistic surveillance of children. Letter to the editor. Journal of the Royal College of General Practitioners 35: 248–250

Wilmot J F 1984 Preparation for paediatric surveillance: a survey of trainee general practitioners. Practitioner 228: 975–977

Wilmot J F, Hancock S, Bush J, Ullyett P 1984 Paediatric surveillance, performance review and the primary care team. Journal of the Royal College of General Practitioners 34: 152–154

13. Cardiac disorders

Kevin Jones

INTRODUCTION

Any chronic or serious disease affecting children is likely to be felt deeply by parents, but the chest has a special place in the spectrum of clinical paediatrics because it carries the emotive organs of life — the heart and lungs. Many of the more severe cardiac abnormalities will have received treatment, often surgical, long before the infants are even registered on general practice lists, making the general practitioner's role one of supporting the parents in the care of their child. However, several cardiac disorders present after the first hours or days of life and are likely to first appear at the primary care level; it is therefore important that general practitioners are aware of which children are more at risk of such disorders, and the steps that can be taken to make the correct diagnosis as rapidly as possible.

With the virtual disappearance of rheumatic fever in the UK, the overwhelming majority of childhood cardiac disorders are congenital, and it is upon this group that the present chapter will focus.

Congenital heart defects occur in approximately 8 in every 1000 live births, with one-quarter of these needing treatment in the first year of life. The average general practice list of 2500 people is likely to contain 10 patients, of all ages, suffering from congenital heart disease, with one new case approximately every 5 years.

GP OBSTETRIC CARE AND CONGENITAL HEART DISEASE

GPs providing total obstetric care may encounter some presentations of congenital heart disease in the first few days of life. The GP should not be too concerned about precise anatomical diagnosis, but should arrange speedy referral to a paediatrician if there is any suspicion of unexplained tachycardia, cyanosis or heart failure. The range of causative lesions is wide, including atrioventricular septal defect, arteriovenous malformations, pulmonary or aortic atresia, severe coarctation, hypoplastic left heart syndrome, total anomalous pulmonary venous drainage and transposition of the great arteries.

LATER PRESENTATIONS OF CONGENITAL HEART DISEASE

In primary care, it is always important to ascertain why a patient is attending on any particular occasion. This is especially important in small children, where all sorts of parental concern may lead to surgery visits. Parents today may be well informed of health risks and may know some of the associations of congenital heart disease. A family history of congenital heart disease is an obvious factor of importance, but others include: preterm delivery, small for dates births, babies of diabetic or epileptic mothers (the latter because of concomitant drug therapy), the presence of other congenital abnormalities and the presence of only one umbilical artery.

Apart from presentations associated with any of these factors, children with congenital heart disease may have any of the following features: heart murmur, cyanosis, heart failure, shock, arrhythmias, fainting episodes, dyspnoea, cough, wheeze, feeding problems or failure to thrive. Examination at any of the routine checks of infancy may also reveal asymptomatic heart murmurs and it is most important to be able to identify those that are likely to be benign and those where early referral is mandatory (Keeton 1985).

THE INNOCENT HEART MURMUR

At least 50% of children have some sort of murmur that does not reflect any cardiac abnormality. These murmurs fall into three categories. A venous hum is a continuous sound in the upper chest, louder on the right in most cases, and is easily quieted by pressure on the jugular vein, or by neck movement or lying down. A vibratory parasternal ejection murmur is a low pitched midsystolic sound, usually localised and loudest at the left side of the midsternum. It gets louder when the child is supine or after exercise, and disappears by the early teenage years. An innocent pulmonary ejection murmur may be heard at the left upper sternal border, and may be easily confused with pulmonary stenosis.

The heart sounds, pulses and cardiac impulses are normal with innocent murmurs. Bruits in the neck are often also of no significance, but murmurs radiating to the back and those in diastole are not innocent.

PRESENTATION OF SPECIFIC CARDIAC LESIONS

Eighty five per cent of congenital heart disease is accounted for by the eight lesions shown in Table 13.1. Rarer lesions will not be considered further, but the presentation of the commoner lesions will be discussed under three headings: cyanosis, heart failure and asymptomatic murmurs.

Cyanosis

Tetralogy of Fallot

The most common form of cyanotic congenital heart disease is tetralogy of Fallot, occurring in 1 in 2000 live births. Some may present in early infancy, even on the first day of life, but other cases may remain undiscovered for some time. Cyanosis may be a continual feature, but some childrens' normal colour may be pink, with cyanosis showing after exercise, coughing, crying or feeding. Fatal attacks preceded by

Table 13.1 Lesions responsible for 85% of congenital heart disease

Defect	Incidence (% of all lesions)
Ventricular septal defect	25
Patent ductus arteriosus	12
Atrial septal defect	10
Pulmonary stenosis	10
Aortic stenosis (including bicuspid valve)	7
Coarctation of the aorta	7
Tetralogy of Fallot	7
Transposition of the great arteries	7

(Reproduced with permission from Hart C (ed) 1982 Child care in general practice, 2nd edn. Churchill Livingstone, Edinburgh)

unconsciousness may follow sudden exertion. Between attacks a heart murmur may be the only obvious abnormality. Squatting attacks are unlikely to be a presenting symptom.

Examination is likely to reveal a systolic thrill and a pulmonary ejection murmur, as well as possible cyanosis and clubbing. The anatomical lesions are ventricular septal defect, right ventricular outflow obstruction, right ventricular hypertrophy and overriding of the interventricular septum by the aorta. Surgical treatment now carries a good prognosis with a low operative mortality (2.5%).

Transposition of the great vessels

Occurring in one in 3000–5000 live births, transposition of the great vessels is the most common cyanotic congenital heart disease presenting in the neonatal period. Most cases present early, with profound cyanosis, no murmur and a single second heart sound. Heart failure in the first month is likely to be the initial sign where a ventricular septal defect (VSD) or patent ductus also occurs. Without treatment, almost all these children die within 2 years, but surgery in stages gives a much brighter prognosis.

Heart failure

Ventricular septal defect

Ventricular septal defect (VSD) is the most common of all congenital heart disease lesions, presenting on its own in 2 in 1000 live births, but often presenting with other abnormalities. It is also the most common cause of heart failure in the months following birth, as the pulmonary vascular resistance gradually falls. The size of the problem is determined by the size of the defect, which is very variable, and by the presence of associated lesions. A history of feeding difficulty and respiratory distress is typical.

The characteristic feature of this lesion is a harsh pansystolic murmur, which is loudest at the left sternal border, although its significance is determined by other clinical features, such as mid-diastolic apical flow murmurs, loud second heart sounds, cardiomegaly, heart failure and growth retardation. Differentiation from respiratory disease is not always easy, but the following features are more suggestive of heart failure: raised respiratory rate (above 50 per minute), breathlessness on feeding, laboured breathing, cyanosis, added sounds in the chest, palpable liver (more than two fingers), easily palpable cardiac impulse, heart murmur and sweating. Liver enlargement may be the sole abnormal physical finding in heart failure. Fever and coryza are, of course, more likely to indicate respiratory disease.

Thirty to sixty per cent of lesions close spontaneously, with many of the smaller ones resolving in the first 18 months of life. Observation and prophylaxis against endocarditis are all that many cases require, but heart failure may necessitate treatment with digoxin and diuretics. Surgery is sometimes needed for larger lesions.

Patent ductus arteriosus

The ductus is likely to be patent in premature infants and may remain open in the first day of life even in term babies. Spontaneous closure is unlikely after 2 weeks. The characteristic feature is a continuous murmur, loudest under the left clavicle, but in the first few months of life only the systolic component may be present. An increased apical pulsation and mitral diastolic flow murmur may also be evident if the shunt is large.

Treatment is by surgical closure, with an excellent prognosis as soon as possible after diagnosis, except in premature infants, where indomethacin may be used to effect closure. Endocarditis is a significant risk if surgery is delayed.

Aortic stenosis

Aortic stenosis is often asymptomatic, but may present with early heart failure. Coarctation of the aorta and patent ductus may be associated and, although the prognosis is generally good, the risk of sudden death must not be forgotten. When stenotic, the valve is usually bicuspid. Severe obstruction may also present with shortness of breath on exertion, angina and syncope.

Those at risk usually have an enlarged heart, a systolic thrill in the carotid or suprasternal notch and an ejection systolic murmur in the aortic area. Severe physical exertion must be banned on suspicion of this lesion until guidance can be obtained from a paediatric cardiologist. Treatment, where required, is surgical.

Asymptomatic murmurs

VSDs, patent ductus and aortic stenosis may present as asymptomatic murmurs, but other causes include atrial septal defect, pulmonary stenosis and coarctation of the aorta.

Atrial septal defect

Atrial septal defect (ASD) occurs in 0.6 in 1000 live births and is twice as common in girls. Several types occur and, in the most common — the ostium secundum variety — the physical signs are subtle and easily missed. There is wide, fixed splitting of the second sound with a midsystolic ejection murmur in the pulmonary area and a tricuspid regurgitant flow murmur if the shunt is large. Surgical repair is indicated in all but the smallest of lesions.

Pulmonary stenosis

Pulmonary stenosis is usually asymptomatic (although cyanosis can develop with right to left shunting) and often no treatment is required. It is associated with congenital rubella. The main physical sign is a fairly loud midsystolic murmur in the pulmonary area, often associated with a thrill and an increased cardiac impulse. Surgical treatment, if needed, carries a good prognosis, but life-long prophylaxis against endocarditis is essential.

Coarctation of the aorta

Coarctation of the aorta occurs in several forms, with early heart failure sometimes a feature, but many cases are a chance finding on examination. It is essential to include palpation of the femoral pulses in the routine examination of the cardiovascular system of children, because the diagnosis is unlikely to be made without feeling the reduced or absent pulses. Other features include an anterior and posterior systolic murmur in the upper chest, left ventricular hypertrophy, upper limb hypertension and sometimes a thrill. Surgery is usually needed and life-long antibacterial prophylaxis is necessary. If diagnosis and treatment are delayed beyond the age of 3 years, systemic hypertension may remain after surgery.

THE WIDER ROLE OF THE GENERAL PRACTITIONER

The screening role of the GP may finish with the referral of a child with suspected congenital heart disease to a specialist, but the GP's major and continuing function is only beginning at that point. Not only must the GP provide relevant clinical surveillance before and after surgical procedures, but they must also support the family through some potentially very traumatic times. It is essential that parents are given time properly to understand the cardiac abnormalities of their child and to ask questions if their doubts remain. Furthermore, they must understand what needs to happen next, why referral is necessary and what the investigations involve. The spectacle of a paediatric cardiac catheterisation laboratory may be rendered less frightening with a little forewarning.

Parents also need to be given a realistic prognosis for their child and how to treat him or her, especially in crises. The need for restriction of activities and drug treatments must be made clear. Antibiotic prophylaxis may well need a lot of explaining.

GPs may be faced with difficult questions, such as the prospects for further babies in the family, the outlook for individual children and their likely educational abilities, and queries as to why the defects have happened at all. With effective communication between the GP and the hospital, this may well prove to be a very satisfying area of primary care.

REFERENCES

Hart C 1989 Child care in general practice, 3rd edn. Churchill Livingstone, Edinburgh

Keeton B 1985 In: Hoskins S, Powell R (eds) Chronic childhood disorders. Wright, Bristol

14. Respiratory disorders

Kevin Jones

Asthma is by far the most common chronic disease of childhood and a considerable part of this chapter is devoted to its consideration. As cystic fibrosis is the most common serious inherited disease, its presentation and diagnosis are of relevance here. Other disorders considered include ciliary defects, immune deficiencies, inhaled foreign bodies and tuberculosis.

CHILDHOOD ASTHMA

It is very difficult to be certain of the true prevalence of asthma in children in the UK because of the differing criteria employed to define the disease. In September 1989, doctors from primary and secondary care met to attempt a new description, rather than a definition, of asthma and placed much greater emphasis on chronicity and inflammation than in previous descriptions. A recent review of studies in this country (Usherwood 1987) reveals lifetime prevalence estimates as widely disparate as 5 and 31%, and even recent prevalence figures (in the previous 2 years) varying from 5 to 17%.

Speight brought the problem of underdiagnosis and therefore of undertreatment in childhood asthma into the literature in 1978 (Speight 1978), but 5 years later showed that a large number of wheezy children in schools had not been properly diagnosed (Speight et al 1983). Marked improvements followed appropriate treatment but even in a practice with a special interest in asthma, on average 16 respiratory consultations were required before the diagnosis was made (Levy and Bell 1984). In the last few years there has been an explosion of interest in asthma in both the hospital and community sectors, but this has not, as yet, been accompanied by reductions in the morbidity and mortality of this common disease. Recent reviews have highlighted this problem and point strongly to primary care as the best level for improvements to occur (Anonymous 1989, Jones 1989). Before better treatment and management can begin to influence the difficulties of asthma, it is essential that underdiagnosis is addressed. This is where screening among children is essential.

It is still a commonly held belief that many children 'grow out of asthma'; this may well lead to a nihilistic attitude to the disease and its cardinal symptoms. The new (1989) description of the illness, developed at a meeting in London of asthma experts and enthusiasts from both primary and secondary care, is as follows:

Asthma is an inflammation of the airways, which is common and persistent.

This inflammation causes variable obstruction and irritability of airways, leading to cough, wheeze and tightness of the chest, often worse at night.

Inappropriate or inadequate treatment leads to continuing symptoms, permanent lung damage or even death.

In most patients, treatment should aim to suppress inflammation and its associated symptoms. Suppressive treatments are inhaled corticosteroids and cromoglycate-like drugs. Breakthrough symptoms may require bronchodilators or oral steroids.

Asthma is more common, more serious and more treatable, than previously thought.

This description may help to reinforce the view that asthma is a long-term affliction with varying symptoms, and therefore lend further weight to the argument for early diagnosis. Recent research has indicated an extremely high prevalence of reversible airways disease in the elderly (Banerjee et al 1987, Holgate & Dow 1988). This gives an all-age perspective to the issue.

Whole practice screening

The first task awaiting primary care teams is to estimate their own rate of childhood asthma diagnosis. This is by no means an easy task, especially in practices without computers, disease registers, age/sex registers or even properly sorted notes. However, a number of methods may be employed to facilitate the exercise. The first, and most simple method, is to get all the doctors to write down the names of the asthmatic children under their care and then to ask other team members to add any further known cases. Unfortunately, this process will identify only a small minority of affected children, and is woefully inadequate.

It is necessary to develop a coordinated approach appropriate to the needs and resources of each practice. Where computerised repeat prescribing exists, it should be easy to search for all children taking any of the asthma-active medications listed in the British National Formulary. This will reveal between one-third and one-half of the likely total number of asthmatics and therefore needs to be augmented by other methods. Reception staff can keep a manual record of repeat prescribing requests over a period of several months — this is clearly paramount in non-computerised practices, but can be a very useful adjunct to the process of computer searches. Additional cases may be found from hospital letters as they are read by GPs and, if notes are still being ordered and summarised, asthmatics may be identified by the noting of key words and events. This can be done by properly briefed clerical staff. Where these tasks are felt to be too difficult or too time-consuming, a significant start may be made by logging those patients presenting with acute asthma attacks both in the surgery and at home.

A combination of the different methods outlined above should produce a percentage of the list known to be asthmatic. Across the whole practice population, a figure between 5 and 10% is to be hoped for, but in children at least 10% should be identified. Anything less than this calls for a re-evaluation of diagnostic criteria by all primary care team members.

The ultimate identification technique must be a detailed examination of all the notes of children in the practice, but this is seldom a realistic proposition. However, all children are seen on multiple occasions by different members of the primary care team, and this opportunity for case-finding must be exploited.

Individual screening and case-finding

Each child in the practice normally receives a 6 week check from the GP, comes four times in the first 18 months for immunisations, has several developmental checks by the health visitor and is also likely to be seen at lease once a year by the GP for a variety of ailments. These contacts give plenty of opportunity both for considering asthma during screening attendances and for opportunistic case-finding during consultations for other reasons. It is clearly helpful to record the family history of each infant so that strong histories of asthma and atopy can be identified, but asthma is so common that all children are at risk. This diagnosis needs to be considered in every childhood consultation for respiratory symptoms.

The majority of asthmatic children can be identified by asking parents one simple question: 'Has your child ever suffered from episodes of wheezing?' However, quite a number of children do not obviously wheeze but suffer from cough, shortness of breath or sleep disturbance. Analysis of tape-recorded cough patterns has, intriguingly, shown that the cough of asthma sufferers may have a different character to other coughs (Toop 1985), although most GPs have to rely on less sophisticated observations. The cough of asthma is classically persistent and worse at night or in the early morning. It is likely to show a variable incidence over time and may also be triggered by upper respiratory tract infections, exercise, emotion, cold air, smoke, dust and pollens. The frequently heard parental statement that their child's 'Colds always go down on to the chest' is a very strong indicator of asthma. There is an interesting group of children who suffer acute bronchiolitis, usually in the first year of life, and then go on to suffer from recurrent episodes of wheeze over the next few years (Wilson 1989). These children are rarely atopic and usually grow out of this problem by the age of 5 years. Their symptoms are asthmatic and they may need anti-asthma treatment, but they are probably not 'proper' asthmatics, at least in the prognostic sense.

Confirmatory tests

Most of the difficulty in making a diagnosis of asthma lies in remembering the possibility, but there are cases in which some doubt remains and confirmatory evidence is thought desirable. The most important diagnostic tool open to the GP is the peak flow meter. There are now several suitable cheap devices admirably suited to home use, and since October 1990 they have been prescribable, a development warmly to be welcomed. The experience of New Zealand has indicated the value of this step — asthma deaths in that country have fallen since the introduction of prescribable meters (Sears 1988).

Peak flow meters can be used at home by children over the age of 5 years for a period of 2–3 weeks, and recordings made of the best of three blows morning and evening. A diurnal variation of 15% or more or a period variation (maximum reading minus minimum

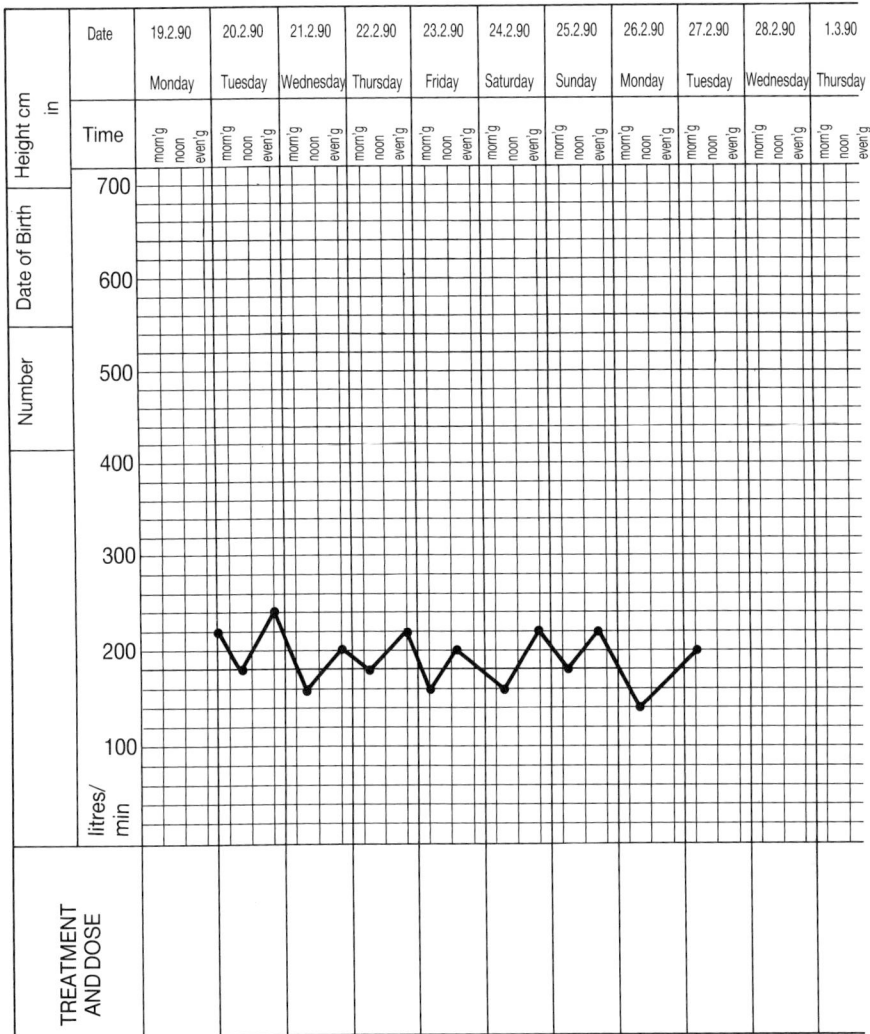

Periodic variation $= \dfrac{240-140}{140} \times 100 = 71\%$

Fig. 14.1 PEFR record in a child.

reading divided by minimum reading x 100) of 20% or more indicate asthma (see Figure 14.1). Quicker diagnostic evidence can be obtained by performing a reversibility test. This entails measuring a best initial peak flow and then administering a suitable dose of inhaled bronchodilator. Ideally this should be by means of a nebuliser to avoid any inhaler technique difficulties, but several puffs of a beta-2 agonist in a large chamber spacer will suffice. Further readings of peak flow are taken after 20 minutes and a rise of 15% is indicative of asthma. However, reversibility in asthma may not be demonstrable at the time of testing.

An exercise test may prove useful in those children where exercise seems to cause possibly asthmatic symptoms, and in others where doubt remains. This again involves a baseline estimate of peak flow but this time is followed by a 6-minute period of steady exercise. Peak flows are recorded at 5-minute intervals after the exercise, and again a drop of 15% is diagnostic. This may also reveal asthmatic tendencies in the health workers performing the test!

One avenue remains in cases of difficulty — the trial of therapy. Indeed, this may be the preferred option in many cases. Courses of inhaled bronchodilator, inhaled cromoglycate, inhaled steroid or high dose oral steroids may all be useful, provided that home peak flow monitoring also occurs. If diagnostic suspicion is suitably high, and some of these confirmatory tests are applied, there should rarely be any great difficulty in correctly identifying asthmatic children.

Many doctors may experience misgivings in recognising asthma in the first 2 years of life. The disease can and does occur at very early ages and is especially hard to treat in small infants. However, as far as making the diagnosis is concerned, the messages cited above still apply. Asthma and its cardinal symptoms should be considered and discussed at every consultation for respiratory disease, particularly in babies with a strong family history.

Asthma surveillance

At present, there is little scope for primary prevention of asthma and measures to reduce antigen exposure, such as attempting to reduce the dust mite population in atopic households, have been disappointing. Making a correct diagnosis is clearly a most important initial step in approaching the disease, but it is in the management of asthma that primary care can most reveal its potential for chronic illness surveillance. Asthma can easily become a problem more of the prescription pad than of the bronchi, because in many cases treatment gets nowhere near its intended target. Fewer than 50% of aerosol inhaler users have a good technique and significant numbers of patients also have difficulties with powder inhalers and with large chamber spacers (Jones & Middleton 1989).

The degree of knowledge of asthma that is beneficial to sufferers and their parents is not yet fully clear, but it is crucially important for three points to be confirmed in all cases. Firstly, the reason for taking each type of inhaler and its medicine, i.e. which is a 'reliever' and which a 'preventer', when suitably explained, will maximise compliance. Secondly, all asthmatics need to know when to take their drugs and in what dosage. Thirdly, and often forgotten, simple guidelines are required for the action to be taken when medications do not have their usual effect.

Performing diagnostic tests, assessing and teaching inhaler technique and giving the necessary education are all part of routine asthma screening and surveillance, but these tasks are time-consuming and do not sit easily in busy general practice, with its average 6-minute consultation. The GP alone will find asthma difficult to manage, but much can be done with teamwork. The practice nurse is the lynch-pin of the primary health care team approach to asthma and can, with training, experience and back up, provide a service to all sufferers, especially children, which can minimise the morbidity of the disease and its impact on life. Detailed consideration of nurse-run care systems in general practice is beyond the scope of this chapter, but the use of accessible, precise and disease-specific records allows the needs and development of asthmatic children to be more easily ascertained.

There are three steps in primary care asthma management and these provide a useful summary. Firstly, a practice needs to know who its asthmatics are. Secondly, all members of the team should agree on protocols for the diagnosis and treatment of asthma. Thirdly, a well documented recall system is required, which should commence by targeting more severe cases and at risk groups, including children.

ALL THAT WHEEZES IS NOT ASTHMA

Asthma is clearly the most common cause of wheeze in children and has rightly occupied a large section of this chapter. However, other pathologies can produce this symptom and should therefore not be forgotten. When cases of asthma and the so-called wheezy bronchitis are combined, 80 wheezers will have this aetiology for every one with another cause. The perspective of the diagnostic problem of wheeze is therefore obvious.

Paediatricians say that it is usually relatively easy to discern those few children with other wheezy illnesses. Wheeze can be monophonic or polyphonic — a useful differentiation factor.

Monophonic wheeze

An expiratory wheeze of constant pitch, often low, of unchanging character and often associated with inspiratory wheeze or stridor, suggests single, fixed obstruction. If this develops acutely, an inhaled foreign body should be considered. This occurs twice as frequently in boys than girls, and 80% occur under the age of 4 years. More than half the instances are caused by nuts, particularly peanuts. The right main bronchus is the most common site of impaction.

Around two-thirds of cases are diagnosed within 1 week of the event, but three factors may contribute to delayed recognition: the inhalation not being witnessed, parents not recognising the importance of apparent choking and doctors failing to appreciate the significance of a history of inhalation. This aetiology of monophonic wheeze may be suggested by an expiratory chest radiograph, but confirmation may well necessitate bronchoscopy.

Other causes are less common, but tuberculous lymphadenopathy may lead to compression of the lower end of the trachea. This is 15 to 20 times more common in children of Asian origin than in the Caucasian population. A Mantoux test is therefore useful where suspicions are raised. Occasionally, congenital lesions such as vascular rings and bronchogenic or enteric duplication cysts are the pathology behind monophonic wheeze and their diagnosis may be aided by barium meal examination. Congenital heart disease may lead to enlargement of the pulmonary artery and thus to carinal compression.

Polyphonic wheeze

Wheezes that vary in timbre and distribution are, of course, typical of asthma and the overwhelming majority of children with this physical sign do have asthma. Asthma may coexist even where other diseases are present, but it should be remembered that the most common presentation of cystic fibrosis in infancy is with wheeze.

Some children, particularly those with symptoms commencing in the perinatal period, may have ciliary disorders such as Kartagener's syndrome. Others may suffer from recurrent aspiration, which has several causes, including tracheo-oesophageal fistula. A number of rarities exist, such as generalised bronchomalacia, but a difficult and more common area of concern includes children with bronchopulmonary dysplasia and post respiratory syncytial virus (RSV) obliterative bronchiolitis. Left ventricular failure may also confuse.

CYSTIC FIBROSIS

Cystic fibrosis (CF) is the most common serious inherited disease. It is an autosomal recessive condition, occurring in approximately 1 in 2500 births, which is characterised by abnormal mucus production leading to disturbances in gut, liver, pancreas, lung and testicular function. About 50% of CF sufferers are diagnosed clinically in the first 2 years of life, but the remainder may not be evident until as late as early adulthood.

The earliest clinical manifestation of CF may be the failure to pass a meconium stool within 24 hours of birth. Typical offensive loose motions may also occur very early. Later gastrointestinal presentations include rectal prolapse, intussusception and non-specific abdominal pain. Pancreatic function drops more slowly, but is severely reduced in 85% of cases. Less than 10% have relatively normal function. Prolonged jaundice may occur in the first weeks of life and liver damage may develop later.

The lungs are normal at birth and there is no histological change in the first few months. However, respiratory symptoms have appeared by the age of 2 in almost all cases, with early severe problems being a poor prognostic sign. Involvement of the upper airways can lead to chronic sinus infection and recurrent otitis media, as well as to nasal polyps. The lungs become colonised by bacteria very early and fungi may also invade the pulmonary tissue.

Probably the most important early symptom is a persistent dry cough; at first this is non-specific but later becomes episodic with vomiting or bouts of choking. A raised respiratory rate with a clear chest is characteristic. More gross and fixed chest abnormalities gradually supervene. CF should be excluded in children with clubbing or persistent thick green sputum. Chest X-rays may be normal in the early stages.

A useful aide-memoire is that 10% of CF patients have no gut symptoms, 10% have no respiratory symptoms and the remaining 80% have the classic combination of steatorrhoea, chest disease and failure to thrive.

Screening for cystic fibrosis

The cystic fibrosis gene was discovered in September 1989 (Kerem et al 1989, Riordan et al 1989, Rommens et al 1989) and diagnosis using gene probes is currently under development. This may have some negative aspects because carriers will also be detectable, possibly to their social detriment. Antenatal diagnosis is already possible using chorionic villus sampling or amniocentesis (see Chapter 10).

The sweat test remains the gold standard of postnatal diagnosis and can be successfully performed from the age of 4 months. Other tests include the estimation of albumin levels in meconium samples and faecal trypsin assays. Neither of these tests is sufficiently reliable to be used for screening, being dependent on reduced pancreatic function. Serum and blood immunoreactive trypsin levels may be more useful. A survey of 20 000 babies using a technique with dried blood samples, as already gathered for phenylketonuria and congenital hypothyroidism screening, identified eight cystic fibrosis cases (Kuzemko & Heeley 1982). There were no false negatives and only one false positive after two specimens were tested, although the first specimen produced 57 false positives. The test is highly sensitive and specific but its predictive value is low. This is not really acceptable, therefore, as a mass screening tool, although it is probably better than many now in use.

THE CHILD WITH FREQUENT UPPER RESPIRATORY TRACT INFECTIONS

Every general practitioner is familiar with the worried parent who is forever bringing a child (or children) to the surgery with respiratory infections. Normally, reassurance that infants suffer on average seven upper respiratory infections per year, combined with advice to reduce parental smoking, will be sufficient. However, abnormalities of host defence, ciliary changes and deficiencies in both specific and non-specific immune systems may occur.

Proper defence of the lungs requires normal cough and sneeze reflexes, balanced ventilation and perfusion, normal mucous membranes and secretions, and functioning cilia. Neuromuscular diseases cause alterations in reflexes and indeed, the most common presentation of myasthenia gravis in childhood is with recurrent respiratory infections. Congenital aberrations of arteries, veins or bronchi may alter the ventilation–perfusion balance, as exemplified by total anomalous pulmonary venous drainage. Cystic fibrosis has already been discussed.

Primary ciliary dysfunction occurs in 1 in 15 000 children, but in 15% of those with dextrocardia. It has an autosomal recessive inheritance and may well present with frequent respiratory infections. Other presentations include neonatal respiratory distress, chronic nasal obstruction or discharge, recurrent otitis media and conductive deafness, chronic productive cough and male sterility.

The diagnosis can be made by examining nasal biopsies under light and electron microscopy, and should be suspected in all children with dextrocardia, neonates with unexplained respiratory distress and infants with either chronic nasal discharge or recurrent lower respiratory tract infections.

Severe combined immunodeficiency occurs in 14 per million births and normally presents early with multisystem problems. Cell-mediated immunity alone may be defective (DiGeorge syndrome) and there are a number of types of antibody deficiency. X-linked agammaglobulinaemia occurs in 1 in 500 000 children, but some immunoglobulin deficiency may be present in 1 in 10 000. Deficiency in IgA is well recognised, and IgG_2 subclass deficiency seems to be related to asthma as well as to recurrent chest infections.

Non-specific immune dysfunctions include many very rare complement disorders, one of which involves reduced opsonisation of bacteria and thus leads to repeated infection. Neutrophils may have reduced numbers as in cyclical neutropaenia, abnormal structure, poor mobility or reduced bacterial killing.

These conditions may seem far removed from primary care, but they are worth bearing in mind when faced with the child with frequent otitis media and suppurative chest infections.

TUBERCULOSIS

Formal screening for tuberculosis (TB) is no longer performed at any age in the UK, but cases do still occur. Children with TB are most likely to be found in families of Asian origin, especially any recent arrivals in this country. Sadly, another group of TB sufferers likely to increase in numbers is those children suffering from AIDS. However, in certain areas of the UK patients do contract TB without being in any special risk category. The role of the GP in identification of this disease is simply to keep the diagnosis in mind when faced with higher risk children.

CONCLUSION

The majority of chest disease in children presenting to the GP is always going to be the frequent, self-limiting upper respiratory tract infections that populate almost every surgery. However, in the continuing care of asthma and the other illnesses discussed in the chapter, the GP may find some of the most taxing and yet fulfilling aspects of family medicine.

REFERENCES

Anonymous 1989 Management of asthma in the community. Lancet 2: 199–200

Banerjee D K, Lee G S, Malik S K, Daly S 1987 Underdiagnosis of asthma in the elderly. British Journal of Diseases of the Chest 81: 23–29

Holgate S T, Dow L 1988 Airways disease in the elderly: an easy to miss diagnosis. Journal of Respiratory Diseases 9: 14–22

Jones K P 1989 Asthma — still a challenge for general practice. Journal of the Royal College of General Practitioners 39: 254–256

Jones K P, Middleton M 1989 Benefits of an inhaler-technique scoring system. Update 38: 1399–1403

Kerem B, Rommens J M, Buchanan J A et al 1989 Identification of the cystic fibrosis gene: genetic analysis. Science 245: 1073–80

Kuzemko J A, Heeley A F 1986 Diagnostic methods and screening. Journal of the Royal Society of Medicine 79: 2–5

Levy M, Bell L 1984 General practice audit of asthma in childhood. British Medical Journal 289: 1115–1116

Riordan J R, Rommens J M, Kerem B et al 1989 Identification of the cystic fibrosis gene: cloning and characterisation of complementary DNA. Science 245: 1066–73

Rommens J M, Ianuzzi M C, Kerem B et al 1989 Identification of the cystic fibrosis gene: chromosome walking and jumping. Science 245: 1059–65

Sears M 1988 Increasing asthma mortality — fact or artifact. Journal of Allergy and Clinical Immunology 82: 957–960

Speight A N P 1978 Is childhood asthma being underdiagnosed and undertreated? British Medical Journal 2: 331–332

Speight A N P, Lee D A, Hey E N 1983 Underdiagnosis and undertreatment of asthma in childhood. British Medical Journal 286: 1253–1257

Toop L J 1985 Active approach to recognising asthma in general practice. British Medical Journal 290: 1629–1631

Usherwood T P 1987 Factors affecting estimates of the prevalence of asthma and wheezing in childhood. Family Practice 4: 318–321

Wilson N M 1989 Wheezy bronchitis revisited. Archives of Diseases of Childhood 64: 1194–1199

15. Disorders of metabolism

Jacqueline Jolleys

NEONATAL SCREENING

For the majority of inborn errors of metabolism the risk of an inherited abnormality is recognised only after the birth of an affected child. Where possible, screening tests have been developed to permit the screening of all neonates for certain inherited and treatable conditions.

Routine screening of newborn infants for metabolic disorders has been in use for more than a quarter of a century. The original blood test was developed by Guthrie for the early detection of phenylketonuria, but the concept has gradually been expanded so that about 50 different conditions can be detected in this way.

Before screening programmes were available, the clinician required a positive family history and a high level of suspicion before considering the diagnosis of metabolic disorder. Screening processes now allow all children equal opportunity to be tested and evaluated, and screening is effective so long as test procedures are carefully followed and results accurately interpreted.

The availability of screening tests is subject to current government legislation and guidelines for screening tests are supplied by the public health departments. Most newborn infants must be screened for hyperphenylalaninaemia (PHP), phenylketonuria (PKU) and congenital hypothyroidism (CH). Additional tests are available for sickle-cell disease and other red blood cell abnormalities, galactosaemia, homocystinuria and maple syrup urine disease. In the future there may be neonatal screening for congenital adrenal hyperplasia, alpha-1-antitrypsin deficiency and hypercholesterolaemia.

A number of criteria have to be considered before a condition is considered suitable for mass screening:

1. The condition should be sufficiently frequent and severe to be a public health concern. Only hypothyroidism and PKU meet this requirement (see Table 15.1) but a case can be made for other, rarer, serious diseases if testing adds little to the cost of the screening programme.
2. The test should be simple, reliable and have a low incidence of false positive and false negative results (high sensitivity and specificity).
3. The condition should be amenable to treatment.
4. Ideally there should be a cost advantage to society. Screening for PKU and hypothyroidism has a favourable cost benefit ratio; other screening tests offer little or no financial incentive and in these cases the benefit is, above all, to the family concerned.

Screening tests are generally performed on small quantities of blood collected on standardised filter paper cards. Specimens are obtained at the time of discharge from the maternity unit and by the general practitioner or community midwife in the case of a home confinement, early discharge or general practitioner maternity unit confinement. A repeat sample for hyperphenylalaninaemia and phenylketonuria is required before the third week after birth if

Table 15.1 Approximate incidence at birth of genetically determined metabolic disease in Caucasians

Disease	Incidence
Cystic fibrosis	1 in 2000
Congenital adrenal hyperplasia	1 in 5000
Neonatal hypothyroidism	1 in 6000
Histidinaemia	1 in 11 000
Phenylketonuria	1 in 12 000
Cystinuria	1 in 17 000
Iminoglycinuria	1 in 17 000
Hartnup disease	1 in 24 000
Glycinuria	1 in 100 000
Hyperglycinaemias	1 in 100 000
Galactosaemia	1 in 120 000
Homocystinuria	1 in 160 000
Maple syrup urine disease	1 in 175 000
Alkaptonuria	1 in 300 000

the first sample was taken at 24-hour disharge, or before sufficient milk intake to allow accurate testing.

Phenylketonuria and hypothyroidism, both of which are treatable if diagnosed early, are routinely tested for in the United Kingdom using the blood spot collected from neonates (Medical Research Council 1981, Grant & Smith 1988). Other tests are not yet carried out routinely, although early screening may be introduced for galactosaemia (Hausen 1988) and hypercholesterolaemia. When suitable screening tests are available and the economic situation permits, routine screening for homocystinuria and maple syrup urine disease would be worthwhile. These diseases, as well as tyrosinaemia and sickle-cell and abnormal haemoglobinaemias, are already screened for routinely in many of the states of America without parental consent, each state having autonomy over public health policy.

All neonates in whom a genetic disorder is suspected or who fail to thrive should be fully investigated. Newborn infants with undiagnosed illness or a serious respiratory acidosis or who fail to thrive need immediate referral to an experienced paediatrician. Neonates with an inborn metabolic disorder may present with similar clinical signs to those with a cardiorespiratory disease or sepsis. Special investigations are immediately ordered in these cases in consultation with specialised, highly experienced laboratory workers. Accurate diagnosis will follow in a proportion of these cases, leading to effective treatment where possible. In others the diagnosis may be less certain and further investigation at central laboratories with special facilities may be indicated. A false negative result is possible, so when there is a strong clinical suspicion the tests should be repeated, or a more sensitive test performed.

Galactosaemia and maple syrup urine disease are both life-threatening soon after birth and the appropriate tests may be urgently ordered when the paediatrician and clinical biochemist work in consultation. Neonates with galactosaemia, keto acid and amino acid disorders die unless early diagnosis is made and treatment is essential if handicap is to be avoided.

Biochemical tests can be conducted on fluid or tissue from the neonate if a genetic condition is suspected. Even in the event of neonatal death, examination of post-mortem material is indicated to confirm the diagnosis, so that the parents may be advised on the risk of subsequent children being affected. In the future there may be emphasis on prenatal diagnosis so that treatment, if available, may begin at birth.

PRENATAL SCREENING

Prenatal diagnosis is important when there is a known risk of a genetic disorder, when there has been a previous affected pregnancy or when one parent has a known genetic abnormality (see also Chapter 10). By analysing the amniotic fluid, either through cell histology or by enzyme and chemical assessment of the amniotic fluid itself, an inborn error of metabolism may be diagnosed. When such a disorder caused by a recessive gene is confirmed in an offspring, the parents may be given accurate genetic counselling on the relative risk of further children being affected and they may choose prenatal diagnosis if an appropriate and sensitive test is available.

Chorionic villous sampling has recently become available. This is performed under direct vision or ultra sound guidance at 8 weeks gestation. Fetal tissue collected in this way can be analysed for abnormal or absent enzymes or their products, normal or abnormal genes recognised by recombinant DNA restriction analysis (Lesch–Nyhan Syndrome) or abnormalities of gene markers (gene mapping analysis) noted when the gene defect itself is not known (phenylhydroxidase or alpha-1-antitrypsin). The recessively inherited conditions — cystic fibrosis and phenylketonuria — are single gene disorders that may be diagnosed prenatally using DNA techniques. There is still a slight risk of miscarriage of a normal fetus subsequent to the test. However, a therapeutic abortion of a fetus affected by a metabolic disorder can thus be offered early in the pregnancy. Prior to this, prenatal diagnosis was limited to the midtrimester — around 18 weeks — when amniocentesis could be performed, and cells cultured for biochemical and cytological diagnosis. A major problem consequent on this examination was that therapeutic abortions were therefore offered during the second trimester, with the risk of severe psychological harm to the mother.

The role of the general practitioner in neonatal screening and prenatal diagnosis

Genetically determined medical conditions not only make considerable demands on the health resources of the community, they also create a psychological and physical health burden on the affected person and the family. There may also be economic pressures consequent on the additional needs of a handicapped person.

Neonatal screening is not normally the responsibility of the general practitioner; the midwife, under the direction of the community paediatricians and regional screening laboratory, usually conducts the tests at the specified time. Parents are not normally given the opportunity to discuss the tests, neither are the implications of the test explored. Parents require increasingly more information so that they can be involved in decision-making. General practitioners are encouraged to do more of the paediatric surveillance currently performed by community paediatricians. As the screening programme is further extended, with the development of cheap and reliable tests, there will be a demand for information and counselling from many parents. It is likely that they will turn to the general practitioner for this, with the result that there will need to be more liaison between the community health services and general practitioners. At the moment the screening takes place without communication with the general practitioner. Even if an abnormal result is found, the general practitioner is not always informed. Referral for further tests to confirm the diagnosis may be made and the first the general practitioner hears of it may be when the concerned parents consult to discuss their fears.

General practitioners may feel able to give advice on genetic problems themselves or may wish to refer the patient for specialist help to a clinical geneticist. Genetic counselling is discussed in detail in Chapter 10.

DISEASES DETECTABLE AT BIRTH

Galactosaemia

Galactosaemia is caused by a genetic deficiency responsible for the synthesis of the enzyme galactose-1-phosphate uridyl transferase, which is involved in the conversion of galactose to glucose. Children with the disease fail to thrive and the accumulation of galactose and galactose-1-phosphate causes mental retardation, liver damage and jaundice, cataracts, renal tubular acidosis, hypoglycaemia and amino aciduria. Routine screening is essential because early diagnosis and immediate life-long treatment on a galactose-free diet can preserve normal mental development and growth. These children can synthesise mucopolysaccharides and lipids containing galactose by an alternative chemical pathway.

Disorders of amino acid metabolism

Phenylketonuria (PKU) and associated conditions of tyrosine metabolism disturbance

Phenylketonuria is caused by a hereditary deficiency of the enzyme phenylalanine hydroxylase, which is responsible for converting phenylalanine to tyrosine by

Table 15.2 Inborn errors of metabolism recorded according to time when the condition is usually recognised and clinical presentation

Birth

Conditions usually recognised perinatally
Cretinism
Albinism
Alkaptonuria
Hurler's syndrome
Congenital adrenal hyperplasia
Congenital hyperbilirubinaemia
Congenital erythropoietic porphyria
Hunter's syndrome
Methaemoglobinaemia

Conditions identified by screening at birth
Phenylketonuria
Tyrosinaemia
Maple syrup urine disease
Galactosaemia
Homocystinuria

First year of life

Conditions that may present as failure to thrive
Cystic fibrosis
Disaccharide deficiencies and intolerances
Hypogammaglobulinaemia
Lysine intolerance
Fructose intolerance
Glycogen storage disease

Childhood
Lesch–Nyhan syndrome
Erythropoietic porphyria
Wilson's disease

Conditions that may present with renal calculi
Cystinuria
Primary hyperoxaluria
Xanthinuria

Conditions that may present with anaemia
Glucose-6-phosphate dehydrogenase deficiency
Acute haemolytic anaemia
Hereditary orotic acidaemia
Chronic non-sperocytic haemolytic anaemia (enzyme deficiency)

Conditions that may present with vitamin D-resistant rickets
Fanconi's syndrome
Tyrosinaemia
Hypophosphatasia
Sex-linked familial vitamin D-resistant rickets
Cholinesterase deficiency
Acute intermittent porphyria

Puberty
Variegate porphyria

hydroxylation in the liver. This causes an accumulation of phenylalanine in the blood and tissues and an excessive excretion of phenylalanine in the urine. It results in severe mental retardation. Treatment with a low phenylalanine diet is started as soon as possible. There are three types of phenylketonuria and recognition of the type is essential to predict the effect of treatment and the prognosis.

1. Mild, physiological, causing no mental retardation. Diet not essential.
2. Classic PKU, which responds to dietary restriction.
3. Malignant PKU, which does not respond to dietary restriction.

Despite early diagnosis and dietary control, malignant PKU progresses to severe cerebral dysfunction. It is not known whether the mental deficiency is caused by the toxic effects of phenylalanine or its derivatives or, as is more likely in malignant PKU, is secondary to a fundamental enzyme abnormality.

In the UK, Government recommendations (HM (69) 72) have meant that all children have been screened for PKU since 1969. This is done by laboratory testing of a heel prick blood sample from newborn infants between the sixth and fourteenth days of life — the Guthrie test. If a raised level of phenylalanine is found, further tests are carried out to make a more precise diagnosis. A recent review of PKV screening in the United Kingdom in 1984–1988 showed almost 100% coverage, with 44.5 cases being identified, an incidence of 11.7/100 000 births (Smith et al 1991).

Homocystinuria

Homocystinuria is an uncommon disorder causing mental retardation and renal failure, although some children affected by the deficiency of the enzyme cystathionine may have normal intelligence but suffer from skeletal abnormalities, such as arachnodactyly, and may later develop dislocated optic lenses. Dietary restriction of selected proteins and amino acids may be beneficial.

Maple syrup urine disease

Maple syrup urine disease is an uncommon disease caused by deficiency of oxidative decarboxylase and resulting in the excretion of excess three-branched chain amino acids and their keto acids. The urine has the odour of burnt sugar or maple syrup as a result. Neurological disturbances develop soon after birth and the affected infant has feeding difficulties and develops spasticity and opisthotonus; there is an absence of the Moro reflex. Death occurs within a few months. If the disease is discovered at neonatal screening, a diet low in three-branched chain amino acids has been shown successful in preventing the manifestations of the disease (Therrell 1987a).

Tyrosinosis

This is a rare condition due to a defect in the enzyme p-hydroxyphenylpyruvate oxidase. The urine gives a positive ferric chloride test, as in PKU, and a positive Benedict's test, and serum tyrosine is raised. It is a serious disease and may result in death. Some infants get diarrhoea and vomiting, haematemesis and melaena, haematuria, abdominal distension due to hepatosplenomegaly and ascites. Others have a more chronic, protracted illness with liver cirrhosis, steatorrhoea and renal tubular defects resulting in rickets. Treatment by a diet low in tyrosine, phenylalanine and perhaps methionine can be successful in preventing the development of the disease.

Hypercholesterolaemia

Familial hypercholesterolaemia (FH II) is an autosomal dominant inherited defect of lipid metabolism, affecting the apolipoprotein B receptor. It occurs in 1 in 500 of the population. The atherogenic low density lipoprotein is increased and this genetic defect accounts for 5% of myocardial infarctions under the age of 60. With early detection, the morbidity and mortality in the fourth and fifth decades are preventable with diet and drug regimes. It is possible to identify those who are at risk and who possibly have this defect by neonatal dried blood spot immunophelometric examination (Therrel 1987b, Ohta et al 1988). This test is not yet available but research is being conducted in several centres around the world. It is anticipated that screening for dyslipidaemias would lead to life-long dietary modification and possible drug treatment for the affected child and the neonatal blood spot would act as a marker for families at risk of premature vascular disease and family-based coronary prevention programmes could then be implemented. This would benefit the parents and other young family members (see also Chapter 20).

Congenital hypothyroidism

The child suffering from congenital hypothyroidism (cretinism) can often be recognised from his/her appearance. The infant has macroglossia, course facies and a short, thick neck. The hands and feet are broad and there is often a small umbilical hernia. The skin is thickened and may feel cool, and the infant has a hoarse cry. Early thyroxine replacement prevents or reduces the associated mental retardation. Any baby found to have a higher than normal serum thyroid-stimulating hormone (TSH) level at 5–7 days on examination of dried blood film must be investigated and treatment must be started immediately. Identification of congenital hypothyroidism late in the first few months of life will delay the start of treatment and will result in permanent mental damage. If congenital hypothyroidism is suspected on clinical grounds, although the neonatal TSH is normal, the TSH test should be repeated — errors can occur.

Congenital adrenal hyperplasia

The adrenogenital syndrome results from the homozygous expression of the autosomal recessive defect responsible for the biosynthesis of adrenal steroid hormones. This results in a deficiency of cortisol and negative feedback stimulates the overproduction of corticotrophin (ACTH) and corticotrophin-releasing hormone (CRH). This, in turn, results in an excess production of steroid intermediates such as 17-hydroxy-progesterone, formed prior to the defect. Virilisation results because androgen synthesis is unaffected. A blood spot filter paper assay for 17-hydroxy-progesterone may soon be available for screening for 21-hydroxylase deficiency in neonates, the most common of these enzyme defects (Therrell 1987c).

Alpha-1-antitrypsin deficiency

A screening test for this condition has been developed and is being evaluated. Cord blood can be analysed for alpha-1-antitrypsin concentration and a deficiency detected. It is an autosomal dominant condition, which plays an important role in the development of early panlobular emphysema and neonatal liver disease. It is also associated with chronic juvenile rheumatoid arthritis, immunological disorders and chronic urticaria. Five per cent of the population have a partial deficiency in its synthesis, so screening may be warranted. Causal treatment is not currently available. Recombinant alpha-1-antitrypsin has been obtained from yeasts and *Escherichia coli* and may become available for treatment in the future (Kimpen et al 1988).

Cystic fibrosis

This is the most common inherited metabolic disease in Caucasians. It is an autosomal recessive condition affecting the exocrine glands in 1 in 3500 live births. Heterozygous parents have a 1 in 4 chance of producing a child with cystic fibrosis. The basic biochemical defect is unknown. Patients with cystic fibrosis may develop obstructive pulmonary disease with recurrent complications due to the increased viscosity of the secretions. Hepatic and renal function may be affected by the development of cor pulmonale and congestive cardiac failure. Much activity is currently focused on screening for this condition, including an assay of immunoreactive trypsin using blood spots similar to those collected for the Guthrie test for PKU (Ryley et al 1988). Cystic fibrosis is discussed in greater detail in Chapters 10 and 14.

DISEASES DETECTABLE IN CHILDHOOD

Diabetes mellitus

Diabetes mellitus is not screened for at birth or at developmental surveillance appointments because the presentation of the disease is acute and there is no detectable presymptomatic phase. Nevertheless, it is quite common: a general practitioner's list with 2000 patients is likely to include two insulin-dependent child diabetics. Diabetes mellitus is a state of chronic hyperglycaemia usually accompanied by glycosuria. It may be caused by an absolute lack of insulin, as in the failure of the B cells of the islets of Langerhans, or by a relative lack of insulin because of an excess of antagonising hormones or insulin-inhibiting substance. For this reason, such a diabetic may require more insulin than a person who has undergone pancreatectomy.

There are two types of diabetes, type 1, or juvenile onset, which is insulin-dependent or requires oral hypoglycaemia agents, and type 2, or maturity onset, which may be controlled by diet or hypoglycaemic drugs. Some young patients develop type 2 diabetes — the aetiology may be genetic or environmental. Type 1 may follow infection with mumps complicated by pancreatitis or Coxsackie B1–B4. Diabetes may be the result of exposure to viruses and chemical agents, whereby the beta cells are destroyed by an immunological process.

Diabetes mellitus in a child is an acute illness with marked thirst, polyuria and loss of weight. Abdominal pain, vomiting and anorexia may occur in the precoma phase. Diagnosis is confirmed by the presence of glycosuria, ketonuria and elevated blood sugar.

Initially the diabetic child is admitted to hospital for stabilisation and correction of the ketoacidosis and dehydration. Renal glycosuria may occasionally be demonstrated in a child presenting with enuresis.

Disorders of storage

Mucopolysaccharidoses

These conditions are due to inherited deficiencies of enzymes required for the normal metabolism of connective tissue mucopolysaccharide, resulting in a deposition of mucopolysaccharides. Patients are characterised by mental retardation, skeletal changes, corneal clouding and visceral involvement.

Hurler's syndrome (gargoylism) is mucopolysaccharidosis type 1, an autosomal recessive condition. It is often recognisable at birth or in infancy by grotesque features, large head, wide set eyes, broad nose with a flattened bridge, short neck, incomplete extension of the fingers and protruberant abdomen, often with an umbilical hernia due to enlargement of the liver and spleen. The skin is dry and coarse. Although there are biochemical tests to confirm the diagnosis, there is no treatment for the condition.

Mucopolysaccharidosis type 2 — Hunter's syndrome — is sex-linked and is less severe than type 1. Clouding of the cornea does not occur, although deafness is common.

Although there is no treatment for these conditions, much can be done to support the parents of affected children. They should, of course, be given genetic counselling.

Lipidoses

The lipidoses include Gaucher's disease, Niemann–Pick disease and Tay–Sach's disease. It may be that these and the mucopolysaccharidoses are not such defined disorders, because cases have been published whereby different members of the same family suffer from various lipidoses or mucopolysaccharidoses. Lipidoses are caused by abnormal intracellular deposition of sphingolipids, both generalised and localised, due to abnormality of specific lysosomal hydrolases. Each condition has different clinical features affecting the brain and nervous system. There is no treatment for these disorders.

Glycogen storage diseases

There are many forms of glycogen storage disease depending on which enzyme is deficient. Diagnosis is confirmed by glycogen and enzyme estimations on liver, muscle or jejunal biopsy. Von Gierke's disease is due to glucose-6-phosphatase deficiency and is suspected when there are hepatosplenomegaly, attacks of hypoglycaemia and ketosis and when the infant fails to thrive.

Disaccharide intolerance and disaccharidase deficiencies

Carbohydrate-induced diarrhoea may be due to congenital or aquired enzyme deficiency. Affected children suffer from malabsorption of a specific carbohydrate, causing enteritis and failure to thrive. Profuse watery diarrhoea starts with milk feeding in lactose deficiency and sucrose in sucrase deficiency. Fructose intolerance is a serious autosomal recessive condition due to fructose-1-phosphate aldolase deficiency in the liver and kidney. The infants become jaundiced, develop hepatosplenomegaly and fail to thrive. Convulsions and coma occur on weaning on to sucrose. If recognised, all these conditions can be treated by dietary manipulation.

PAEDIATRIC SURVEILLANCE

Suitably trained general practitioners can provide and are increasingly encouraged to provide child health surveillance for the under 5-year-olds on their lists. The District Health Authorities specify a surveillance schedule broadly based on the recommendations of the Joint Working Party on Child Health Surveillance (Hall 1989, see also Chapter 12). A typical schedule would be:

Neonatal;
10 days;
6 weeks;
8 months;
21 months;
39 months.

Many of the metabolic disorders are noted at birth or perinatally at one of the screening examinations. Others manifest during the first year of life, often with repeated respiratory illness or gastroenterological signs. Despite negative neonatal screening, if a condition is suspected on clinical grounds rescreening is advisable because laboratory or reporting errors can occur and delay in diagnosis can have serious sequelae.

A disorder of metabolism may be suspected if the infant is failing to thrive — falling behind on the centile chart for height and weight. Another early manifestation of metabolic disease may be the retention of primitive reflexes, or delay in attaining developmental milestones. The child's appearance may arouse suspicion — an unusual facies or bearing no

resemblance to either parent. As parents are often the first to comment on the child's slow development or differences between the baby and its siblings, their concerns should not be ignored.

REFERENCES

Grant D B, Smith I 1988 Survey of neonatal screening for primary hypothyroidism in England, Wales, Northern Ireland 1982–4 British Medical Journal 296: 1355

Hall D M B 1989 Health for all children: a programme for child health surveillance. Oxford University Press, Oxford

Hansen T 1988 Galactosaemia — to screen or not to screen? Paediatrics 81: 327

Kimpen J, Bosmans E, Raus J 1988 Neonatal screening for alpha-1-antitrypsin deficiency. European Journal of Pediatrics 148: 86

Medical Research Council Steering Committee for MRC/DHSS Phenylketonuria Register 1981 Routine screening for phenylketonuria in the United Kingdom 1964–78. British Medical Journal 282: 1680

Ohta T, Masahiro M, Yasutake T, Matsuda I 1988 Enzyme linked immunosorbant assay for apolipoprotein B on dried

blood spot derived from newborn infant: its application to neonatal mass screening for hypercholesterolaemia. Journal of Paediatric Gastroenterology and Nutrition 7: 524

Ryley H C, Deam S M, Williams J et al 1988 Neonatal screening for cystic fibrosis in Wales and the West Midlands. 1. Evaluation of immunoreactive trypsin test. Journal of Clinical Pathology 41: 276

Smith I, Cook B, Beasley M 1991 Review of neonatal screening programme for phenylketonuria. British Medical Journal 303: 333–335

Therrell B L 1987a Advances in neonatal screening. Excerpta Medica International Congress Series 741. p. 217

Therrell B L 1987b Advances in neonatal screening. Excerpta Medica International Congress Series 741. p 325

Therrel B L 1987c Advances in neonatal screening. Excerpta Medica International Congress Series 741. p 273

16. Orthopaedic disorders in childhood

Nicholas M P Clarke

INTRODUCTION

Screening is 'the presumptive identification of unrecognised disease or defect by the application of tests, examinations or other procedures which can be applied rapidly' (Commission on Chronic Illness 1957). In the context of deformity and disability in paediatric orthopaedics it may appear that screening programmes are ideal methods of reducing morbidity. Nevertheless, in practice, formal screening in paediatric orthopaedics relates primarily to the detection of congenital dislocation of the hip (CDH) and scoliosis. Several factors must be considered in the assessment of a screening programme for any disorder (see also Chapter 2). The screening test must be accurate and safe, and this particularly applies to congenital dislocation of the hip. The treatment of cases diagnosed at screening should be effective and its indications agreed — for instance, there is considerable controversy about the place of early or delayed splintage in the management of CDH. The disease for which the population is to be screened should be important, have a known natural history and should be better treated before the usual time of clinical presentation — scoliosis and CDH may well not fulfil these criteria because of diverse opinions relating to the natural history of the disease. The screening programme should also be practical and economical.

This chapter will consider the role of screening in relation to CDH, scoliosis and atlanto-axial instability in Down syndrome.

CONGENITAL DISLOCATION OF THE HIP

Congenital dislocation of the hip (CDH) has been defined as 'a spectrum of deformation of the hip joint present at birth in which the head of the femur is, or may be, displaced from the acetabulum. The term embraces secondary hip joint dysplasia, whether or not instability or dislocation persists' (The Standing Medical Advisory Committee 1986a). Indeed, congenital 'displacement' of the hip is probably a better term.

The reported incidence of CDH varies widely from 2 to approximately 50 per 1000 births. This wide variation occurs mainly as a result of the subjective nature of the tests on which the diagnosis depends. Additionally, ethnic and geographical differences, and the age at which the infant is first examined, contribute. The publication by Von Rosen (1956) commenced a new era in the management of CDH and early splintage of unstable hips in abduction remains the basis for current treatment programmes. It was the confidence in diagnostic tests for CDH introduced by Barlow (1962) and Ortolani (1937) that led to the belief that most cases could be treated without recourse to later surgery. Indeed, it is still generally accepted that most cases of CDH are more easily treated in the neonate by splintage rather than by the surgery that is often required in the older infant. For this reason considerable effort is expended in screening for hip abnormalities at birth.

Aetiology and incidence

CDH is closely associated with congenital postural deformities, such as torticollis, scoliosis and foot deformities. These deformities in turn are related to primiparity, oligohydramnios and breech presentation (Dunn 1976). CDH is four times more common in girls, probably as a result of induced hormonal laxity of joints. Nearly 20% of all hip dislocations occur with a breech presentation and it has been estimated that the incidence of CDH at birth is doubled in a first pregnancy (Dunn 1987). A female infant delivered in the breech position has a risk of CDH of 1 in 35.

A positive family history of CDH is an additional risk factor and may be obtained in up to 33% of patients. A second child has a ten-fold increase of the risk of CDH if the first child is affected. Postnatal factors also contribute: swaddling the hips in extension as performed by certain ethnic groups may adversely affect normal hip development.

The incidence of late presentation of established CDH remains at approximately 1 to 2 per 1000 births, despite neonatal screening programmes.

Diagnosis and terminology

Ortolani described the reduction manoeuvre that bears his name in 1937. Barlow (1962) subsequently described a modification of the clinical tests to provoke hip displacement. The Ortolani and Barlow tests form the basis of the clinical examination that is currently used to detect CDH in neonates.

The clinical examination is performed with the infant lying quietly and relaxed whilst supine. The knee is flexed and the middle finger is placed over the greater trochanter. The examiner's thumb and index finger grasp the anterior aspect of the knee. The level of the greater trochanter is assessed to ensure that it is symmetrical. The Ortolani test is performed by gently lifting the trochanter towards the acetabulum as the leg is abducted. As the manoeuvre is performed a dislocated hip reduces with a palpable clunk (Ortolani positive). In the Barlow test the leg is gently held in the same way. One hip is tested at a time as the other hand steadies the pelvis. The leg is gently adducted past the midline and gentle downward pressure results in provoked displacement of a 'dislocatable' hip, i.e. a located hip dislocates.

Terms of abnormality correlate with the tactile interpretation of the tests. Hips may thus be described as dislocated, dislocatable or subluxable. Similarly, a hip may be said to 'click' on examination. This may imply uncertainty on the part of the examiner about the stability of the hip or may describe the tactile subjective sensation of a click in a stable hip.

The detection of a 'clicking' hip at a clinical examination is common. Most hip clicks are innocent, although displaced hips may be more frequent in this group (Cunningham et al 1984).

The Ortolani and Barlow tests should be performed within the first 24 hours of life, as resolution of clinical instability may occur rapidly without the hip necessarily becoming normal (Clarke 1986). Tests may reveal hip instability up to about 6 weeks of age, thereafter the clinical examination places more emphasis on limitation of hip abduction, thigh shortening and asymmetry. After about 3 months of age the dislocated hip becomes stable in the dislocated position and the Ortolani sign disappears. However,

secondary changes occur with tightness of hip abduction. Finally, after walking age, a unilateral hip dislocation will give rise to a limp; a waddling gait is associated with bilateral dislocation.

A dislocated hip in a newborn occasionally presents with severe restriction of hip abduction and a dislocated hip that cannot be reduced by the Ortolani manoeuvre. Such a dislocation is usually termed 'teratologic' and may be due to arthrogryposis, sacral agenesis and other rare disorders.

Effectiveness of neonatal screening programmes

Doubt has recently been cast upon the efficiency of neonatal screening for CDH, because the incidence of late established cases has not been reduced. Barlow originally stated that 60% of unstable hips at birth would be clinically normal at 1 week of age without any intervention. Accordingly, Leck (1986) has estimated that there is a high incidence of false positive results. He has also stated that the prevalence of false negatives averages about half as much as the prevalence of CDH in unscreened populations. Difficulties in ensuring the efficiency of screening programmes arise from the two basic premises upon which the programme depends:

1. It is assumed that adequately trained personnel can detect all abnormal hips at birth by clinical examination. Clinical examiners often vary in status and expertise and medical staff may often be required to perform the clinical test without ever having examined an abnormal hip.
2. There is an implicit assumption that all abnormal hips are indeed abnormal on clinical testing.

Early management of neonatal hip instability

Uncertainty in this area creates furthur difficulties. The early splintage of the unstable hip with an abduction device is regarded as the most successful method of early treatment. However, given that many unstable hips resolve spontaneously in the first week, such a policy means that many neonates are probably treated unnecessarily. Additionally, immediate rigid abduction and splintage may be associated with a risk of compressive vascular injury to the vulnerable femoral head, resulting in avascular necrosis. For this reason, delayed splintage may be performed. Thus, there are three components to the therapeutic dilemma:

1. Which of the hips, unstable at birth, will spontaneously resolve and thus not require treatment?

2. Does resolution of clinical hip instability necessarily mean that the hip has become normal?
3. Should splintage be immediate or delayed?

Knowledge of the natural history of hip instability in the first weeks of life would considerably assist those who are confronted with these problems.

Ultrasound

Ultrasound is becoming a useful adjunct to the clinical examination of the infant hip in experienced hands (Clarke et al 1985). It is non-invasive and can provide an accurate picture of the joint; a dynamic examination may provide evidence of instability on provocation. Consequently, ultrasound examinations can provide scientific data on which to base the management of a displaced unstable hip (Clarke 1986). The natural history of the suspect hip can be sonographically documented. At present the place of routine ultrasound screening of the hips has not been determined in terms of cost or practicability.

Recommendations

There remains some controversy about the effectiveness of neonatal screening programmes for CDH for reasons stated above. However, most criteria for successful screening would appear to be satisfied in respect of CDH. It is generally accepted that the earlier the treatment is instituted the more favourable the outcome. Certainly, splintage after the age of 6 weeks becomes more difficult as restriction of hip abduction becomes more established. For this reason there is a therapeutic 'window' and the aim should be to detect all cases of hip displacement by 6 weeks at the latest. Late diagnosis results in more complex and often surgical treatment and a high incidence of late onset osteoarthritis.

A Department of Health and Social Security report has made a recommendation for screening for CDH (The Standing Medical Advisory Committee 1986a):

1. *When to screen*
   a. Neonatal
      (i) Within 24 hours of birth,
      (ii) On discharge from hospital (within 10 days).
      The Barlow and Ortolani test should be performed at this stage. The early examination is particularly important as early instability may resolve spontaneously.
   b. At 6 weeks of age. At this stage the hip may present limitation of abduction but the conven-

tional tests for hip instability (Barlow and Ortolani) may still remain positive.
   c. 6–9 months of age. Limb shortening and restriction of hip abduction are now important clinical signs.
   d. 15–21 months of age. At this time abnormalities of gait may present.

The child's gait should be reviewed at 2½ years. Immediate referral to an experienced consultant should be made whenever an abnormality is suspected.

2. *At-risk groups*
   All infants at high risk for CDH, i.e. those with: (i) a family history; (ii) breech presentation; (iii) other congenital postural deformities, e.g. clubfoot; or (iv) oligohydramnios, should be double checked and examined frequently.

3. *Who should screen*
   A successful neonatal screening programme relies on a sustained multidisciplinary approach. Many medical and paramedical staff may be involved, but all should be proficient and education and training are of great importance.
   There should be a clear policy to ensure that those responsible for undertaking the examinations at the relevant ages communicate with the General Practitioner.

The goal of neonatal screening for CDH is to detect cases early and to treat them successfully and conservatively. A multidisciplinary approach is necessary to reduce the number of children requiring complex surgery and subsequently suffering early degenerative osteoarthritis of the hip in later years.

SCOLIOSIS

Screening for scoliosis appears to fulfil all the criteria necessary for a successful programme. It was first introduced in 1947 in Minnesota for the detection of spinal curvatures after epidemics of poliomyelitis, and subsequently in 1963 for idiopathic scoliosis (Lonstein 1977). Most subsequent programmes have used the 'one minute' screening test to detect scoliosis in schools. Children, usually between the ages of 9 and 14 (Lancet 1981) are examined standing and leaning forward. Any evidence of spinal asymmetry and particularly rotational prominence is noted.

The continuing late presentation of adolescents with severe spinal deformity requiring complex surgery seems to support those who enthusiastically screen school children with a view to detecting spinal curvatures earlier. The principal intended outcome of these screening programmes is to identify children with scoliosis who have progressive curves that can be arrested with early conservative management, which is essentially the use of a light-weight moulded cosmetic brace.

There are, however, important issues at the heart of the continuing debate on this issue.

The natural history of the disease must be known in order to understand how to screen for it. In general it is not possible to predict which children with minor curves will have progressive scoliosis. This is critical as it is important to know which children will need treatment or follow-up. Additionally, this raises questions concerning the effectiveness of brace treatment, which is used to obviate the necessity for surgery.

The basis for scoliosis screening is the forward bending test, which locates rotational assymetry or a rib hump. The quick visual examination has proved effective in detecting spinal asymmetry, which has, however, been shown to be a common feature in adolescent males (Burwell et al 1983). About 15% of adolescents show evidence of asymmetry of the trunk on inspection and when X-rayed and, although many adolescents may have a measurable scoliosis, it is commonly due to a tilted pelvis (Dickson 1983). About 2% of children screened have a spinal curve measuring $10°$ or more (Dickson 1983). Consequently, the proportion of children referred to hospital after school screening for scoliosis varies between 2% and 15% (British Orthopaedic Association and the British Scoliosis Society 1983) and it has been reported that the ratio of referred children to those who are managed conservatively is 10 to 1. More sophisticated tests for spinal asymmetry, such as Moire topography (a photostereometric system) have not met with universal success.

The high rate of false positives is the major issue confronting advocates of school screening programmes for scoliosis. This is in part related to the status and training of the screeners and in part to the validity of the tests.

The uncertainty about the efficacy of early conservative management in preventing the need for later surgery and the lack of knowledge of the natural history have resulted in a call for cessation of school screening programmes (Morrissy 1988).

Dickson (1984) has drawn attention to the benign cause of most instances of scoliosis of late onset that would be detected by screening adolescents. He has recommended earlier examinations at 3 months and 5 years to exclude the more sinister infantile progressive scoliosis.

Among the many points made in the 1983 British Orthopaedic Association and British Scoliosis Society report on school screening for scoliosis were:

(i) Twenty-five per cent or more of healthy children examined in a recent study (Burwell et al 1983) had asymmetry of the torso on forward bending. The forward bend test is too sensitive and creates an unacceptably high number of false positive results.

(ii) Whether it is worth screening adolescent boys (who have established idiopathic scoliosis less frequently than girls) has to be determined.

(iii) Criteria need to be defined to determine which children should be sent to hospital for radiography and an orthopaedic opinion.

(iv) A problem is whom to treat: screening may lead to unnecessary treatment of some children.

(v) The natural history of idiopathic scoliosis is not fully known.

(vi) Further study of the morbidity associated with untreated scoliosis is essential.

(vii) The dividing line between normal truncal asymmetry and scoliosis (in both clinical and radiological terms) has yet to be defined.

(viii) The cost of screening in terms of money and anxiety needs to be assessed.

The report concluded that it should not be national policy to screen children for scoliosis routinely throughout the United Kingdom. Nevertheless, it did recommend a programme of education so that potentially deformed children are detected and treated before their condition becomes irretrievable.

It seems clear that a reappraisal of screening programmes for scoliosis is in progress. However, the education of doctors and paramedical personnel in the examination of the spine and referral of spinal deformity remains paramount.

ATLANTO-AXIAL INSTABILITY IN DOWN SYNDROME

Atlantoaxial instability in children with this distinct chromosomal entity was first described by Tishler & Martel (1965). Since then many reports of C1–C2 instability in Down syndrome have been published. It is estimated that 14–22% of children with Down syndrome display atlanto-axial instability. Neurological complications may occur if the odontoid process causes spinal cord compression and pyramidal tract signs may become apparent. Accordingly, it has been suggested that all children with Down syndrome should undergo radiological investigation. In terms of screening, however, an effective treatment for positive cases must be available. In this context the Chief Medical Officer issued a statement from the Standing Medical Advisory Committee in 1986 (Standing Medical Advisory Committee 1986b). The Committee made a number of recommendations but did not support a formal screening programme to detect possible atlanto-axial instability. Amongst the recommendations were that:

1. Examination of the central nervous system should form an integral part of the medical examination of all people with Down syndrome. Neurological abnormalities should be investigated radiologically to exclude atlanto-axial instability.
2. Where instability is demonstrated consultant advice should be sought.
3. Individuals with Down syndrome should continue to participate in sport but if the activity is vigorous the neck should be X-rayed.

OPPORTUNISTIC SCREENING

Opportunistic screening plays an important part in detecting unrecognised paediatric orthopaedic path-ology. The regular radiological and clinical examination of the hips in cerebral palsy children may prevent neurological dislocation. Similarly, awareness of the association of moulding deformities with CDH may lead to the detection of covert hip dysplasia in metatarsus adductus or torticollis. Spinal dysraphism and neurological disorder may be the cause of progressive foot deformity or leg length discrepancy in a young child. Many orthopaedic conditions may first come to light during regular screening examinations in childhood. Therefore 'consultation-based' screening in paediatric orthopaedic disorders is an important adjunct to the well-defined screening programmes in, say, CDH. This concept is illustrated well when the causes of limp in childhood are considered. The cause may be neurological, e.g. cerebral palsy, associated with the spine or with a neurological lesion. Spinal lesions in general and all hip lesions, such as Perthes' disease or slipped upper femoral epiphysis, may be responsible. Osteochondritis of the knee, tumours, bone cysts or fractures (traumatic, stress or pathological) may present with a limp. Finally, the affected limb may be short.

As in other areas of medicine, a great deal can be gained by alertness and familiarity with pointers to possible future problems.

REFERENCES

Barlow T G 1962 Early diagnosis and treatment of congenital dislocation of the hip. Journal of Bone Surgery 44B: 292–310

British Orthopaedic Association and the British Scoliosis Society 1983 School screening for scoliosis. British Medical Journal 287: 963–964

Burwell R G, James N J, Johnson F et al 1983 Standardised trunk asymmetry scores. A study of back contour in healthy school children. Journal of Bone and Joint Surgery 65B: 452–463

Clarke N M P 1986 Sonographic clarification of the problems of neonatal hip instability. Journal of Paediatric Orthopaedics 6: 527–532

Clarke N M P, Harcke H T, McHugh P et al 1985 Real time ultrasound in the diagnosis of congenital dislocation of the hip. Journal of Bone and Joint Surgery 67B: 406–412

Commission on Chronic Illness 1957 Secondary prevention through screening examinations in chronic illness in the United States, Vol 1. Harvard University Press, Cambridge, Massachusetts

Cunningham K T, Moulton A, Beningfield S A, Maddock C R, 1984 A clicking hip in a newborn should never be ignored. Lancet i 668–670

Dickson R A 1983 Scoliosis in the community. British Medical Journal 286: 615–8

Dickson R A 1984 Screening for scoliosis. British Medical Journal 289: 269–270

Dunn P M 1976 Perinatal observations on the aetiology of congenital dislocation of the hip. Clinical Orthopaedics and Related Research 119: 11–22

Dunn P M 1987 Screening for congenital dislocation of the hip. In: Macfarlane J A (ed) Progress in child health, Vol 3. Churchill Livingstone, London, pp. 1–13

Lancet 1981 School screening for scoliosis. Lancet ii: 345–346

Leck I 1986 An epidemiological assessment of neonatal screening for dislocation of the hip. Journal of the Royal College of Physicians 20: 56–62

Lonstein J E 1977 Screening for spinal deformities in Minnesota schools. Clinical Orthopaedics and Related Research 126: 33–42

Morrissy R T 1988 School screening for scoliosis. A statement of the problem. Spine 13: 1195–1197

Ortolani M 1937 Un segno noto e sue importanza per la diagnosi precoce di prelussazione congenita dell'anca. Pediatria 45: 129–36

Pueschel S M, Hernoon J H, Gelch M M et al 1984 Symptomatic atlanto-axial subluxation in persons with Down's syndrome. Journal of Paediatric Orthopaedics 4: 682–688

The Standing Medical Advisory Committee for the
Secretaries of State for Social Services and for Wales 1986a
Screening for the detection of congenital dislocation of the
hip. HMSO, London

The Standing Medical Advisory Committee for the
Secretaries of State for Social Services and for Wales 1986b

Atlanto-axial instability in people with Down's syndrome
CMO(80)9. HMSO, London

Tishler J M, Martel W 1965 Dislocation of the atlas in
mongolism: preliminary report. Radiology 84: 904

Von Rosen S 1956 Early diagnosis and treatment of
congenitial dislocation of the hip joint. Acta Orthopaedica
Scandinavica 26: 136–40

17. Developmental screening

Tom Hutchison   Leon Polnay

INTRODUCTION AND HISTORY

The broader issues of preschool surveillance have been discussed in Chapter 12; this chapter will focus in greater detail on developmental screening.

The tradition of mass screening for health problems in the UK started with the introduction of a school health service in 1908. This was established following the 1904 report of the Government Interdepartmental Committee on Physical Deterioration, which in turn followed the recognition of the poor state of health of recruits for the Boer War, and recommended that improvement could be made by screening and health promotion. Emphasis was on physical health, as this was the major problem of the day. In the early 1900s infant welfare clinics staffed by health visitors and community doctors oversaw some preschool children. Maternal and child health services were closely linked.

Developmental testing scales became available during the 1930s through the work of Gesell (1925, 1938), Stutsman (1931), Buhler & Hetzer (1935) and Cattell (1940). These authors were mostly interested in providing the first descriptions of normal development and assigning some form of numerical quotient to children in the first 2 years of life. Various types of Binet scale served the same purpose for the over 2-year-olds (Terman and Merrill 1961). The 1950s and 1960s saw an enthusiasm for general measures to improve the health of the population in many countries — the spirit in which the NHS was born. The idea of systematically testing all children for abnormalities of development became almost irresistible. The jump was made from description to diagnostic tool and, by simplification, from a tool to a test that had predictive value. Under the title 'developmental screening' these examinations fitted into schemes of physical checks and immunisations epitomised by the M&CW 46 (Maternal and Child Welfare) schedule. The M&CW 46 is a document designed by the Society of Community Medicine for the recording of the periodic preschool medical examination of children.

More complex tools, such as the Griffiths (1967) scales, required specific training courses to teach their administration, and used special equipment in strictly controlled circumstances. This made them unsuitable for mass testing, but for many years they have been used as part of diagnostic assessments and as a gold standard for the calibration and validation of other simpler testing tools. (Eu 1986).

The true cost of administration of the 'tests' was not calculated and the effectiveness of developmental screening was not measured; it was assumed to be of value. It was also assumed that parents would not notice their child's problem or would not seek appropriate help early enough. The delivery of this service could also become mechanical and unproductive, as shown by Newsholme (1916), in a quote that would still be relevant 50 years after it was first made:

The work of medical inspectors of schools largely consists in filling up answers to the numerous questions on these schedules and completing forms for treatment, re-examination, and other objects arising out of them. There is little time for careful observation, and insufficient time to form a clear picture of each child as a whole, so that the doctor soon resigns himself to noting the isolated signs on cards.

Early diagnosis was the main reason given for these screening measures — early to start more effective treatment; early to provide genetic counselling where inherited problems, such as muscular dystrophy, existed; early to prevent secondary problems, such as contractures, following cerebral palsy; early to mobilise support for a family with a developmentally disabled child, or to help those parents with a developmentally delayed child who might otherwise be said to be 'naughty'. Finally, early to prevent the disaster of an unrecognised child turning up, aged 5, for a school system that cannot meet its needs.

DEVELOPMENTAL TESTING TOOLS

Paediatricians in the UK have relied most heavily on the published texts of Illingworth (1953, 1960) and, most of all, Sheridan, whose book *Developmental Progress of Young Children* was first published by the Department of Health and Social Security in 1960, and was widely acclaimed as the bible of child development (Sheridan 1960). Based on many years of her own work in developmental paediatrics, Sheridan produced the STYCAR materials (Standard Tests for Young Children and Retardates) (Sheridan 1968). Sheridan has always insisted that her charts were not intended to produce a quotient or a pass/fail scale, but that they should be used as a tool to aid an experienced examiner, who would take into account all the information available from a full history and examination before formulating conclusions. In spite of these warnings, her sequences were assembled in a modified form as a step graph in the Woodside developmental screening test (Barber et al 1976), which was used in a pass/fail way. The sequences were also assembled to give numerical scores (Bellman et al 1985), so that computer processing would be possible when the new scales were used to evaluate children in the National Childhood Encephalopathy Study.

The most widely used instrument in the USA is the Denver developmental screening test (Frankenburg & Dodds 1967, Frankenburg et al 1971). This is a battery of 105 milestones between birth and 5 years of age in the four main areas of development, which are identified as: gross motor, fine motor/adaptive, language and personal/social. The test was standardised on more than 1000 children and was designed to be administered in 15 to 20 minutes, according to a strict protocol, by a trained health aide; there were clear pass/fail criteria leading to further assessment. It was created in response to a climate of national concern about early identification of children with school problems in the USA, with the prospect of a mandatory national screening programme. The UK, with its universal health visitor, community doctor and family practitioner provision, had no need for such mechanistic technician-operated screening systems. The Denver chart is, however, valued for the clear way in which it presents the range of children's abilities. Each item is presented with a percentile bar indicating the percentage of children by age who are able to perform the task. A Cardiff version (Bryant et al 1974) has been published and standardised on British children. Some differences were found in the ages at which motor and language items were achieved by children from Denver and Cardiff, but these were not sufficient to make a difference in the pick-up of severe problems. The Cardiff work has never been made commercially available because of copyright problems. The Denver chart has been incorporated wholesale into the community records of some British District Health Authorities, and will certainly be being used by staff who have not been trained in the way Frankenburg intended. It is often used in child development centres to this day as a tool in the further assessment of a child who is known to have problems, much in the way Mary Sheridan envisaged, although a recent study has shown the Denver to be weak in the identification of children with speech and language impairment (Borowitz & Glascoe 1986). The test has also been shown to be a poor detector of children with mild delays (Nugent 1976, Carmichael & Williams, 1981, Harper & Wacker 1983) and to be a poor predictor of future school problems (Cadman et al 1984).

LOCAL DEVELOPMENT CHARTS

Many health districts and organisations have produced charts for their own staff. The Nottingham charts (Fig. 17.1) are an example and are reproduced here to serve as a reference for normal development. These are a modification of the Woodside system (Barber 1976), which mainly uses items that can be found from parental history, and are not strongly dependant upon culture. They have long since ceased to be used in a pass/fail way but instead are used as an aide-memoire for professionals, as a teaching tool with parents and as a substitute for time-consuming written descriptions of normal milestones that have been passed.

ABNORMAL DEVELOPMENT

Although published normal values set absolute standards, parental, cultural and other expectations may influence the frame of reference and the perception of what is normal. Any single achievement will be attained over a range of ages by any group of children. Abnormal development is a matter of degree. One strength of the Denver test is that data are presented visually as a range of normal.

Three terms commonly applied to abnormal growth and development are often used incorrectly. They are:

1. *Impairment*, which is a problem or lesion at a physiological or anatomical level, e.g. a squint, talipes or cerebral damage after meningitis.
2. *Disability*, which is the way an impairment affects performance, e.g. visual difficulties, mobility problems, or slow learning.

4½ years (range 3–5 years) Descends stairs — one foot per step — can hold on Hops either foot	
3 years (range 2½–4 years) Climbs stairs — alternate feet Stands on one foot/walks on tip-toe	
2 years (range 18/12–2½) Up and down stairs — holding on Kicks ball	
18/12 (range 14/12–22/12) Climbs stairs, hands held, two feet per step Kneels without support	
12/12 (range 8/12–15/12) Pulls to standing, on furniture Cruises round furniture	
9/12 (range 8/12–12/12) Sits steadily on floor and can turn to reach toys Stands holding on to furniture	
6/12 (range 5/12–8/12) Sits against wall — no lateral support Can roll over	
3/12 (range 3/12–6/12) Pull from lying — no head lag Holds head above plane of body	GROSS MOTOR
6/52 Head in plane of body — ventral suspension	

0 6 12 26 36 52   1½   2   2½   3   3½   4   4½
Weeks   Years

4½ years (range 4–5½ years) Copies squares Draws a man with head, trunk and legs/builds stairs	
3 years (range 2½–3½ years) Copies a circle Builds a bridge of 3 cubes when shown/tower of 8 bricks	
2 years (range 18/12–3) Imitates vertical line when shown Turns pages singly/tower of 6 bricks	
18/12 (range 12/12–24/12) Scribbles on paper Turns pages in a book 2 or 3 at a time/tower of 3 bricks	
12/12 (range 7/12–14/12) Pincer grasp Bangs cubes together when shown	
9/12 (range 7/12–12/12) Looks for toys falling off end of table or pram Pokes at small sweets with index finger	
6/12 (range 5/12–8/12) Picks up spatula from hand Transfers spatula from hand to hand	
3/12 (range 2/12–4/12) Holds rattle briefly Follows moving person with eyes	FINE MOTOR
6/52 Follows dangling object with eyes (12″ away through 45°)	

0 6 12 26 36 52   1½   2   2½   3   3½   4   4½
Weeks   Years

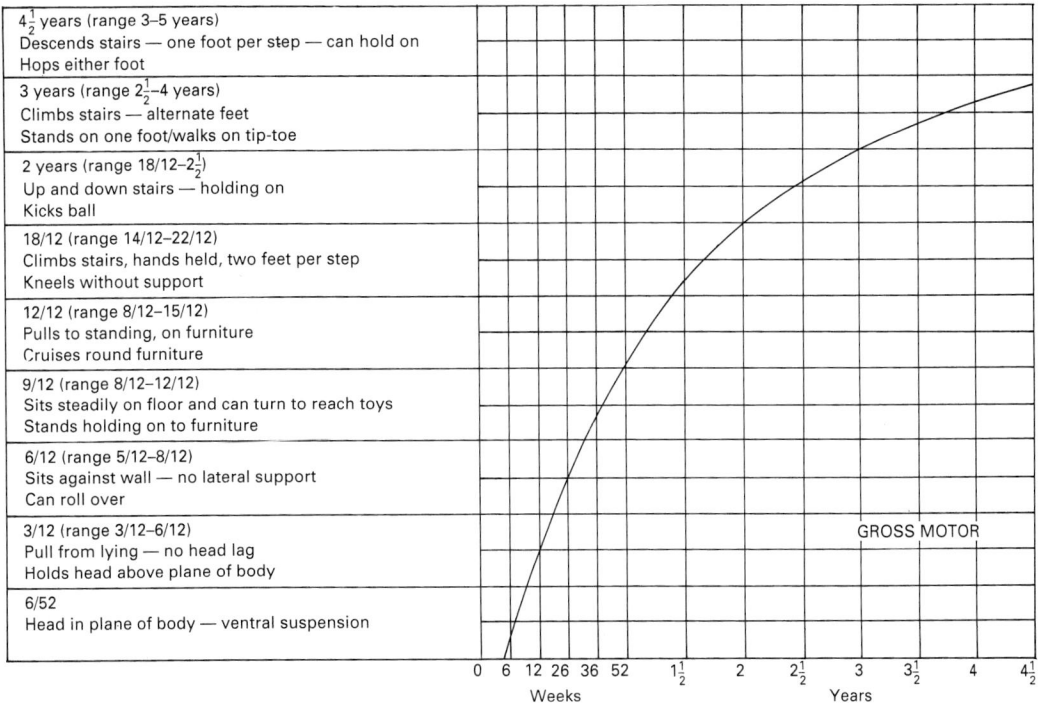

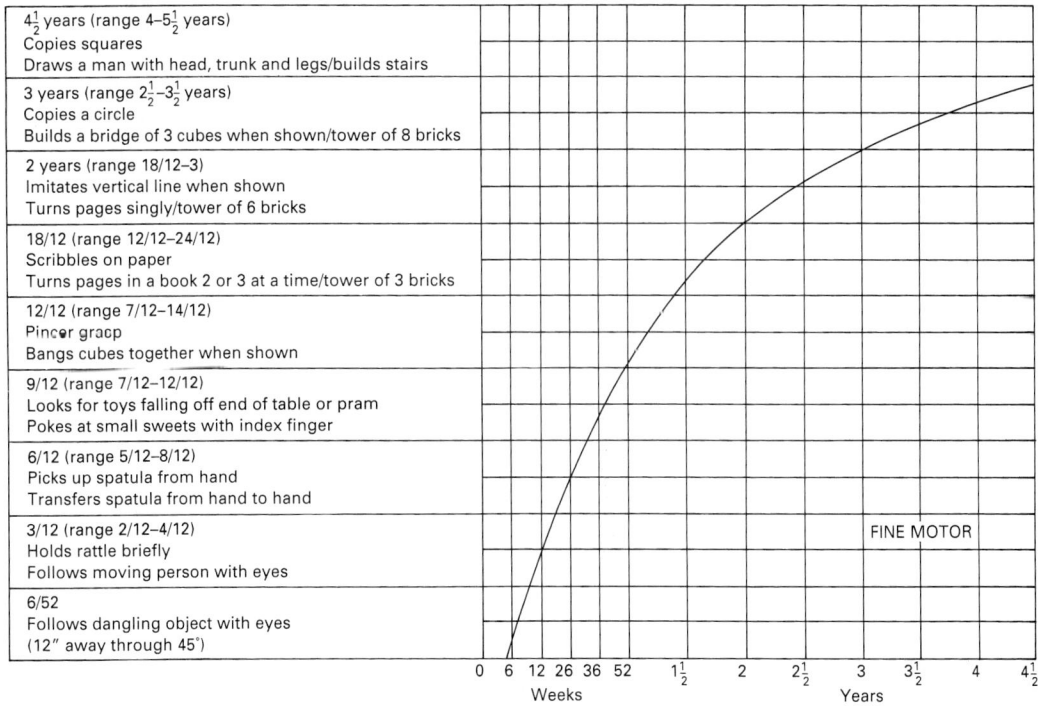

Fig. 17.1a The Nottingham charts of child development.

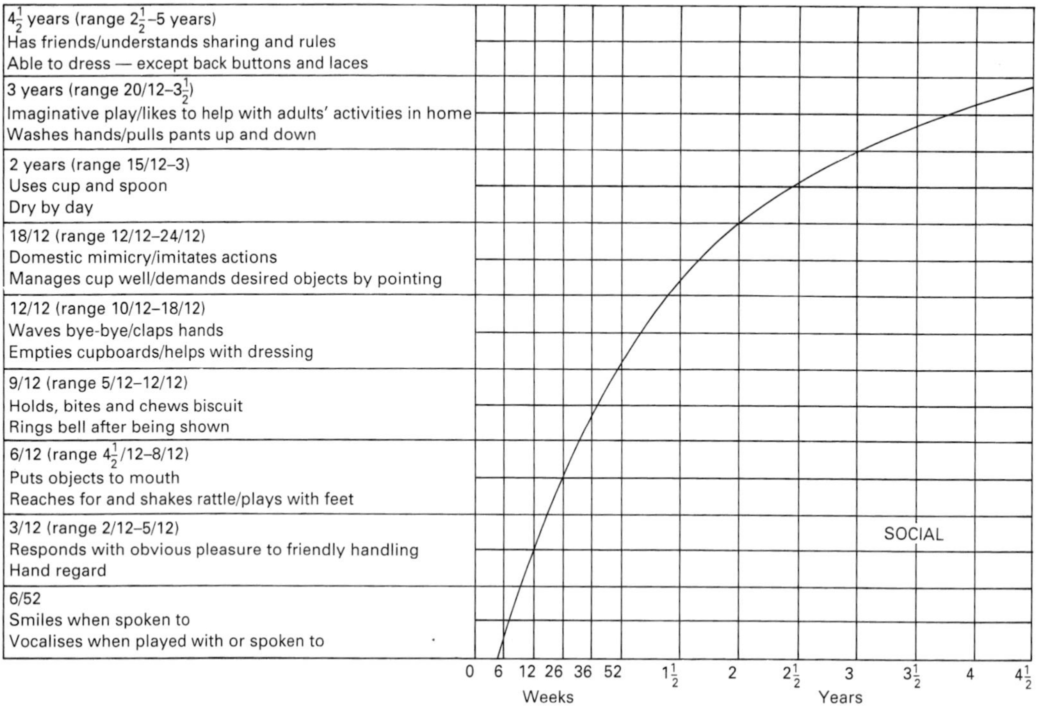

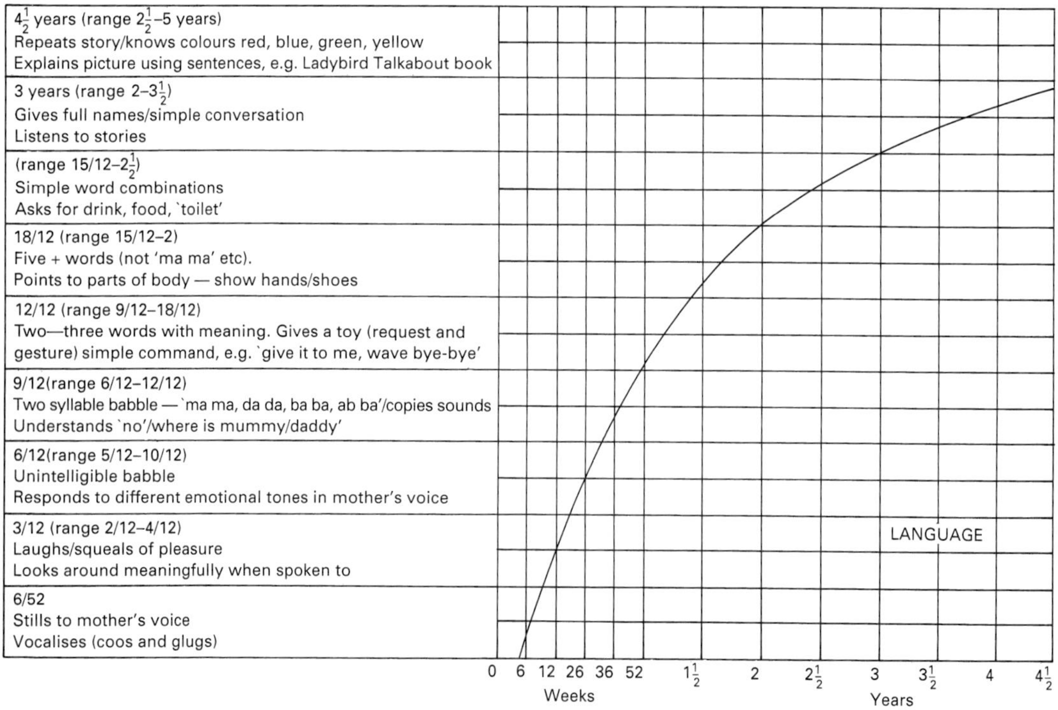

$4\frac{1}{2}$ years (range $2\frac{1}{2}$–5 years)
Has friends/understands sharing and rules
Able to dress — except back buttons and laces

3 years (range 20/12–$3\frac{1}{2}$)
Imaginative play/likes to help with adults' activities in home
Washes hands/pulls pants up and down

2 years (range 15/12–3)
Uses cup and spoon
Dry by day

18/12 (range 12/12–24/12)
Domestic mimicry/imitates actions
Manages cup well/demands desired objects by pointing

12/12 (range 10/12–18/12)
Waves bye-bye/claps hands
Empties cupboards/helps with dressing

9/12 (range 5/12–12/12)
Holds, bites and chews biscuit
Rings bell after being shown

6/12 (range $4\frac{1}{2}$/12–8/12)
Puts objects to mouth
Reaches for and shakes rattle/plays with feet

3/12 (range 2/12–5/12)
Responds with obvious pleasure to friendly handling
Hand regard

6/52
Smiles when spoken to
Vocalises when played with or spoken to

SOCIAL

0 6 12 26 36 52 $1\frac{1}{2}$ 2 $2\frac{1}{2}$ 3 $3\frac{1}{2}$ 4 $4\frac{1}{2}$
Weeks   Years

$4\frac{1}{2}$ years (range $2\frac{1}{2}$–5 years)
Repeats story/knows colours red, blue, green, yellow
Explains picture using sentences, e.g. Ladybird Talkabout book

3 years (range 2–$3\frac{1}{2}$)
Gives full names/simple conversation
Listens to stories

(range 15/12–$2\frac{1}{2}$)
Simple word combinations
Asks for drink, food, 'toilet'

18/12 (range 15/12–2)
Five + words (not 'ma ma' etc).
Points to parts of body — show hands/shoes

12/12 (range 9/12–18/12)
Two—three words with meaning. Gives a toy (request and
gesture) simple command, e.g. 'give it to me, wave bye-bye'

9/12 (range 6/12–12/12)
Two syllable babble — 'ma ma, da da, ba ba, ab ba'/copies sounds
Understands 'no'/where is mummy/daddy'

6/12 (range 5/12–10/12)
Unintelligible babble
Responds to different emotional tones in mother's voice

3/12 (range 2/12–4/12)
Laughs/squeals of pleasure
Looks around meaningfully when spoken to

6/52
Stills to mother's voice
Vocalises (coos and glugs)

LANGUAGE

0 6 12 26 36 52 $1\frac{1}{2}$ 2 $2\frac{1}{2}$ 3 $3\frac{1}{2}$ 4 $4\frac{1}{2}$
Weeks   Years

Fig. 17.1b   The Nottingham charts of child development.

3. *Handicap*, which is the way a disability disrupts progress towards full achievement of potential and independent adult living.

Abnormal development is a disability due to an impairment, which may cause handicap.

CAUSES OF ABNORMAL DEVELOPMENT

Table 17.1 Diagnosis of 450 children with severe learning problems (born 1968–77) (from the Oxford Mental Handicap Register, Elliot et al 1981)

Problem	Children with problem (%)
Down syndrome, other chromosomal abnormalities	26.5
Non-chromosomal abnormalities of the CNS	9.0
Cerebral palsy	6.5
Birth injury	2.0
Infection, postinfection, immunological causes	2.0
Nutritional, metabolic	2.0
Psychiatric syndromes	4.0
Cerebral anoxia	1.5
Cultural, familial	1.0
Heredofamilial, degenerative	1.5
Epilepsy	1.0
Recognised syndromes of unknown aetiology	1.5
Other conditions	3.0
Subnormality (not elsewhere classified)	4.0
No known cause	34.5

These genetic, intrauterine or perinatal catastrophes may make developmental impairment obvious at birth to a skilled examiner, if not to the parents, and disability and future handicap may be predicted.

However, it is sometimes not until the second or third year of life that failure to achieve expected milestones provokes a search for early causes.

It is only under the pressure of formal education that some milder developmental disabilities cause handicap. For example, degrees of motor clumsiness, specific difficulties in perception, writing and reading unrelated to intelligence.

While children attending schools for severe learning difficulties have parents in all socio-economic groups and a clear medical diagnosis in about 60% of cases, schools for moderate learning difficulties have a preponderance of children from low income and deprived family backgrounds (Fig. 17.2).

Identifiable familial disorders play a small part here (see also Chapter 10). For example fragile X syndrome has been reported in 5% of a Swedish population with moderate learning difficulties (Blomquist et al 1983). It is otherwise difficult to disentangle the effects of de novo chromosomal abnormalities from the results of polygenetically determined lack of intellectual ability. It is a real challenge to the medical model to cope with the effects of poor parenting in the form of lack of stimulation and lack of consistent discipline or the effects of emotional and sexual abuse.

HOW HAS SCREENING BEEN IMPLEMENTED IN THE UK?

Developmental examination at birth is carried out by midwives, GPs and hospital obstetric and paediatric staff. At 10 days of age the midwife hands over responsibility for the child to the health visitor. Thereafter health checks are carried out through clinics provided either by

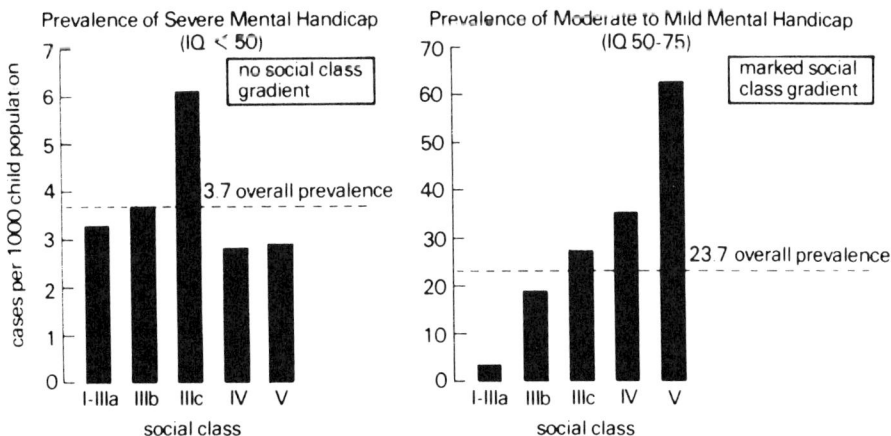

Fig. 17.2 Prevalence and social class distribution of mental handicap (after Birch et al 1970).

District Health Authorities or by general practitioners.

A survey in 1985 (Department of Health and Social Security 1987) showed that 54% of clinic sessions in England were held by community paediatric doctors, 34% by health visitors, 11% by GPs working for the health authorities on a sessional basis and 1% by hospital doctors.

General practitioners have run a wide range of parallel services, from simply offering opportunistic screening to those who consult for other reasons, through specific clinics for 6-week checks, to complex systems of routine interval checks with or without a nurse or health visitor doing specific parts of the work. Various studies quote 20–40% of GPs working in this way (Powell 1985, Burke & Bain 1986). Considering GP practices rather than individuals, it has been estimated that 37% of all GPs were in practices that hold paediatric screening sessions (Burke & Bain 1986).

Health visitor involvement nationally has been very variable, both in the Health Authority and in the GP setting. A study of 88 Area Health Authorities (Connolly 1982) showed that 22% followed a policy incorporating hearing tests but no developmental testing, while 17% had only a general brief to oversee children's progress. The remaining 61% worked with doctors to complete a specific programme of developmental tests. Across the UK approximately 33% of community child health clinics are run by health visitors (Department of Health and Social Security 1987), with a wide range of 2–91% between districts (Macfarlane & Pillay 1984). In a literature review Butler (1989) estimated that between 15 and 25% of health visitor time is spent on home visits to the under 5-year-olds, and of this time only about one-quarter was actually spent on screening procedures. In working with GPs Burke (quoted in Butler 1989) reports that health visitors were wholly responsible for the developmental examinations in about 10% of practices. Apart from 6-week checks, which are mostly done by doctors, it seems that there is no consistent pattern in division of labour between doctors and health visitors at older ages.

At the time of writing (1991), the new GP contract has already made major changes in the division of responsibility between GP and Health Authority.

GPs who are accredited in Child Health Surveillance may claim £10 per year for every child whose parent has registered for surveillance with the practice. Over 90% of practices, nationally, appear to have sought accreditation. This has forced FHSAs to join with local community paediatricians to run training courses and devise accreditation procedures.

The 10% who chose not to offer these services, plus the few who do not pass accreditation will force local authorities to continue to operate primary care clinics as a safety net.

In order to provide a service the GP is usually asked to follow the guidelines of the local Child Health Surveillance Policy. These are likely to be based closely on the 'Health for All Children' recommendation (Hall 1989).

GPs are also expected to have suitable premises and to be accessible to health visitors and parents, usually in the context of a practice baby clinic, for any referrals which may arise. The bulk of the work will remain with nursing staff and good liaison is essential.

Even now these new arrangements have inbuilt difficulties. The GP may feel ultimately answerable for the completion and quality of the surveillance programme and yet feel helpless because the nursing staff are neither employed nor professionally accountable to the practice. This is in some ways similar to the situation in midwifery. Problems have arisen for example, when the Health Authority has been unable to resolve staff shortages, or when the GP has failed to co-operate in liaison and support for nursing staff.

Evaluation of a screening programme

The aim of a developmental screening programme must be to identify from the total population those children whose condition requires treatment or observation. Such children are cases and, immediately, there is a basic problem (in milder conditions, such as clumsiness or expressive language delay) of defining just who is a case. In evaluating the results of a test it is important to know the sensitivity, specificity, predictive value and yield of the test. These terms are all defined in Chapter 2.

The paediatric literature contains many studies of individual child health surveillance and its outcome but these use such a variety of methods that they are hard to compare. All but a few have ignored the difference between true and false screening results, so that specificity and sensitivity cannot be measured. Predictive value cannot be measured when yield is expressed in terms of *all* positives rather than *true* positives.

Only two studies give some idea of the productivity of screening for developmental disorders.

1. Roberts & Khosla (1972) studied 386 children aged 11–13 months who had an initial neurological screening examination. Twelve were found to be abnormal and eleven of these were confirmed as true positives at detailed follow-up examination. *Yield* here was 2.8% and *predictive value* was 92%.

2. The Dundee study (Drillien & Drummond 1983, Drillien et al 1988) studies 5334 children born in 1974 and 1975. They were examined for neurological and developmental disorders on a programme of checks at 8, 20 and 29 weeks and at 15, 24 and 36 months. In all, 22 070 screening examinations were carried out at the six target ages. The yield in this study was 1.6% and the predictive value was 83.8%. The sensitivity could not be measured because there was no information about false negatives. In a smaller, later, study of 128 children a sensitivity of 50% was found along with a yield of 8.2% and a predictive value of 80%. It seems fair to suppose that examination in the field rather than as part of a research study would produce less impressive results.

DEVELOPMENTAL SCREENING SCHEDULES

At what age should children's development be checked? Butler (1989) reviewed the literature and found 35 authors who had described model screening programmes. There were 24 different combinations of recommended ages, and only 10 authors gave explicit reasons for their choices. The most commonly mentioned was that these ages were critically related to certain milestones; they would give a maximum opportunity for intervention but minimise the number of false positive findings. Other reasons were the suitability of the age for certain pieces of anticipatory guidance of parents, that the chosen ages were practical or convenient or fitted well around the immunisation programme or, in the case of 'birthday checks', were more likely to be remembered by parents. Finally, Butler noted evidence that screeners select ages based upon their own clinical skills, and quotes one author as realising that he advised against a 3-year check because he found difficulty in establishing rapport with this age group.

Developmental testing is only one aspect of individual paediatric surveillance and so selected ages must be a compromise with the requirements of other types of screening test. While key ages for hip checking or distraction testing of hearing can be defined by scientific criteria, no such evidence has been forthcoming for pure developmental tests. Butler (1989) quotes Hall (1988) and Smith & Jacobson (1988) in suggesting not that optimal screening ages have yet to be established, but that they do not actually exist.

The term 'developmental screening' has been used for many years, likening it to other early detection procedures. However, for a long time scientists much more than practitioners have felt that these programmes do not fulfil some of the screening pro-

gramme criteria described by Wilson & Jungner (1968) (see Chapter 2), namely:

1. There is not actually one single condition being sought. Developmental delay, although it can exist alone, is most often a symptom or consequence of a wide variety of other pathologies. Many of these certainly do meet the criteria of being important health problems for the individual and the community.
2. The treatments for many of these conditions are in no sense curative, they are often supportive and palliative.
3. In many cases there is no recognisably distinct latent early stage and the natural history of the condition may be unpredictable.
4. There are no agreed policies on whom to treat as a case.
5. Nobody has shown developmental screening programmes to be cost-effective.

The available screening tests likewise do not fit any of the ideals characterised by Cochrane and Holland (1971). They are not simple, quick and easy to interpret and although they are generally acceptable to the public they are hardly accurate measurements. There is considerable interobserver variability. Evidence of their sensitivity is scarce and what there is ranges between 50 and 90%. There are no studies giving figures for specificity. The yield is low — about 2% — although other well established programmes such as phenylketonuria have an accepted lower yield (see Chapter 15).

Use of the term 'developmental surveillance' has been promoted to avoid the problems inherent in the use of the word screening. The word surveillance itself, besides its connotations of policing, has been used to mean a variety of different things since it was used in *Fit for the future* (Court Committee 1976) to mean all aspects of primary prevention including immunisation and health education. This broad usage is to be found most recently in *Health for all children* (Hall 1989). Butler (1989), in his timely and scholarly review of the literature, suggests that, under the title *Preventive child health care*, surveillance be used to mean secondary prevention. Developmental tests are then a part of the list of tests available for individual surveillance. To those of us who found it semantically uncomfortable to describe immunisation as a surveillance activity this is a welcome publication, and we hope it finds wide acceptance (see Chapter 12, Fig.12.1).

CURRENT RECOMMENDATIONS

A working party of paediatricians, general practitioners, health visitors and other doctors and nurses has published a review of child health surveillance in *Health for all children* (Hall 1989). They concluded: 'That the routine developmental examination of all children as a means of detecting impairments is unnecessary in the case of serious disorders such as cerebral palsy and severe learning difficulties, and we doubt its relevance to the detection of developmental impairments such as delayed language acquisition' (Hall 1989 p. 77).

The alternative they propose is that all children be included in a programme of health surveillance that will succeed if all the professionals in contact with families, routinely and opportunistically, have a detailed knowledge of child development. Judgement will determine when a formal developmental investigation is warranted. Rigid referral rules are undesirable, as is the routine keeping of detailed developmental attainment charts.

INTERPRETING ABNORMAL FINDINGS

Information about a child's development may be obtained by history, observation or examination. All three may be subject to error if they are carried out without training and without awareness of the limitations and weaknesses of the exercise. Common errors leading to incorrect conclusions are:

1. Poor history-taking with incorrect use of open, closed and leading questions.
2. Confusion over unwillingness as opposed to inability to perform developmental items.
3. The child who is frightened, shy or does not display his/her best in a strange environment.
4. Failure to take account of prematurity.
5. Mistaken cultural assumptions; perhaps English is not the main family language.
6. Although general practitioners may be the first to notice a child's developmental problem they are far more likely to be consulted by a health visitor or by the family directly. What should be done?
7. Taking action without gathering a detailed medical, social, family and developmental history, and without co-ordinating with other staff who have had time to form an opinion about the child. A quick referral may be inappropriate and hasty reassurance may be facile.
8. Overinterpretation on a single consultation. The child's progress monitored over time is a great assistance in formulating the problem.

Part of the art of developmental surveillance comes in helping parents. Anxiety is the product of caring, although it may seem disproportionate. It is best tackled by time, patience and honesty.

Once it seems that a problem is likely, the GP or nurse should refer the child for more detailed assessment. This may be to a local community or hospital paediatrician, to a specific therapist or expert, or to a local child development centre. Familiarity and good communication with the local referral network is as important to a GP as knowledge of normal development.

The job of this second tier is to confirm or exclude a problem, to investigate its cause and to institute remedy, therapy and support. There may be a District Handicap Team overseeing the co-ordination of services or providing full multidisciplinary assessments and based in a child development centre. There may be a computerised register of children with special needs held by the Health Authority. The District Health Authority has a legal duty to inform the education department of any child with problems likely to require special educational provision. The education department may initiate a Statement of Special Educational Needs, which is compiled by seeking opinions from parents, the Health Authority and an educational psychologist.

DEVELOPMENTAL SURVEILLANCE INTO THE 1990s

There will be increasing financial pressure for all practices to offer child health surveillance.

Some who cannot, because of poor premises or for personal reasons, have already opted to subcontract services to the health authority, dividing the payments to benefit both parties.

The emergence of budget holding general practices may or may not survive politically. A budget holding practice unhappy with, for example, the health visiting time or quality provided by the health authority may wish to hire its own nursing staff and enter negotiations to obtain a top slice of the community nursing budget to do this. Screening and surveillance could then be undertaken by whatever grade of nurse the practice sees fit.

Such a piecemeal approach could foster patches of excellence, and similarly pockets of very old fashioned, mechanistic or simply inadequate practice.

As long as nursing services are provided on a district-wide basis, resources can be channelled to areas of greatest need, classically the inner cities. Available resources are in reality rationed by the NHS. The combination of general underfunding with the emergence of pockets of strong self contained budget holding primary care in predominantly rural middle class areas threatens to widen the divide between rich and poor and make two tier health care a reality.

By the end of 1991 one in five newborn children has a parent-held record. This trend is likely to continue though many health districts have not yet found funding for this approach.

This is not a professional record held by the parent. Professionals will need to keep separate records of their activities, though the form of these, particularly in health visiting, may change. The parent-held record is unlikely to diminish the amount of paperwork burying doctors but has great promise for improving the transfer of essential information. The use of, for example, carbonless copies of key health checks done by GP and health visitor or health authority doctor promises to give all four parties updated and succinct information about health surveillance on each child. The main purpose of the record is undoubtedly to educate and empower parents, putting them more in charge and in touch with their child's development.

It is a paradox of the 1990s that in the midst of increasing concern about the recognition and correct management of child abuse, the very idea that improper parenting is likely is becoming less and less the lowest common denominator for which surveillance programmes are designed.

As ideas of mechanistic screening of development are being replaced by the more modern concepts of surveillance, so these practices are being replaced in many health authorities by an innovative type of health visiting known as the Child Development Programme (Barker et al 1987). This offers a cost-effective solution for health visitors working in socially-stressed areas, who find themselves faced with the choice of leaving for a less stressed area or being remorselessly swamped by crisis work.

The programme seeks to empower parents and enable them to build their child-rearing skills. It uses intensive visiting of first-time mothers, and selected second- and third-time mothers, with an education programme focusing on diet, children's health, behaviour and development, maternal health and depression, engaging fathers in child rearing, and many other areas. It claims achievements such as immunisation rates close to 100%, reductions in child abuse and cot death, improved parental self-esteem and reduced rates of children's hospital admission. In addition to this type of programme, many health authorities are reviewing health visitor services in general. New working practices are being tried as alternatives to rigid systems of fixed age checks and caseloads. One approach is the allocation of priority to high-risk families and the curtailment of checks on those who do not need them. Others include running groups for parents with children of a certain age, or doing health checks by post. These changes may frustrate general practitioners and increase their desire to employ their own health visitors to achieve control of the surveillance programme. It is far more likely that rearrangements of this sort will occur where a health authority has difficulty in providing sufficient staff to fulfil its part of the surveillance programme.

The appointment of Consultant Community Paediatricians should continue until there is one for every 100 000 population. There will then be the local facility to evaluate many of the children presenting to the primary care surveillance team without needing referral to a more distant hospital.

REFERENCES

Barber J H, Boothman R, Paget-Stanfield H 1979 A new visual chart for pre-school developmental screening. Health Bulletin 34: 80–91

Barker W, Rowe G, Sutcliffe D 1987 Community health and the child development programme. Early Childhood Development Unit, Bristol

Bellman M H, Rawson N S B, Wadsworth J et al 1985 A developmental test based on the STYCAR sequences used in the National Childhood Encephalopathy Study. Child: Care Health and Development 11: 309–323

Birch H G, Richardson S A, Baird G, Illsley R 1970. Mental subnormality in the community. A clinical and epidemiological study. In: Polnay C, Hull D 1985 Community Paediatrics. Churchill Livingstone

Blomquist H K, Gustavson K H, Holingren G 1983 Fragile X syndrome in mildly mentally retarded children in a northern Swedish county. Clinical Genetics 24: 293–298

Borowitz K C, Glascoe F P 1986 Sensitivity of the Denver developmental screening test in speech and language screening. Pediatrics 78(6): 1075–78

Bryant G M, Davies K J, Newcombe R G 1974 The Denver developmental screening test. Achievement of test items in the first year of life by Denver and Cardiff infants. Developmental Medicine and Child Neurology 16: 475–484

Buhler C, Hetzer H 1935 Testing children's development from birth to school age. George Allen and Unwin, London

Burke P, Bain D J G 1986 Paediatric developmental screening: a survey of general practitioners. Journal of the Royal College of General Practitioners 36: 302–306

Butler J 1989 Child health surveillance in primary care, a critical review. HMSO, London

Cadman D, Chambers L W, Walter S D et al 1984 The usefulness of the Denver developmental screening test to predict kindergarten problems in a general community population. American Journal of Public Health 74: 10

Carmichael A, Williams H E 1981 Developmental screening in infancy — a critical appraisal of its value. Australian Paediatric Journal 17: 20–23

Cattell P 1940 Measurement of intelligence of infants and young children. Psychological Corporation, New York

Cochrane A L, Holland W W 1969 Validation of screening procedures. British Medical Bulletin 27: 3–8

Connolly P 1982 An enquiry into child health surveillance procedures undertaken by health visitors in England. In: Health visiting principles in practice. Council for the Education and Training of Health Visitors, London

Court Committee 1976 Fit for the future. Report of the Select Committee on Child Health Services. HMSO, London

Department of Health and Social Security 1987 Health and personal social services statistics for England. HMSO, London

Drillien C, Drummond M 1983 Developmental screening and the child with special needs. Spastics International Medical Publications, London.

Drillien C M, Pickering R M, Drummond M B 1988 Predictive value of screening for different areas of development. Developmental Medicine and Child Neurology 30: 294–305

Elliot D, Jackson J M, Groves J P 1981 The Oxfordshire mental handicap register. British Medical Journal 282: 289–292

Eu B S L 1986 Evaluation of a developmental screening system for use by child health nurses. Archives of Diseases of Childhood 61: 34–41

Frankenburg W K, Dodds J B 1967 The Denver developmental screening test. Journal of Pediatrics 71: 181

Frankenburg W K, Goldstein A D, Camp B W 1971 The revised Denver developmental screening test: its accuracy as a screening instrument. Journal of Pediatrics 79: 988–995

Gesell A 1925 Mental growth of the pre-school child. Macmillan, New York

Gesell A 1938 Psychology of early growth. Macmillan, New York

Griffiths R 1967 Griffiths mental development scales for testing babies and young children from birth to eight years of age. The Test Agency, High Wycombe, Buckinghamshire

Hall D M B 1988 Delayed speech in children. British Medical Journal 297: 1281–1282

Hall D M B (ed) 1989 Health for all children: Report on the Joint Working Party On Child Health Surveillance. Oxford University Press, Oxford

Harper D C, Wacker D P 1983 The efficiency of the Denver developmental screening test with rural disadvantaged children. Journal of Pediatric Psychology 8: 3

Illingworth R S 1953 The normal child. Churchill Livingstone, London

Illingworth R S 1960 The development of infants and young children: normal and abnormal, 1st edn. Churchill Livingstone, Edinburgh

Macfarlane J A, Pillay U 1984 Who does what, and how much in the preschool child health services in England. British Medical Journal 289: 851–852

Newsholme 1916 School hygiene, the laws of health in relation to school. George Allen and Unwin, London

Nugent J H 1976 A comment of the efficiency of the revised Denver developmental screening test. American Journal of Mental Deficiency 80: 5

Powell P V 1985 A survey on attitudes to preventive medicine in general practice. Health Bulletin 43: 288–295

Roberts C J, Khosla T 1972 British Journal of Preventive and Social Medicine 26: 94–100

Sheridan M D 1960 The developmental progress of infants and young children. DHSS Reports on Public Health No. 102, London

Sheridan M D 1968 Manuals of instruction for STYCAR tests of vision and hearing. NFER, Windsor

Smith A, Jacobson B (eds) 1988 The nation's health. King Edwards Hospital Fund for London, London

Stutsman R 1931 Mental measurement of pre-school children. World Book Co, New York

Terman L M, Merrill M A 1961 Manual for Stanford Binet intelligence scale. Harrap, New York

Wilson J M G, Jungner G 1968 Principles and practice of screening for disease. Public Health Papers No. 34. World Health Organization, Geneva

18. The identification and management of deafness in children

John Tuke

INTRODUCTION

Normal hearing is essential, not only for the acquisition of speech and language but for the child's interaction with its parents and for its all round development (Martin 1972). Severe sensorineural hearing loss (SNHL), rare as it is, may be detected too late to apply the very beneficial effects of specialized early help. The less disabling, but very common, conductive problems associated with middle ear disorders can result in social, behavioural and educational difficulties, which can be modified by timely detection and proper management (Zincus et al 1978).

GPs are well placed through their relationship with families, awareness of the family's particular risk factors, facilities for screening and, in particular, the much underused ability to coordinate and oversee the sometimes complex help available for the impaired or disabled child. The family doctor now also understands that if parents suspect a hearing deficit they are usually correct (World Health Organization 1980, McCormick 1983).

Reassurance can only follow valid testing carried out either within the GP's own team or through appropriate referral. Accurate measurement of the type and degree of hearing defect will provide only a guide to the likely effects on the child's development and behaviour, this being also modified by intrinsic personal qualities and environmental factors.

SENSORINEURAL HEARING LOSS

Bilateral (due to damage to the cochlea or nervous pathway) SNHL can result in profound deafness. It is usually permanent or progressive and the majority are present at birth. About 40% of cases are unexplained and assumed to be genetically determined; the remainder are due to intrauterine, infective or perinatal problems; to central nervous system maldevelopment or are associated with low birth weight (Newton 1985, Cremers et al 1989).

Whilst that proportion allocated to a genetic aetiology has declined, and perhaps will continue to do so as other factors are revealed, it may be appropriate to assume a risk of 1 in 4 for siblings of those in this group (Newton 1985). Families in this category therefore deserve the offer of genetic counselling (see Chapter 10). The advice given in turn will depend upon the results of postnatal investigation, including viral studies, in an attempt to exclude an infective origin. As the rubella seronegativity rate in the United Kingdom drops towards 1% in pregnant women, this disease, although now a much less frequent cause of congenital deafness, remains the most common single infective origin, with cytomegalovirus (CMV) infection and toxoplasmosis as relatively rare aetiologies. CMV is excreted by 0.5% of neonates and, of these, some 10% are found subsequently to be deaf (Peckham et al 1987). Perinatal causes include low birth weight, hyperbilirubinaemia and anoxia, a history of any of these identifying the infant as at risk.

Some 10% of severe childhood deafness is due to bacterial meningitis, although in many the hearing loss will gradually improve following the acute episode (Lancet 1986a). The incidence of congenital SNHL in the UK is between 1 and 2 per 1000 live births. This figure compares with an estimate for EEC countries of 0.9 per 1000 (Bock & Iurato 1988); 80% of cases are manifest by the first birthday and 95% by the third. The disability in some of these late onset children is due to progressive infection, including the congenital rubella syndrome and CMV. The rarity of this handicap in practice population terms may result in a very low level of suspicion.

SNHL, then, is usually present at birth and is more likely when the history includes:

1. Infection during pregnancy — rubella, CMV, toxoplasmosis, measles.

2. Perinatal problems and low birth weight.
3. Bacterial meningitis.
4. Family history of severe hearing loss.

The above at-risk groups merit extra surveillance for hearing loss throughout infancy and, when a child's records are identified as 'at-risk', this can be done on an opportunistic basis.

CONDUCTIVE HEARING LOSS

Otitis media, glue ear (secretery otitis media, otitis media with effusion — OME), eustachian problems and adenoidal enlargement are all associated with the pathophysiology of conductive hearing loss, which is usually a transient condition. OME has been defined as an effusion of variable viscosity behind an intact eardrum. If the condition is recurrent or prolonged — 3 to 6 months in both ears — the impairment will be significant in terms of its effect on learning and development (Bock & Iurato 1988). The condition peaks at around 2 and again at 5 years of age, with a wide-ranging prevalence according to various studies, from 5.6 to 59% in the early school years (Nietupska & Harding 1982), depending on the locality and social status of the study population. In one survey, involving a relatively deprived inner city population, nearly 3/4 of a group of 8-year-olds showed various degrees of ear pathology and hearing loss.

IDENTIFICATION OF DEAFNESS IN CHILDREN

Sensorineural hearing loss detection

Early detection of SNHL is vitally important because the first year of life is a critical period of sound reception and there is evidence suggesting that the lack of antenatal auditory stimulation is a significant loss (Ockleford et al 1988). During the first year, children are 'ready to hear' and this is the preparation for the second year when they are 'ready to speak'. Studies in developing song birds, where auditory experience is stored and later used in vocal expression, may have relevance here (Leppelsack 1986).

Perhaps the most important advance in the diagnosis of early deafness has been the formal introduction of the simple concept of involving parents in detection by guiding their observation and by completion of a questionnaire. This has been shown to be successful and is now being used extensively in the UK and elsewhere (Hitchings & Haggard 1983, McCormick 1983, Lancet 1986b)(Fig. 18.1). An infant arousing such parental concern deserves early referral for full audiological assessment and this should be possible without delay (Fig. 18.2).

Much has been written about neonatal screening for hearing using a computerised auditory response cradle (ARC). This may have some potential for the future but at present can be recommended only for the screening of infants at risk. The levels of sensitivity and specificity reported suggest the need to continue the more traditional methods of screening. The present consensus is that further debate is needed (Hall & Garner 1988, McCormick et al 1984).

Another test suitable for children over 2 years of age, which appears reliable, standardised and operator-friendly and is at present in the development stage, is the Automated Toy Discrimination Test (McCormick 1989).

An objective physiological estimate of hearing, especially useful in difficult cases and in children with other handicaps, can be achieved using the auditory brain stem response, now available in most ENT departments. A better understanding of cochlear function and simple objective testing without the use of electrodes is also likely to be readily available in the near future. This method is being increasingly used for screening in some neonatal populations (Kemp 1991).

Accurate diagnosis and management may be far from easy in both the relatively rare SNHL and the very common conductive deafness of childhood. Whilst parental doubts about a child's hearing cannot be discounted until adequate and repeated scrutiny reveals normal function, parents will occasionally resist the suspicion of deafness. Older children are often skilled in devices to mislead the examiner, e.g. lip-reading and by maximum use of residual hearing at close range. They may also use self-deception and deny any deficiency. In quiet surroundings they can concentrate and mislead the speaker using simplistic and unreliable test methods.

Behavioural problems can result at any age from hearing deficit but the doctor should be aware of the family's natural inclination to explain more profound and multiple problems involving failure to achieve and emotional disturbances as resulting simply from deafness.

In the congenital form, there is a marked tendency to find accompanying problems, especially visual disturbances (Snashall 1988). This is an example where full investigation of the child should precede any statement of future expectations. Premature conclusions may lead to frustration and anger when the complex clinical picture fails to resolve on dealing simply with the hearing impairment.

Age at first diagnosis of SNHL in western European countries has fallen remarkably in the last decade but

West Suffolk Health Authority

Test Your Baby's Hearing

(*DELETE AS APPROPRIATE)

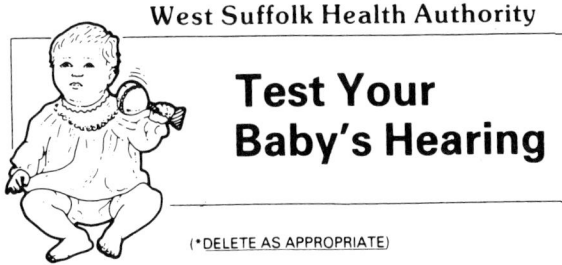

In the First Weeks:-
Is your baby startled by a hand clap , door slamming or other loud noise ?
Do these sounds make him blink or look startled ?

* YES/NO

At 1 Month.
Does your baby appear to notice the noise of the hoover or telephone when they start ?

* YES/NO

At 4 Months.
Does your baby smile or calm down at the sound of your voice even when he cannot see you ? Does he turn his eyes or face to you when you speak to him from the side, having come from behind him ?

* YES/NO

At 7 Months.
In a quiet room when he is not too engrossed by a toy (for example) does he turn to quiet sounds made at a short distance to the side, or to your gentle voice across the room ?

* YES/NO

At 9 Months.
Does he appear to listen with concentration to common familiar sounds, and look around for them ?

* YES/NO

At 1 Year.
Does he respond to his own name, and common words such as 'no' and 'bye bye' even when you make no gesture.

* YES/NO

Your Health Visitor will be testing your baby's hearing at about 7 months.

If at any time you think your baby is not hearing normally, either as a result of your own observation or because you cannot answer YES to one of the above questions, you should get in touch with your Health Visitor or Doctor.

It is important that any hearing problems are discovered and treated as soon as possible.

Fig. 18.1 Questionnaire for parents (Adapted with permission from the original by Dr Barry McCormick, Children's Hearing Assessment Centre, General Hospital, Nottingham).

still averages over 2 years. In (West) Germany it fell from 38 months in 1981 to 13 months in 1988 and in the UK the age of first diagnosis is probably similar (Aust et al 1989).

In the UK, hearing screening of all infants is carried out before 12 months of age, usually at 7-8 months. This is done by health visitors using a distraction hearing test. A trained operator presents sounds of different frequencies and intensity at specific locations while an assistant distracts the child's attention, with care being taken to avoid the acceptance of an invalid response to secondary cues such as shadows and smells. Everyday sounds are used, but they are manufactured, for example, by a special rattle

Advice and guidance to
Parents and Teachers
(What to look for)

↓

Listen closely to
their observations

↓

Offer high quality
assessment facility quickly
at primary care or community leve

↓

Refer to specialist
service if required

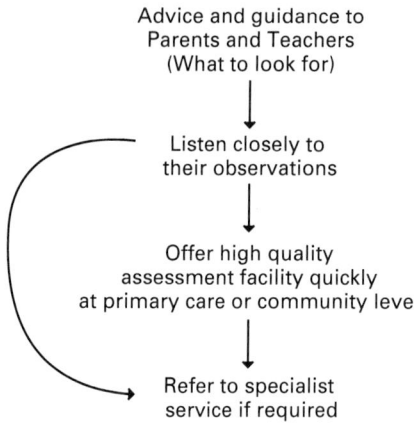

Fig. 18.2 Parents are good observers.

producing a delicate high frequency equivalent to the spoken 'S', 'F' and 'SH', and produced at a specified distance from the infant's ear (Fig. 18.3). The effectiveness of this approach is reduced by poor sensitivity and specificity, compounded in some inner city areas by the difficulties of locating the individual within a moving population. To be successful the test requires careful and regularly repeated retraining of the operators and monitoring of their own hearing. Also necessary are quiet, unhurried conditions and a good deal of patience in all concerned.

Doctors responsible for child health surveillance will need to be familiar with this very important technique, so that they can continually monitor standards and the criteria for its success.

Any suspicion of failure in this test will require a repeat in 2–3 weeks. A second failure or doubtful result indicates an immediate referral to a clinic, where an experienced audiologist will carry out detailed assessment. Ideally this audiology centre operates in association with a developmental paediatrician and teacher for the hearing-impaired or social worker for the deaf. Referrals would normally be received from general practitioners, health visitors, paediatricians,

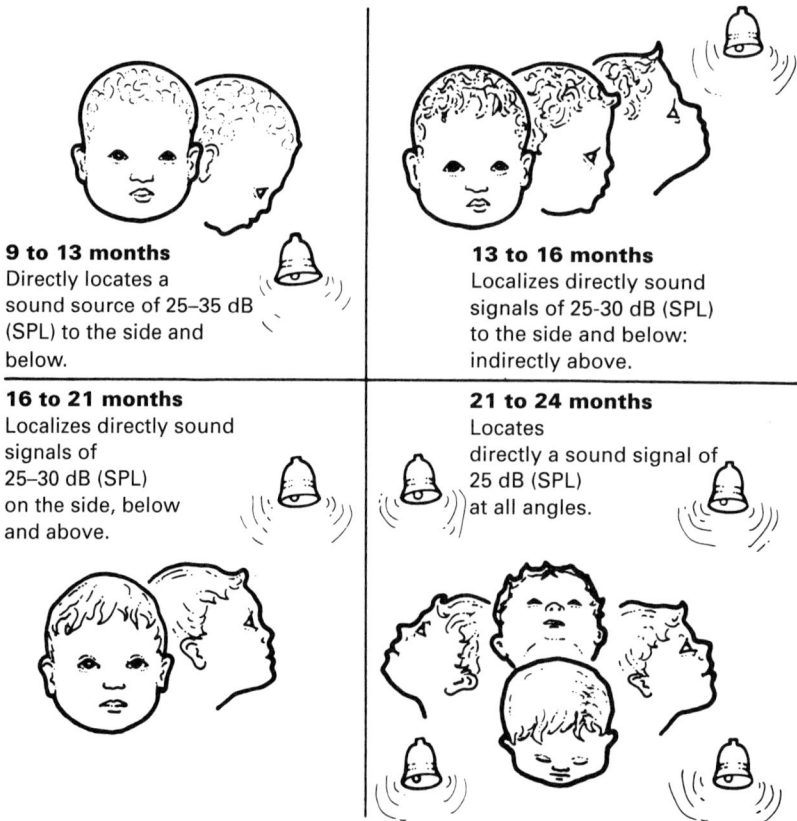

9 to 13 months
Directly locates a
sound source of 25–35 dB
(SPL) to the side and
below.

13 to 16 months
Localizes directly sound
signals of 25-30 dB (SPL)
to the side and below:
indirectly above.

16 to 21 months
Localizes directly sound
signals of
25–30 dB (SPL)
on the side, below
and above.

21 to 24 months
Locates
directly a sound signal of
25 dB (SPL)
at all angles.

Fig. 18.3 Infant responses to sound.

ENT surgeons, speech therapists and community health doctors. A simple and time-saving system depending upon trust and good relationships allows direct referral by these agencies but this requires prior approval and agreement.

As mentioned above, congenital handicap frequently involves more than one system and hearing loss is no exception. Whilst this is the most common result of a fetal rubella viraemia in the first trimester, cardiac problems, intellectual impairment, visual anomalies and motor and other disturbances may also occur. The Child Development Centre style of multi-assessment clinic is therefore appropriate for such a child.

Conductive deafness

Other than hearing loss, otitis media with effusion (OME), the common cause of conductive deafness, will often be quite symptom-free, although the origin in most cases can be traced back to one or more painful inflammatory episodes (Sade et al 1989).

The hearing loss may involve a varying proportion of the speech frequency range, i.e. 250–8000 Hz. A mild deficiency of 20–30 dB, evenly distributed over this range, is commonly found in acquired conductive

deafness, causing some loss of discrimination for speech, even if this is only unilateral. This loss will be observed by use of a pure tone audiometer, indicating the minimum intensity at which the sounds are heard on testing and will be graphically expressed as shown in Fig. 18.4. Ability to detect sounds over the 400–4000 Hz range, with a loss of up to 20 dB, constitutes normal hearing for speech. The more severe central neuronal deafness usually involves the higher frequencies (Fig. 18.5). A total absence of low frequency residual hearing is rare.

The usual screening technique employs pure tone audiometry, a simple test of each ear in which sounds are applied frequency by frequency at reducing intensity until the hearing threshold is reached. More information about the flexibility or compliance of the tympanic membrane, partly dependent on middle ear condition, can be gained by use of an impedance audiometer, which produces a tympanogram — a recording of the eardrum responses to air pressure and applied sound at different frequencies. Whilst useful as a diagnostic tool for revealing middle ear disturbances, and perfectly appropriate for primary care use and as a measure of progress in a defective ear, the impedance audiometer is not sufficiently specific for mass screening purposes.

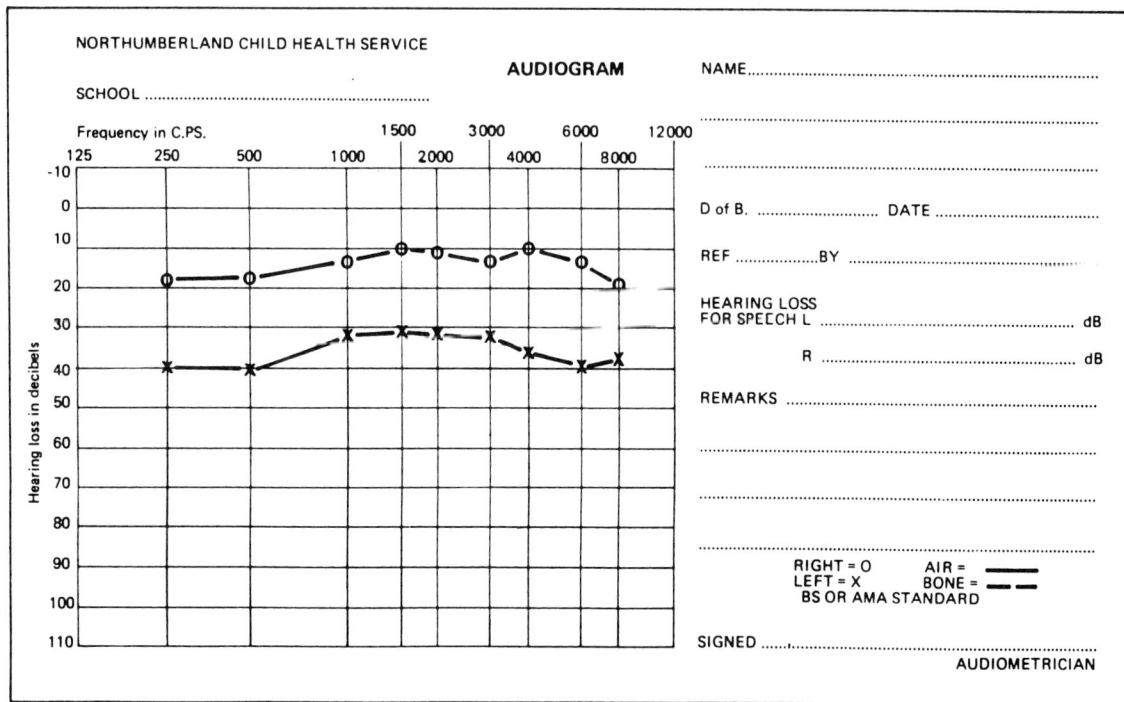

Fig. 18.4 Example of conductive hearing loss in the left ear.

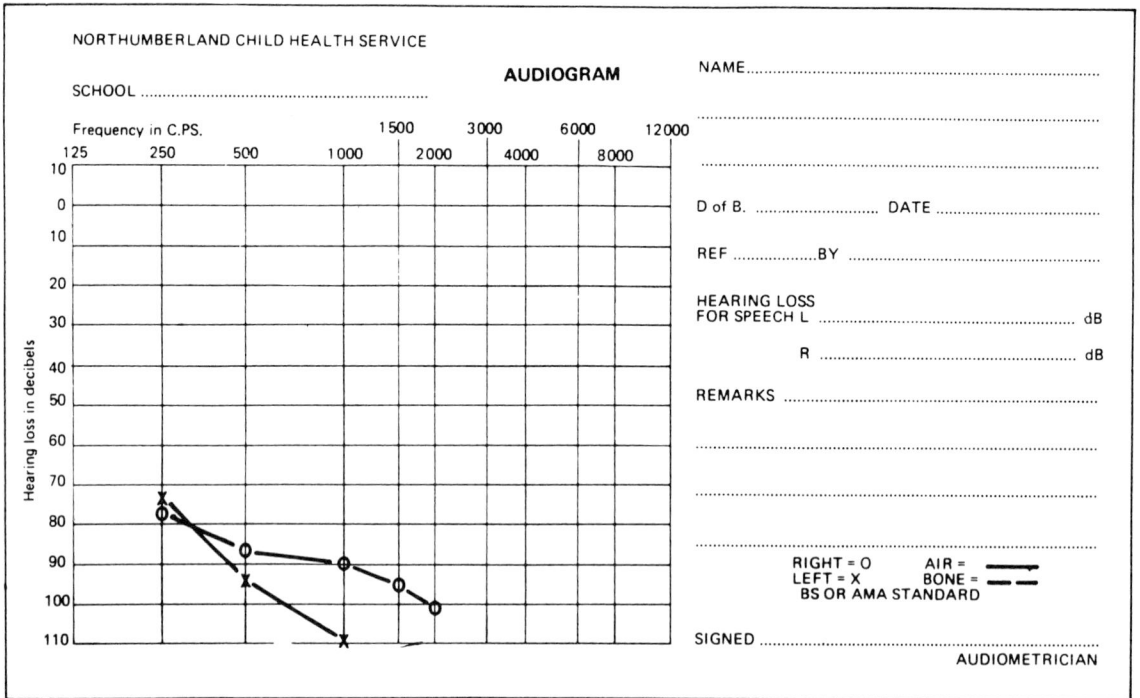

Fig. 18.5   Example of bilateral sensorineural hearing loss.

Language delay beyond 2¹/₂ years merits consideration of hearing deficit and at this age the STYCAR picture hearing test can be used (Sheridan 1976). Another indication for interval testing in the older age group is a history of intercurrent bacterial meningitis.

There is now a tendency not to recommend hearing screening between the first year test and school entry at about 5 years of age, which is the second and last hearing screening test, when audiometry is performed. In addition, at this time a full assessment of the child in conjunction with information obtained from the school teacher about speech, language development and behaviour, is required (O'Callaghan & Colver 1987).

The prevalence of OME might appear to justify frequent screening of school-age children (see Table 18.1) but the natural history of the condition and the long-term ineffectiveness of available treatment call this into doubt when the accepted prerequisites for any screening programme are considered (see Chapter 2).

This view is taken by the report of the Joint Working Party on Child Health Surveillance (Hall 1989) and is supported by much literature, which questions the routine surveillance of children and of hearing in particular (Drillien & Drummond 1983). Swedish, Canadian, North American and UK studies have been

critically reviewed by Professor John Butler (Butler 1989). There is little evidence to indicate any long-term improvement in hearing problems in older children through screening. This is probably due to the failure of commonly used interventions to produce other than temporary benefit (Bluestone et al 1988, Skinner et al 1988, Zielhuis et al 1989).

Table 18.1   A question of screening — children 6–14 years

Prerequisites for screening	Intermittent hearing impairment
Is the defect important?	Yes — usually temporary
Is it common?	Yes
Can it be reliably detected by a test?	Yes
Is the test acceptable?	Yes
Is effective treatment available?	Doubtful
Is the treatment harmless?	Not always
Is the screening cost-beneficial (worthwhile) — including treatment cost?	Probably not
Is the screening cost-effective (cheapest for same result)?	Evidence lacking

However, local needs must sometimes be considered. The dismantling of existing screening programmes, developed in equilibrium with local needs, may destroy more than the opportunity to detect the occasional deaf 3-year-old who has 'slipped through the net' — it may represent lost contact with a needy family.

A child with substantial sensory hearing impairment may also suffer a superimposed middle ear defect, which profoundly increases the disability and, although very easily overlooked, requires special attention.

Parents are inherently good observers of their child and reinforcement of this ability by guidance in looking for deviation, will produce better results in revealing problems than routine surveillance. This has now been stated by many organisations, including the World Health Organization, The Council of Europe (1985), The National Children's Bureau in the UK and in the USA by Palfrey et al (1987).

At the same time, as we have seen, a prolonged hearing loss during the school years, especially common in primary school children, can be damaging. Suspicion of persistent partial deficit should be assessed, so that arrangements can be made in school and elsewhere to assist the child during this phase and to act as a baseline to monitor progress.

In conclusion, screening for conductive deafness at times other than infancy and school entry probably does not influence the outcome, but if parents and teachers are alert to the indicators, and if children are referred for audiological assessment when doubts are raised, then appropriate social and educational assistance can be provided for the duration of the problem. Teachers and others should have an especially high level of suspicion of children from deprived families and localities with an unstable population.

Management of sensorineural hearing loss

The expansion of primary medical care towards primary health care, encourages a family doctor to take the lead in the role of prevention, detection and management of a child with SNHL. Early discovery, rapid input of expert help from the education service, audiologists and others can be rewarding. Following diagnosis, the doctor's role is in secondary prevention. Deaf children are especially vulnerable to the dynamics of the day-to-day changes in their development and environment and to succeed in coping with these they will require more than the usual quota of understanding, affection and the skills of various professionals. In the European collaborative study only 32% of 8-year-old deaf children had achieved satisfactory reading skills (Bock & Iurato 1988).

Adolescence is a crucial period requiring special attention, when evolving self-identity results in poor esteem, unhappiness and underachievement. Integration in mainstream education is a great deal to ask at this time and understanding support from the family doctor may be crucial.

In our steps towards a truly satisfactory primary health care system, we should look towards a primary preventive role that considers the avoidable aspects in the aetiology of congenital deafness: infections in pregnancy, low birth weight with its socio-economic association, antenatal smoking and family history of deafness.

Early suspicion, careful whole-child assessment and understanding help for the family can result in near normal speech and communication. Sound amplification using every scrap of residual hearing, together with teaching methods now available, can enable a deaf child to integrate into society as a literate and whole personality.

There is a need for the coordination of this help, which changes as the child develops. This role may be successfully taken by a teacher for the deaf, audiologist or community paediatrician. Alternatively, the family doctor may wish to undertake this.

The teacher for the deaf is primarily concerned with speech and communication development but will also encourage the parents to develop their own skills in offering the child maximum stimulation through other senses and with the help of hearing aids. In the United Kingdom the National Deaf Children's Society can give valuable help from an early stage — the weeks and months following diagnosis when families repeatedly ask for support (Lawson & Carnegie-Smith 1980). This includes information about future expectations, equipment, financial aid available, educational toys and self-help groups.

The hearing-impaired child is increasingly integrated into normal schooling, partly in response to the 1981 Education Act, which places upon professionals the obligation to identify children with disability and handicap as soon as possible and to offer appropriate help, not simply in formal educational terms. It also encourages the placement of children within the normal education system wherever possible. This trend is reflected in other European countries and on the North American continent where, for example, a Canadian review shows the number of schools dedicated to the hearing impaired reduced from 20 in 1977 to 14 ten years later, with a 40% reduction in pupils (Williams et al 1989). This study also reveals an apparent international trend — a three-fold increase in paraprofessional staff, such as speech therapists. This

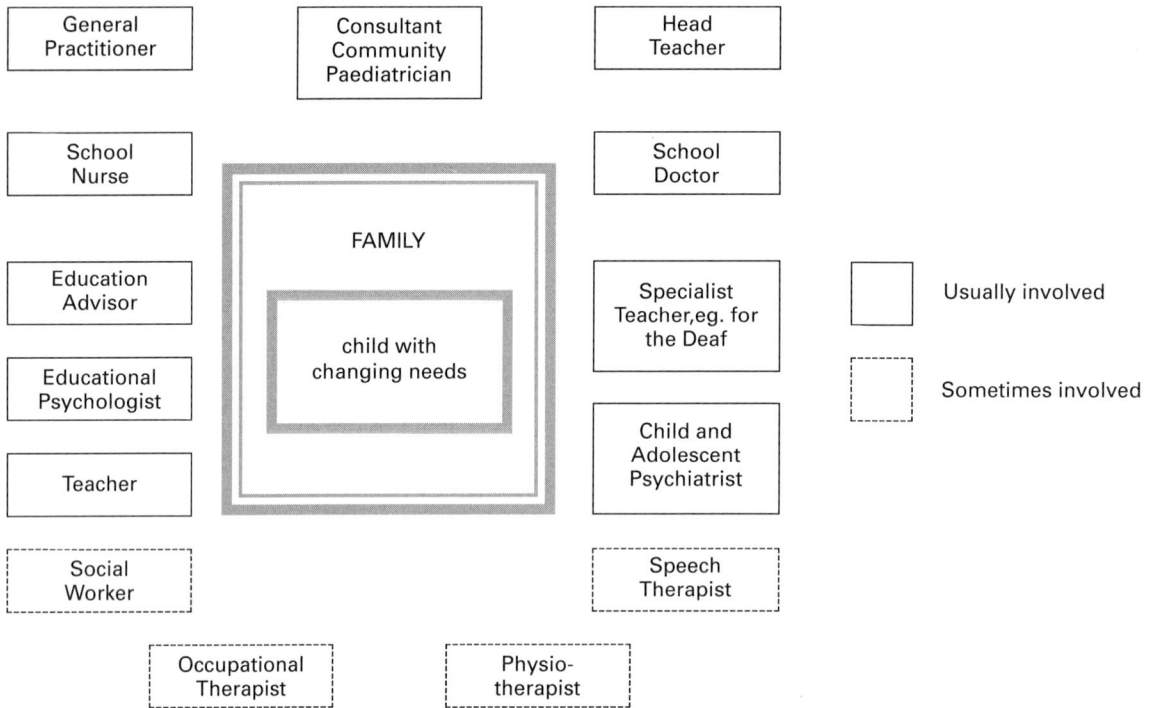

Fig. 18.6   The child's needs change through time. Professional help requires co-ordination.

displays a paradox: the increasing specialised input in such institutions with individualised programmes and support, against the attempt to offer, in a small unit within a normal school, adequate provision in the interest of integration in a normal environment.

General practitioners may consider their few handicapped children consumed by the hospital paediatric service, the community paediatricians and the education department. Whilst many agencies will be necessarily involved, at a rate that is inversely proportional to the child's age, the concerned involvement of the family doctor in a constructive and coordinating role can only be helpful and should be welcomed (Fig. 18.6).

The profoundly deaf school leaver requires much support in the years before leaving school, in readiness for the move into employment or further education. The child's own doctor will wish to monitor, from an early stage, the adequacy of these arrangements. This is surely the GP's role.

Management of conductive hearing loss

Otitis media with effusion is subject to spontaneous recovery. Treatment with antihistamines, deconges-

tants, antibiotics and pressure equalisation tubes (grommets) do not appear to change its natural history in the long term (Cantekin et al 1983, Froom et al 1990). While it may be quicker to insert a grommet with some immediate benefit, however short-lived, than to argue the case at length for endurance and patience, the doubtful long-term results and possible complications should not pass without mention. For example, otorrhoea followed in 18% of 309 T-tube insertions in a recent French study (Francois et al 1988). Further well designed trials of different methods of treatment, using large numbers of children, would be required before existing methods were entirely free of conjecture (Skinner & Lesser 1990).

In the more protracted and severe cases, selection for surgery is a matter for the ENT surgeon; this also applies to the two special at-risk risk groups — those with Down syndrome and those with a cleft palate. Myringotomy and grommet insertion, with or without adenoidectomy, continues to be performed throughout the western world but substantial evidence to justify this in terms of eventual outcome is hard to find.

It is clearly helpful to children, their parents, teachers and peer group to be aware of the limiting effects of this temporary disability. Compensatory arrangements can be made, which largely overcome these limitations. It is therefore useful to carry out serial pure tone audiometry and tympanometric tests in affected children, as only in this way can hearing ability be objectively studied and progress measured.

CONCLUSION

Most childhood illness is related to socio-economic status. Otitis media with effusion is more common in relatively deprived inner city populations and within households where there is at least one cigarette smoker (Hinton 1989). Generalisation about the health needs of a nation's people can be dangerous and some would argue that the regular observation of some groups, more at risk through behavioural and environmental disadvantage, is intrinsically worthwhile because of the many, often interconnected, problems that may be revealed. The difficulty in satisfying a 'lust for proof' or a paucity of available studies proving efficacy through identified outcome measures, does not necessarily justify the dismantling of screening and surveillance programmes (Zusman & Bissonette 1973, Marmot 1986). Within the UK, inequalities in health and in available services, both primary and secondary, do exist and arrangements for the detection and management of a hearing impaired child will need to be constructed accordingly.

Many profoundly deaf young people leave school socially well adjusted, with easily intelligible speech and with prospects for an otherwise relatively normal future. Many do not. Of all the factors involved in this disparity, the role of the general practitioner is considerable. Retrospective review of one school leaver requiring help from the social services department comes too late because there may not be a further opportunity to apply the lessons learned.

REFERENCES

Aust G, Foll U, Lutt B, Schaffrath R 1989 Hearing handicap in childhood — responsibilities of public health, early diagnosis. Das Oeffentliche Gesundheitswesen 51(1): 2–6
Bluestone C D, Gates G A, Paradise G L, Stool S E 1988 Controversy over tubes and adenoidectomy. Paediatric Infectious Diseases Journal 7(11) Supp: 146–149
Bock G R, Iurato S 1988 EEC hearing impairment programme: collaboration in Europe, 1974–1988. Otorhinolaryngology 50: 349–354
Butler J 1989 Child health surveillance in primary care. A critical review. HMSO, London
Cantekin E I, Mandel E M, Bluestone C D, et al 1983 Lack of efficacy of a decongestant – antihistamine combination for otitis media with effusion in children. Results of a double blind randomised trial. New England Journal of Medicine 308(6): 297–301
Council of Europe 1985 Child health surveillance. Council of Europe, Strasbourg
Cremers C W R J, van Rijn P M, Haggeman M J 1989 Prevention of serious hearing impairment or deafness in the young child. Journal of the Royal Society of Medicine 82: 484–487
Drillien C M, Drummond M B 1983 Developmental screening and the child with special needs. Spastics International, London
Francois M, Laccourreye O, Margo J N, et al 1988 Short term complications of transtympanic aerators. Annales d'oto-laryngologie et de Chirogie Cervico-faciale (Paris) 105(5): 349–353
Froom J, Culpepper L, Grob P et al 1990 Diagnosis and antibiotic treatment of acute otitis media: Report from international primary care network. British Medical Journal 300: 582–86
Hall D M B 1989 Health for all children. Report of the Joint Working Party on Child Health Surveillance. Oxford University Press, Oxford
Hall D M B, Garner J 1988 The feasibility of screening all neonates for hearing loss. Archives of Disease in Childhood 63: 652–653
Hinton A E 1989 Surgery for otitis media with effusion in children and its relationship with parental smoking. Journal of Laryngology and Otology 103(6): 559–561
Hitchings V, Haggard M P 1983 Incorporation of parental suspicions in screening infants. British Journal of Audiology 17: 71–75
Kemp D T 1991 Early detection of peripheral hearing disorders using otoacoustic emissions. Presentation at Section of Otology at Royal Society of Medicine Feb 1991, London
Lancet 1986a Deafness after meningitis (Editorial) Lancet i: 134–135
Lancet 1986b Developmental surveillance (Editorial) Lancet i: 950–952
Lawson G R, Carnegie-Smith K 1980 Audit of the services available to deaf children under the age of 11 years. Report to Northumberland Health Authority, unpublished data
Leppelsack H J 1986 Critical periods in audiological development. Acta Otolaryngologica (Suppl): p 57–59
McCormick B 1983 Hearing screening by health visitors: a critical appraisal of the distraction test. Health Visitor 56: 449–451
McCormick B 1989 Automated toy discrimination test — description and initial evaluation. British Journal of Audiology 23: 249–254
McCormick B, Curnock D A, Spavins F 1984 Auditory screening of special care neonates using the auditory response cradle. Archives of Diseases in Childhood 59: 1168–1172
Marmot M G 1986 Epidemiology and the art of the soluble. Lancet i: 887–890
Martin J A M 1972 Hearing loss and human behaviour. In: Rutter M, Martin J A M (eds) The child with delayed speech. Clinics in developmental medicine No. 34. Heineman 87–93

National Children's Bureau 1987 Investing in the future. National Children's Bureau, London

Newton V E 1985 Aetiology of bilateral sensorineural hearing loss in young children. Journal of Laryngology and Otology (Suppl 10)

Nietupska O, Harding N 1982 Auditory screening of school children: fact or fallacy? British Medical Journal 284: 717–720

O'Callaghan E M, Colver A S 1987 Selective medical examination on starting school. Archives of Disease in Childhood 67: 1041–1043

Ockleford E M, Vince M A, Layton C, Reader M R 1988 Responses of neonates to parents and others voices. Early Human Development 18(1): 27–36

Palfrey G S, Singer J D, Walker D K, Butler J A 1987 Early identification of children's special needs: A study in five metropolitan communities. Journal of Paediatrics 111: 651–659

Peckham C S, Stark O, Dudgeon J A et al 1987 Congenital cytomegalovirus infection: a cause of sensorineural hearing loss. Archives of Diseases of Childhood 62(12): 1233–1237

Sade J, Luntz M, Pitashny R 1989 Diagnosis and treatment of secretory otitis media. Otolaryngology Clinics of North America 22(1): 1–14

Sheridan M S 1976 Manual for the STYCAR hearing test. National Federation for Education Research, Slough

Skinner D W, Lesser T H, Richards S H 1988 A fifteen year follow-up of a controlled trial of the use of grommets in glue ear. Clinical Otolaryngology 13(5): 341–346

Skinner D W, Lesser T H 1990 Surgery for Glue Ear. British Medical Journal 301:290

Snashall S 1988 Deafness in childhood. In: Ludman H (ed) Mawson's diseases of the ear. Edward Arnold, London, p 245

Williams D M L, Hopman W M, Latimer J 1989 Support services in Canadian schools for the hearing impaired. Journal of Otolaryngology 18(7): 386–389

World Health Organization 1980 Early detection of handicap in children. EURO Reports and Studies, 30. Regional Office for Europe, World Health Organization, Copenhagen, pp 15 and 25

Zielhuis G A, Rach G H, van-den-Broek P 1989 Screening for otitis media with effusion in pre-school children. Lancet i: 311–314

Zinkus P W, Gottleib M I, Schapiro M 1978 Development and psycho educational sequelae of chronic otitis media. American Journal of Diseases of Childhood 132: 1100

Zusman J, Bissonette R 1973 The case against evaluation. International Journal of Mental Health 2: 112–125

19. The identification and management of visual impairment

Carol Church

This chapter is written from a paediatric rather than an ophthalmological point of view. It concentrates on suggestions for practice that have been found useful in the primary care setting, and in particular in child health surveillance. As vision is the most common reason for referral from these programmes (Curtis Jenkins et al 1978), and similarly from the School Health Service, a thorough knowledge of this topic is essential.

THE DEVELOPMENT OF VISION

The visual apparatus is not completely developed at birth and, unlike the ear, is without experience. The visual cortex develops in the early months but the retina is not fully developed until 18 months of age and the lateral geniculate body until 20 months. Input is critical to visual development and deprivation of the stimulus in the early months, e.g. opacity in the media, complete ptosis, etc. affects vision seriously. It follows that such conditions require urgent action.

The normal sequence

1. *'Fix and follow'* is present in 80% of normal babies by 1 month of age and in 100% by 3 months of age. Any delay beyond this requires investigation.
2. *Accommodation* is present in 80% of normal babies by 1 month of age. By 6–8 months there is full accommodation.
3. *Convergence* is demonstrable by 3–4 months of age. Both accommodation and convergence are necessary for the development of hand-eye coordination.
4. *Binocular single vision* is developed by 4 months of age and therefore any squint, even if intermittent, is considered to be abnormal from that age.
5. *Visual fields* are virtually full by 6–7 months of age.
6. The *sphere of interest* during the first year extends from 3 metres at 6 months of age to 6 metres at 12 months. It must be noted, however, that scanning requires an understanding of something to look for. Mentally handicapped children tend to give low visual acuity results because of lack of drive and because they are recumbent for longer during the first year. Looking at the ceiling for many months can induce bilateral amblyopia. Both mentally and physically handicapped children need to be seated upright and have toys to look at, both near and far.
7. *Visual acuity* improves during the first year from the equivalent of 6/60 at 3 months to 6/24 at 6 months and 6/6 by 8–12 months.

Vision and general development

Most of a child's development in the first year of life depends on vision. One only needs to follow the progress of a visually handicapped infant to appreciate the profound effect it has in all fields of development:

1. *Social smile* at 6 weeks of age, surprisingly, is not dependent on vision. It can be triggered by the sound of the mother's voice, smell of the breast pads, etc.
2. *Hand regard* may be a neurological rather than a primary visual phenomenon.
3. *Hand–eye coordination*, as shown first by 'batting' at about 3 months of age, and then soon after by finger play, is a visually directed behaviour. Blind babies must wait until about 4 months of age — when a toy placed in the hand can be held and then mouthed — before starting to learn about size, form, texture, etc.
4. *Motor milestones* and the development of secondary responses are dependent on visual feedback for the appreciation of the position of the body in space.
5. *Hearing responses* are difficult to interpret in visually handicapped babies because there is no reinforcement in turning to a sound source that cannot be seen. Hence the adage that vision should always be tested before hearing.

183

6. *Speech and language* development is delayed in blind and partially sighted children because even the acquisition of first word labels is difficult when relying on other special senses.

EXPLANATION OF TERMS

Refractive errors

Emmetropia (normal sight)

In the normal eye, parallel rays of light are brought to a focus at the fovea by refraction at the cornea and lens (Fig. 19.1). When looking at near objects, accommodation by the lens keeps the image in focus.

Hypermetropia (long sight)

Hypermetropes have a slightly shorter eyeball than normal so that parallel rays of light are brought to a focus behind the retina (Fig. 19.1). This can be overcome by accommodation by the lens so that mild degrees of bilateral hypermetropia can be tolerated.

In high degrees of hypermetropia, the lens cannot accommodate sufficiently and therefore both near and far vision are reduced. If it is bilateral, the accommodative effort tends to induce excessive convergence and squint. If it is unilateral, the visual cortex relies on the good eye, and amblyopia develops in the other.

Axial length and refractive error (schematic)

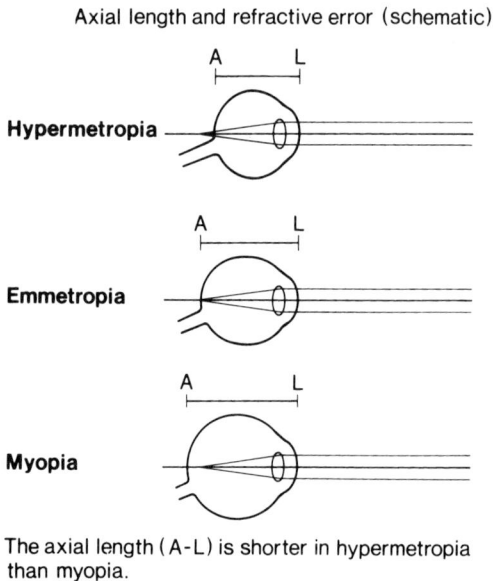

Hypermetropia

Emmetropia

Myopia

The axial length (A-L) is shorter in hypermetropia than myopia.

Fig. 19.1   Axial length and refractive error (schematic).

Myopia (short sight)

The eyeball is slightly longer than normal in myopes, so that parallel rays of light are brought to a focus in front of the retina (Fig. 19.1), therefore distant vision is reduced. Myopes see well for near and they do not use accommodation.

Anisometropia

A marked difference in refraction between one eye and the other is known as anisometropia. It is an important error because it may cause amblyopia.

Astigmatism

Astigmatism occurs when the cornea has an uneven curvature. There is difficulty focusing the image in the different meridia simultaneously and the effect is blurring in one axis, and distortion. Mild degrees of astigmatism occur during growth of the eyeball or skull, and this can be tolerated. The eyeball virtually reaches adult size by the age of 2 years, the axial length having increased from 18 mm at birth to 24 mm. High degrees of astigmatism can cause meridional amblyopia.

How to tell the refractive error from spectacles

It is useful to know the type of spectacle correction a child's relatives are wearing and the age at which they were first prescribed when assessing risk of visual problems. It is also important in adult patients to know what error they have, because of the association with a number of ocular disorders occurring later in life, e.g. hypermetropia with narrow angle glaucoma, myopia with retinal detachment.

The eyes of a myope will appear small when viewed through the spectacles because concave lenses are used for correction and the profile of the face appears recessed when viewed through the spectacles (Fig. 19.2). If print is then observed through the spectacles held horizontally over a page, it will appear smaller. If the spectacles are then moved backwards, forwards and sideways above the page, the print will appear to move in the same direction. The eyes of a hypermetrope will appear large because convex lenses which magnify are used and the profile of the face will seem to be displaced outwards. When the print test is carried out, it appears larger, and moves in the opposite direction to the movement of the spectacles.

Astigmatism may be associated with either myopia or hypermetropia and is easiest to diagnose from the

Appearances of spectacle correction for refractive error

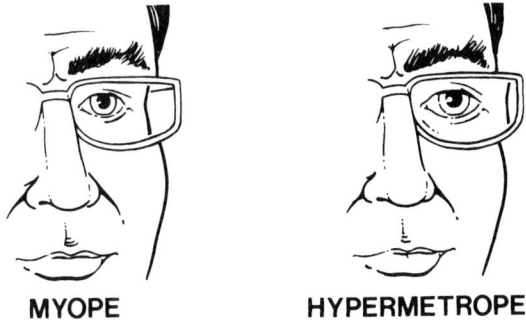

MYOPE   **HYPERMETROPE**

Fig. 19.2   Appearances of spectacle correction for refractive error.

lenses while doing the print test. The speed of movement of the print will be different in the two planes, and if the spectacles are rotated the print appears to twist.

Anisometropia can be diagnosed in the same way because the size of the print when viewed through each lens, and the speed of movement, will be different, and can be directly compared.

Amblyopia

Amblyopia can be defined as defective visual acuity in a healthy eye which cannot be made normal with spectacles. It occurs early, the most sensitive period being the first few months of life (Barlow 1975). It does not develop after the visual sensory system is no longer plastic, i.e. after about 8 years of age. The causes are squint, anisometropia, high astigmatism and stimulus deprivation.

The time interval between onset of amblyopia and treatment is crucial to prognosis.

Squint

Squint is present when the two eyes are not looking at the same object. Thus the central fusion mechanism for the images is not functioning and there is no stereopsis. There are numerous terms used to describe squint:

Concomitant, a deviation which is constant regardless of the position of gaze. Non-paralytic.
Incomitant, the angle of deviation varies with the position of gaze. Paralytic.
Esotropia, convergent squint.
Exotropia, divergent squint.
Hypertropia, visual axis of deviating eye is directed too high.

Hypotropia, visual axis of deviating eye is directed too low.
A&V pattern, angle of squint alters on elevation and depression.
Manifest, evident at the time of examination, demonstrated by the cover test.
Latent, underlying tendency to squint demonstrated by the cover/uncover test.
Alternating, either eye can take up fixation.
Accommodative, evident when accommodating. Can be influenced by use of spectacles.

Squint occurs in 5% of children. The most common type is convergent accommodative, with a peak incidence at 2–3 years. Divergent squint is less common and usually has a later onset. If divergent squint occurs in the first year of life, it may be due to low vision with a number of possible serious causes. At any age it is important to remember that squint may be symptomatic of severe eye disease, e.g. cataract, retinoblastoma or toxoplasmosis.

The mainstays of treatment for squint are spectacles, occlusion and surgery.

CHILDREN VISUALLY AT RISK

Before embarking on the visual content of child health surveillance programmes, it is helpful to know that there are some categories of children who are at greater risk of a visual problem than the general population. Such 'at-risk' lists can be used to formulate preschool vision screening policy (Table 19.1).

Family history

1. *Visual handicap* has a genetic cause in about 50% of cases.
2. *Squint*. In one series, 55% of patients with a squint and/or hypermetropia had a positive family history (Ingram 1973).

Table 19.1   Risk factors for visual problems

Family history of
 Visual handicap with possible genetic cause
 Squint
 Amblyopia
 Eye surgery in childhood
 Hypermetropia
 Early spectacles

Prematurity (of < 2200 g birthweight)

Twins

Other handicap

3. *Amblyopia* is also called lazy eye. Two thirds of amblyopes are squinters and one third are straight-eyed (Ross et al 1977). The latter group are usually due to uniocular refractive error.
4. *Eye surgery* in childhood is usually for squint. Other rare, but important, reasons might be retinoblastoma, cataract or congenital glaucoma, all of which can be genetically determined.
5. *Hypermetropia* is the most common and most important refractive error of infancy (Atkinson et al 1984). It increases the risk of developing squint, and hence amblyopia, by twenty-fold (Ingram et al 1979). Bilateral hypermetropia is likely to cause accommodative squint but, if the error is unilateral, it may cause straight-eyed amblyopia.
6. *Glasses* worn by first degree relatives for a refractive error originating in infancy are significant. Again, hypermetropia is the most important cause, but it is possible for high astigmatism, whether unilateral or bilateral, to cause meridional amblyopia. Myopia is of less importance, especially the common acquired type, which develops after school entry and has a peak incidence between 11 and 13 years. This is because myopia rarely causes amblyopia, near vision being good. Hypermetropia and astigmatism, on the other hand, cause reduced vision for both near and far, making amblyopia more likely. However, there is a rare type of congenital high myopia, often genetically determined, which would necessitate glasses in the preschool years. First degree relatives of these patients should be screened early. Parents often do not know what type of refractive error family members have, but it is possible to tell from their glasses (see Fig. 19.2) so that a judgement about risk can be made.

Prematurity

Babies weighing less than 1500 g at birth and/or those of less than 32 weeks gestation and those that have been nursed in oxygen are usually referred directly to an ophthalmologist from the Special Care Baby Unit for assessment and follow-up. Babies of between 1500 and 2200 g birthweight are also visually at risk (Gardiner 1982). Premature infants have an increased prevalence of optic atrophy, retrolental fibroplasia, myopia, squint and postnatal cataract.

Twins

As well as overlapping with the premature group, twins are said to be visually at risk in their own right (Gardiner 1977).

Handicap

Children with a handicap, particularly of neurological type, e.g. cerebral palsy, spina bifida, mental handicap, are at greatly increased risk of visual disorder. The prevalence of refractive error in this group is of the order of 30–40%, commonly hypermetropia and hence squint (Gardiner et al 1969). Children with Down syndrome, cyanotic congenital heart disease and physical handicap, e.g. muscular dystrophy, are at increased risk of myopia.

Other categories

Under some circumstances, a child may become visually at risk later.

Parental concern

If parents express concern about their child's vision this must be taken seriously. Parents rarely suspect acuity problems in preschool children and, if they do, they are likely to be right. Squint is often diagnosed by parents first. Nothing short of a specialist opinion will do.

Deafness

Children with bilateral neurosensory hearing loss should have their vision assessed at an early age because they are more dependent than the general population on good eyesight.

Severe behaviour problems

The special senses should always be tested if there are serious behaviour problems. This applies even more to hearing than to vision.

VISION TESTING

Background and recent developments

Interest in vision screening is quite recent. It has been known for some time that most visual defects, with the exception of visual handicap and manifest squint, were not identified until school entry (Court 1976). STYCAR tests for measuring visual acuity were developed during the 1960s and introduced in the 1970s without published validation (Sheridan 1976). In the 1980s it was found, by careful comparison against Snellen testing, that these tests were not sufficiently sensitive to identify common acuity defects (Hall et al 1982) (Table 19.2)

Table 19.2 Sensitivity and specificity of STYCAR tests of visual acuity

Test	Sensitivity for Detection (%)		Specificity
	Moderate defects (6/12–6/36)	Severe defects (≤6/60)	
Fixed balls	5	68	100
Rolling balls	12	70	100
Miniature toys	58	95	91
Matching letters	98	100	64

(Reproduced with the kind permission of Professor D M B Hall)

With the exception of letter matching, the STYCAR tests measure the minimum observable rather than the minimum separable and cannot be equated to visual acuity (Reinecke 1978). Because the STYCAR letter matching test is single optotype there are important pitfalls with this test too (Brant & Novotny 1976). It underestimates amblyopes such that the diagnosis may be missed altogether.

There are three prerequisites for the identification of amblyopia.

1. 6 metre test.
2. Linear format.
3. Crowding of letters.

These criteria are most satisfactorily fulfilled by the Snellen test and the minimum age for population screening using this chart with clue cards and occlusion is about 4 years, although some individual children are able to carry it out when younger. It is important to know whether identification of visual defects at this age produces better ultimate results than at school entry, and Ingram suggests that it does not (Ingram et al 1986).

A more recent approach to screening is the use of refraction, but it has been found that even correction with spectacles from the age of 1 year does not alter the subsequent incidence of squint or severe amblyopia (Ingram et al 1985). Younger children still are now being screened, in some cases by photorefraction (Atkinson et al 1984). This apparatus can be operated by paramedical personnel, and may thus be a population screening method for the future. Some encouraging results are being obtained from identifying and treating 6–9 month-olds.

VISUAL CONTENT OF THE CHILD HEALTH SURVEILLANCE PROGRAMME

It has been recommended by the Joint Working Party on Child Health Surveillance that screening for visual

Table 19.3 Vision screening in child health surveillance

Age	Content	Equipment
Neonatal	Inspection of eyes	
	Window test	
	Pupillary responses	
	Blink to light	Pencil torch
	Red reflexes	Ophthalmoscope
6 weeks	Visually at risk?	
	Parental concern	
	Inspection of eyes	
	Pupillary responses	Pencil torch
	Red reflexes	Ophthalmoscope
	Visual alertness	Face or suspended ball
8 months and 3 years	Parental concern	
	Visual behaviour	
	Inspection of eyes	
	Eye movements	Small toy
	Squint tests	Pencil torch
4½ years/ school entry	Parental concern	
	Inspection of eyes	
	Eye movements	Small toy
	Squint tests	Pencil torch/ Keystone machine
	Visual acuity	Snellen chart/ clue cards

defects in preschool children should be confined to history and observation (Hall 1989, Johnson et al 1989). Not all ophthalmologists agree with this, the main area of contention being whether anyone other than orthoptists can carry out cover testing adequately. Certainly, any health personnel doing this work would need to be trained by an orthoptist and it is doubtful whether this is feasible for all the necessary general practitioners. There is agreement on the absence of a satisfactory screening test for visual acuity and the following suggested schedule will only stand until the new population screening methods currently being researched are generally available. The cover test is included for the sake of completeness. The ages chosen are widely used in surveillance programmes (Table 19.3).

Neonatal examination

Inspection of the eyes

It is possible to detect many severe visual defects by simple inspection of the eyes around the time of birth. This is important because some defects are surgically treatable and many have genetic implications.

Some conditions to be aware of that require referral.

Constant squint is abnormal at any age.

Nystagmus may be congenital (jerk type), secondary to low vision (pendular type), or spasmus nutans.

Congenital cataract may be seen as a white pupil or as an absent or reduced red reflex.

Congenital glaucoma (buphthalmos): the cornea is large and hazy, which causes dimming of the red reflex. There is photophobia and lacrimation.

Retinoblastoma usually presents later (average 18 months) but occasionally at birth. The chief signs are white pupil, absent or reduced red reflex and, later, squint.

Ptosis demands immediate action only if the lid is sufficiently low to cover the pupil on down gaze. This also applies to any other lesion that obstructs vision, e.g. cavernous haemangioma.

Ophthalmia neonatorum is conjunctivitis presenting in the first 12 days of life, and is a notifiable disease. The usual organisms are chlamydia, gonococcus, streptococcus, staphylococcus and pneumococcus. Such infants are best admitted for investigation and treatment, which requires frequent instillation of drops.

Window test

From the first week of life, if the baby is held supine at 90° to a window, he will turn his head towards the light. If the baby is then turned through 180°, the head should turn the other way towards the light.

Pupillary responses

The pupils should respond to light from birth. It is not necessary to use a torch to test this because it may induce blinking. It is sufficient to shade the open eye with the hand for a moment or two and then withdraw it. Infants' eyes respond less briskly than adults'.

Blink to light

A sudden bright light shone into the eyes causes blink from birth.

Absence of any of the above three responses requires investigation.

Red reflexes

This is best tested with an ophthalmoscope at a distance of about 30 cm with a +3 setting. Cataract may be seen as a black silhouette against the red reflex.

If the infant will not open his or her eyes, change the position to upright, sitting. The vestibulopalpebral reflex will usually make the eyes open. Absence, inequality or any diminution of the red reflex demands immediate ophthalmological referral.

6 weeks

Visually at risk

Birth and family history will determine whether the baby is visually at risk. If there is a family history of visual handicap with possible genetic causes, or if it is already known that the infant has a neurological handicap, a specialist opinion is necessary.

The question of how to manage other visually at-risk infants, who have no observable abnormality, arises. They need screening by 6–9 months of age, and this depends on local arrangements. Most eye hospital out-patient departments are too overstretched to see such cases. Some districts employ community orthoptists (MacLellan & Harker 1979) and it has been suggested that they might learn to refract (British Medical Journal 1977). In Southampton, a Preschool Vision Screening Clinic has been running since 1982. It is staffed by an ophthalmic medical practitioner and two orthoptists. Here, a selected population is examined, either on the basis of being visually at risk or if there is a query about vision from health personnel or parents (Hughes, unpublished data). As an interim measure, this is probably the best way forward until a satisfactory, cost-effective, total population screening method for infants is found.

Parental concern

At every surveillance contact the parents should be asked whether they have any concerns about the baby's vision. At this age there should be a specific enquiry as to whether the baby fixes on their faces, and follows their movements nearby. This has to be distinguished from response to voice. If squint has been noticed, is it constant?

Inspection of the eyes

Any morphological abnormality, constant squint, nystagmus, photophobia or ptosis should be referred.

Other rare conditions that may be more obvious now.

Coloboma of the iris causes keyhole pupil. Its significance lies in the fact that the retina, including the macula, may also be involved, in which case very low vision results.

Aniridia is partial absence of the iris. Nystagmus occurs and there may be cataract and glaucoma. There is an association with Wilm's tumour and other renal abnormalities.

Albinism may be either ocular or oculocutaneous. The red reflex may appear as a pink glow through the iris. There is nystagmus, photophobia and often squint or high refractive error.

Pupillary responses

The pupils should respond to light both directly and consensually. It may be necessary to darken the room to carry out the test.

Red reflexes

These should be repeated as in the neonatal examination.

Visual alertness

This is a specific test. The examiner makes sure that the baby's eyes are fixed on his/her own, and then silently moves his/her head slowly from side to side; the baby's eyes should follow. A suspended ball can be used instead but in general, babies prefer faces. Most babies are visually alert by 6 weeks but if not, and the eyes themselves appear normal, then the baby should be re-examined at 12 weeks. If there is still no response the baby should be referred for a specialist opinion. If it transpires that no ophthalmological problem is found, then late acquisition of visual alertness is a useful early sign of developmental delay. The rest of the neurodevelopmental examination may confirm this suspicion, and the vision under these circumstances may improve with time. In general, visual development proceeds in line with chronological, rather than gestational, age.

Some minor conditions to be aware of.

Epicanthus. Many children have a fold of skin at the medical canthus and a rather flat bridge to the nose. It disappears during growth, but its importance lies in the fact that it causes pseudosquint. Remember, however, that children with epicanthus can also have a true squint.

Blocked tear ducts cause watery eyes. The obstruction is usually at the lower end of the nasolacrimal duct. Infection should be treated by the use of antibiotic drops and the parents should be taught how to massage the tear sac. This expresses mucopus from the lower punctum and is a diagnostic test. The condition nearly always resolves spontaneously during the first year. Ophthalmologists are therefore reluctant to probe, especially as the procedure itself carries the risk of stenosis.

8 months and 3 years

As there is no universally satisfactory visual acuity test for 3-year-olds, the procedure for these two age groups can be dealt with together, as they are almost identical.

Parental concern

The parents must again be asked if they have any concerns about vision, either near or far, and if they ever see a squint.

Visual behaviour

Visual behaviour can either be observed by the examiner during the fine manipulation tests of developmental screening, or reported by the parents. The baby should not have to hold toys close to the eyes or alter the head position to get a view. Head tilt may be caused by vertical squint, and face turn by horizontal muscle paresis. Chin elevation or depression may be caused by ptosis or A&V pattern squints, i.e. squints that vary with position of gaze. Children with nystagmus may also adopt an abnormal head posture because there is a null point at which the amount of eye movement is damped.

Eye movements

Check that the eyes are straight when directly facing the examiner, and that they remain aligned in all eight positions of gaze (Fig. 19.3), using a small bright toy to obtain fixation.

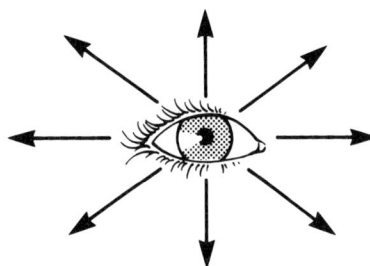

Fig. 19.3 Positions of gaze.

Inability to abduct the eye causes incomitant squint in lateral positions of gaze. In 3-year-olds check the ability of each eye to follow separately. Poor fixation or resistance to occlusion may indicate amblyopia.

Squint tests

Corneal reflections. Shine a pencil torch directly at the eyes and check that the corneal light reflexes are in a symmetrical position in both pupils. NB Small angle squints can be missed if only this test is used.

Cover tests. Use a small toy at a distance of about 30 cm to obtain fixation.

1. *Cover test.* Each eye is covered in turn using the back of the hand or a piece of card. If each eye remains stationary when its fellow is covered, then no squint is present.

   If, on covering one eye, the other has to move to take up fixation, this eye was originally squinting (manifest squint). This may be observed in one eye only (uniocular squint) or in both eyes (alternating squint).
2. *Cover/uncover test.* If no manifest squint has been found, next observe each eye in turn as the cover is removed from it. If the eye moves to take up fixation when the cover is removed, then this eye was squinting under cover (latent squint).
3. *Alternate cover test.* In practice, an infant's attention can be held for such a short time that only a quick alternate cover test may be possible. Here the hand is moved to cover first one eye and then the other in rapid succession several times. If either eye moves then squint is present, either latent or manifest.

It may be possible, in 3-year-olds, to carry out the cover tests in near and far positions, by using a rotating toy or small wall picture in the far position. Convergent squints are usually maximal near, and divergent squints are maximal far.

All children with squints should be referred for a full orthoptic and ophthalmological assessment immediately after the squint is discovered — the time interval between onset and treatment affects outcome. The earlier the onset of squint, the worse is the prognosis, but this does not mean that children should not be referred with the utmost speed (Catford et al 1984).

If the parents think they see a squint, but this cannot be demonstrated, it is still essential that an orthoptic opinion is obtained (Reinecke 1983). This is for medicolegal reasons, and in fact parents often prove to be right. If possible this should be arranged in the community, provided that a suitable clinic exists, so as not to overload out-patients with false positive cases.

$4\frac{1}{2}$ years/school entry

The parents are again asked for any concerns about vision and family history should be reviewed. The doctor carrying out the preschool medical examination is not necessarily the same one who has been carrying out the surveillance programme, and new eye disorders may have been discovered in siblings. The eyes are inspected and pupillary reactions, ocular movements and squint tests carried out as before.

Keystone test of muscle balance

The Keystone machine may be used to test for squint. It is limited by the child's ability to use a binocular device and knowledge of colours. It is a useful adjunct to the cover test, and for school nurses working alone.

Visual acuity

The Snellen test is the most accurate method of testing visual acuity at school entry. It is essential to use a test that will identify amblyopia (see p. 185). Although it may be considered late to make this diagnosis, some useful gains in acuity can be made through occlusion therapy, largely dependent on the age of onset (Catford et al 1984). Even if the visual acuity in the amblyopic eye regresses again after stopping occlusion, because cortical function has been improved, it remains as a potential skill that can be redeveloped in the event of an accident to the good eye later in life (Gardiner 1982).

Tips on testing

So many technical errors are made on Snellen testing that it is worthwhile describing the method used for non-literate children.

It is best to have the child seated at a low table, next to the mother. If possible, siblings should be excluded from the room. The clue card is usually 7-letter, but 5-letter can be used for very immature children. The chart is brought to the table and the child asked to match a few letters. The chart chosen must have enough of the clue letters on it, especially on the 6/9 and 6/6 lines. If the child is successful, the chart is pinned on the wall at the child's eye level, a measured 6 m away, in good light. The child is asked to match a few letters binocularly. The left eye is then occluded, preferably using dermicel because it is easily applied and removed, and is usually well tolerated. If the child refuses this, then a crumpled tissue or mother's palm can be used, but this is not ideal. The child is then asked to match just one central letter from each line working downwards to the point of failure. It is important to reach the end-point as quickly as possible to maintain concentration. The letters must be indicated by using a finger, pointing from below so as not to obscure other letters on the same line. A horizontal rider may be used to indicate the line, but never a vertical one, because it would isolate letters. On the line of failure the child is then asked to match an edge letter, and, if successful, another central letter. If successful again, move on down. The visual acuity is recorded as the best achieved. The test is repeated for the left eye.

A result of 6/9 or better in each eye is considered to be normal. A result of 6/12 or worse in either eye should be referred for full orthoptic and ophthalmological assessment.

It is not considered necessary at this time to test near vision (Hall 1989). There have been some studies into the possible educational significance of isolated near vision defect (Stewart-Brown 1987, Williams et al 1988). Children with this defect are usually mild hypermetropes and were shown to be reading less well than expected. However, a small group that had been treated with spectacles were doing no better educationally than the untreated group. More research is needed on larger sample sizes before a conclusion can be reached.

Individual assessment

Outside the surveillance programme, parents may express doubt about their child's vision at any age. It is possible to reassure parents in the surgery setting only when:

1. The child is mature enough to carry out a distance visual acuity test, as described for school entry, and achieve a result of at least 6/9 in each eye. This may be possible from the age of 3 years onwards.
2. The cover test is negative, carried out by a trained examiner, confident of the result.
3. Fundoscopy is normal, using mydriasis if necessary.

If it is impossible to carry out all three tests, either because of age, immaturity or non-cooperation, then a referral should be made, either to a visual assessment clinic, or to out-patients if there is no other suitable facility.

A word about school children

There is wide variation in vision screening programmes for school children nationally (Stewart-Brown & Haslum 1988). At present it is recommended that

distance visual acuity is tested every three years throughout school life (Hall 1989). Some authorities have questioned the need to test at all after the age of 8 years because this detects only acquired myopia (Cross 1985). All other significant refractive errors will be identified earlier and their prevalence alters little during the school years (Kohler & Stigmar 1978). There is no educational benefit from diagnosing acquired myopia (Peckham et al 1977, Stewart-Brown 1987) and indeed adolescents have been shown to be reluctant to wear spectacles unless they themselves recognise a visual difficulty (Peckham et al 1979).

Some authorities prefer to test annually for the first three years of school and include the Keystone muscle balance test because both convergent and divergent squint can develop after the age of 5 years (Kohler & Stigmar 1978). The incidence of abnormal vision at school entry is 10%, rising to 16% by the age of 16 years (excluding minor errors), mainly through the rising incidence of acquired myopia (Tibbenham et al 1978). Up to the age of 8 years, all referrals require full orthoptic and ophthalmological assessment. After this, distance vision need only be tested once in Middle/Junior school at the age of 10 years, and once in secondary school at the age of 12/13 years, to combine this last screen with the Ishihara colour vision test. This timing allows careers guidance to be given to children with varying degrees of colour blindness before subject options are decided. Referrals for acuity failures over the age of 8 years can be to opticians, as the vision is no longer plastic and therefore orthoptic assessment is not mandatory.

VISUAL HANDICAP

Blindness is defined as a corrected visual acuity of 3/60 or less in the better eye. Partial sightedness is a corrected visual acuity of between 4/60 and 6/24 in the better eye. There is some flexibility in definition depending on the visual fields. Prevalence figures vary according to the precise age taken, but between 0.1 and 0.2 per 1000 of the population will develop serious visual problems in early life (Baraitser 1981). The Director of Social Services registers the child as blind or partially sighted on the advice of the consultant ophthalmologist, and this confers certain benefits.

50% of the disorders are genetically determined (Table 19.4). Vision is the only handicap in half of blind and partially sighted children, but in the other half there is at least one additional handicap, the most common of which is mental retardation.

The presentation of visual handicap in children depends on the age of the child, the severity of the loss,

Table 19.4   A classification of visual handicap

Type	Aetiology	Percentage	Examples
Genetic	Primary ocular	38	Retinitis pigmentosa
	Complex	12	Albinism
Acquired	Prenatal	6	Rubella
	Perinatal	33	Retinopathy of prematurity
	Postnatal	11	Measles keratitis Ophthalmia neonatorum

whether it is unilateral or bilateral and whether there are other associated handicaps. Many are diagnosed in the first few weeks of life by simple inspection, but in general the visual loss has to be severe and bilateral for parents to notice (Table 19.5).

Unilateral visual loss often presents later because visual behaviour is normal (Table 19.6).

The rarity of visual handicap in children is such that few general practitioners will have such a child on their lists. However, the prevalence is rising, due to increasing survival of very low birthweight infants. The assessment of visually handicapped children is highly specialised and requires close cooperation between ophthalmologists, paediatricians, genetic counsellors, the Education Authority and Social Services. Antenatal diagnosis is now available for X-linked retinitis pigmentosa, choroideraemia and retinoblastoma (Jay 1987) (see also Chapter 10).

Management in the community is greatly assisted by Advisory Teachers for the Visually Handicapped, who are employed by the Education Authority and visit on a domiciliary basis from the early weeks. They advise on handling the baby, feeding, toys and early learning. The contact continues throughout the preschool and school years and includes the provision of educational aids. Low vision aids are prescribed by the ophthalmologist.

Table 19.5   Presentation of bilateral visual loss

Morphological abnormality of the eyes
Abnormal visual behaviour
Nystagmus
Photophobia
Eye poking
Squint — the worse eye may deviate

Table 19.6   Presentation of unilateral visual loss

Squint
Morphological abnormality of the eye
White pupil
Routine vision screening

Before nursery education, many parents appreciate attending an Opportunity Group or a similar alternative. It is wise for visually handicapped children to be assessed by an educational psychologist prior to nursery placement. Many of the children manage well in normal nurseries with full time Special Needs Assistants. Multiply handicapped children may already have been attending child development or assessment centres, and will then require special nursery placement. Reassessment by an educational psychologist before school entry is essential because an Educational Statement of Special Needs (1981 Act) must be made. All professionals involved with the care of the child are asked for a contribution. Many partially sighted children cope well in mainstream education, at least initially. Schools for the blind are few and far between and this usually means weekly boarding at least. School entry is sometimes deferred until the child is thought to be mature enough to go away on this basis.

SOME USEFUL ADDRESSES

Royal National Institute for the Blind
224 Great Portland Street
London W1N 6AA
Tel: 071 388 1266

Partially Sighted Society
Queens Road
Doncaster
South Yorkshire
Tel: 0302 68998

SENSE (National Association for the Deaf/Blind and Rubella Handicapped)
311 Grays Inn Road
London WC1
Tel: 071 278 1005

REFERENCES

Atkinson J, Braddick O, Durden K et al 1984 Screening for refractive errors in 6–9 month old infants by photorefraction. British Medical Journal of Ophthalmology 68: 105–112

Baraitser M, 1981 The genetics of blindness. Hospital Update 7: 516–527

Barlow H, 1975 Visual experience and cortical development. Nature 258: 199

Brant J, Novotny M 1976 Testing of visual acuity in young children; an evaluation of some commonly used methods. Developmental Medicine and Child Neurology. 18: 568–576

British Medical Journal 1977 Screening children for visual defects (editorial). British Medical Journal 2: 594

Catford J, Absolon M, Millo A 1984 Squints — a sideways look In: Macfarlane J (ed) Progress in Child Health, vol 1. Churchill Livingstone, Edinburgh

Court S D M 1976 Committee on Child Health Services. Fit for the future. HMSO, London

Cross A 1985 Health screening in schools, Part 1. Journal of Pediatrics 107: 487–493

Curtis Jenkins G, Collins C, Andren S 1978 Developmental surveillance in general practice. British Medical Journal 1: 1537–1540

Gardiner P 1977 Vision screening in pre-school children. British Medical Journal 2: 577

Gardiner P 1982 The development of vision In: Studies in developmental paediatrics 3. MTP Press, Lancaster

Gardiner P, Mackeith R, Smith V (eds) 1969 Aspects of developmental and paediatric ophthalmology. In: Clinics in developmental medicine 32. Spastics International Medical Publications, London

Hall D M B (ed) 1989 Health for all children. Joint Working Party on Child Health Surveillance. Oxford University Press, Oxford

Hall S, Pugh A, Hall D M B 1982 Vision screening in the under 5's British Medical Journal 285: 1096–1098

Ingram R 1973 Role of the school eye clinic in modern ophthalmology. British Medical Journal 1: 278–280

Ingram R, Trayner M, Walker C et al 1979 Screening for refractive errors at age 1 year: a pilot study. British Journal of Ophthalmology 63: 243–250

Ingram R, Walker C, Wilson J et al 1985 A first attempt to prevent amblyopia and squint by spectacle correction of abnormal refractions from age 1 year. British Journal of Ophthalmology 69: 851–853

Ingram R, Holland W, Walker C et al 1986 Screening for visual defects in pre-school children. British Journal of Ophthalmology 70: 16–21

Jay B 1987 Causes of blindness in school children. British Medical Journal 294: 1183–1184

Johnson A, Stayte M, Wortham C 1989 Vision screening at 8 and 18 months. British Medical Journal 299:545–549

Kohler L, Stigmar G 1978 Visual disorders in 7 year old children with and without previous vision screening. Acta Paediatrica Scandinavia 67: 373

MacLellan A, Harker P 1979 Mobile orthoptic service for primary screening of visual disorder in young children. British Medical Journal 1: 994–995

Peckham C S, Gardiner P A, Goldstein H 1977 Acquired myopia in 11 year old children. British Medical Journal 1: 542–545

Peckham C S, Gardiner P A, Tibbenham A 1979 Vision screening of adolescents and their use of glasses. British Medical Journal 1: 1111–1113

Reinecke R 1978 Vision, amblyopia and strabismus. In: Feman S, Reinecke R (eds) Handbook of paediatric ophthalmology. Ghune & Stratton, New York

Reinecke R 1983 Ophthalmic examination of infants and children by the pediatrician. Pediatric Clinics of North America 30: 995–1002

Ross E, Murray L D, Stead S 1977 Prevalence of amblyopia in grade 1 school children in Saskatoon. Canadian Journal of Public Health 68: 491

Sheridan M 1976 Manual for the STYCAR vision tests, revised edn. NFER, Windsor

Stewart-Brown S 1987 Visual defects in school children: screening policy and educational implications. In: Macfarlane J (ed) Progress in child health, vol 3. Churchill Livingstone, Edinburgh

Stewart-Brown S, Haslum M 1988 Screening of vision in school: could we do better by doing less? British Medical Journal 297: 1111–1113

Tibbenham A D, Peckham C S, Gardiner P A 1978 Vision screening in children tested at 7, 11 and 16 years. British Medical Journal 1: 1312–1314

Williams S, Sanderson G, Share D et al 1988 Refractive error, IQ and reading ability: a longitudinal study from age 7 to 11. Developmental Medicine and Child Neurology 30: 735–742

The younger adult

20. Risk factors for ischaemic heart disease

John Coope

Ischaemic heart disease is by far the most common cause of death and, more relevantly, of early death. About half of deaths under retirement age are due to heart attacks, and of these about one-third die so suddenly that medical assistance is not available. In addition, there is a huge amount of disability and unemployment due to the symptoms of the late stages of coronary narrowing and resulting heart failure. No condition, not even cancer, approaches this in the challenge to preventive medicine or more fully meets the criteria of Table 2.3 (p. 22), in that it has a substantial effect on the length and quality of life, a high prevalence and a natural history that is well understood.

Identifying patients who are prone to heart attacks depends on the presence of so-called risk factors. Knowledge of these factors has accumulated from insurance statistics, epidemiological studies and intervention trials and a list of these can be seen in Table 20.1. Some of these factors, such as gender, stature and race indicate a genetic disposition and are unalterable, although many environmental factors may interact in the case of racial susceptibility. Others, such the level of the blood pressure, may be markers for some other common factor and may not be causal. Some risk factors, such as family history, are easy to ascertain and others, like clotting factor VII, need complicated and expensive tests to measure. They also differ considerably in their predictive power and some, such as weight, are poor predictors when allowance is made for other factors that are associated with them. On the other hand, multiple risk factors increase the overall liability by a greater amount than the summation of their individual risks. This means that an individual with a moderate level of a number of factors may be at a higher risk than another with a high level of one. Identification of these patients is not possible without using some scoring system that takes into account the interaction of the risk factors. Even with such devices, and using the known risk factors that are easily measured, those classified in the top fifth of risk will suffer just over half of all the events in a population in a 5-year period (Shaper et al 1986). Most of the events will occur in the large number of individuals exposed to moderately increased risk (Kannel & Gordon 1970). For this reason, a population approach has been advocated to prevent ischaemic heart disease and this has a further advantage that it can be targeted at families and at influencing social factors, such as food availability and attitudes to smoking. Doctors in general practice need to be aware of such population strategies and help to implement them within their communities, as well as screening for individuals with high risks for personal intervention. Posters in waiting areas, literature on diet and smoking cessation, and videos at medical centres

Table 20.1 Risk factors for ischaemic heart disease

Age
Male gender
Asian birth
Low stature
Personality type
Stress
Family incidence
Social class 3, 4 or 5
Familial hypercholesterolaemia
Familial combined hyperlipidaemia
Remnant hyperlipidaemia
Polygenic hypercholesterolaemia
Raised fibrinogen
Raised clotting factor VII
Raised blood viscosity
Diabetes and impaired glucose tolerance
Smoking and exposure to smoking
Systolic and diastolic blood pressure
Overweight
Alcohol excess
Lack of physical exercise
Hyperuricaemia
Oral contraceptive use
Soft water supply
Previous cardiovascular disease

197

help to reinforce national education. More active intervention in the community, such as putting pressure on local shops to refuse cigarette sales to minors, or to encourage the distribution of skimmed milk, has been successfully pursued by general practitioners.

I will now take each of the major risk factors that are amenable to alteration and consider in each case the strength of the association with ischaemic heart disease, the evidence that the association is causal and that the risk can be reversed by lessening the factor concerned, before discussing the strategy for implementing such a reduction in practice.

THE BLOOD LIPIDS

The scientific evidence

Blood total cholesterol and low density lipoproteins are strongly related to the development of coronary artery disease. There is a progressive rise in incidence over the whole range above the bottom fifth of cholesterol; the rise increases exponentially (Fig. 20.1). This relationship is probably causal as it can be reversed by lowering the cholesterol whether by diet or drugs (Mann & Marr 1981). It holds for variations between nations, where it underlies a seven-fold difference in the incidence of ischaemic heart disease (Keys 1970),

Relation Between Serum Cholesterol and Risk of CHD

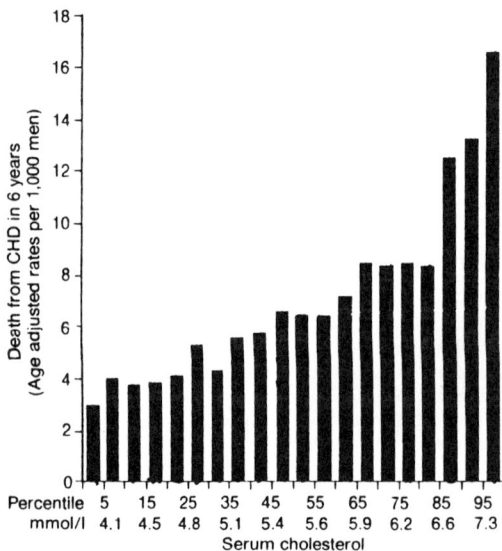

Fig. 20.1   The relation between serum cholesterol level and risk of coronary heart disease (from Martin et al 1986).

and for differences within single countries. The British Regional Heart Study found that, in British men aged 40–50, those in the top fifth of cholesterol level have 3.5 times the risk of those in the lowest fifth. The level of high density lipoproteins is inversely related to risk, although the slope is not as steep as with total cholesterol, with a two-fold increase of risk across the range (Shaper et al 1986). Triglyceride levels do not make an independent contribution to risk once other factors have been taken into account (Hulley et al 1980).

Interaction of lipids with other risk factors

In countries with very low levels of total cholesterol, like Japan, other factors such as smoking and hypertension do not have much effect on the incidence of ischaemic heart disease. This may indicate that lipids constitute a 'final common path' for other risk factors in the causal chain. On the other hand high lipid levels on their own, without the presence of either smoking or hypertension, are not nearly as powerful at predicting liability, a fact that is used to support selective screening by cholesterol testing (Tunstall-Pedoe 1989).

Lipid levels, age and total mortality

With increasing age the strong positive relationship of serum total cholesterol to cardiovascular disease wanes, especially in men (Kannel & Gordon 1978). All-cause mortality is related to cholesterol in a J-curve with increased mortality at the lower end of the range (Martin et al 1986). This is almost certainly in part the result of 'reverse causation', due to the effect of underlying disease, including cancer, on the cholesterol level (McMichael et al 1984). Two recent reports, however, have indicated that this is not the whole story. In a long-term follow-up of men in Scotland, the J-curve persisted after 5 years, making 'reverse causation' implausible (Isis et al 1989). A French study of older women has reported a five-fold increase in all-causes mortality in subjects with low cholesterols; this was independent of the incidence of cancer (Forette et al 1989). Clearly, more prospective work needs to be done on this important subject. Until further evidence is forthcoming screening for raised lipids should not be performed above the age of 60.

Variability in cholesterol levels and the establishment of cut-off points

Like blood pressure, cholesterol levels show a continuous distribution in the population and also considerable fluctuations in the same individual. This makes for two difficulties in establishing cut-off points. First, with the exception of familial hypercholestero-laemia, there is no biological marker to assist decision-making, which must be, as with hypertension, on the basis of a calculation of risk versus benefit. Secondly, to avoid misclassification, treatment decisions should be made on the basis of a minimum of two measure-ments at different times. For instance, if a cut-point of 7 mmols/litre is adopted, 1 in 5 of those found to be above this level on a single measurement will be found to be below it on repeat.

The effect of selecting a different cut-point can be shown by the following example. The chance of a middle-aged man (aged 40–59) having a major heart attack over the next ten years will be 1 in 20 if his serum total cholesterol is 6 mmols, 1 in 10 if it is 6.5 mmols and 1 in 7 if it is above 7.2 mmols. The risk of coronary heart disease in women is much less than that in men and the absolute risk of any given level of cholesterol is less. Therefore cut-off points for intervention should be 0.5 mmol/litre higher in women than men.

Genetic control of serum lipids

The range of lipid levels found in different individuals and across different countries reflects a complex interaction between genetic and environmental factors. So called 'polygenic' hypercholesterolaemia is, rather like 'essential' hypertension, the upper end of this range of normality. About 54% of the variance of serum cholesterol is accounted for by genetic factors. More specific types of inheritance, however, are shown by a group of disorders, the principal of which is familial hypercholesterolaemia. This is a single gene abnormality in which the homozygous form has cholesterol levels of 15–25 mmol/litre and severe cardiovascular disease, with an expectation of life of about 20 years. The heterozygous form is found fairly frequently, affecting 1 in 500 of the population. Therefore a practice of 10 000 patients would expect 20 cases of this condition. Affected men have cholesterol levels usually as high as 9–12 mmols/litre and at least an eight times greater risk of ischaemic heart disease than normal. Tendon xanthomas may occur in the patients or relatives, as may premature arcus senilis or xanthelasmas around the eyes. One way of picking up cases of this condition is to screen relatives of patients with early heart attacks who also have high lipid levels. Most affected patients will need active treatment with diet and drugs with regular follow-up. Other genetic conditions are remnant hyperlipidaemia with xanthomas and a high incidence

of cardiovascular disease, particularly in the peripheral arteries, and familial combined hyperlipidaemia, in which a very strong family history is combined with moderate increase in lipid levels (cholesterol and/or triglyceride) and in which the abnormality lies in the excessive production of apolipoprotein B, the struc-tural protein of LDL and VLDL.

Lipid levels and diet

Between nations there is a strong positive relationship between serum cholesterol and the proportion of total energy requirements obtained from saturated fat (Keys 1970). Such a relationship is difficult to demonstrate within countries with high average cholesterol levels and relatively similar dietary patterns. However, if sub-jects with quite different diets, e.g. vegans, vegetarians, fish eaters and meat eaters are studied, there is a gradient of over 1 mmol/litre (Thorogood et al 1987). That dietary intervention can effectively reduce serum cholesterol was demonstrated in a large American study where levels were lowered by 7% over a 4-year period (Caggiula et al 1981). The effort put into modifying eating habits in this trial was considerable and involved ten education sessions, with advice on shopping and cooking, as well as close follow-up. If such changes are to be achieved in general practice this is going to mean much more time spent with the patient and the family and the training and employ-ment of many more ancillary helpers.

Polyunsaturated fats lower the total serum chol-esterol, and these may be used to substitute partially for saturated fats. Fibre of vegetable origin, including pulses, also has a pronounced cholesterol-lowering effect; these effects are additive to the reduction of total fat (Lewis et al 1981). A reduction of 7.5% can be expected from adding conspicuous amounts of fibre.

Monounsaturated fats, such as olive oil, may increase the level of HDL, as may consumption of fish. The effect of dietary cholesterol is controversial. One large study in the US showed a relationship between chol-esterol intake and the incidence of heart attacks but this was independent of serum cholesterol levels (Shekelle et al 1981). Another study in Oxford showed that adding five eggs to a diet that was already low in satu-rated fat and high in fibre made no significant dif-ference to the serum cholesterol (Edington et al 1987).

Other factors affecting serum cholesterol

Obesity of any degree is associated with raised cholesterol levels and reduction of excess weight is accompanied by an impressive reduction of serum cholesterol (Caggiula et al 1981). Exercise reduces the serum cholesterol and elevates HDL levels but the exercise needed to produce these effects is 8 miles of jogging each week (Haskell 1986). Alcohol does not affect the cholesterol level, although it raises the triglyceride level.

Several drugs may cause disturbances in blood lipid levels. These include oral contraceptives (Wallace et al 1977), diuretics (Williams et al 1986) and beta-blockers (Northcote 1988). Combined contraceptives cause a small increase in cholesterol (5%) and a much larger increase in triglycerides (48%). Diuretics used over a long period cause a temporary rise in serum cholesterol, which returns to normal after two years. Beta-blockers, without intrinsic sympathomimetic activity, lower HDL and increase triglyceride levels.

Some disease states are associated with raised cholesterol levels and these should be borne in mind in assessing patients. They include diabetes, hypothyroidism, chronic renal failure and nephrotic syndrome.

Treatment of hyperlipidaemia

If raised levels of serum cholesterol and LDL are associated with increased risk of ischaemic heart disease, what is the evidence that reduction of high levels will reduce this risk? Three intervention trials using lipid lowering agents: clofibrate (Oliver et al 1978), cholestyramine (Lipids Research Clinics Program 1984) and gemfibrazil (Frick et al 1987), have shown a reduction in the incidence of heart attacks by about 20%. Unfortunately, these drugs were not without side-effects and, in the case of clofibrate, there was an excess of deaths in the treatment group that was probably drug-related. These studies, however, provide convincing evidence that reduction of cholesterol, at least for those with levels above 6.5 mmols/litre, will reduce consequent heart attacks. The fact that this effect was produced over the short period of a clinical trial gives hope that a more substantial time-scale would increase the protective effect. There is no reason to think that dietary reduction of cholesterol of the magnitude achieved by drugs would not achieve a similar result. A controlled trial to test whether dietary intervention would be successful has proved too expensive to mount but a number of multiple risk factor trials have included a dietary component. The Oslo Heart Study (Hjerman et al 1981) combined dietary advice with smoking cessation and achieved a significant 40% reduction in coronary mortality. We know from the British Regional Heart Study that substantial reduction in mortality from

stopping smoking would take much longer than the duration of this trial (Cook et al 1986) and therefore most of this effect was probably due to dietary intervention. The very large Multiple Risk Factor Intervention Trial (MRFIT) in the United States is very difficult to evaluate because the 'control' group were told their cholesterol levels and referred to their doctors for 'usual care' (Multiple Risk Factor Intervention Trial Research Group 1982). The result was that the difference between the two groups in cholesterol was only 2% and the consequent reduction in CHD deaths was small.

The European Multifactorial trial in the Prevention of Coronary Heart Disease, sometimes called the European Factory Study, randomised factories to intervention on smoking, cholesterol lowering advice and reduction of weight and blood pressure or no intervention (WHO European Collaborative Group 1983). The reduction in cholesterol in the UK part of the trial was only 0.4%, so it is perhaps not surprising that no beneficial effects were observed on coronary heart disease. In the trial as a whole the reduction in fatal heart attacks was proportional to the effective reduction of cholesterol.

A recent trial of changes of diet, smoking and exercise on the progress of coronary heart disease as measured by quantitative angiography showed regression of the atheromatous narrowing in the treatment group after 1 year (Ornish et al 1990). This is the first demonstration of regression of atheroma in human subjects on lifestyle changes without the use of lipid lowering agents and is a very important finding. It was achieved by a low fat vegetarian diet containing 10% of calories as fat. The fact that significant regression was achieved after only 1 year should give fresh impetus to energetic dietary treatment of cardiovascular disease.

Adverse effects from lowering serum cholesterol

The presence of adverse effects in trials using drugs to lower cholesterol has already been referred to. Even comparatively rare or small side effects either on the body physiology or on the quality of life of the recipient may outweigh any benefit in a drug being used to treat large numbers of symptomless members of the public. However, lipid lowering drugs are perhaps in the same stage of development as anti-hypertensive agents were 20 years ago and, with intensive research in hand, a more acceptable range of agents is likely to emerge. Large-scale clinical trials will then be needed to make sure that they are free from side-effects.

Could there be adverse effects from dietary control of cholesterol? The presence of J-curves in total mortality (although not in cardiovascular mortality) has already been referred to but this increase is at least in part due to the effect of diseases that reduce the serum cholesterol level. Furthermore, the level at which it occurs is well below that at which intervention is likely to be targeted.

Is screening for raised lipids worthwhile in general practice?

Having presented the scientific evidence it is necessary to address the questions of whether screening is advised in the context of general practice today, who should be screened and how?

The benefits may be summarised as follows. Levels of serum total cholesterol above 6.5 mmol/litre in patients below the age of 60 carry with them seriously increased risk of heart attack, particularly if combined with other risk factors, such as hypertension, smoking or diabetes. Higher levels are not uncommon, including a few patients with an urgent need for treatment because of familial hypercholesterolaemia. Some of these patients should be treated with lipid lowering drugs.

Dietary modification is capable of reducing high levels of cholesterol and lowering the attendant risk. These patients also need counselling on smoking and obesity. The improvement that is noted in the trials could possibly be greater if intervention was begun earlier and continued for longer.

On the other hand, universal screening of all the adults in the community 'preferably before the age of 30', as was advised by the British Hyperlipidaemia Association (Shepherd et al 1987), would place a considerable strain on the capacities of the average practice team. Because of the very high mean level of cholesterol (5.7 mmols/litre) in this country the cut-off points used for intervention would have to be higher than in the United States. Follow-up would be costly and would need to be planned. As is the case with blood pressure, sufficient time has to be given to advising patients and reassuring those with anxiety. Taking repeat measurements is a considerable additional work-load to the practice. Altering lifetime eating habits cannot be done by a few words at the end of a consultation, but probably requires sessions with a trained nurse and should involve members of the family.

The Coronary Prevention Group (Scientific & Medical Advisory Committee 1987) and other writers (Hart 1986) have advised selective screening on the basis of other risk factors, taking into account the multiplicative nature of risk combinations and with the intention of keeping the work task down to manageable levels. There is disagreement over exactly what these risks are. For some it is existent coronary disease (Tunstall-Pedoe 1989), for others a family history of coronary disease or the presence of hypertension, diabetes, obesity or smoking (Study Group of the European Atherosclerosis Society 1987).

A sensible approach would seem to be to start by screening all those with existing signs or symptoms of ischaemic heart disease, a positive family history, hypertension or borderline blood pressure, diabetes or considerable obesity (body mass index > 30). A positive family history means a definite myocardial infarction before age 60 in a first degree relative (parent, sibling, offspring) or before the age of 50 in a second degree relative (uncle or aunt); or a cholesterol greater than 7.8 mmol/litre in a first degree relative. Increasingly, patients in our practice are either asking to have their blood lipids measured or coming to us with measurements that have been made elsewhere. In practice, therefore, we may well slowly progress to a stage when we know the lipid levels of most of our patients. Whether a decision is made to accelerate this process will depend on the resources and other priorities in the tasks facing the medical centre. In any case, a protocol needs to be prepared to manage the follow-up of patients with hyperlipidaemia and the implications of this need thorough discussion or, as in the case of hypertension, the presence of critical information will not be acted upon and another 'rule of halves' will be generated.

Patterns of screening for hyperlipidaemia in practice

As in the case of hypertension, values for blood lipids will be collected over time in a variety of ways. Some patients will already know their levels or will have had them measured at hospital visits or commercial screening clinics. It is important that such information, when it is known, is easily available in a structured record card along with other coronary risk factors, such as weight for height, blood pressure and smoking habit. Extending the screen to cover patients with other high levels of coronary risks can be done opportunistically at consultations, by running a coronary risk clinic or by a combination of these approaches. Enquiry about the incidence of heart attacks under the age of 60 in first degree relatives only takes a minute and a positive family history should be recorded on the problem list. Known hypertensives or diabetics, whether on pharmacological treatment or surveillance, may have had their cholesterol measured at the initial work-up. The same is true of patients under 60 with evidence of atherosclerotic target organ damage, angina, myocardial infarction, claudication or stroke. Some, however, will have slipped through the net and should be referred for cholesterol measurement when they attend. Finally, some patients will ask for their blood lipids to be measured. In the first place a total cholesterol in the non-fasting state should be done. If the result is between 5.2 and 6.9 mmol (5.7 and 7.4 mmol in women) the patient should be told that their cholesterol is somewhat elevated but that this is a common condition and all they need to do is to modify their diet. Detailed dietary advice on a suitable low fat, high fibre diet should be given and the patient should be given a booklet to take home. (The *Guide to healthy eating*, published by the Health Education Council, is available free.) No future follow-up is needed for this group. If the result is above 7.0 mmol/litre (7.5 mmol/litre in women) a further sample should be sent and a total and HDL

cholesterol measured before any action is taken. The further follow-up and treatment of high-risk hyperlipidaemia patients in general practice must follow a protocol with defined targets and a graduated series of therapeutic manoeuvres, such as are used in the treatment of hypertension. A suggested protocol is shown in Figure 20.2. This flow diagram may seem complicated at first sight but, used as a reference chart by our practice nurse, it has not been difficult to follow. Without such an aid to decision-making there is every likelihood that goal levels will not be achieved. On the other hand, like using a route map when out walking, the actual decisions will be guided by immediate common sense. In particular, patients' willingness or ability to moderate their lifestyle or take therapy must obviously be taken into account.

Card index files or computer-generated registers are necessary for the adequate follow-up of hyperlipidaemic patients. These are needed to check whether patients are continuing to attend and also to make audit of results possible. Regular reviews of the degree to which targets are being met should be done. An

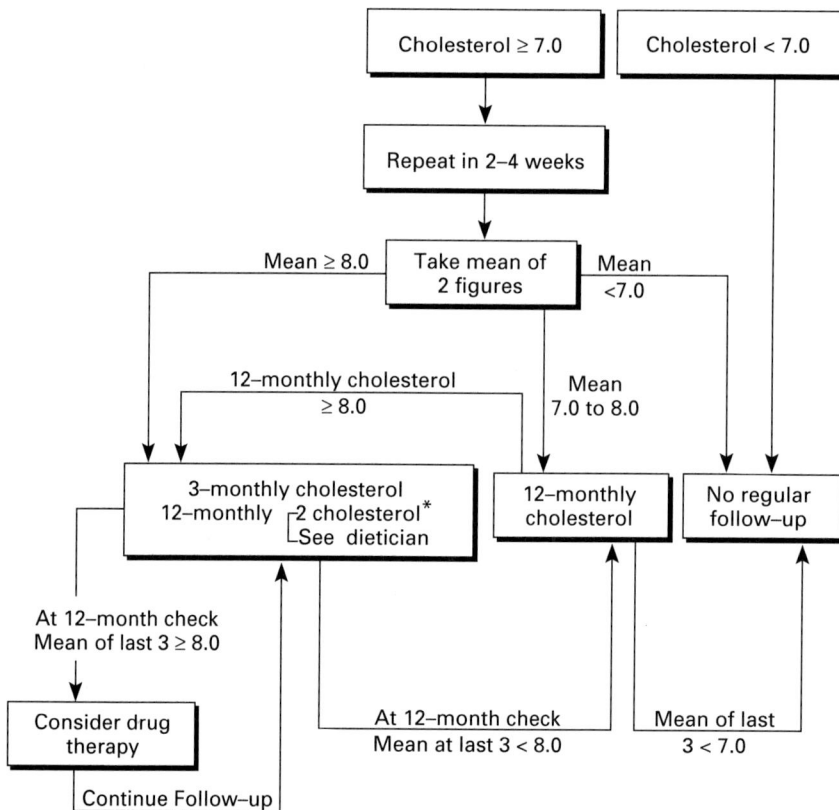

Fig. 20.2   Cholesterol follow-up. Suitable for middle-aged.
(* mean of 2 cholesterol)

Table 20.2 Audit of cholesterol reduction in the Bollington practice

	n	C1 (mmol/1)	C2 (mmol/1)	Percent reduction
Drug-treated patients	9	8.60	7.20	16.3
Diet-treated patients	75	8.04	7.27	9.6

example of a simple audit in our practice of initial and most recent cholesterol level is shown in Table 20.2. All the patients currently being followed-up after presenting with serum total cholesterols greater than 7 mmol/litre are included in the audit. The mean of all baseline measurements (C1) was calculated, and the mean of the last recorded measurement (C2). Those patients who did not attend for any further measurements after the initial screening are excluded.

Practice measurement of serum cholesterol

Commercial desktop analysers that can perform a serum cholesterol estimation in a few minutes on capillary blood are now available. Used with meticulous care they give reliable results, but a survey of measurements made with one of these in general practices and occupational health departments showed that although many of the participants obtained

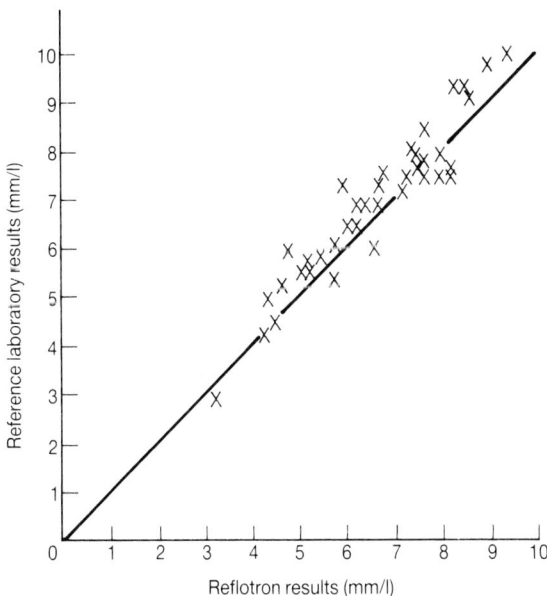

Fig. 20.3 Correlation of serum cholesterol values obtained in author's practice and values obtained in the quality control laboratory.

satisfactory results, in 8.6% they differed by more than 1 mmol/litre from the target value (Broughton et al 1989). Nurses who use these machines need special training in the technique and regular comparison with an external standard is mandatory. Figure 20.3 shows the correlation of values obtained in the Bollington practice with those from the quality control laboratory.

OBESITY, ALCOHOL AND LACK OF EXERCISE

Although obesity, expressed as body mass index (the weight in kilograms divided by the height in metres squared) is clearly related to the incidence of major cardiovascular occurrences, with a two-fold increase from those in the lowest to those in the highest fifth, if allowance is made for the cholesterol and the blood pressure, both of which are weight related, this relationship disappears (Shaper 1987). Reduction of excess body weight, however, is the first stage in correcting hyperlipidaemia and hypertension, as well as reducing the incidence of maturity onset diabetes, so this risk factor is clinically important. It is, moreover, easily measured both in the surgery and at home. Unfortunately, pessimism is the order of the day in most practices and only a minority of patients have a record of weight and even fewer a record of height in their notes (with the advent of new terms of service for general practitioners, this situation may change in future years). Most weight-watching classes have a great predominance of women who are conscious of their figures and a dearth of men who should be conscious of the increased risk of heart attack. As with all the other major risk factors, a structured record system allowing the immediate reminder that a patient sitting with you has an obesity problem (BMI of 30 or greater) is important if a check is to be kept on an opportunistic basis. Leaflets giving general advice on weight reduction should be available but some patients may need more detailed counselling and follow-up; we run group therapy sessions from time to time. In the absence of adequate support within the practice it is preferable to refer patients to a Weight Watchers group in the area than to give vague advice on 'getting some weight off' (see also Chapter 33).

Alcohol consumption is related to the risk of heart disease in two ways. It increases the blood pressure (Saunders 1987) and, in large amounts, is directly toxic to the myocardium and may precipitate cardiac failure. It is associated with an increased incidence of sudden death (Lilhell et al 1987). Most surveys have shown a U-curve in the relation of alcohol intake and total mortality. This phenomenon is almost certainly due to the presence of a few high risk ex-alcoholics and other serious diseases in the group of total abstainers (Shaper et al 1988). Alcohol consumption should be recorded as the number of units drunk in the previous 7 days. A unit is a half pint of beer, a glass of wine or a 'single' of spirits. Consumption of over 20 units a week indicates moderately heavy drinking that needs restricting. Over 35 units a week indicates a serious drinking problem; about 14% of men and 3% of women have a serious drinking problem by this criterion. A well conducted randomised trial of intervention offered to such patients in British general practices, selected by questionnaire, showed that advice on two occasions with selective follow-up resulted in a reduction of 18.2 units/week in the intervention group as against 8.1 units/week in the control group after a year (Wallace et al 1988)(see also Chapter 34).

Physical activity has been suggested by a number of studies as having a protective effect on ischaemic heart disease (Morris et al 1973). The mode of action is controversial. In one Australian study it did not appear to alter any of the known risk factors (Sedgwick et al 1980). Another report suggested a beneficial effect on lipids (Haskell 1986). This 'training effect' on the cardiovascular system is only apparent on regular use of vigorous exercise, corresponding to that of a heavy industrial worker, or several physical workouts per week.

The triad of increasing weight, heavy alcohol intake and decreasing exercise commonly found in middle-aged men and often associated with smoking, is best described (to the patient) as going to seed. Some of these men have been athletic in the past and can be made to feel ashamed of their lack of physical fitness. An energetic programme to change their lifestyle and improve their self-image may be more effective than warnings about early death because vanity may be a stronger suit with many of them than forward planning. The 'Look After Yourself' courses may be an appropriate start if there is one in your area.

SMOKING

Smoking is a causative risk factor for coronary heart disease. The mechanism of the cardiovascular damage is not fully understood. There may be activation of platelets leading to the production of thromboxane B2, which in turn leads to coronary occlusion (Lassila et al 1988). Atheroma is more pronounced in smokers, who also have narrowed arterioles in the myocardium (Auerbach et al 1976). Tobacco smoke contains carbon monoxide, which leads to the formation of carboxyhaemoglobin and a compensatory poly-

cythaemia. Finally, there is an increase in cholesterol and a reduction of HDL in smokers, which may account for some of the increased risk (Craig et al 1989).

The relative risk of smoking for heart attack mortality declines with increasing age from 14.8 at under 45 to 3.3 at 45–50 and to 1.9 at 55–64. Because of the increased number of heart attacks in older patients, however, the absolute impact of smoking on heart attacks is probably maintained (Doll & Peto 1976). Smoking is also a risk factor for peripheral arterial disease, for stroke and particularly for subarachnoid haemorrhage (Shinton & Beevers 1989). I shall not deal here with the many non-cardiovascular diseases that are related to smoking.

Does stopping smoking reduce the risk of ischaemic heart disease?

It used to be stated that the risk will reduce to that of the normal population about 4 years after the cessation of smoking. The evidence on which this idea was based was drawn from the postinfarction situation where the direct effect of continuing to smoke is particularly dangerous. Evidence from the British Regional Heart Study suggests that the risks to the heart from smoking are related to the number of years that the person has spent smoking and although there was some reduction in risk 6 years after stopping smoking this was relatively small and the main benefit from stopping smoking was not adding further risk (Cook et al 1986).

Can patients' smoking habits be changed and how?

In the pitifully small number of studies that have looked at the effectiveness of intervention against smoking, a small but worthwhile change in smoking habits was achieved by general practitioners by intervening in the course of consultations. One study using 2 minutes of firm advice followed by a leaflet advising the patient how to stop and the promise of follow-up achieved a 5.5% success rate after 1 year (Russell et al 1979). Another more extended intervention with six visits over 6 months resulted in a 22% abstention rate at 3 years (Richmond et al 1986). The critical elements in a strategy to reduce smoking would seem to be: ask about smoking habits and record in a structured way, advise the patient to stop smoking and offer advice and support with follow-up visits, give a booklet to reinforce the advice. The occasion of attendance for respiratory infections and other smoking-related illnesses should be used to reinforce the message. The use of nicotine chewing gum, although it has worked in special smoking cessation centres, does not seem to have been very successful in general practice (Lam et al 1987). Transdermal patches are now being tested and may be more successful (Abelin et al 1989).

Audit of the results of advice against smoking in the Oxford Prevention of Heart Attack and Stroke Project showed only a 2.3% stoppage of smoking, but only half of the patients had any documented follow-up (Mant et al 1989).

HYPERTENSION

Screening for hypertension is dealt with in Chapter 21. Here I will consider raised blood pressure in its contribution to the risk profile for heart disease.

Systolic and diastolic blood pressure are both major risk factors for ischaemic heart disease. There is a similar J-curve relationship to overall mortality to that found with cholesterol. As with cholesterol, the relative risk declines with advancing age but the absolute risk is maintained (Coope & Warrender 1988). Hypertension, however, is different in that the incidence of heart attacks is not reduced by lowering the blood pressure (Report of British Hypertension Society 1989). This suggests that the relationship may not be causative but depend on some other common factor. Another hypothesis is that lowering blood pressure to a moderate degree does indeed cause a reduction in heart attacks but that this is counterbalanced by an increase in deaths from excessive lowering in some patients (Cruickshank et al 1987). The situation is quite different from that of stroke, which can be reduced 40–50% by lowering the blood pressure.

The combination of any degree of hypertension or smoking with a raised cholesterol greatly increases the overall risk. All hypertensive patients, including borderline blood pressures under surveillance, should therefore have a non-fasting cholesterol measurement performed. Although the presence of hypertension increases the urgency of treating hyper-cholesterolaemia, the converse does not hold. This follows from the lack of effect of antihypertensive therapy on heart attacks.

DIABETES

Non insulin dependent diabetes is a potent risk factor for ischaemic heart disease, which is the usual mode of death in diabetics. In the Whitehall study of civil servants, impaired glucose tolerance without frank diabetes was associated with a doubling of coronary heart disease mortality (Fuller et al 1983). All diabetics must therefore have cholesterol, blood pressure and smoking habit assessed and acted upon. The unique concentration upon blood glucose levels, which characterises many diabetic clinics, is certainly not justified. It has been argued that an underlying metabolic hyperinsulinaemia may account for many of these patients with glucose intolerance, obesity, hypertension and hyperlipidaemia and that early treatment with diet and exercise might reverse this trend (Anonymous 1989). In insulin dependent (type 1) diabetes, aggressive treatment of hypertension will reduce the incidence of diabetic nephropathy and renal failure (Parving et al 1987)(see also Chapter 22).

FAMILY HISTORY

A positive family history may be due to genetic hypercholesterolaemia, which has been referred to above. Some of the family aggregations that are seen are not related to cholesterol levels. They may be caused by unknown genetic factors or, more likely, by shared lifestyles (smoking, eating habit). Whatever the cause, it is relatively easy to screen for and familial cardiovascular disease should figure prominently on the problem list of affected patients.

SCREENING CLINICS FOR ISCHAEMIC HEART DISEASE RISK FACTORS

In addition to utilising patient attendances for other reasons, sometimes called 'opportunistic screening', some practices hold sessions to which patients are invited for risk factor screening. A good example of what can be achieved is the programme organised by Dr Alan Jones and his partners at Swansea (Jones et al 1988). Family Health Services Authorities have taken the initiative in organising a call and selective recall system on the same basis as has been used for cervical screening. Whatever method is used, the identification of patients at risk will be totally wasted if the considerable resources and motivation needed to follow-up and treat these patients are not in place. The employment of peripatetic facilitators with the remit to assist practices in the organisation necessary for screening and recording results is a critical advance.

In our practice we have a nurse-run cardiovascular risk clinic and send a card to all men who will be 40 years of age in the year. They are questioned about smoking, alcohol intake and diet and family history, and asked about angina. Weight, height and blood pressure are measured. A specimen of blood for serum cholesterol is taken if there is a positive family history, current smoking, hypertension or diabetes, or at the patient's request. The cholesterol is estimated immediately using a Reflotron analyser. Advice is given on diet, smoking and alcohol intake and arrangements made for follow-up.

The pioneering work of the Oxford Prevention of Heart Attack and Stroke Project, who have set up screening services in a number of general practices in Oxford, is a model that many areas have since adopted (Fullard et al 1987). Here patients are offered a screening examination when they attend and an appointment is made for them to attend the screening nurse at a mutually convenient time. Each screening examination takes about 20 minutes. About 30% of the patients will need a follow-up visit and a further 15 minutes should be allowed for this.

A recent retrospective audit of this scheme looked at changes in smoking habit, blood pressure and body weight (Mant et al 1989). After 3 years there was only a 2.3% change in smoking habits and 2% reduction in those with body mass index greater than 30. There was

a reduction of 7.7% in the number of patients with diastolic blood pressure in excess of 100 mmHg. Follow-up was not good in the smokers and the obese. The authors of the report comment: 'the results emphasise the need to develop formal protocols for dietary and antismoking interventions and to evaluate formally the effectiveness (and cost effectiveness) of health checks.'

Changing lifelong habits is never going to be easy and we need to discover new and more effective ways of getting good results. Most studies have shown that the more time that is devoted to the work, the greater the number of repeat attendances and the higher the success rate. This means that many more ancillary workers of all kinds will have to be drawn into the primary care teams. With the large number of initiatives of different kinds being started it is important for those involved to audit the outcomes, successful and unsuccessful. Only in this way can progress be made in evolving the new style of anticipatory care that is needed for ischaemic heart disease.

REFERENCES

Abelin T, Buehler A, Muller P et al 1989 Controlled trial of transdermal nicotine patch in tobacco withdrawal. Lancet i: 7–10

Anonymous 1989 Type 2 diabetes or NIDDM: looking for a better name. Lancet i: 589–591

Auerbach O, Carter H W, Garfunkel L, Hammond E C 1976 Cigarette smoking and coronary heart disease, macroscopic and microscopic study. Chest 70: 697–705

Broughton P M G, Bullock D G, Cramb R 1989 Quality of plasma cholesterol measurements in primary care. British Medical Journal 298: 297–298

Caggiula A W, Christakis G, Farrand M et al 1981 The multiple risk factor trial (MRFIT) iv: intervention on blood lipids. Journal of Preventive Medicine 10: 443–475

Cook D G, Shaper A G, Pocock S J, Kussick S J 1986 Giving up smoking and the risk of heart attacks. Lancet ii: 1376–1379

Coope J, Warrender T S 1988 The prognostic significance of blood pressure in the elderly. Journal of Human Hypertension 2: 79–88

Craig W Y, Palomaki G E, Haddow J E 1989 Cigarette smoking and serum lipid and lipoprotein concentrations: an analysis of published data. British Medical Journal 298: 784–788

Cruickshank J M, Thorp J M, Zacharias F J 1987 Benefits and potential harm of lowering high blood pressure. Lancet i: 581–584

Doll R, Peto R 1976 Mortality in relation to smoking: 20 years observation on male British doctors. British Medical Journal 4: 1525–1536

Edington J, Geekie M, Cartet R et al 1987 Effect of dietary cholesterol on plasma cholesterol concentration in subjects following reduced fat, high fibre diet. British Medical Journal 294: 333–336

Forette B, Tortrat D, Wolmark Y 1989 Cholesterol as risk factor for mortality in elderly women. Lancet i: 868–870

Frick M H, Elo U, Haapa K et al 1987 Helsinki Heart Study. Primary prevention trial with gemfibrazil in middle-aged men with dyslipidaemia. Safety of treatment, changes in risk factors and incidence of coronary heart disease. New England Journal of Medicine 317: 1237–1245

Fullard E, Fowler G, Gray M 1987 Promoting prevention in primary care; controlled trial of low technology, low cost approach. British Medical Journal 294: 1080–1082

Fuller J H, Shipley M J, Rose G et al 1983 Mortality from coronary heart disease and stroke in relation to the degree of glycaemia: the Whitehall study. British Medical Journal 287: 867–870

Hart J T 1986 Reduction of blood cholesterol in the population: can it be done? Journal of the Royal College of General Practitioners 36: 538–539

Haskell W L 1986 The influence of exercise training over plasma lipids and lipoproteins in health and disease. Acta Medica Scandinavica 711 (Suppl): 25–37

Hjerman I, Holme I, Byre K V, Leren P 1981 Effect of diet and smoking intervention on the incidence of coronary heart disease. Lancet ii: 1303–1310

Hulley S B, Roseman R H, Bawol R D, Brand R J 1980 Epidemiology as a guide to clinical decisions. The association between triglyceride and coronary heart disease. New England Journal of Medicine: 302: 1383–1389

Isis C G, Hole D J, Gillis C R et al 1989 Plasma cholesterol, coronary heart disease and cancer in the Renfrew and Paisley Survey. British Medical Journal: 298: 920–924

Jones A, Davies D H, Dove J R et al 1988 Identification and treatment of risk factors for coronary heart disease in general practice: a possible screening model. British Medical Journal: 296: 1711–1714

Kannel W B, Gordon T (eds) 1970 Some characteristics related to the incidence of cardiovascular disease and death: the Framingham study, 16 year follow-up, Section 26. United States Government Printing Office, Washington D C

Kannel W B, Gordon T 1978 Evaluation of cardiovascular risk in the elderly: the Framingham study. Bulletin of the New York Academy of Medicine: 54: 573–592

Keys A (ed) 1970 Coronary heart disease in seven countries. American Heart Association Monograph 29

Lam W, Sze P C, Sacks H S, Chalmers T C 1987 Meta-analysis of randomised trials of nicotine chewing-gum. Lancet ii: 27–30

Lassila R, Seyberth H W, Naapanen A et al 1988 Vasoactive and atherogenic effects of cigarette smoking: a study of monozygotic twins discordant for smoking. British Medical Journal 297: 955–957

Lewis B, Hamnett F, Katan M, Kay R M 1981 Towards an improved lipid-lowering diet: additive effects of changes in nutrient intake. Lancet ii: 1310–1313

Lilhell H, Aberg H, Selimus I Hedstrand H 1987 Alcohol intemperance and sudden death. British Medical Journal 294: 1456–1458

Lipid Research Clinics Program 1984 The lipid research clinics coronary prevention trial results 1. Reduction in incidence of coronary heart disease. Journal of the Americal Medical Association 251: 351–364

McMichael A J, Jensen O M, Parkin D M, Zaridze D G 1984 Dietary and endogenous cholesterol and human cancer. Epidemiological Review 6: 192–216

Mann J I, Marr J W 1981 Trials of cholesterol reduction In: Miller N E, Lewis B (eds) Lipoproteins, atherosclerosis and coronary heart disease. Elsevier, North Holland, 197–210

Mant D, McKinlay C, Fuller A et al 1989 Three year follow-up of patients with raised blood pressure identified at health checks in general practice. British Medical Journal 298: 1360–1362

Martin M J, Hulley S B et al 1986 Serum cholesterol, blood pressure and mortality: implications from a cohort of 361 662 men. Lancet ii: 933–936

Morris H M, Chave S P W, Adam C et al 1973 Vigorous exercise in leisure-time and the incidence of coronary heart disease. Lancet i: 334–339

Multiple Risk Factor Intervention Trial Research Group 1982 Risk factor changes and mortality results. Journal of the American Medical Association 248: 1465–1477

Northcote R J 1988 β blockers, lipids and coronary atherosclerosis: fact or fiction. British Medical Journal 296: 731–732

Oliver M F, Heady J F, Morris J N, Cooper J 1978 A cooperative trial in the primary prevention of ischaemic heart disease using clofibrate. British Heart Journal 40: 1069–1118

Ornish D, Brown S E, Scherwitz L W et al 1990 Can lifestyle changes reverse coronary heart disease? Lancet ii: 129–133

Parving H, Anderson A R, Smidt U M et al 1987 Effect of antihypertensive treatment on kidney function in diabetes nephropathy. British Medical Journal 244: 1443–1447

Report of British Hypertension Society Working Party treating mild hypertension 1989. British Medical Journal 298: 694–698

Richmond R L, Austin A, Webster I W 1986 Three years evaluation of a programme by general practitioners to help patients stop smoking. British Medical Journal 292: 803–806

Russell M A H, Wilson C, Taylor C, Baker C D 1979 Effect of general practitioners' advice against smoking. British Medical Journal 2: 231–235

Saunders J B 1987 Alcohol: an important cause of hypertension. British Medical Journal 294: 1045–1046

Scientific and Medical Advisory Committee of the Coronary Prevention Group 1987. Risk assessment : its role in the prevention of coronary heart disease. Coronary Prevention Group, London

Sedgwick A W, Brotherhood J R, Harris-Davidson A et al 1980 Long-term effects of physical training programmes on risk factors for coronary heart disease in otherwise sedentary men. British Medical Journal 7: 7–10

Shaper A G, Pocock S J, Phillips A N, Walker M 1986 Identifying men at a high risk of heart attacks: a strategy of use in general practice. British Medical Journal 293: 474–479

Shaper A G 1987 Risk factors for ischaemic heart disease. Health Trends 19: 3–8

Shaper A G, Wannamethee G, Walker M 1988 Alcohol and mortality in British men: explaining the U-shaped curve. Lancet ii: 1267–1273

Shekelle R B, Shrylock A M, Paul O et al 1981 Diet serum cholesterol and death from coronary heart disease. The Western Electric Study. New England Journal of Medicine 304: 65–70

Shepherd J, Betteridge D, Durrington P et al 1987 Strategies for reducing coronary heart disease and desirable lipids for blood lipid concentration: guidelines for the British Hyperlipidaemic Association. British Medical Journal 295: 1245–1246

Shinton R, Beevers G 1989 Meta-analysis of relation between cigarette smoking and stroke. British Medical Journal 298: 789–793

Study Group of the European Atherosclerosis Society 1987 Strategies for the prevention of coronary heart disease: a policy statement of the European Atherosclerosis Society. European Heart Journal 8: 77–88

Thorogood M, Carter R, Benfield L et al 1987 Plasma proteins and lipoprotein cholesterol concentration in people with different diets in Britain. British Medical Journal 295: 351–353

Tunstall-Pedoe H 1989 Who is for cholesterol testing? British Medical Journal 298: 1593–1594

Wallace R B, Hoover J, Sandler D et al 1977 Altered plasma lipids associated with oral contraceptive or oestrogen consumption. Lancet ii: 11–14

Wallace P, Cutler S, Haines A 1988 Randomised controlled trial of general practitioner intervention in patients with excessive alcohol consumption. British Medical Journal 297: 663–668

Williams W R, Schneider K A, Berhani N O et al 1986 The relationship between diuretics and serum cholesterol in hypertension detection and follow-up programme. American Journal of Preventive Medicine 2(5): 248–255

World Health Organisation European Collaborative Group 1983 Multifactorial trial in the prevention of coronary heart disease. European Heart Journal 4: 141–147

21. Screening for hypertension in general practice

Ralph H Burton

Until the methods of science are made satisfactory for all the important distinctions of human phenomena, our best approach to many problems in therapy will be to rely on the judgements of thoughtful people who are familiar with the total realities of human ailments.

Feinstein (1972)

Hypertension would seem to be the archetype of a condition ideal for screening (Wilson 1966). It has everything — a diagnostic test that is easy to perform, a protracted presymptomatic phase and a large number of acceptable treatments. It was the first of the modern screening procedures to be widely adopted and having knowledge of a patient's blood pressure has become axiomatic of good clinical practice.

Given these advantages it is surprising that it remains controversial and is still subject to great debate, despite vast resources being invested in trying to prove its worth. Why is it that hypertension screening is perceived as largely failing to have lived up to its promise and are there lessons to learn for other promoted screening procedures?

HYPERTENSION — DOES IT MATTER?

In discussing hypertension, I will be concentrating on essential hypertension of mild to moderate degree, which is normally symptomless. Malignant hypertension is rare and probably a different condition in which no-one doubts the need for treatment. Blood pressure is otherwise distributed unimodally in the population leading to differences of opinion as to whether it should be labelled as a disease.

The history started with the actuarial studies in the United States (Actuarial Society of America 1941). It was followed on through the large population studies such as Framingham (Dawber et al 1962), which suggested disadvantages from a raised blood pressure. The exact levels of blood pressure that constituted risk remained doubtful and further large studies, notably in Australia (Australian Therapeutic Trial 1980) and the

UK (Miall 1977) have attempted to define them, but most non-academic observers and, I suspect, a considerable number of academic ones, have ended up rather more confused than they were before.

The best-known study in the UK was the MRC trial of mild hypertension, the principal results of which were published in 1985 (Medical Research Council 1985). Its main aims were to determine whether drug treatment of mild hypertension (phase V diastolic of 90–109) reduced strokes and coronary events in men and women aged 35–64. A secondary aim was to compare the effectiveness and tolerability of thiazide diuretics and propranolol. The study was general practice-based and involved 17 354 patients (85 572 patient years). There was random allocation to placebo, bendrofluazide or propranolol on entry, methyldopa being used as a second-line drug.

The results were presented as all groups and then with various subgroup analyses. The all-group results showed a reduction in the stroke rate in the active treatment group, the number of strokes being more than halved. Treatment made no difference to the overall rates of coronary events. The subgroup analyses showed that the all-cause mortality was reduced in men on active treatment by about 13%, but increased in women by about 20%. Comparison of the two active drugs showed that the reduction in stroke rate was greater with bendrofluazide than with propranolol. This was true for smokers and non-smokers, and only non-smokers showed any benefit from propranolol. Coronary event rate was not reduced by bendrofluazide whatever the smoking habit, nor was it reduced in smokers taking propranolol. It was reduced in non-smokers taking propranolol.

The message seems to be that treating mild hypertension reduces stroke but has little impact on cardiac disease. Although this is disappointing, it is no reason for therapeutic nihilism. It highlights the importance of looking at hypertension in the context of other risk factors, particularly smoking, (see also Chapter 20).

The level of blood pressure at which treatment should start is a matter of great controversy. All sorts of factors are taken into account including the patient's age, sex, lifestyle, other known risk factors and how the doctor feels that day. What has occurred is that the goal posts have constantly shifted and even slight shifts in policy can alter the number of patients treated, on a global scale, by millions. In a brave attempt to clarify this for the practising clinician, the British Hypertensive Society (Swales et al 1989) have issued the guideline that any person under the age of 80 with a diastolic blood pressure confirmed to be over 100 mmHg should have it reduced. This takes into account evidence from the European Working Party report on hypertension in the elderly (Amery et al 1985) which, to some surprise, showed unequivocal benefit in older patients (so much so that the study had to be abandoned before completion); it it the only study to do so.

IDENTIFICATION OF HYPERTENSION

The method of recording blood pressure in the UK is not standardised and it is still possible for half the medical students graduating from a British school to take the blood pressure by recording the fourth sound (softening) and for the other half to record the fifth sound (disappearance). It would therefore be possible for a good number of patients, who have had their hypertension diagnosed by fourth sound recording doctors, to have their condition cured by merely finding themselves a doctor who records the fifth sound. The position of a doctor taking over the care of a hypertensive patient already under treatment is also complicated by this dilemma. It is often impossible to find the original criteria by which the diagnosis was made, either by level or method. In any case the treatment policy may have changed since the original diagnosis was made. Often the only way of clarifying the situation is to stop the treatment and start again — sometimes a little difficult in patients who have been told that they must continue their treatment for life.

The recommendation now is that the blood pressure should be taken in the resting patient using the right arm and recording the fifth sound. A raised level should be confirmed on two further occasions and a large arm cuff should be used if necessary (Lancet 1980). Certainly, the exact criteria used in deciding upon treatment should be recorded in the notes.

Nearly all hypertension diagnosed by general practitioners is essential. Debate exists as to how much effort should be made to find secondary causes. To most general practitioners the textbook lists of Cushing's disease, hyperaldosteronism and renal artery stenosis are esoteric rarities and most will spend little or no time looking for them. This is probably a correct decision, bearing in mind their extreme rarity and the huge numbers of patients who would have to be processed (Mayhew 1982). However, clinical acumen still counts for a lot — it does not take long to rule out coarctation of the aorta by feeling the femoral pulses, or to listen for a bruit over the renal arteries. If there is any suspicion a consultant referral is sensible. A readily identifiable cause of reversible hypertension is drug treatment and the non-steroidal anti-inflammatory group is probably the most common. Care should be taken when confirming mild to moderate hypertension in a patient taking these drugs.

A similar debate exists about how much investigation is appropriate to identify end-organ damage due to hypertension. Fundoscopy and urinalysis are probably good starting points, and there may be an argument for chest radiography, electrocardiography and measurement of blood urea. Some doctors may use these investigations in their decision on whether to treat, arguing that the case for treatment would be stronger if there was evidence of damage. Others may include investigations to look at the spectrum of risk factors for coronary artery disease, often including a blood cholesterol estimation. With the development of well-person clinics this approach is increasingly common but, as the relevance of these other screens is under doubts of the same sort as I have described for hypertension, knowledge of their results does not always clarify! I tend to take a reductionist approach to these matters, arguing that it is the control of the blood pressure that is important, regardless of other findings. If there were evidence of end organ damage I would wish to minimise it, and if not I would wish to prevent it. My knowledge may have some minimal prognostic use but does not influence my decision to treat. I would take a similar view about monitoring a treated patient by these methods.

I will spend little time on treatment itself, as this is outside the scope of this book, but it is nearly always possible to find a suitable therapy. This is almost invariably drug therapy but good evidence exists for non-drug treatment in some patients. Vastly greater resource has gone into investigating drugs because of the obvious vested interests of the drug companies. However, refinements do occur and sometimes clear advantages of one drug over another are demonstrated, so patients should not necessarily expect to be on one therapy for the whole of their hypertensive career. With care, treatment can be achieved without producing damage to the psyche of an essentially well patient who may only have attended to have his passport form signed (Gill & Beevers 1983).

The drug treatment of hypertension has seen a number of quantum leaps and vast numbers of 'me too' drugs. The significant changes of recent years have been through the sequence of rauwolfia compounds, ganglion blockers, methyldopa, beta-blockers, calcium channel blockers and angiotensin-converting enzyme inhibitors. Thiazide diuretics have survived more or less throughout. Whether to use single or combination therapy has depended on changing fashion.

SCREENING AND CASE FINDING

Having negoitiated this minefield and defined your criteria, the method by which blood pressure is to be recorded, the appropriate investigations and the treatment programme, you now have to discover the patients — there are many of them. Several years ago at St George's we decided to investigate the most efficient means of detection. First, hypertension is a disease of general practice and it is in this context that it must be considered. Community medicine can detect but not treat and hospital medicine can treat but not detect. General practice should be in a position to do both but is often critised for inefficient detection and inadequate treatment (Heller & Rose 1977, Relman 1980). The oft quoted 'rule of halves' summarises these criticisms. This states that, in a given population, only half of the patients with the condition will have been detected; of these, only half will be treated and finally, of those treated, only half will be adequately controlled. If this rule still holds true then only one-eighth of those likely to benefit will have their blood pressure successfully treated. Treatment cannot start without detection (unless we add antihypertensives to the tap water) so we sought to compare formal screening and case finding. As has been stated elsewhere (see Chapter 2) screening implies identifying those at risk (in this case the entire population under 80) and offering them the detection procedure. Case finding brings the detection procedure into the normal consultation as opportunistic health care (Stott & Davies 1979). We limited our study to men and women between the ages of 40 and 64.

Four group practices were recruited and nurses were employed to do the screening, which was unusual then but much more commonplace now. An initial note search revealed a group of 7871 patients whose blood pressure status was unknown. These patients formed the study group and were randomly allocated to screening and case finding groups. Those who failed to attend after screening invitations were tagged for case

finding and those who either did not attend surgery during the study period or who attended but, for various reasons, were not offered the procedure, were subsequently sent a screening invitation. We thus had a primary and secondary screened group and a primary and secondary case-found group. In other words we were able to examine our non-attenders to both procedures. Our first finding was that during the time available, 20% more of the screened group were examined. However, we were in for a surprise.

Within both groups, a proportion of patients were examined. Of those examined some were found to be abnormal. Of those found to be abnormal some established satisfactory treatment. From these numbers we were able to calculate the rates of those examined, those abnormal and those treated from those allocated. When this was done the initial marked preference for screening was eliminated and, in fact, there was a swing in favour of case finding — the rates of those allocated and found abnormal and the rates of those abnormal who established treatment, being significantly higher.

The conclusion from this is that people attending for consultation have a higher incidence of hypertension than those who do not. This could mean that hypertension is not a symptomless condition after all but is linked to a symptom pattern yet to be described, or is possibly linked to the personality type of people who attend doctors. However, case finding is more efficient than screening, providing over twice the proportions for treatment; it is also clearly cheaper and easier (Buchan & Richardson 1973). Formal screening would not seem to have much to recommend it (although giving the patient the opportunity to refuse may arguably be the more ethical approach). Indeed, if formal screening is substituted for systematic case finding, it will be counter-productive. Doctors who are running screening clinics (often conducted by nurses) by invitation should continue to case-find at every opportunity. Perhaps the nurse clinics would be better run as referral clinics, sorting out those found to be abnormal.

LENGTH OF TREATMENT

One further dilemma lies in wait for those who undertake this work — the length of the treatment. Conventional wisdom suggests that treatment continues for ever but with many patients starting therapy in their 20s to 30s this is, to say the least, daunting. One reason for stopping may be redefinitions of the levels of blood pressure at which treatment is judged to be beneficial. Each such redefinition, depending on which way it goes, leaves either screened patients judged now to be normal in need of treatment or some patients now on treatment who would be judged normal. A practice will need to be in a position to review the blood pressure status of its patients in the light of changing knowledge. It is a dynamic affair and clearly an efficient computer system would greatly aid this process.

Hypertension does seem to get better in some individuals — even allowing for the well known phenomenon of regression to the mean – and treatment may be reduced or stopped. The justification for considering this comes from the Australian Therapeutic Trial (1980) and the MRC (1985) study. In the former, at the end of 3 years of follow-up, no less than 48% of the placebo group had a blood pressure below the entrance criteria. In the MRC study, between one-third and one-half of the placebo population had blood pressures below 90 phase V diastolic on one of the anniversary visits and 18% had values below this at the end of their first three anniversary visits.

The subject of hypertension continues to fascinate and infuriate. It is relatively easy to record but difficult to interpret. This seeming impossibility in calculating individual risks and benefits leaves doctors swinging between evangelical zeal and therapeutic nihilism, as report after report apparently contradict each other. There seems little doubt that there is some benefit, but not as much as was initially claimed, in the detection and treatment of hypertension. It is not a number crunching exercise but depends upon thoughtful doctors making sensible decisions for their patients, as stated in my quote from Feinstein at the beginning of this chapter.

REFERENCES

Actuarial Society of America and the Association of Life Insurance Medical Directors 1941 Supplement to blood pressure study. Actuarial Society of America and the Association of Life Insurance Medical Directors, New York

Amery A, Brixho P, Clement D et al 1985 Mortality and morbidity results from the European Working Party on Hypertension in the Elderly Trial. Lancet i: 1349–1354.

Australian Therapeutic Trial in Mild Hypertension 1980 Lancet i: 1261–1267

Buchan I C, Richardson I M 1973 Time study of consultation in general practice. Scottish Health Service Study No.27. Scottish Home and Health Department, Edinburgh

Dawber T R, Kannel W B, Revotzkie N, Kagan A 1962 The epidemiology of coronary heart disease — the Framingham enquiry. Proceedings of the Royal Society of Medicine 55: 265–271.

Feinstein A R 1972 The need for humanised science in evalulating medication. Lancet ii: 421–423

Gill J S, Beevers D G 1983 Hypertension and wellbeing. British Medical Journal 287: 1490–1491

Heller R F, Rose G 1977 Current management of hypertension in general practice. British Medical Journal i: 1442–1444

Lancet 1980 The pressure to treat (editorial). Lancet i: 1283–1284

Mayhew S R 1982 Hypertensive screening. General Practice International 3: 129–130

Medical Research Council 1985 Trial of treatment of mild hypertension: principal results. British Medical Journal 291: 97–105

Miall W E 1977 Medical Research Council working party on mild to moderate hypertension: design and pilot study. British Medical Journal i: 1437–1440

Relman A S 1980 Mild hypertension: no more benign neglect. New England Journal of Medicine 302: 293-294

Stott N C, Davis R H 1979 The exceptional potential of each primary care consultation. Journal of the Royal College of General Practitioners 29: 201–205

Swales J D, Ramsay L E, Coope J R et al 1989 Treating mild hypertension: report of the British Hypertension Working Party. British Medical Journal 298: 694–698

Wilson J M G 1966 Some principles of early diagnosis and detection. In: Teeling-Smith G (ed) Surveillance and early diagnosis in general practice. Proceedings of Colloquium held at Magdalen College, Oxford, 7th July 1965. Office of Health Economics, London

FURTHER READING

Hart J T 1987 Hypertension, 2nd edn. Churchill Livingstone, Edinburgh

22. Screening and surveillance of disorders of metabolism in adults

Katharine Orton

INTRODUCTION

Screening

There is no metabolic disease that justifies the screening of all the adults on a general practice list. No disease in this group is prevalent enough, serious enough or responsive enough to treatment, in the asymptomatic phase, to justify the costs. Even diabetes mellitus does not overcome these objections, although epidemiological studies using different screening techniques continue to be done.

It has been suggested (Nusynovitz 1980) that any laboratory-based screening procedure should meet a number of criteria before a screening programme is started:

1. The disease must affect the quality or duration of life.
2. Effective treatment must be available.
3. Treatment in the asymptomatic phase must reduce morbidity or mortality.
4. The test must be cheap and easily performed.
5. The test must be highly sensitive.
6. The disease prevalence must be sufficiently high so that the case finding cost is low.

Subgroups of the adult population particularly at risk of non-insulin dependent diabetes and impaired glucose tolerance, hypothyroidism, hyperlipidaemia, osteoporosis and hyperuricaemia may be considered as candidates for selective screening. Family clusters of metabolic diseases occur because of shared genetic and environmental factors.

There is a group of rare, inherited, metabolic diseases (including cystinuria, porphyria, cholinesterase deficiency, haemochromatosis and Wilson's disease) that present in adulthood and that should be screened for in the families of sufferers. Identifying these high-risk groups is a task that may well fall to the general practitioner.

Surveillance

There is a need for long-term surveillance of a number of the conditions listed above and also of some closely allied diseases. For most general practitioners the surveillance of diabetes, thyroid disease and gout is a part of each day's work. It is becoming generally accepted that this surveillance should take on a more structured form and be undertaken by a multidisciplinary team within the practice. The prime example of this is the diabetic mini-clinic, which is now established as a valuable alternative to hospital diabetic clinics, principally for non-insulin dependent diabetics.

A follow-up programme for any chronic disease is only as effective as the manual or computer-based disease index from which it is run. The organisation of surveillance programmes is covered in Chapters 5 and 6.

The metabolic diseases that may be supervised are diabetes, hyperthyroidism, simple goitre, hyperlipidaemia, haemochromatosis, hyperuricaemia and other forms of urinary calculi. Some of the aims of surveillance for each condition will be discussed under each disease heading.

DIABETES

Screening for diabetes in general practice

Diabetes is a common disease, present estimates of prevalence in the UK being between 2–5% of adults (WHO Study Group 1985) and in our ageing, industrialised population the figure is expected to increase further.

Screening for diabetes applies only to adult onset or non-insulin dependent diabetes (NIDDM). A number of cases of NIDDM will go on to require insulin, but the group name implies an insidious onset, with an asymptomatic stage during which screening would

Table 22.1   Criteria for diagnosis (from WHO Study Group 1985)

	Criteria
Diabetes mellitus	Fasting venous plasma glucose > 7.8 mmol/litre Venous plasma glucose 2 h after 75g glucose load > 11.1 mmol/litre
Impaired glucose tolerance (using the oral glucose tolerance test)	Fasting venous plasma glucose < 7.8 mmol/litre Venous plasma glucose 2 h after 75g glucose load 7.8–11.1 mmol/litre

alert the patient and GP to the additional risks. As well as this asymptomatic diabetic state, there is now increased awareness of the risks attached to impaired glucose tolerance (IGT) (see Table 22.1 for definitions of diabetes and IGT).

Why screen for diabetes and impaired glucose tolerance?

Patients with impaired glucose tolerance show a 2–4% deterioration to unequivocal diabetes annually. There is a similar percentage who return to normality. Both IGT and non-insulin dependent diabetes have been shown to cause a doubling in the incidence of large vessel disease, such as coronary heart disease, cerebrovascular disease and peripheral vascular disease.

In the Whitehall Study of 18 000 male civil servants age 40-64 (Fuller et al 1980), coronary heart disease mortality over the $7\frac{1}{2}$ year follow-up period was compared with the blood glucose response 2 hours after a glucose load. Coronary heart disease mortality was approximately doubled for subjects with a blood sugar of above the 95th centile (> 96 mg/dl), i.e. subjects who had impaired glucose tolerance. There was no trend in heart disease mortality below this point. Within the IGT group age, systolic blood pressure and ECG abnormality were all significantly predictive of subsequent coronary heart disease mortality (Fuller et al 1980).

Patients identified as being in this group of IGT, as well as those with NIDDM, can be regarded as having an additional risk factor for coronary heart disease. Once identified they can be advised to reduce weight, increase exercise and stop smoking. Follow-up of their glycaemic state and control of blood lipids and hypertension may improve outcome (Keen 1989).

The duration of diagnosed disease in NIDDM seems to have little predictive value on the severity of large vessel disease, suggesting that diagnosis and pre-

ventative action taken in the asymptomatic stage, or in impaired glucose tolerance, may be the only way to reduce the resulting mortality and morbidity.

A higher risk of small vessel disease occurs only in the full diabetic state. The clinical risk of retinopathy is negligible over periods of up to 10 years with IGT.

Whom do we screen?

Total population screening for diabetes and IGT is as yet undertaken only in epidemiological studies. However the increasing commitment of general practice to the prevention of coronary heart disease, a major cause of morbidity and mortality in the UK, has increased the feasibility of screening those over 45 years, male and female, for asymptomatic NIDDM and IGT as part of heart disease screening. Women with NIDDM and IGT have the same risk of coronary heart disease as men with these conditions — the relative immunity due to being female is lost.

Family history is a vital clue to those most at risk. HLA-typing in insulin-dependent diabetes can detect especially susceptible normal siblings (DR3 and/or DR4 in Caucasians). As there is no preventative action that can be taken, this is a research field only.

The genetic link in NIDDM is more important, although HLA-typing is no help. Virtually all the identical twins of affected individuals have the disease, as opposed to 50% in IDDM. The strong genetic predisposition is added to by shared environmental effects such as obesity, exercise and dietary habits.

Obesity has a well recognised association with NIDDM although the relationship is not simple. Both may be due to insulin resistance.

Parity is probably not a risk factor, although even mild glycosuria is a risk to the successful outcome of a pregnancy. Screening for glycosuria is part of normal antenatal care (see Chapter 11). Women who bear a baby over 4.5 kg (10 lb) also have an increased risk of NIDDM.

Routine screening for diabetes using urine testing is part of many pre-employment and insurance medicals. It is also part of the clinical examination of presenting problems as varied as urinary tract infection and myocardial infarction.

Good practice dictates that we keep diabetes in the forefront of our minds, so that any chance of opportunistic screening can be taken. The target groups to be observed are:

Those over 45 years of age
Those with a family history of diabetes
Those with premature atherosclerosis

Individuals with other risk factors for coronary heart disease:

a. hypertension
b. hyperlipidaemia
c. smoking

Obese individuals

Pregnant women

Women with a previous baby weighing > 4.5 kg (10 lb)

Screening methods

As screening tests have become more sensitive and the understanding of the natural history of NIDDM and IGT has improved, estimates of the prevalence of these conditions in the community have increased.

Despite the recognised insensitivity of urine glucose estimation, even after a meal (see Table 4.1, p.40), it is still the mainstay of opportunistic and clinical screening for diabetes. It is, of course, useless for the detection of impaired glucose tolerance. It is not appropriate for case-finding in the general population (WHO Study Group 1985).

Fasting blood glucose testing is limited by the difficulty in ensuring the fasting state. Also patients with IGT have, by definition, a normal fasting glucose level.

Random blood glucose estimation may strongly suggest NIDDM but many cases fall into an uncertain zone, even if there is a careful history of food intake prior to testing.

An effective screening procedure, which can be applied to the general population, is still being sought. All new tests have to be compared with the 2 hour postload blood glucose level (2hBG), as advocated by the WHO for prevalence studies and screening purposes. This is usually applied as a single capillary or venous sample taken 2 hours after a 75 g glucose or equivalent load. Supervision of the patient when the glucose is given and for the intervening 2 hours is expensive and time-consuming. The full oral glucose tolerance test (OGTT) remains the reference standard for the diagnosis of diabetes but it is too cumbersome for large-scale use (WHO Study Group 1985).

The Islington diabetes survey (Forrest et al 1988) performed in a North London general practice in 1986, compared estimates of prevalence of diabetes and IGT by the OGTT and the 2hBG methods and was able to support the WHO Study Group recommendation. Both tests showed a similar variability on repeat testing of individuals and in and out of impaired glucose tolerance.

The same survey found that a blood glucose reflectance meter, which tested 2hBG samples, per-formed well. Compared with a glucose–oxidase method it required a smaller blood volume, no transport and the results were available in 2 minutes. It became less expensive after 143 subjects had been tested (Forrest et al 1987).

Glycosylated haemoglobin (HbA1c) has been studied as a possible screening test, with the advantage that the preparation of the patient does not have to be standardised. Unfortunately, it is too insensitive, as there is considerable overlap between the blood levels in normal glucose tolerance, IGT and diabetes (Orchard et al 1982).

Serum fructosamine has recently been introduced as a cheaper, more easily automated measure of mean blood glucose concentration. However, it is not able to detect the very small increment in mean blood glucose that is required of a screening test for diabetes and IGT. (Swai et al 1988).

In summary

The only effective way to screen at-risk patients is to subject them to a 2 hour post-glucose load blood glucose test, which will detect asymptomatic diabetes and the almost equally damaging state of IGT. The next best thing would be a casual or random blood glucose estimation: this would be followed by a fasting blood glucose where the random glucose exceeds 5.5mmol/l, and by a full oral glucose tolerance test in those with a fasting figure in excess of 5.5mmol/l.

Surveillance of diabetes in general practice

Why establish follow-up care for diabetes?

Once diabetes has been diagnosed it must be assumed that this is only the beginning of a lifetime of follow-up and screening for serious causes of morbidity and mortality. It is also the start of a long-term relationship with a patient who has a life-long disease that requires daily modification of behaviour.

An important point is that doctors, nurses and all the other professionals involved have first to share care with patients, who will decide for themselves whether the care provided is worthwhile.

As with all chronic diseases, the general practitioner is in an extremely good position to supervise continuing care in diabetes. He or she has not got the problems of rapidly changing junior hospital staff and lack of knowledge of the patient and family. With suitable planning and staffing most non-insulin dependent diabetics, and many insulin dependent diabetics, can be managed in the community.

The increasing emphasis in the new contract on service provision and proof of good management, linked to financial reward in general practice, should mean that those who undertake these 'extra' tasks will be rewarded. Those who leave chronic disease surveillance to the hospital will be poorer in many ways.

Diabetic mini-clinics

The care of diabetic patients can be arranged in a number of ways (Table 22.2). It is no longer acceptable to see diabetics in the middle of busy surgeries. A group practice may decide that doctors should see their own cases or that one or more should specialise in diabetic care. Either way a commitment must be made to continuing education in diabetic surveillance.

To ensure adequate opportunity for other professionals to be available for diabetic patients it is probably necessary to arrange a separate time for a diabetic mini-clinic. This gives clerical staff the chance to operate a manual or computer-based diabetic register. Patients can be called and recalled and non-attenders can be followed-up.

The practice nurse is a vital part of the mini-clinic set-up. The nurse will want to be involved in the assessment of the patient in the form of weight, blood pressure, urine testing and measurement of visual acuity. The taking of capillary blood specimens for use in a glucometer can fall to the nurse. If the clinic is arranged so that the doctor sees the patient after the nurse then the pupils may be dilated in preparation for fundoscopy.

In all cases nurses are able to provide invaluable continuity, support and education, providing time and opportunity for problems and worries of all sorts to be discussed informally.

Access to dietetic advice is essential, either through specially trained nurses or a practice-based dietitian. Schemes for reimbursement of dietitian salaries are available through many FHSAs.

Table 22.2 Care of diabetes — the options (from Alberti 1986)

Hospital-based diabetes clinic

Hospital-based general medical clinic

General practice-based diabetes clinic (mini-clinics):
    Run by general practitioners
    Run by visiting hospital diabetologists

Individual patient care by general practitioner

Shared care schemes

Chiropody must be available either in the mini-clinic or through close liaison with hospital-based chiropodists.

For this system to succeed there should be close communication between the practice-based team and the local hospital diabetic clinic. A good relationship between the local consultant in charge and the general practitioner will ensure rapid treatment of complications and advice on the management of difficult problems.

Shared care

Some diabetics will benefit most from shared care between the primary care run mini-clinic and perhaps yearly visits to a hospital for review by a consultant. This review clinic must include access to other specialist consultants — ophthalmologists, cardiologists and nephrologists. This arrangement means that even the more difficult NIDDM patient and many IDDM patients can be jointly under the care of their general practitioner who, after all, has to know and understand their problems when called on in an emergency.

Communication

Diabetic care collapses when communication between the hospital and the general practitioner, between the general practitioner and the diabetic primary care team or between the members of the diabetic primary care team fails. More important still is the relationship with the patient, on whom the burden of self-care falls. Co-operation cards held by the patient are very valuable, particularly if all entries are fully understood by the patient.

The application of computers to a protocol for diabetic management, perhaps shared by both the hospital and general practice and including up-to-date pathological data, would be a way to further integrate diabetic care.

Those who have opted out

A number of diabetic patients opt out of every system that is on offer. Some will respond to individual care and support even if no form of clinic can hold them. As with all services for patient care, effort must be made to cater for each individual. Attention to the allocation of enough time by the doctor and/or nurse to each patient, so that special needs and fears can be understood, will reduce the number of non-attenders.

Table 22.3 Diabetic complications

Glucose control	Associated mental states
Hyperglycaemia	Depression
Hypoglycaemia	Rebellion
	Self-abuse
Macroangiopathy	Microvascular disease
Cardiovascular disease	Retinopathy
Cerebrovascular disease	Nephropathy
Peripheral vascular disease	
Neuropathy	Mixed problems
Sensorimotor	Diabetic foot
Autonomic	Impotence
Mononeuropathy	

Associated risk factors partly the result of the diabetic state
  Hypertension
  Obesity
  Hyperlipidaemia

What is worth doing?

It is now known to be more than mere clinical impression that careful control of blood sugar can and does delay the onset of diabetic complications. The complications of both IDDM and NIDDM are shown in Table 22.3

Glucose control

There are now better methods of blood glucose control available, both in the clinic and at home, allowing more stringent control to be achieved. The advent of HbA1c (glycosylated haemoglobin) estimations for the assessment of control over the previous 3 months, and of more widespread home blood glucose monitoring has meant that targets can be set and progress monitored.

The change to insulin in previously NIDDM patients is inevitable in some, with time. Some authors quote that 10% of NIDDM are no longer satisfactorily controlled after 1 year and 90% after 5 years on diet and sulphonylureas alone.

Hypoglycaemia is probably the inevitable consequence of adequate insulin therapy. It engenders a lot of fear in patients and relatives. Blood glucose monitoring can reduce episodes to a minimum.

In NIDDM hypoglycaemia is a danger only in elderly diabetics who can have prolonged and life-threatening attacks on the longer acting sulphonylureas.

The prevention of hyperglycaemia in intercurrent illness, can be achieved by checking that the need to continue medication and even increase insulin dosage is understood by the patient and the relatives. Urine tests for ketones can help the patient predict when to seek help.

How often should glucose control be checked?

The first requirement is to help patients to start a system of home monitoring that suits the severity of their disease and allows them to live as normal a life as possible. IDDM patients need blood glucose testing using sticks or glucometers. Once or twice a day is adequate as long as the times are spread pre- and postprandially. Urine testing may still be satisfactory for most NIDDM patients but this must be kept under review in each case.

Urine glucose can be checked on each attendance at the clinic. The frequency of random capillary or blood glucose estimations and HbA1c will vary from one patient to another, 6 monthly blood glucose and yearly HbA1c may be recommended. The availability of a glucometer eases the burden of the transport of specimens.

Microvascular disease

An almost linear relationship exists between the duration of diabetes and the severity of microvascular disease.

Retinopathy

Diabetic retinopathy is the chief cause of blindness in people aged 30–65 years, despite effective treatment being available for more than a decade. Treatment has also been shown to be long-lasting in its effect (British Multicentre Research Group 1977, ETDRS 1985), thereby justifying screening.

Non-proliferative or 'background' retinopathy carries a risk of blindness of < 3% in 5 years for those under 60 years, whilst proliferative retinopathy, with new vessel formation, brings a risk of 50% in 5 years (Caird et al 1969).

In a population-based study carried out in Wisconsin, USA, in 1984, the prevalence of non-proliferative retinopathy after only 5 years in individuals diagnosed with IDDM before the age of 30, was 17% of nearly 1000 patients (Klein et al 1984). More surprising was that non-proliferative retinopathy was found in 28.8% of over 1300 diabetics diagnosed after the age of 30 years (NIDDM), again only 5 years after diagnosis. This suggests that damage was being done prior to clinical diagnosis. The prevalence of proliferative retinopathy, with its greater risk of

Table 22.4   Prevalence of retinopathy (from Klein et al 1984)

	Duration of diabetes (years)	Retinopathy (%)	Proliferative retinopathy (%)
IDDM (996)	< 5	17.0	0.0
	< 10	97.5	25.0
NIDDM (1370)	< 5	28.8	2.0
	15+	77.8	15.5

blindness, was 25% of IDDM by 10 years from diagnosis and 15.5% of NIDDM after at least 15 years (Table 22.4).

Effective action first entails screening; patients are generally unaware of changes until late in the disease. Secondly, good glycaemic control must be exercised because poor control has been shown to speed retinal changes. Thirdly, referral for photocoagulation, cryotherapy and, where necessary in severe disease, vitreoretinal surgery to limit damage.

Whom do we screen? All diabetics should have fundoscopy at annual review. Those most at risk of retinopathy are those with the longest duration of illness, those poorly controlled, either through the disease or through non-compliance, those with hypertension, those with a positive family history, those with proteinuria suggesting generalised microvascular damage and the obese. Pregnancy may accelerate established lesions.

Who should screen? It falls to the doctor supervising the general management of the practice's diabetics to screen for retinopathy. Careful assessment should be made of visual acuity and then the fundi should be examined with dilated pupils. This is essential for the diagnosis of peripheral new vessel formation. The risk of congestive glaucoma following dilatation is overstated. Ophthalmic opticians (optometrists) offer their diabetic patients a yearly check-up, including retinoscopy. This is a very useful additional check (Rohan et al 1989).

Nephropathy

There is evidence that nephropathy is progressive from diagnosis in NIDDM but is unusual until after 10 years of IDDM. The first sign of trouble is microalbuminuria, defined as proteinuria > 30 mcg/minute. Dipsticks cannot detect proteinuria at this level, but until the natural history is known and some method of reversing the process has been found, microalbuminuria levels have relatively low management

value. Renal function deteriorates slowly, with end-stage renal failure occurring 7–10 years after the appearance of persistent dipstick-positive proteinuria. Those with proteinuria almost always have proliferative retinopathy.

Careful glycaemic control, blood pressure control and examination for macrovascular disease, including renal artery stenosis, are all important in the management of diabetic nephropathy. These patients will be under the care of a hospital but will require regular support and supervision by their general practitioners.

How often should we screen? All diabetics on each visit, be it 3- or 6- monthly, should have their urine checked for protein. Blood urea and creatinine should be monitored once a year.

Macroangiopathy

Cardiovascular disease, cerebrovascular disease and peripheral vascular disease carry a 2–3 times increased mortality and morbidity in diabetics. A number of newly diagnosed NIDDM patients present with quite advanced large vessel disease. Management should be by prevention by the usual measures. Those most at risk are younger diabetics, those with hypertension, those with dyslipoproteinaemia (the importance of which is not known), those with hyperinsulinaemia and those with obesity. Female diabetics have an equal risk with males.

Renal artery stenosis must be remembered when hypertension supervenes in an atherosclerotic, diabetic patient.

Systematic examination of the patient at least once a year, at a review appointment, should ensure that large vessel disease is detected as early as possible.

Neuropathy

Sensorimotor neuropathy is the most common of the chronic complications of diabetes. In one study, it was present in 7.5% of all diabetics at diagnosis and in 50% after 25 years (Macleod 1989). However, figures vary because of the lack of standardised diagnostic criteria. The prevalence is greater in those with poor glycaemic control and can be shown to improve with intensive insulin therapy. Neuropathy benefits from tight glucose control. Screening for early changes, the first being decreased vibration sense in the great toe and absent ankle jerks, is necessary to focus on those most at risk of foot ulcers.

Autonomic neuropathy is unlikely to be clinically important unless there is a marked sensorimotor loss.

Postural hypotension and impotence are the most important problems.

Assessment of the patient for neuropathy is also best performed systematically once a year.

Mixed problems

Feet

All diabetic patients need to be helped to care for their feet and to know when to seek attention between clinic appointments. The patient is best placed to detect the first signs of trouble, i.e. colour change, swelling, throbbing or discharge. The function of the doctor and nurse in clinic is to screen for the earliest signs of neuropathy, ischaemia or infection. A chiropodist must be available for advice and treatment of some cases.

Impotence

At least 25% of male diabetics have some form of problem with sexual function. In one study with age-matched controls, this compared with 9% of non-diabetics (Macleod 1989). This embarrassing subject needs to be discussed openly and a careful sexual history taken. Diabetic impotence is a diagnosis of exclusion. Medication may well be the cause or a factor. In the absence of autonomic neuropathy, arterial disease in the pudendal vessels may be the problem and require an arteriogram. Endocrine and psychological causes must not be ignored.

Other risk factors

Hypertension

Hypertension in a diabetic patient is an important additional risk factor in retinopathy, nephropathy and large vessel disease. The management is much the same as in the non-diabetic patient, with treatment recommended at the same levels. Secondary hypertension due to rare conditions such as acromegaly, Cushing's disease and phaeochromocytoma must at least be considered, as should renal artery stenosis in individuals with generalised atherosclerosis. Other risk factors, such as smoking and hyperlipidaemia, should be dealt with where possible.

There is no evidence in favour of any particular group of antihypertensive drugs so, as in essential hypertension, medication is tailored to the individual patient, although the theoretical hyperglycaemic effects of thiazide diuretics should be borne in mind.

Obesity

The management of any obesity is of vital importance in the control of NIDDM. The only diet necessary, in many, is energy restriction to reduce weight to normal. Compliance with any weight reduction regime is poor; between 50–93% of patients do not comply. A dietitian who is skilled at communication can motivate the patient towards weight reduction combined with healthier eating. Follow-up appointments will be needed to keep up morale, monitor progress and continue the process of informing the patient on the best management of his/her illness.

Hyperlipidaemia

Raised blood fats constitute an additional risk factor in macroangiopathy and should therefore be controlled in diabetes. The exact value of this management is unknown and specialist advice is needed prior to instituting more than dietary treatment.

Associated mental states

Depression, rebellion and possible self-abuse through diabetic medication have been seen by all physicians who treat diabetic patients. A vital part of the diabetic care team's work is to monitor patient morale as it affects self-care. Some workers have included a psychologist in the team for this reason. We must all have had experience of the non-compliant adolescent IDDM patient, but have to be more aware of rebellion and lack of self-esteem in the resistant, obese NIDDM patient.

In summary

The aims of long-term care of NIDDM with applications to all diabetes have been described (Gatling & Hill 1988) as follows:

1 To maintain patient morale.
2 To maintain the patient's determination to continue self-care.
3 To continue education and revision.
4 To monitor glycaemic control.
5 To monitor weight.
6 To detect long-term complications at an early stage.
7 To identify risk factors.
8 To advise on treatment.
9 To arrange an appointment and recall system.

HYPERLIPIDAEMIA

Screening and surveillance of hyperlipidaemia

Blood lipids are assuming an increasingly important role in the prevention of coronary heart disease. The basis for this is discussed in detail in Chapter 20.

OSTEOPOROSIS

Screening for the risk of osteoporosis

Osteoporosis is the major bone disease of the western world and will affect the majority of women by the end of their lives. Indeed, half of all women will sustain a significant osteoporotic fracture. Prevention is more effective than treatment and the early identification of those at risk has assumed great importance.

Osteoporosis is a reduction in bone mass per unit of bone volume. There is an underlying defect that causes an uncoupling of bone formation and resorption. This allows a decrease in formation with an insufficient decrease in resorption or, in other cases, an increase in resorption without a sufficient increase in formation.

There are many causes of osteoporosis in adults (Stevenson 1988) including:

Postmenopausal.
Age-related (senile).
Hyperparathyroidism.
Metastatic carcinomas.
Reticuloendothelial disorders.
Connective tissue disorders.
Hypercortisolism.
Hyperthyroidism.
Hypogonadism, oöphorectomy.
Immobilisation.
Drugs — corticosteroids
        — heparin
        — alcohol.
Myelomatosis.

As already suggested, postmenopausal osteoporosis is the most important of these conditions. It depends on two major factors. First, the peak adult bone mass achieved prior to the menopause and secondly, the amount of bone lost due to loss of ovarian function.

Both genetic and environmental factors have a part in determining peak bone mass. The genetic influence is the most important, but factors such as nutrition and exercise also have some effect. The effect of calcium is controversial. It is important for skeletal growth but different calcium intakes have an incomplete or absent effect on postmenopausal bone loss.

Osteoporosis can be prevented by delaying the onset of bone loss with oestrogen therapy, plus progestogens to protect the endometrium where necessary The mechanism of action of oestrogen is not understood but there are possible oestradiol receptors in human osteoblasts. Interestingly, calcitonin levels are low in women, relative to men, throughout adult life. Levels of secretion fall with age but are increased by exogenous oestrogens.

Target group

Postmenopausal osteoporosis does occur in some women who seem to have no predisposing factors. However, a subgroup of the premenopausal female population is more at risk. The risk factors for osteoporosis include:

Early menopause.
Artificial menopause.
Race — white or oriental women are more at risk than black races.
Family history of postmenopausal osteoporosis.
Nulliparity — the pill may be protective.
Amenorrhoea or prolonged oligomenorrhoea.
Other skeletal disease, osteogenesis imperfecta, coeliac disease.
High alcohol intake.
Underweight — obesity seems to protect.
Inadequate childhood nutrition.
(Possibly smoking).

How should we screen?

That the prevention of osteoporosis in postmenopausal women reduces morbidity and mortality is not in doubt. It also saves money in terms of working days lost and the costs of hospitalisation for major fractures. Other than clinical awareness and patient interest, we need to have a programme that will alert the doctor and patient to individual levels of risk. Such a programme, of careful history-taking to assess risk, could form part of cervical smear screening of family planning in older women. The practice nurse could extend this part of well-women screening, referring those at risk to the general practitioner.

Assessment of bone mass is not freely available but can be used to confirm or refute those most at risk. Photon absorptiometry and quantitative computer tomography are now allowing measurement of bone density. X-rays and X-ray densitometry are not sensitive enough, only diagnosing severely affected individuals.

Surveillance of those at risk from osteoporosis

Arguably, those groups listed above should be considered for hormone replacement therapy (HRT), and some would suggest that all perimenopausal women should be given hormone replacement therapy as a right. This debate continues and this issue is discussed further in Chapter 30. The detailed use and follow-up of hormone replacement therapy is beyond the scope of this chapter, although a few points are worth making. Firstly, hormone replacement therapy is almost mandatory for women losing their ovarian function before the age of 40 years, and perhaps before 45 years. Secondly, exercise does not prevent bone loss due to hormonal changes and is not an alternative to hormones. Thirdly, as mentioned before, the preventive role of calcium once bones have stopped growing is still controversial. Fourthly, the increased rate of bone loss starts just before cessation of the periods. Hormone replacement needs to be continued for at least 5 years, thereby delaying the age of onset of the majority of fractures, which starts 10 years later.

THYROID DISEASE

Hyperthyroidism

Should we screen anybody?

Hyperthyroidism was found to occur in 19 in 1000 women (this figure rising to 27 in 1000 if possible cases were included) in a community study in Whickham, County Durham in 1977 (Tunbridge et al 1977). This compares with 1.6–2.3 in 1000 men. The figures would be higher if a thyroid-stimulating hormone (TSH) assay with a low detection limit were used.

The diagnosis of hyperthyroidism should, of course, be made as early as possible, but population screening is not justified at present. Symptoms are present at least 6 months prior to diagnosis in most cases. Clinical suspicion must be enough for GPs to check for hyperthyroidism in patients with a large number of different presenting complaints (Toft 1989).

Other than in those with overt disease, opportunistic screening may be of value in the anxious and agitated young woman, in pregnancy and in the long-term follow-up of simple diffuse goitre. This latter may progress over 20–30 years to have areas of autonomous function and eventually hyperthyroidism. Unexplained atrial fibrillation in middle-aged and elderly men and women should also arouse suspicions.

Surveillance of patients with hyperthyroidism

The immediate follow-up of patients will fall primarily to the specialist in charge of treatment of the disease. Unfortunately, a number of patients are lost to follow-up but the general practitioner, if using a well maintained manual or computer-based disease index, is well placed to help with continuing care. In particular, patients with Graves' disease follow a relapsing and remitting course and may assume too early that treatment is complete.

The thyroid status of a patient cannot be properly assessed for up to 6 months after subtotal thyroidectomy because thyroid failure is often temporary. Thereafter, annual review of patients treated surgically is necessary, due to the gradual development of hypothyroidism and the possible recurrence of thyrotoxicosis many years after apparently successful surgery.

The rate of hypothyroidism after radio-iodine treatment rises with treatment dosage. It may be temporary if it occurs within 6 months of treatment. Thereafter, annual review with thyroxine (T_4) and TSH levels are required as hypothyroidism develops at a rate of 2–4% per year to a level of 80% at 15 years (Toft 1989). Some treatment centres prefer to give a higher dose so that permanent hypothyroidism is induced earlier and patients are less likely to be lost to follow-up prior to the development of their hypothyroidism.

Hypothyroidism

Screening for hypothyroidism

The question as to whether there should be screening for hypothyroidism remains unsettled. In developing countries and in areas of known dietary iodine deficiency, there are compelling reasons to screen. The common, primary form of hypothyrodism due to atrophy of the thyroid gland, for whatever reason, is a graded condition (Table 22.5).

In the Whickham survey (Tunbridge et al 1977), the prevalence of overt hypothyroidism was 14 in 1000 women, rising to 19 in 1000 when possible cases were included; this compared with less than 1 in 1000 men. If all iatrogenic cases were excluded, the prevalence dropped to 10 in 1000 women.

Some information about the progression of the disease was found in a follow-up study 4 years later. Only in those with 'mild disease' (normal T_4, raised TSH and positive antibodies) did the TSH level rise significantly. Of these 40 patients (30 women and 10 men) 3 became overtly hypothyroid in under 3 years and 7 in under 4 years.

Table 22.5 Grades of hypothyroidism (from Evered et al 1973)

Grade	Symptoms and signs
Overt disease	Clinically and biochemically abnormal Low T_4 Raised TSH Positive antibodies
Mild disease	Non-specific symptoms and signs Responsive to thyroxine T_4 may be normal Raised TSH Positive antibodies
Subclinical	Clinically normal Normal T_4 Raised TSH
Euthyroid	Positive antibodies

T_4, thyroxine; TSH, thyroid-stimulating hormone

Even if screening were to find cases of subclinical disease, it is by no means certain that early treatment with thyroxine confers any benefit in terms of morbidity and mortality.

No link between raised TSH and ischaemic heart disease has been proved especially as there is no proven link between overt hypothyroidism and coronary atheroma.

At present widespread population screening is not justified.

Target groups

Screening of elderly hospital in-patients has been advocated because hypothyroidism is an eminently treatable cause of general deterioration. The cost of screening a high-risk group, such as postmenopausal women, as part of a wellwoman clinic programme may be justified. Patients who have been treated for hyperthyroidism with surgery or radio-iodine do require yearly follow-up. For the rest, a high index of suspicion in patients presenting with any of the numerous clinical features of hypothyroidism is all that is required at present.

Surveillance of hypothyroidism

Surveillance of hypothyroidism consists of supervision of thyroid replacement therapy. It is now realised that doses necessary to suppress TSH secretion may be associated with hyperthyroidism in other tissues. The possible adverse effects include an increased incidence of postmenopausal osteoporosis, sodium and water retention, raised nocturnal heart beat and changes in liver metabolism. The recent introduction of the sensitive TSH assay may help to alert the clinician to excessively low levels of TSH and should be more reliable during intercurrent illness.

Those who still advocate clinical assessment alone as the arbiter of euthyroid status, need to prove that excess T_4 does no harm. For now we must manage our hypothyroid patients on the lowest dose of T_4 that keeps TSH in the normal range.

Compliance with long-term thyroid replacement therapy can be a problem. One series of cases who had become hypothyroid after surgery for thyrotoxicosis showed that 15% had stopped treatment and 54% were on inadequate doses. A computer-based follow-up programme in general practice with yearly recall of patients is one obvious solution to this problem. The compliant patient can probably be left longer between blood tests for thyroid function as there is no great change in dosage requirement with age.

Surveillance of goitre

The simple diffuse goitre found most commonly in young women requires review every few years, once the diagnosis has been confirmed. In the second and third decades thyroid function tests are normal and tracheal compression is rare. In the fourth and fifth decades early formation of hot spots may reduce TSH levels. In the sixth decade the patient may present with the complications of thyrotoxicosis, usually with some signs of thyroid compression. These patients are at risk of atrial fibrillation and congestive cardiac failure, even with relatively small increases in circulating T_4. Early diagnosis due to careful surveillance can be expected to reduce morbidity.

Goitre caused by autoimmune thyroiditis may eventually end in hypothyroidism; some degree of supervision is therefore desirable. If the goitre is large then T_4 will be prescribed earlier to shrink it.

GOUT

Screening for hyperuricaemia and gout

Hyperuricaemia

Hyperuricaemia, defined as a plasma uric acid level of > 0.42 mmol/l (> 7 mg/100 ml), is found in 5% of the adult male population, and in fewer than one-tenth of this number of females, whose uric acid levels rise slowly through life but do not reach male levels, even after the menopause. These figures originate from a long-term population study in Framingham, Massachusetts (Hall et al 1967).

Table 22.6 Causes of hyperuricaemia (from Dieppe and Calvert 1983)

1. Increased intake of purines in the diet
   Alcohol intake of great importance

2. Overproduction of uric acid
   Primary
   1. idiopathic
   2. rare enzyme disorders

   Secondary
   1. myeloproliferative diseases
   2. haemolysis
   3. carcinomatosis

3. Renal undersecretion of uric acid
   Primary
   1. idiopathic

   Secondary
   1. chronic renal failure
   2. hyperparathyroidism
   3. lactic acidosis
   4. starvation
   5. lead poisoning
   6. diuretics and other drugs
   7. Down syndrome
   8. myxoedema

4. Gut undersecretion of uric acid

Much higher prevalence figures have been found in routine screening of male hospital in-patients. Paulus et al (1970) found that 13.2% of 4148 male in-patients had > 7 mg/100 ml serum urate values. Of the 200 patients studied more closely, the vast majority had secondary hyperuricaemia due to serious illness. Chronic renal failure, acidosis and diuretics accounted for 20% each. Eighty per cent did not require treatment and only 20% had gout or sustained hyperuricaemia that warranted drug treatment. In the Framingham study, only 3% were found to have secondary hyperuricaemia, but this study was done before the widespread use of diuretics in the community. Surveys in general practice in the UK show a preponderance of diuretic therapy causing hyperuricaemia (Table 22.6).

Gout

Gout is far less prevalent than hyperuricaemia, occuring in 0.3–0.5% of the population. A single attack does not warrant treatment; indeed a commitment to long-term management, of any sort, has to be considered very carefully. The risk of gouty arthritis increases gradually with uric acid levels and is variable from one individual to another.

The risk of renal damage due to parenchymal deposition of urate has been overstated. The natural history of hyperuricaemia has been studied only in hospital in-patients.

At the present time, the small numbers who would actually benefit from screening in general practice do not justify a screening programme. It is worth considering a subgroup in who any chance for opportunistic screening should taken.

Target groups

Hyperuricaemia is associated with plenty. The caricature of a typical patient is of a male of high social class and IQ who drinks to excess and may be obese. He would be prone to hypertension, hypertriglyceridaemia and cardiovascular disease. The relationship between diet, obesity, hypertriglyceridaemia, alcohol and hyperuricaemia is not fully understood but individuals deserve that we should be aware of the disease complex.

Those on chronic diuretic therapy should be screened for raised serum urate and their medication reviewed if this is found.

There is a positive family history in 30-50% of cases of hyperuricaemia.

Patients with urate stones or calcium salt stones have an increased risk of being hyperuricaemic.

Surveillance of hyperuricaemia and gout

Once it has been confirmed, on two or more readings, that the patient has a blood urate of 0.42 mmol/l, some management decisions need to be taken, based on the history and examination of the patient. As hyperuricaemia is far more prevalent than gout, joint pain often has a non-gout cause even in such patients.

The medical management of hyperuricaemia and gout requires a life-long commitment by the patient and the doctor. It is justified only where there are recurrent attacks of gout, renal disease or calculi, tophi or a persistent serum urate level > 0.6 mmol/l.

Treatment consists first of removing any possible cause, such as unnecessary use of a diuretic. Secondly, the patient should be helped to lose weight, reduce alcohol intake and avoid a high purine diet. A practice-based dietition or nurse would be of benefit in this context. Lastly it must be considered whether drug treatment is necessary.

If drug treatment is commenced, the xanthine oxidase inhibitor, allopurinol, is the usual agent. Safeguards to prevent the precipitation of gout have to be in place in the form of non-steroidal anti-inflammatory drugs.

Annual review of the uric acid level, renal function and the cardiovascular system is necessary. The dosage of allopurinol needs to be adjusted so that the uric acid level falls below 0.42 mmol/l. Regular checks of blood pressure, weight, diet and alcohol intake are made and the fasting lipid levels should be known, in case additional dietary management is necessary. The amount of chronic joint damage needs to be assessed so that pain control and the need for exercise and physiotherapy can be assessed. Periodic X-rays of the hands and feet may be needed. A history suggestive of ureteric calculi requires an intravenous urogram, as urate stones are not radio-opaque. Figures vary, but between 5 % and 25% of gout sufferers get renal calculi.

Careful surveillance can improve the lot of hyper-uricaemic patients.

METABOLIC CAUSES OF URINARY CALCULI

A number of metabolic diseases, including hyper-uricaemia, present with urinary calculi. Screening for a metabolic cause of stones is mandatory in all patients, as the recurrence rate of all stones is variously put at between 75 and 90%, depending on the follow-up period of the study.

Follow-up and treatment of metabolic stones have been shown to reduce recurrence. Prevention of recurrence in turn reduces the risk of infection and renal damage.

Screening for metabolic stones

Of a series of 120 patients with urinary stones, who were followed up for a mean of 5 years, 60% were found to have a treatable metabolic abnormality. The most common causes were idiopathic hypercalciuria and incomplete renal tubular acidosis, i.e. patients who were unable to acidify their urine but had no systemic acidosis. The rate of recurrence of urinary stones in metabolic stone formers was twice that of patients with normal metabolic study results (Williams and Chisholm 1976).

Some baseline investigations for metabolic causes of stones can easily be performed by the general practitioner prior to referral to a urologist. A full set of such investigations would be:

1 Midstream urine (MSU) microscopy, culture and sensitivity.
2 Random urine for cystine screening.
3 Random urine for pH.
4 Full blood count.
5 Erythrocyte sedimentation rate (ESR).
6 Blood for urea, electrolytes, creatinine, calcium, phosphate, alkaline phosphatase, uric acid and total proteins.
7 24 hour urine collections for calcium and uric acid excretion, also cystine and oxalate excretion and creatinine clearance.
8 Stone examination can prevent some of the above.

A full metabolic screen is necessary even when urinary tract infection is thought to be the cause of the stone formation, as the two causes may well coexist.

Family screening is important when one family member has cystine stones (see below).

Surveillance of metabolic stone formers

With the difficulties and cost of out-patient treatment, metabolic stone formers are best followed up in general practice, once surgical treatment and investigation are complete and as long as a system for recall and identification of non-attenders is in position.

The aetiology of stone formation is often multiple. From Table 22.7 it may be seen what treatment and supervision is necessary in each case.

In some of the causes of stones the treatment methods are also employed to prevent recurrence. The majority, however, are dealt with by a urologist with the help, increasingly, of interventional radiology.

In all cases, the patients are asked to monitor their urine output and to record the results on a weekly to 3-

Table 22.7   Aetiology of stones (from Kincaid-Smith 1986)

Stone type	Causes	% of all stones
Calcium oxalate or phosphate	Hypercalciuria Hyperuricosuria Hyperoxaluria High urine pH Low urine volume	70.6
Infection	Urinary infection with bacteria that possess urease and cause the combination of high pH and high ammonia concentration	21.5
Uric acid stones	Low urine pH Hyperuricosuria Low urine volume	5.4
Cystine stones	Cystinuria	3.5

monthly basis. This will then alert the patient and the doctor to any drop off in urine volume. The patient can then be encouraged to take more fluid. If the 24-hour urine volume can be kept in the region of 2.5–3.5 litres, recurrences can often be prevented even without further action. For this approach to work the patient must maintain a high night volume. This entails drinking enough on going to bed to necessitate voiding 2–3 times during the night, and drinking the same volume again after emptying the bladder each time.

Dietary restrictions either for oxalate stones or uric acid stones are not effective and life-long compliance is unlikely. If calcium intake is excessive then it is reasonable to ask for a modest reduction. Calcium restriction does increase oxalate absorption from the bowel, therefore is of dubious benefit.

The specific management of metabolic causes of urinary stones rarely effects a cure, except for the removal of a parathyroid adenoma, present in 3% of the 120 cases in a study by Williams and Chisholm (1970).

Idiopathic hypercalciuria

Calcium reabsorption in the distal tubule may be enhanced by prescribing a thiazide diuretic, e.g. bendrofluazide 5 mg, best taken at night to further increase urine flow. In a few cases it may be necessary to give potassium citrate (20–30 mmol/per day) to correct hypokalaemia.

Hyperuricosuria

Uric acid and calcium oxalate stones are associated with hyperuricosuria. In many cases alkalinisation of the urine with potassium citrate (40–60 mmol/day) may be prophylactic, as will reduction of any hyper-uricaemia, (see gout, above).

Renal tubular acidosis

This may be found where there are calcium phosphate stones and an alkaline urine. Careful evaluation is needed as to whether the condition is primary or secondary. Thereafter the patient may be advised to take potassium citrate to reduce calcium excretion and increase urinary citrate.

The diagnostic criteria used vary between series, causing different incidences to be found.

Cystinuria

Cystinosis is an inborn error of metabolism that causes failure of reabsorption of amino-acids, including cystine, from the urine. The cystine crystallises out, causing stones, which often present in teenagers. Without intervention patients progress to renal failure following multiple episodes of obstruction and surgery. Inheritance may be either completely or incompletely recessive. Heterozygotes have increased excretion of amino acids, but are not affected.

Cystine stones will dissolve spontaneously if patients are able to excrete between 3 and 5 litres of fluid per day. In addition, penicillamine contributes to stone dissolution and prevents recurrence. Many patients find it impossible to stick to this regime and stones continue to form.

Hyperoxaluria

Primary oxalosis is an extremely rare cause of calculi. It is inherited as an autosomal recessive.

Secondary oxaluria is seen after gut resection and disease of the small intestine; it is due to excessive absorption of oxalate. Dietary restriction is not used as most of the oxalate is endogenous in origin. Pyridoxine, phosphate and magnesium supplements can help in prevention of calculus formation.

SCREENING AND SURVEILLANCE OF RARE INHERITED METABOLIC DISEASES IN ADULTS — FAMILIES OF INDEX CASES

Cystinuria

See above — urinary stones.

Porphyria

The great majority of prophyrias are inherited as autosomal dominants. The gene for acute intermittent porphyria is carried by 1 in 20 000 of population of northern Europe and the USA. However, some ethnic groups have a higher rate, for example 1 in 400 of white South Africans have variegate porphyria.

The importance of screening family members of index cases is that it may be possible to prevent precipitation of latent disease, or at least recognise that porphyria is the problem.

Surveillance of known cases aims at reducing the attacks by helping the patient to avoid precipitating factors.

Acute porphyrias

These diseases all cause abdominal and neuro-psychiatric disorders. Photosensitivity is seen in two forms.

Blood relatives should be tested for latent disease, although urinary and faecal excretion may be normal out of an attack.

Alcohol and drugs can precipitate attacks, sulphonamides, oral contraceptives and anticonvulsants being most commonly involved. Some female sufferers have regular premenstrual attacks and pregnancy may provoke an exacerbation.

Stringent dieting, below 800 kcal (3360 kJ) per day, must be avoided. Vigilance is necessary in diagnosing and treating infections, as these too can precipitate an attack.

Barrier creams and avoidance of sunlight are all that can be offered to those with photosensitivity. However, the skin manifestations do settle between attacks.

For detailed, up-to-date drug advice consult the British National Formulary or The Porphyria Research Unit, Western Infirmary, Glasgow G11 6 NT.

Cutaneous porphyrias

Porphyrins are deposited in the upper epidermal layer in all cutaneous porphyrias. They are photosensitising and the eruptions are scarring.

The liver is affected in cutaneous hepatic porphyria, hepatomegaly occuring particularly where there is a high alcohol intake. Alcohol is also the most common precipitating factor. Chemicals such as fungicides have been implicated in severe outbreaks. Other causes include oral contraceptives and occasionally a primary or secondary liver tumor.

Cholinesterase deficiency

A relative deficiency in serum cholinesterase causes increased sensitivity to the anaesthetic muscle relaxant, succinylcholine. Under normal circumstances succinylcholine is short-acting, due to its rapid hydrolysis by cholinesterase. When this fails the first indication is that the patient suffers prolonged apnoea for several hours after anaesthesia.

The deficiency of serum cholinesterase is due to various abnormal forms with low activity. These are inherited in a complex manner and at least six different recessive genes have been found. The estimated frequency of any degree of sensitivity is 4 in 100.

The importance of this inherited sensitivity is in women of child-bearing age, as serum cholinesterase is depleted in normal pregnancy and succinylcholine is used in obstetric anaesthetic practice.

If a sensitive individual is discovered, screening is offered to all close relatives and warning cards are issued to all homozygotes. The only heterozygotes given cards are women of child-bearing age (Milligan et al 1986).

Haemochromatosis

Inherited haemochromatosis is an autosomal recessive trait with the gene locus on the short arm of chromosome 6. In Anglo-Saxon and Celtic populations the carrier (heterogyzote) rate is 10% and the disease frequency 0.3%.

It is mandatory to screen families of recognised cases because the disease is asymptomatic in the early stages and complications can be prevented and the life expectancy of treated patients, before cirrhosis develops, is probably no shorter than that of the general population.

The transferrin saturation and serum ferritin level are the most cost-effective tests. If all tests are normal they should be repeated in 2 years.

Human leucocyte antigen (HLA) is helpful in determining the risk of first degree relatives (HLA-A3 is seen in 70% of cases). A liver biopsy should be offered to all siblings with the same HLA status as the sufferer, and to any first degree relative with abnormal iron storage tests. If a normal iron content is found in the liver, patients should be re-examined every 2 years (Halliday and Powell 1986).

The surveillance of haemochromatosis is usually under the care of the local haematologist. However, the treatment is life-long, consisting of phlebotomy every 3 months or so once the serum ferritin and iron concentration have been brought into the low normal range. Shared care and support from the general practitioner can greatly help these patients and their families. The 5-year survival, after venesection, rises from 18% to 66%.

Wilson's disease

Wilson's disease in an autosomal recessive disorder that results in excess storage of copper in the tissues, most importantly the liver and the brain. It presents at any age from 6 to 50 years with hepatitis. Early diagnosis can prevent the progressive, irreversible liver, neurological and psychiatric disease, and death.

The homozygous disease state is rare but should be considered in those under 35 years who present with unexplained liver disease, persistently raised transaminases, unexplained neurological disease of the motor system or unexplained psychiatric disease, or who are blood relatives of Wilson's sufferers and offspring of consanguinous matings. Heterozygous carriers — 1% the population — are not at risk.

When Wilson's disease is suspected, and when screening relatives, a low serum caeruloplasmin level and raised urinary copper are very suggestive. If these tests are abnormal then liver biopsy is necessary. A raised hepatic copper content is diagnostic. Definite Kayser–Fleischer rings and deposits of copper in the

margin of the cornea further confirm the diagnosis.

If the disease has not reached a terminal stage at diagnosis then removal of excess copper will be life-saving. Treatment with penicillamine must be started, even if the patient has no symptoms. It is thus mandatory that all siblings of the patient are screened.

REFERENCES

Alberti K G M M 1986 The diabetic clinic and shared care: a hospital physician's view. Treating Diabetes No. 5. Servier Laboratories Ltd,

British Multicentre Research Group 1977 Proliferative diabetic retinopathy: treatment with xenon-arc photocoagulation. British Medical Journal 1: 739–742

Caird F I, Pitie A, Ramsell T G 1969 Diabetes and the eye. Blackwell, Oxford pp 72–100

Dieppe P, Calvert P 1983 Crystals and joint disease. Chapman and Hall, London, p12

Early Treatment Diabetic Retinopathy Study Research Group 1985 Photocoagulation for diabetic macular oedema. Archives of Ophthalmology 103: 1796–1806

Evered D C, Ormston B J, Smith P A, Hall R, Bird T 1973 Grades of hypothyroidism. British Medical Journal 1: 657–662

Forrest R D, Jackson C A, Yudkin J S 1987 Screening for diabetes mellitus in general practice using a reflectance meter system. The Islington diabetes survey. Diabetes Research 6: 119–122

Forrest R D, Jackson C A, Yudkin J S 1988 The abbreviated glucose tolerance test on screening for diabetes: the Islington diabetes survey. Diabetic Medicine 5: 557–561

Fuller J H, Shipley M J, Rose G et al 1980 Coronary heart disease risk and impaired glucose tolerance: the Whitehall study. Lancet i: 1371–1376

Gatling W, Hill R D 1988 The long-term care of non-insulin dependent diabetes. Bailliere's clinical endocrinology and metabolism, vol 2, no. 2 pp 507–526

Hall A P, Barry P E, Dawber T R, McNamara P M 1967 Epidemiology of gout and hyperuricaemia. American Journal of Medicine 42: 27–37

Halliday J W, Powell L W 1986 Haemochromatosis. Medicine International 29: 1186–1187

Keen H 1989 The nature of the diabetic state. Medicine International 65: 2672

Kincaid-Smith P 1986 Urinary calculi. Medicine International 33:1358–1362

Klein R, Klein B E K, Moss S E et al 1984 The Wisconsin epidemiologic study of retinopathy II and III. Archives of Ophthalmology 102: 520–532

Macleod A 1989 Diabetic neuropathy. Medicine International 65: 2700–2703

Milligan K R, Hayes T C, Huss B K D, Beattie B 1986 Atypical plasma cholinesterase. Anaesthesia 41: 841–843

Nusynovitz M L 1980 Screening tests and the free thyroxine index. Archives of Internal Medicine 140: 1017

Orchard T J, Daneman D, Becker D J et al 1982 Glycosylated haemoglobin: a screening test for diabetes mellitus. Preventative Medicine 11: 595–601

Paulus H E, Coutts A, Calabro J J, Klinenberg J R 1970 Clinical significance of hyperuricaemia in routinely screened hospitalised men. Journal of the American Medical Association 211: 277–281

Rohan T E, Fiost CD, Wald NJ 1989 Prevention of blindness by screening for diabetic retinopathy: a quantitative assessment. British Medical Journal 6709. Vol 299: 1198–1201

Stevenson J C 1988 Bailliere's clinical endocrinology and metabolism, vol 2, no. 2 : 87–101

Swai A B M, Harrison K, Chuwa et al 1988 Screening for diabetes: does measurement of serum fructosamine help? Diabetic Medicine 5: 648–652

Toft A 1989 Hyperthyroidism. Medicine International 63: 2588–2595

Tunbridge W M G, Evered D C, Hall R et al 1977 The spectrum of thyroid disease in a community: the Whickham survey. Clinical Endocrinology 7: 481–493

WHO Study Group on Diabetes Mellitus 1985 Diabetes mellitus — a report of the WHO study group. Technical report series No. 727. World Health Organization, Geneva

Williams G, Chisholm G D 1976 Stone screening and follow-up are necessary? British Journal of Urology 47: 745–750

23. Breast cancer

Christopher Hinton

BREAST CANCER — THE PROBLEM

Over 12 000 women die from breast cancer in England and Wales every year. It is the cause of death in more women in the UK than any other cancer and is the most common single cause of death in women between the ages of 35 and 60 (Office of Population and Census Surveys 1982). In recent years there appears to have been an increase in both incidence and mortality from breast cancer (Office of Population and Census Surveys 1971, 1974.).

As the cause of breast cancer is not known and no treatment is effective once the disease has become disseminated, the only hope of reducing the mortality from breast cancer lies in early detection and treatment.

CAN EARLIER DETECTION AND TREATMENT HELP?

The idea that attempts at early detection and treatment of breast cancer may lead to a reduced mortality from the disease is not new. When Halsted described his radical mastectomy (Halsted 1894) it was believed that breast cancer proceeded in a logical sequence from local growth to lymphatic infiltration and lymph node involvement before producing disseminated metastases. Although local lymph node involvement has now been shown to be an indicator of, rather than a necessary prerequisite to, distant metastases, the concept of a quiescent period of local growth during which time the tumour is amenable to surgery prior to dissemination may still apply in many cases.

Based on a comparison of studies of untreated breast cancer with those in which patients were treated at a relatively early stage of the disease, it can be concluded that local treatment is in many cases successful in limiting the progression of the disease and prolonging survival. The form of local treatment used does not appear to influence long-term survival provided that at least total (simple) mastectomy is performed (Phillips 1959, Bloom et al 1962, Brinkley & Haybittle 1975, Cancer Research Campaign Working party 1980). A few studies have associated more radical treatment with marginal improvements in survival but the effect is small. More conservative treatment by excision of the lump and irradiation of the 'intact' breast has been shown to be equally effective for certain subgroups of patients with small tumours (Pierquin 1976, Levene 1978), but further work and longer follow-up are required before this can be accepted without reservation.

EVIDENCE FOR THE EFFICACY OF BREAST SCREENING

The published results of programmes of examination of asymptomatic women show that such programmes are effective in detecting breast cancer at an earlier point in the progression of the disease. Results from controlled and uncontrolled trials have consistently shown a reduction in tumour size and lymph node involvement when compared with patients presenting through existing medical channels. This has been associated with an apparent improvement in survival.

The 1940s and 1950s saw studies that attempted to seek out breast cancer in its early stages by examination of asymptomatic women instituted in several centres in the USA. The results of these studies showed considerable promise in terms of improved survival for patients with breast cancer, although it remained doubtful whether this finding reflected merely the detection of the cancer at an earlier point in the course of the disease, thus producing an apparent survival advantage (lead-time bias), or whether there was a genuinely increased rate of cure. Randomised studies which looked at mortality from breast cancer in the population rather than survival from the time of diagnosis were required to resolve this. Several large randomised trials have now been reported or are in progress. In response to these favourable reports the

Department of Health and Social Security in the UK set up the Trial of Early Detection of Breast Cancer to compare different methods of early detection.

The early studies

Shahon et al (1960) reported the 12-year result of a programme of annual clinical breast examination in asymptomatic women from the Cancer Detection Center, Minneapolis, Minnesota. Although only a small number of women were involved (4956) and only 53 cancers were detected, the survival of these patients was markedly better than that being reported from other centres for symptomatic women. Indeed, the reported 5-year survival rate for patients who were asymptomatic at the time of detection of their breast cancer was 100%. Gilbertsen subsequently reported the 17-year experience from the same unit and the encouraging early results were confirmed (Gilbertsen 1966) — 70% of the patients had no evidence of nodal metastases at the time of mastectomy. The overall 5-year survival for patients whose tumours were detected at the centre (as opposed to interval cancers) was 91% and the 10-year survival was 77%. This was in contrast to the 40% 10-year survival reported from the National Cancer Institute for symptomatic cases (National Cancer Institute 1964). Further encouraging data from New York were provided by Holleb et al (1960), but again this was an uncontrolled study.

Conclusions drawn from these studies needed to be verified with reference to mortality from breast cancer in the population at large, and to do this a controlled study was essential.

The Health Insurance Plan Study

In 1963 the Health Insurance Plan of New York, under the sponsorship of the National Cancer Institute, USA, began a long-term, randomised trial aimed at determining whether periodic screening would result in a reduction in mortality from breast cancer in the female population (Shapiro et al 1972).

At the outset of the study, 62 000 women aged 40 to 64 were allocated to two carefully matched groups of 31 000. All had been enrolled in the Health Insurance Plan of Greater New York for at least 1 year. The groups were comparable in all demographic and epidemiological factors (Shapiro 1977). Women in the study group were offered a screening examination on entry and three additional examinations at annual intervals. Each screening examination consisted of clinical examination and two-view mammography. Women in the control group were given no special

instructions. No effort was made to encourage or discourage the women from having general physical examinations (which were part of the benefit of HIP membership). Of those invited for screening, 65% appeared for the initial examination but only 39% underwent all four examinations. Careful records were kept of all cases of breast cancer occurring in the study group (whether or not they attended for screening) and in the control group and an exhaustive search was made to identify all deaths from breast cancer.

Similar numbers of breast cancers were identified in the two groups — 296 in the study group and 284 in the control group. This is important because it implies that all detected tumours were of clinical relevance. However, encouraging differences between the cancers detected in the study group and those detected in the control group were found. An increased proportion in the study group were under 2 cm in diameter (57% of study, 27% of control), node negative (57% of study, 46% of control) and there was a greater proportion of in situ carcinoma (9% of study, 5% of control) (Shapiro 1977). All of these findings, however, are secondary to the fact that after 5 years only 40 women in the study group had died from breast cancer compared with 63 controls. This represents a reduction in mortality of more than 30% and is statistically significant ($0.01 < P < 0.05$). Follow-up beyond 5 years has been limited to those patients who had breast cancer diagnosed during the period of the study. Results to 12 years have been presented (Shapiro et al 1982), at which time there was still a significant survival advantage to those patients in the study group. This advantage takes account of a lead-time in diagnosis of cancer in the screened group, which has been calculated to be 1 year (Shapiro et al 1974). This difference is entirely accounted for by women whose cancer was detected on screening. Survival rates for patients who failed to attend for screening or whose cancer was detected in the intervals between screening were not significantly different from those of the control group. It seems that the Health Insurance Plan Study has thus been successful in demonstrating a reduction in mortality from breast cancer as a result of breast cancer screening.

Some subsequent studies

Following the Health Insurance Plan Study many breast screening services were introduced on an experimental basis. In the United States this lead to the development of the Guttman Institute in New York and 27 breast cancer detection demonstration projects under the guidance of the National Cancer Institute and the American Cancer Society. This programme involved 280 000 women in a 5-year screening effort (Beahrs et al 1979). This was not a controlled trial, participants being self-selected. For these reasons, data on mortality have not been presented and interpretation of the data must be circumspect because the self-selected participants appear to constitute a high risk group whose incidence of breast cancer exceeded both that of the Health Insurance Plan Study and that reported elsewhere. This may in part relate to the fact that some of the participants were symptomatic at the time of their examination. In spite of these problems, the available results are very encouraging. A large proportion of the breast cancers detected were localised. Over 70% were without lymph node metastases and one-third of all the detected cancers were described as 'minimal' (less than 1 cm in diameter or non-invasive tumours). The incidence of these 'minimal cancers' was greatest in women aged over 45 years and most were detected by mammography. The work of Lundgren in Sweden using single-view oblique mammography alone as a screening procedure provides further evidence for the efficacy of breast cancer screening in a large controlled trial (Lundgren 1981).

These encouraging results suggest that lives may be saved by annual mammographic screening. Repeated mammography may not be without potential danger, however, and this has led to the investigation of other possible modalities of screening.

HAZARDS OF MAMMOGRAPHY

It has long been recognised that irradiation of breast tissue is carcinogenic. Evidence of this comes from studies of the survivors of the atomic bombs in Hiroshima and Nagasaki (Wanebo et al 1968), patients with tuberculosis examined by repeated fluoroscopy (McKenzie 1965) and women treated for benign conditions by radiation therapy (Mettler et al 1969, Simon 1977). In all of these groups there has been a marked excess in the observed numbers of breast cancers developing in the years following irradiation beyond natural expectation. Extrapolation of the effects of these high radiation exposures to the low levels of exposure associated with mammography has led to some debate on the safety of mammographic screening. In a report in 1976 the American College of Radiation suggested that there was a threshold below which radiation could be considered entirely safe, but this view has been challenged (Bailor 1977, Upton et al 1977). Upton et al estimated that exposure to 1 rad would raise the lifetime risk of breast cancer by 1%.

Strax (1978) has estimated from consideration of the mid-breast radiation dose received during the Health Insurance Plan study that if 40 million women at risk were screened annually for 20 years, 120 lives would be lost due to induced breast cancer, although he contrasts this with the 12 000 lives that might be saved as a result of this screening. Since the Health Insurance Plan study, modern mammographic techniques have produced a marked reduction in radiation dose. Using single-view oblique mammography, Lundgren and Jakobsen have reported average skin exposure of only 0.1 rad (Lundgren and Jakobsen 1976). Despite this reduction, there remains real concern that mammography may carry a small but significant risk and attempts have been made to find alternative means of early detection using imaging techniques that do not rely on breast irradiation. To date these efforts have been disappointing.

OTHER BREAST IMAGING TECHNIQUES

Lawson (1956) demonstrated that most breast cancers generated more heat than normal tissue, resulting in an increase in the overlying skin temperature. This led to the investigation of thermography as a means of detection of breast cancer. Thermography makes use of the fact that the intensity of infra-red radiation from the breast surface depends upon the heat produced in the tissues beneath, and records the pattern of this infra-red emission from the breast surface. Images can be studied directly from an oscilloscope screen or as a permanent photographic record. In this way the presence of most breast cancers can be recognised (Forrest & Gravelle 1969, Stark and Way 1974, Dodd 1977). The great advantage of thermography is that it relies on the natural infra-red emissions from the breast surface and is therefore non-invasive. To be of value as a screening tool, however, it would have to be able to detect clinically occult lesions. Gauthrie and Gros (1976) have studied thermography in 50 000 women over a 10-year period. Their results have shown a high number of apparent false positive results (some of which are associated with inflammatory lesions) and a high number of false negative results in subclinical and non-invasive tumours. For these reasons it seems unlikely that thermography will be useful in isolation as a means of early detection. With refinement, it may, however, have a role, because a significant number of women with apparently false positive thermograms have subsequently developed breast cancer (Gauthrie and Gros 1980).

More recently, ultrasound has been investigated as a means of providing a breast image. There are no known hazards from ultrasound and it is therefore an attractive proposition as a screening tool. Ultrasound detects interfaces of different acoustic density, which produce different patterns of transmission and reflection of sound waves. Carcinomas of the breast produce a heterogeneous pattern of echogenicity with a high acoustic impedance and poor transmission of the ultrasound. They thus cast an acoustic shadow. Conversely, cysts transmit ultrasound readily, produce an enhancement of the image behind them and generate no echoes. Benign breast disease and fibroadenomata produce homogeneous patterns of echogenicity without shadowing or enhancement when compared with the surrounding breast tissue. In the early studies breast ultrasonography was time-consuming (Baum 1977) and not capable of the fine resolution of mammography (Dodd 1977), with a sensitivity in the diagnosis of subclinical carcinoma of less than 60% (Kobayashi et al 1974). Even today it is unsuitable in isolation as a screening tool. It may have a role in the investigation of clinically or mammographically detectable lesions by further clarifying their nature and providing helpful information when planning clinical management.

BREAST SELF-EXAMINATION

Breast self-examination (BSE) has been widely advocated for many years but has received little critical evaluation. It is known that patients whose presentation with breast cancer is delayed have a worse prognosis than those who seek immediate medical attention (Ellwood and Moorehead 1980) and it has been suggested that a sufficient drive towards educating the population to detect their own breast cancer and present immediately would go some way to achieving the results of mammography without the expense (Baum 1981). Experience in Canada has shown that education in self-examination has resulted in a reduction in delay in presentation (Phillips 1978). Retrospective studies on patients with breast cancer have suggested that tumours detected by self-examination are of reduced size and have a decreased incidence of node involvement. Foster et al (1978) were able to show that women who practised self-examination presented with tumours with fewer lymph node metastases than those who did not. This reduction in the presence of positive nodes at mastectomy was confirmed by Feldman et al (1981) who showed a reduction of 30% in node involvement in those women regularly carrying out self-examination. They suggested that this could result in a reduction in mortality from breast cancer of 10–17%. Greenwald et al (1978), in another retrospective study, suggested that regular self-

examination could reduce mortality from breast cancer by nearly 20%. A programme of education and self-examination in Finland has been reported to show an apparent reduction in mortality but no control group was provided (Gastrin 1980). In an attempt to improve detection of interval cancers, i.e. cancers that become manifest in the interval between screenings, self-examination was included as a formal part of the Minneapolis Cancer Detection Centre study. These interval cancers accounted for one-third of the total in the early part of the study. The introduction of self-examination resulted in the detection of these cancers, with a markedly reduced rate of nodal involvement (Gilbertsen 1969). In a mathematical model of early detection methods Kirch and Klein (1978) calculated that self-examination would significantly contribute to a reduction in the overall rate of nodal metastases when performed in conjunction with conventional screening methods, claiming that it could reduce nodal involvement at presentation by up to 29%. Hugaley and Brown (1981) reported a series of 719 cases of breast cancer in patients who practised breast self-examination. Although they found that only 45% of these patients had found their cancer at the time of regular self-examination they reported that self-examiners who had found their tumour by chance, i.e. between regular examinations, still presented with cancers of a more favourable stage than patients who did not practise breast self-examination. They suggested that this was a result of better awareness of the significance of changes in the breast and of the importance of early presentation. Not all such studies have shown a favourable impact. Smith et al (1980) and Senie et al (1981) have reported series of patients with breast cancer in whom the stage of disease at presentation was apparently unaffected by breast self-examination.

THE UK TRIAL OF EARLY DETECTION IN BREAST CANCER

In 1971, with the support of the DHSS, pilot studies were set up in the United Kingdom. The purpose of these studies was to investigate the feasibility of routine screening of women over the age of 40 by clinical examination, mammography and thermography. These studies reported encouraging rates of response to invitations for screening (up to 75%) (Thomas et al 1981) and provided further evidence that mammography and clinical examination contributed independently to detection (Chamberlain et al 1975, Owen et al 1977). They further provided evidence of the efficacy of non-medical staff in clinical examination and mammographic interpretation in a screening unit (George et al 1976). The findings of these studies led to the design of the UK Trial of Early Detection of Breast Cancer.

In view of the evidence suggesting that the mortality from breast cancer might be reduced by an early detection programme, pressure was brought to bear on the National Health Service to provide breast cancer screening in the UK. The efficacy of breast cancer screening had never been tested in the UK and it was not known, particularly in the context of the NHS, whether the results from other countries could be applied to the UK. Furthermore, while it has been shown that breast screening using such sensitive means of detection as mammography can be effective, no large study had ever shown whether such investigations are necessary or cost-effective (an important consideration in the context of a national breast screening programme). It is of note that, although mammography was an integral part of the Health Insurance Plan study, only 20% of all cancers detected in the screened population would have been missed had mammography been omitted (Shapiro et al 1972) whereas 41% arose as interval cancers. In 1979, the UK Trial of Early Detection of Breast Cancer was initiated with the aim of evaluating the cost-effectiveness of the early detection of breast cancer by either:

1. annual clinical examination with mammography in alternate years;
2. educating women in breast self-examination (BSE).

Each of these means of early detection was tested in two Health Districts and, in addition, a further four Health Districts acted as controls. The study involved a total of over 200 000 women between the ages of 45 and 64 at entry (UK trial of Early Detection of Breast Cancer Group 1981).

At the time of writing data collection is still in progress and definitive mortality statistics will not be available for many years. Nevertheless, early results give cause for optimism. Women in both the breast self-examination and mammographically screened arms of the trial have presented with smaller tumours and with a reduced incidence of lymph node involvement. In both of these aspects mammography has produced a greater effect than breast self-examination. Furthermore, there has been a distinct increase in the numbers of in situ (non-invasive) cancers presenting in the group undergoing mammographic screening. All of these changes lead to a hope of a substantial reduction in mortality. The earliest results for mortality published at the end of 7 years tend to bear this out, with a reduction of mortality of 14% in the group offered mammographic screening. There has as yet been no observable reduction in mortality in the breast self-examination group (U.K. Trial of Early Detection of Breast Cancer Group 1988).

THE FORREST REPORT

In July 1985 a working group was set up under the chairmanship of Professor Sir Patrick Forrest to consider the case for the provision of breast screening in the UK and to make recommendations regarding the implementation of such a programme.

After due consideration of the evidence available to them from overseas trials and the early results of the UK trial of early detection, they published their recommendations in November 1986 in the form of a report to the Health Ministers of England, Wales, Scotland and Northern Ireland (Forrest 1986).

They concluded that there was sufficient evidence to suggest that mortality from breast cancer in women between the ages of 50 and 64 could be reduced by a programme of breast screening and that such a programme should be introduced on a national scale for women in this age group. The preferred investigation was single-view oblique (mediolateral) mammography and, in the absence of evidence to the contrary they recommended a screening interval of 3 years.

They further made specific recommendations for the organisation of screening programmes. These included the recommendations that every women in the age group should receive an invitation to screening from her general practitioner, that there should be a fail-safe mechanism to ensure that action was taken in reponse to every positive result, that each screening unit should have access to a specialist team for the assessment of screen detected lesions and that arrangements should be made for stringent quality control both within and between units.

The Forrest report was accepted in its entirety by the Department of Health and each Health Authority has now established a breast screening programme.

THE ROLE OF THE GENERAL PRACTITIONER IN THE EARLY DETECTION OF BREAST CANCER

Despite initial difficulties screening units are now operating throughout the country. General practioners will have a vital role in the success of these units.

The role of general practitioners in the early detection of breast cancer does not end there. They have an important role to play in the management of women outside the targeted age group.

GENERAL PRACTITIONERS AND THE SCREENING PROGRAMME

Accurate identification of the target group

The central role of general practitioners in the success of the breast screening programme begins before the first mammogram. The success of the programme relies on a high rate of acceptance of invitation to screening. This in turn is possible only if the invitations reach the targeted population. Invitations to women are sent out by the local screening office based on information obtained from the Family Health Services Authority. In many parts of the country these FHSA records contain errors and omissions because of their tendency to lag behind population movements and because of the time taken for address changes to be notified. Thus, regular reporting to the local FHSAs of changes in patient details is a first important step.

Prior to the sending of invitations, the screening office sends a list of women to be invited to the general practitioner so that he or she may correct any errors or omissions and can remove the names of anyone whose invitation would be inappropriate (for instance patients who are already undergoing treatment for breast cancer). Prompt and careful scrutiny of these lists in essential.

Compliance

The Forrest commission has estimated that about 70% of women will attend for screening in response to an invitation. This should be considered a minimum requirement. The reduction in mortality achieved by the Swedish trials was based on a take-up of greater than 90%. Take-up depends on a number of factors. The first, the accuracy of information supplied to the screening office, has been outlined above. Of the other factors which determine a woman's decision to attend most, if not all, can be influenced by her general practitioner.

Attendence relies on a balance of anxieties. All women are aware of the risk of breast cancer. Many have misconceptions about treatment and the likely outcome. Most have no clear idea of the aims, effectiveness and limitations of breast cancer screening. The media can play some role but information of a much higher quality should be available from a woman's general practitioner and other health care professionals with whom she comes into contact. Good quality information regarding the benefits of sceening is the single most important factor in determining response to an invitation.

General practitioners have a particular ability to reach and influence non-attenders. It has been estimated that over 90% of patients will consult their general practioners in any 5-year period. The opportunity will, therefore, usually arise to discuss a woman's reasons for non-attendance, provided that the general practitioner has been notified and the patient's records flagged.

The assessment clinic

Whilst in most cases general practitioners will have no direct involvement in the assessment clinic, it is likely that many women will consult their general practitioner in the event of their being recalled for further mammography or for assessment of a screen-detected lesion. At this time it will be appropriate to disscuss with the woman the procedures that she is likely to undergo in the assessment unit and to reassure her that recall for assessment does not mean that cancer has been diagnosed.

Between 7 and 10% of all women screened will be recalled. In early studies about one-third of these were because of technical deficiencies in the initial mammograms. (The technical quality of mammograms is improving rapidly.) These women will have further mammography and, provided that no lesion is seen, will be reassured and recalled for screening after the usual interval.

The remainder will have been found to have abnormalities that require further clarification. These women will have further mammography, clinical examination and, in many cases, ultrasound examination of the breasts. Some will undergo fine needle aspiration cytology of the detected lesion. The results of these investigations should be available to the woman at the time of her attendance and will, in most cases, result in a diagnosis of benignity. About one in ten assessment clinic attendances will result in a recommendation that the woman undergoes open surgical biopsy. In all such cases the decision will be discussed with the patient's general practitioner. It is the aim of the screening services to minimise the rate of open biopsy of benign lesions by providing a level of expertise in the assessment clinics such that most benign lesions can be confidently diagnosed without surgery. It is likely then that over 50% of women undergoing open biopsy will be found to have breast cancer.

Women with screen detected breast cancer

When a women is diagnosed as having breast cancer she will, in most cases, be given some choice in how it is to be managed. All assessment units will be staffed by a clinician with a special interest in breast cancer and a specialist nurse counsellor. Initial discussion of treatment options and the implications of the diagnosis will take place in the assessment unit with these members of the team. Many women will also wish to discuss these matters with their general practitioner, who will have a much more intimate knowledge of their personal circumstances, and such discussion should be encouraged. The psychological impact on women diagnosed as having breast cancer after screening may be quite different to that of women diagnosed in the usual way because such women often have no symptoms suggestive of any disease. They may feel resentful towards the whole screening system and have more than usual difficulty in coping with the disease and its treatment. They may require persistent sympathetic support.

Interval cancers

A negative screening examination may be reassuring but it does not, of course, confer immunity. Mammography will miss some breast cancers (perhaps as many as 10%) and more will arise in the intervals between screening. The latter tend to be more rapidly growing and aggressive than cancers detected at screening. It is therefore all the more important to be alert to the possibility of interval cancers so that they may be detected and dealt with at as early a stage as possible. They will present through the conventional channels provided by general practitioners and the hospital service. It is essential that, as part of the screening process, women are encouraged to report changes that occur in their breasts and to seek medical advice promptly. Referral to a specialist breast unit will then be appropriate.

THE ROLE OF GENERAL PRACTIONERS OUTSIDE A FORMAL SCREENING SERVICE

Most breast cancer presenting in the UK will occur in women not included in the national breast screening programme. Although trials of breast screening have failed to show any significant reduction in mortality for younger women accruing through screening efforts, there is certainly evidence that there are benefits for all age groups from early treatment. More conservative methods of treatment such as excision of the lump and 'intact' breast irradiation or subcutaneous mastectomy are less effective in dealing with cancers that are large at presentation. Breast self-examination remains controversial and may in some cases lead to an increase in anxiety. Its practice, however, is effective in encouraging earlier presentation and can be recommended to all women.

The most important aspect of the management of breast disease is that breast cancer, when it arises, is promptly and effectively treated. The management of breast cancer requires access to specialised equipment and a multidisciplinary approach. There is little doubt that it is managed best in specialist units where there is easy access to mammography, ultrasound, cytological and pathological expertise and counselling services. General practitioners can help greatly by encouraging the development of such units to serve their patients.

REFERENCES

Bailor J V III 1977 Screening for early breast cancer: pros and cons. Cancer 39: 2783–2795

Baum G 1977 Ultrasound mammography. Radiology 122: 199–205

Baum M 1981 Breast cancer: the facts. Oxford University Press, Oxford

Beahrs O H, Shapiro S, Smart C, McDiunt R W 1979 Report of the working group to review the National Cancer Institute — American Cancer Society breast cancer detection demonstration projects. General issues related to breast cancer screening. Journal of the National Cancer Institute 62: 641–698

Bloom H J G, Richardson W W, Harries E J 1962 Natural history of untreated breast cancer. British Medical Journal 2: 213–221

Brinkley D, Haybittle J L 1975 The curability of breast cancer. Lancet ii: 95–97

Cancer Research Campaign Working Party 1980 Cancer Research Campaign (Kings/Cambridge) trial for early breast cancer: a detailed update at the tenth year. Lancet ii: 55–60

Chamberlain J, Roger P, Price J L et al 1975 Validity of clinical examination and mammography as screening tests for breast cancer. Lancet ii: 1026–1030

Dodd G D 1977 Present status of thermography, ultrasound and mammography in breast cancer detection. Cancer 39: 2796–2805

Ellwood J M, Moorehead W P 1980 Delay in diagnosis and long term survival in breast cancer. British Medical Journal 280: 1291–1294

Feldman J G, Carter A C, Nicastri A D, Hosat S T 1981 Breast self examination, relationship to stage of breast cancer at diagnosis. Cancer 47: 2740–2745

Forrest A P M 1986 Breast cancer screening. Report to the health ministers of England, Wales, Scotland and Northern Ireland. By a working group chaired by Professor Sir Patrick Forrest. HMSO, London

Forrest A P M, Gravelle I H 1969 The diagnosis of cancer of the breast with special reference to mammography and thermography. The Practitioner 203: 137–145

Foster, R S Jr, Lang SP, Costanza M C et al 1978 Breast

self-examination practices and breast cancer stage. New England Journal of Medicine 299(6): 265–267

Gastrin G 1980 Programme to encourage self-examination for breast cancer. British Medical Journal 2: 193

Gauthrie M, Gros C M 1976 Contribution of infra-red thermography to the early diagnosis, pretherapeutic prognosis and post irradiation follow-up of breast cancer. Medica Mundi 21(3): 135–147

Gauthrie M, Gros C M 1980 Breast thermography and cancer risk prediction. Cancer 45: 123–9

George W D, Gleave E N, England P C et al 1976 Screening for breast cancer. British Medical Journal 2: 858–860

Gilbertsen V A 1966 Survival of asymptomatic breast cancer patients. Surgery, Gynaecology and Obstetrics 122: 81–83

Gilbertsen V A 1969 Detection of breast cancer in a specialised cancer detection centre. Cancer 24: 1192–1195

Greenwald P, Nasca P C, Lawrence C E et al 1978 Estimated effect of breast self-examination and routine physician examinations on breast cancer mortality. New England Journal of Medicine 299(6): 271–273

Halsted W S 1894 The results of operations for cure of cancer of the breast performed at the John Hopkins Hospital from June 1889-January 1894. Annals of Surgery 20: 497–555

Holleb A I, Venet L, Day E, Hoyt S 1960 Breast cancer detected by routine physical examination. Three year survey of the Strang Cancer Prevention Clinic. New York State Journal of Medicine 60: 823–870

Hugaley C M, Brown R L 1981 The value of breast self-examination. Cancer 47: 989–995

Kirch R L A, Klein M 1978 Prospective evaluation of periodic breast examination programmes: interval cases. Cancer 41: 728–736

Kobayashi T, Takatoni O, Hattori N 1974 Differential diagnosis of breast tumours. Cancer 33: 940–951

Lawson R N 1956 Implication of surface temperatures in the diagnosis of breast cancer. Canadian Medical Association Journal 75: 309

Levene M B, Harris J R, Hellman S 1978 Primary radiation therapy for operable carcinoma of the breast. Surgical Clinics of North America 58: 4: 767–776

Lundgren B 1981 Breast screening in Sweden by single oblique-view mammography. Reviews of endocrine-related cancer (Suppl. 10) 67–70

Lundgren B, Jakobsen S 1976 Single view mammography. A simple and efficient approach to breast cancer. Cancer 28: 1124–1129

MacKenzie I 1965 Breast cancer following multiple fluoroscopies. British Journal of Cancer 19: 1–18

Mettler F A, Hempelmann L H, Dutton A M 1969 Breast neoplasias in women treated with X-rays for acute post-partum mastitis. Journal of the National Cancer Institute 43: 803–822

National Cancer Institute 1964 End results in cancer. Reports No. 2. U.S. Department of Health Education and Welfare. Bethesda, Maryland

Office of Population and Census Surveys 1971 Cancer statistics. Series MBI: 1–4

Office of Population and Census Surveys 1974 Mortality statistics. Series DH2: No. 1.

Office of Population and Census Surveys 1982 Mortality statistics. Series DHA 2: No. 9

Owen A W, Forest A P M, Anderson T I et al 1977 Breast screening and surgical problems. British Journal of Surgery 64: 725–728

Pierquin B, Baillet F, Wilson J F 1976 Radiation therapy in the management of primary breast cancer. American Journal of Roentgenology 127: 645:648

Phillips A J 1959 A comparison of treated and untreated cases of cancer of the breast. British Journal of Cancer 13: 20–25

Phillips A J, Brennan N E 1976 Reactions of Canadian Women to PAP tests and breast self examination. Canadian Family Physician 22: 1261–1264

Senie R T, Rosen P P, Lesser M L, Kinne D W 1981 Breast self-examination and medical examination related to breast cancer stage. American Journal of Public Health 71: 585–590

Shahon D, Santoro B, Wangensteen O 1960 Periodic examinations of the breast for cancer. Proceedings of the 4th National Cancer Conference. J B Lippincott, Philadelphia, pp 225–227

Shapiro S 1977 Evidence on screening for breast cancer from a randomised trial. Cancer 39: 2772–2782

Shapiro S, Strax P, Venet L, Venet W 1972 Changes in 5-year breast cancer mortality in a breast cancer screening program. Seventh National Cancer Conference Proceedings. American Cancer Society Inc. pp 663–678

Shapiro S, Goldberg J, Hutchinson G 1974 Lead time in breast cancer detection and implication for periodicity of screening. American Journal of Epidemiology 100: 357–366

Shapiro S, Venet W, Strax P et al Ten to fourteen year effects of breast cancer screening on mortality. Journal of the National Cancer Institute 62: 340–354

Simon N 1977 Breast cancer induced by radiation. Journal of the American Medical Association 237: 789–790

Smith E M, Francis A M, Polinar L 1980 The effect of breast self-examination practices and physician examinations on the extent of disease at diagnosis. Preventive Medicine 9: 409–417

Stark A M, Way S 1974 The use of thermovision in the detection of early breast cancer. Cancer 33: 1664–1670

Strax P 1978 Evaluation of screening programmes for the early diagnosis of breast cancer. Surgical Clinics of North America 58(4): 667–679

Thomas B A, Price J L, Boulter P 1981 Breast cancer population screening by single view mammography and selective clinical examination. A pilot study. Clinical Oncology 7: 201–204

UK Trial of Early Detection of Breast Cancer Group 1981 Trial of early detection of breast cancer. Description of method. British Journal of Cancer 44: 618–627

UK Trial of Early Detection of Breast Cancer Group 1988 First results on mortality in the UK. Trial of early detection of breast cancer. Lancet ii: 411–420

Upton A L, Beebe G W, Brown J W et al 1977 Report of NCI ad hoc working group on the risks associated with mammography in mass screening for the detection of breast cancer. Journal of the National Cancer Institute 59: 479–493

Wanebo C K, Johnson K G, Sato K, Thorslind T W 1968 Breast cancer after exposure to the atomic bombings of Hiroshima and Nagasaki. New England Journal of Medicine 279: 667–671

24. Screening for carcinoma of the cervix

Leone Ridsdale

In 1990 Dr Kay Farnham was invited to join her training practice as a partner. During her first month in practice the following four patients came to see her:

1. Mrs Dodds, aged 45, complaining of bleeding after intercourse. Inspection of her notes showed she had never had a cervical smear.
2. Mrs Afshar, who received a letter inviting her for cervical screening. Having met Dr Farnham when she was a trainee, Mrs Afshar decided to come and ask about it.
3. Mrs Smart-Jones, who came to ask 'What is mild dyskaryosis?' She had been asked to have a repeat smear in 6 months. She had private insurance and asked if it would be better for her to see a gynaecologist now.
4. Mrs Mary Joe Manson, aged 30, who asked for a cervical smear. Her last one had been done 1 year previously in the United States and it was normal.

Each of these four patients have problems that raise complex issues. To make informed judgements the GP needs to bring together knowledge from several disciplinary perspectives (Fig. 24.1).

The purpose of this chapter is to present the necessary evidence for GPs to consider the answers to the following questions:

1. How has the provision of cervical screening developed in Britain?
2. To what extent does cervical screening satisfy criteria of effectiveness?
3. What are the obstacles to effective screening?
4. What potential improvements can be made?

THE DEVELOPMENT OF CERVICAL SCREENING PROVISION IN THE UK

Cervical screening was first offered in the 1960s. The main providers were the Family Planning Association (FPA) and Local Authority Clinics. These clinics were staffed almost entirely by female receptionists, nurses and doctors. Although all staff were paid, the co-operative user–provider style was not unlike that observed in self-help groups. GPs performed a small minority of cervical smears at this time.

The number of smears taken increased in the 1970s, although the FPA and Local Authority Clinics were still the major providers. Some innovative GPs (Scaife 1972, Dixon & Morris 1974) set up call and recall programmes for all women registered with them. A national recall system was started, and abandoned in the early 1980s.

In the 1980s GPs began providing the greatest number of smears. Most GPs provided smears on demand, or when they remembered to offer one, e.g. in the context of family planning or antenatal care. As might be expected, middle class and young women were the main users of this service. An increasing number of GPs initiated systematic screening for all patients on their lists, but a few GPs persistently refused to do cervical smears at all (Havelock et al 1988). In the late 1980s Family Practitioner Committees began computer-assisted call and recall of women for cervical screening in cooperation with local practitioners.

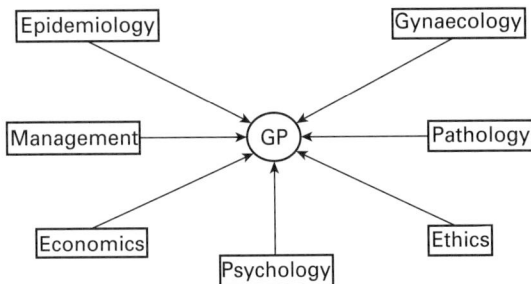

Fig. 24.1 Disciplinary perspectives.

TO WHAT EXTENT DOES CERVICAL SCREENING SATISFY CRITERIA OF EFFECTIVENESS?

Wilson's screening criteria are listed in Chapter 2. They provide a useful framework to assess the effectiveness of a screening method. Each criterion will be discussed with reference to cervical screening in order critically to assess the value of cervical screening in practice.

Is cervical carcinoma an important health problem?

The extent to which a disease poses a health problem can be measured in at least two ways. The frequency of mortality is one such indicator. In 1984, 1899 women in England and Wales died of cervical carcinoma, 94% of whom were aged 35 and over (Office of Population Census and Surveys 1985). This is the equivalent to three patients on the average GP's list dying of cervical carcinoma during the GP's working life.

Death is the ultimate measure of ill-health but some women will be diagnosed and cured: not all women will die of their disease. In 1984, 4043 new cases of carcinoma of the cervix were diagnosed (Office of Population Census and Surveys 1988) — approximately twice as many women are diagnosed with the disease as die of it (see above). More women have non-invasive

lesions — in 1984, 8423 women were reported to have carcinoma in situ (Office of Population Census and Surveys 1988), i.e. four times the number who were dying of invasive disease.

Is the natural history of the disease well understood?

The natural history of cervical carcinoma is not well understood. Evidence derived by association suggests that cervical carcinoma is linked to an agent transmitted during sexual intercourse (Campion et al 1986). The first changes occur at the transformation zone, which lies between the squamous epithelium of the ectocervix and the columnar epithelium of the endocervix (Fig. 24.2).

Cells superficial to the basement membrane in the transformation zone may undergo neoplastic change. Histopathologists classify cervical intraepithelial neoplasia (CIN) on the basis of severity as CIN 1, 2 and 3. When neoplastic changes are found to extend deep to the epithelial basement membrane, invasive carcinoma is diagnosed.

CIN and carcinoma in situ are most frequently diagnosed in women aged 25–44; invasive carcinoma and deaths occur most frequently in women over 60 years of age, but it is difficult to make inferences about the natural history of the disease because:

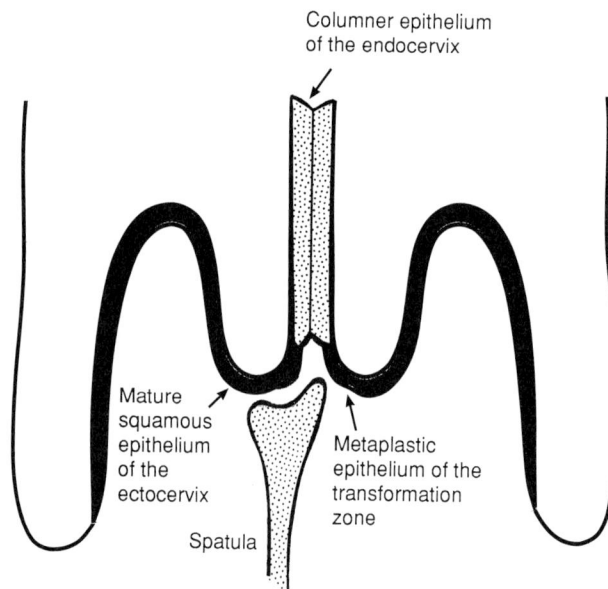

Sampling the cervical transformation zone

Fig. 24.2 Sampling the cervical transformation zone. (C B Woodman et al, Lancet 1989 with permission.)

Table 24.1 Identification of cervical intraepithelial neoplasia

Cytologist's report		Likely histology
Mild dysplasia	predicts	CIN 1
Moderate dysplasia	predicts	CIN 2
Severe dysplasia	predicts	CIN 3 or carcinoma in situ

1. The identification of preclinical disease depends on the intensity of screening. It is likely that more CIN and carcinoma in situ will be identified in groups of women who have been more extensively screened, for example young women.
2. The natural history of cervical cancer has been affected by preclinical identification and by medical management. Cook and Draper (1984) found that in some age groups there is evidence of a large increase in carcinoma in situ of the cervix, but mortality has remained stable. They infer that it is likely that a potential increase in cervical cancer incidence and mortality has been partially prevented as a result of the screening programme.

Is there a recognisable early stage?

The purpose of screening is to identify women before they reach the stage of clinically invasive carcinoma. Screening, therefore, would ideally identify all women with carcinoma in situ or CIN 3. The ideal diagnostic technique to identify CIN 3 would be colposcopy, with histological examination of clinically suspicious areas — this test is the gold standard. Screening involves the examination of a sample of exfoliated cervical cells. Cytologists make a prediction from this about the likely histological abnormality (Table 24.1).

As cells beneath the basement membrane do not normally exfoliate, severe cytological dysplasia does not exclude the possibility of there being invasive carcinoma on histology (Evans et al 1986).

The finding of severe dysplasia is a recognisable early stage, identifiable through screening. It is likely that not all carcinoma in situ invades the basement membrane, and a small proportion may regress. As clinicians believe that the risk of invasion is high, women with this condition are generally treated with laser therapy or other destructive therapy.

Is treatment of the disease at an early stage of more benefit than treatment started at a later stage?

One outcome measure of benefit is avoided mortality. A randomised controlled study of cervical screening has not been undertaken, but some populations have been offered systematic cervical screening over the past few decades, whilst others have not. Provided that risk factors for cervical cancer do not act differentially between countries, then changes in mortality will indicate the benefit of early identification and treatment.

In Iceland there is a nationwide programme with a wide target age range. Between 1965 and 1982 mortality has fallen by 80% (Laara et al 1987). Finland has a smaller target age range and less frequent screening intervals; there has been a 50% reduction in mortality over the same period. In Norway, with only 5% of the population covered by organised screening, mortality fell by only 10%. During the same period the decline in mortality from cervical cancer in Britain was 21%. This evidence supports the concept that the presence and extent of screening is associated with a decrease in mortality from cervical carcinoma.

Screening for carcinoma in situ could also prevent morbidity from clinically invasive disease. A systematic screening programme to detect preinvasive carcinoma of the cervix was started in British Columbia in 1949. Between 1955 and 1985 the incidence of invasive squamous carcinoma of the cervix fell by 78% (Anderson et al 1988). This was during a time in which there was an appreciable increase in carcinoma in situ. This evidence suggests that morbidity can also be prevented.

A third way to assess the potential benefit of screening (or loss to women not identified) is examination of the screening status of women who have developed cancer. La Vecchia and colleagues (1984) found that women who had undergone two or more smears were more likely to have had their cancer diagnosed at an early stage, and lack of screening was associated with more advanced cancers. In a study of women who died, 90% had never been screened (Spriggs & Boddington 1976).

Is there a suitable test?

The initial diagnosis of cervical carcinoma is made by the histological examination of a biopsy specimen. Subsequent clinical staging depends on the degree of spread. The screening test involves visualizing the cervix and collecting exfoliated cells by rotating a spatula twice over the surface. The sample is examined cytologically. Inevitably there is loss of accuracy in using a simple test. The reasons for this are:

1. Small localised CIN lesions may fail to exfoliate sufficient abnormal cells (Giles et al 1988).

Spatula with extended tip

Endocervical brush

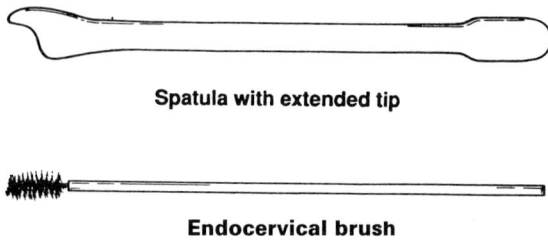

Fig. 24.3   Spatula with extended tip and endocervical brush. (M R Wolfendale et al 1987 with permission.)

2. The adequacy of samples is dependent on the presence of metaplastic and columnar cells of endocervical origin (Woodman et al 1989). Gynaecologists, general practitioners and nurses vary in their ability to submit adequate smears (Duguid 1986).

3. The transformation zone in older women moves into the os. To reach this area a spatula with a pointed and extended tip (Wolfendale et al 1987) or a spatula together with an endocervical brush (Taylor et al 1987) should be used (Fig. 24.3).

These instruments are more effective in older women who are also at greater risk from cervical carcinoma.

4. The recognition and grading of cell samples may vary from one cytologist to another and when cytologists are given the same samples to report on a second time.

For these reasons smear tests tend to underestimate the presence of disease (Chomet 1987). A single smear has a false negative rate of about 40%. However, after two independent tests, on average only 16% of lesions will be negative on both occasions (IARC Working Group 1986).

Is the test acceptable?

Some women do not accept the invitation to attend for cervical screening. The reasons for non-acceptance are practical, cognitive, attitudinal and emotional.

1. There is a higher uptake of screening if a specific appointment time is given (Wilson & Leeming 1987). But some women find the time allocated inconvenient because of work or domestic commitments or because they have a period on that date. The service requires built-in flexibility to allow women to telephone and change their appointment time.

2. Some women do not know or understand the reasons for cervical screening. Where there is genuine medical uncertainty, patients will also be uncertain. Some patients think they are ineligible because they associate the disease with promiscuity, when they themselves have had only one sexual partner (Meadows 1987) or believe they need a current sexual partner to be at risk. They may not realise that there is a need for continued monitoring, or they may be confused about the varying intervals recommended.

3. Refusal may be attitudinal. Some people dislike medical intervention of any kind. Some have a fatalistic attitude or fear the discovery of cancer (Nathoo 1988).

4. Embarrassment about an internal examination deters some women. When women have never had a smear most of them express a preference for the procedure to be done by female personnel (Standing and Mercer 1984). This preference is more strongly held by ethnic groups such as Asian women (McAvoy & Raza 1988). This kind of response has been recorded by interviewing non-responders:

'No, I did not go — I just keep putting it off and putting it off. It is embarrassing. You see the last time I had it done — my doctor is a man doctor, and I just don't feel it is right that a man should be doing that kind of thing — I don't think men should do it... it is just too embarrassing' (Elkind et al 1988).

Reasons for non-acceptance, when known by the providers, can be circumvented. Non-acceptance is sometimes assumed to be a major obstacle to cervical screening but provided that patients' practical, cognitive and emotional needs are met, only about 10% of women will refuse (Standing & Mercer 1984, Ridsdale 1987).

Are there adequate facilities for the diagnosis and treatment of detected abnormalities?

Bottle-necks in the provision of services can occur from the GPs surgery, when patients find telephone lines engaged, through to waiting lists for colposcopy clinics and for admission to hospital. The extent to which facilities are judged adequate also depends on clinical opinion about the appropriate stage at which cytological abnormalities require further investigation. There is concensus that severe dysplasia on cytology requires referral for diagnosis and treatment.

The management of patients whose smear is reported as mild or moderately dysplastic is more controversial. If cytologists recommended that GPs refer all women for cytology when moderate dysplasia was first reported then there would be even further bottle-necks in the system. Cytologists therefore base their recommendations on pragmatic considerations locally. Patients with moderate dysplasia may be asked to return for a repeat smear in a prescribed period or they may be referred for colposcopy straight away (BSCC Working party 1986).

Reducing pressure on colposcopy clinics increases pressure on the provision and organisation of cytology services. To link information obtained on sequential smears and inform doctors and patients of the results, laboratories need computer systems. If results are not linked, a patient with a normal smear may be asked to return in 3 years when a smear done previously showed moderate dyskaryosis.

If all women in the UK with mild dyskaryosis were referred for colposcopy, then present NHS facilities for diagnosis and treatment would not be adequate.

At what intervals should screening be repeated?

The purpose of screening is to identify abnormalities before they become clinically apparent. The duration of the detectable preclinical phase is known as the sojourn time. Ideally, monitoring would occur at sufficiently frequent intervals to detect abnormal cytology during this sojourn time.

Data from European and North American studies have been pooled to assess the optimal frequency of screening. It has been estimated from these data that if all women had at least one screen prior to the age of 35, and were then rescreened at 5-year intervals, there would be an 84% reduction in the cumulative incidence of invasive cervical cancer. Screening at 3-year intervals would reduce the cumulative incidence by 91% (IARC Working Group 1986).

A more difficult question is, 'At what intervals should women be rescreened when the cytologists report moderate dyskaryosis?' Fox (1987) argues that if colposcopy services were freely available, then all women with these abnormalities would benefit from the service. As cytological predictions tend to underestimate abnormalities found on colposcopy, if moderate dyskaryosis is reported, the patient should be referred for colposcopy.

The natural history and management of mild dyskaryosis are controversial. Follow-up of these women shows that up to 26% will progress to CIN 3 in 2 years (Campion et al 1986). But in the same period up to half can revert to normal (Robertson et al 1988). In view of the high frequency of this abnormality, the variable outcome and scarce resources, recommenda-

tions vary from colposcopy to a repeat smear in 6 months or 1 year.

Are the chances of physical and psychological harm less than the chance of benefit?

This general question was raised in Chapter 4. The doctor has a duty to do no harm (or non-malificence) and a duty of beneficence, which involves prevention and removal of harm. Two other basic principles are respect for autonomy and the principle of justice (Beauchamp & Childress 1983).

Illich (1976) argued that western societies are undermining personal autonomy by medicalising life. Skrabenek (1988) argues that screening for cervical cancer, in particular, is an act of unwarranted medicalisation. Whether it is warranted depends on an estimate of the benefit that has been, or may be, achieved. Systematic cervical screening in Iceland and British Columbia has been associated with an 80% reduction in mortality from cervical cancer and invasive disease. If this were achieved in Britain, approximately 1600 out of 2000 lives might be saved and 3200 out of 4000 invasive cancers might be prevented each year. Without systematic screening the mortality rate fell by only 20% in 25 years.

Against benefits and potential benefits, physical and psychological harms need to be weighed. Patients with mild and moderate dysplasia are made anxious (Reelick et al 1984) and treatment may cause physical and psychological harm (Britten 1988, Posner and Vessey 1988). Unsystematic screening may incur harm without sufficient benefit. The reductions in mortality and morbidity were achieved in Iceland and British Columbia with systematic screening. If this outcome is possible with systematic screening in the UK, then it would be unjust not to inform each woman in the population and offer her screening. Benefits are more likely to rise when all women are systematically informed and invited.

Can the cost be balanced against the benefits the service provides, and against other opportunity costs and benefits?

There have been very few attempts to measure the costs and benefits of cervical screening. In the mid-1980s the Department of Health estimated the cost of undertaking and reporting smears to be between £5 and £15.40. Assuming an average cost of £10, 4.5 million smears would cost £45 million. In 1984, 94% of deaths and 45% of the screening occurred in the over 35s; 6% of deaths and 55% of the screening occurred in the under 35s. Translating this into figures of investment for avoidable mortality, approximately £20 million was spent in an attempt to prevent 1785 deaths in the over 35s, whilst £25 million was spent attempting to avoid 114 deaths in the under 35s.

Because of the high cost to benefit ratio, economists (Roberts et al 1985) have argued that the same investment would prevent more deaths in other areas of the National Health Service. However, the high cost per life saved in the 1980s reflects the fact that the group with the lower risk were screened most intensively and frequently. High cost and low effectiveness are not an inevitable outcome of cervical screening, only of an unplanned and poorly distributed service. Using a computer simulation model, Parkin and Moss (1986) suggest that 5-yearly testing of women aged over 35 is the most cost-effective option. Extension of screening to women in lower risk groups or an increase in the frequency of screening leads to a progressive reduction in the marginal benefit per unit cost.

WHAT ARE THE OBSTACLES TO EFFECTIVE SCREENING?

Wilson and Jungner's (1968) criteria have been used to examine the performance of cervical screening. There

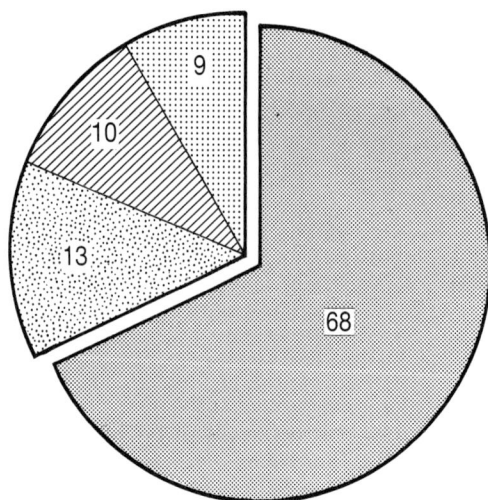

68% — no screening
13% — suspicious smear repeats — not followed adequately
10% — last smear normal over 5 years previously
9% — normal smear in previous 5 years

Fig. 24.4 Pie chart showing review of 100 invasive cervical cancer cases.(After Ellman and Charmberlain 1984.)

is a lack of scientific knowledge about the epidemiology and pathology of cervical carcinoma, which makes clinical decision-making difficult. However, the complexity of this area need not lead to reductive or nihilistic thinking, but to clinicians continuing to evaluate new evidence with an open mind. An immediate challenge is to identify obstacles to a systematic service and find solutions for them. One hundred cases of invasive cervical cancer were reviewed by Ellman and Chamberlain (1984) to assess how screening might be improved (Fig. 24.4). They found that no screening had been undertaken in 68 cases; suspicious cervical smear reports in 13 cases had not been followed up adequately; in 10 cases the last smear had been reported as normal over 5 years previously; a normal smear had been reported in 9 cases in the last 5 years.

The care of these groups will be considered in turn:

No screening

Sixty-eight per cent of women with invasive cancer had never received screening. How can this be explained? In the 1980s there were no national figures for screening rates but regional surveys (Charney & Lewis 1987, Coulter & Baldwin 1987) showed 50–75% of women reported having had a smear in the previous 5 years. Women with invasive carcinoma, however, were more likely to be older, widowed or divorced (Sansom et al 1971) and living in more deprived areas (Johnson et al 1987), and women whose age, civil status and class put them at greater risk are less likely to be screened. A survey in one region illustrates the two ends of the spectrum — 90% of women in social class 1 and 2 aged 25–34 reported having smears in the previous 5 years, whilst 44% of women in social class 4 and 5 aged 55–64 had had a smear in the previous 5 years (Coulter and Baldwin 1987).

Charny and Lewis (1987) asked a group of women why they had never been screened. The most frequent response was that they had not been asked. A useful model of utilisation of screening services has been developed by Eardley et al (1985) (Fig. 24.5).

Self-initiators are likely to be middle class and knowledgeable about the potential of screening to prevent cancer. In the context of the failure of spontaneous screening to reach a large proportion of women at risk, the decision to adopt a universal programme to invite women was a significant advance, but operating this system has identified other barriers. In urban areas it has been found that up to one-half of patients are no longer at the address they gave when registering (Beardow et al 1989). In addition, when

Attendance for cervical screening

Potential users
influenced by the system

| Self-initiators uninfluenced by the system | Attenders | Non-attenders | Refusers uninfluenced by the system |

Population of women eligible for cervical screening

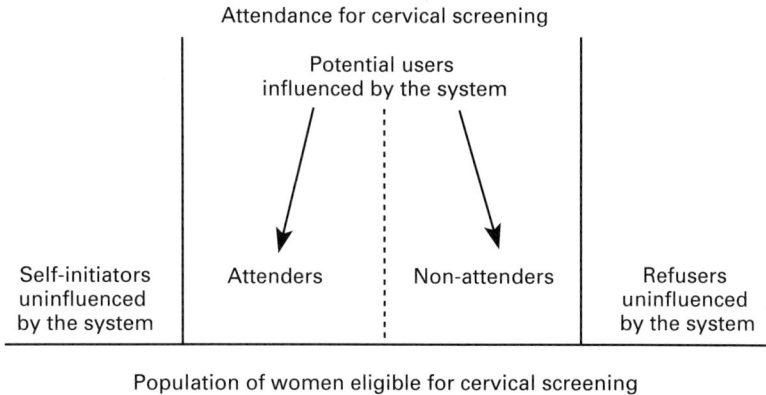

Fig. 24.5   Model of utilisation of cervical screening. The broken line indicates that the proportion of screened women will increase in size in relation to the extent that the system offered incorporates the principles of provider-initiation and user-orientation (from Eardley et al 1985).

invitations are sent without women having sufficient information about their eligibility and the purpose of the test, the response rate may be low.

Standing and Mercer (1984) found 60% of women prefer to see a female health professional for cervical screening but in 1987 over 10 000 GPs serving over 20 million patients had no woman partner (Department of Health 1989, personal communication). Some practices may have had a salaried woman doctor or nurse available, but those who did not would be likely to have a lower response, particularly from some ethnic groups and from women who had never had a cervical smear.

Inadequate follow-up

In Ellman and Chamberlain's study, 13% of women with invasive carcinoma had had suspicious smears reported but these had not been adequately followed up. The most frequent reason for poor follow-up was that the patient had moved to a new and unknown address. Lack of computer systems that can link patients' results with previous smears and facilitate communication between the laboratory and GPs was another cause of failure of follow-up.

Normal smears more than 5 years before

Ten per cent of women with invasive carcinoma had had normal smears performed more than 5 years previously. It is likely that these women did not know that they required repeat monitoring, and that they had not been recalled by the system then in operation. In an analysis of the national recall system Pye (1988)

estimated that only 3% of the appropriate population were effectively recalled by the national recall system!

Normal smears within 5 years

Nine per cent of patients had had normal smear reports within 5 years of their diagnosis of invasive cancer. It was estimated that half of these might have been due to false negative reports.

WHAT POTENTIAL IMPROVEMENTS CAN BE MADE?

1. The introduction of a universal call and recall scheme based on FHSA (Family Health Services Authority) computer systems was a major step forward. There is evidence that systematic invitations increase the use of the service by those who have not previously been screened (Pierce et al 1989).
2. It has been shown that patients are more likely to respond if offered specific appointment times. FHSAs therefore need to improve communications with local practices, and practices need to provide flexibility for those wishing to change their appointments.
3. Women who are invited should receive information booklets about the purpose of the test and its applicability to the recipient (Eardley et al 1988) (Fig. 24.6).
4. In view of patients' expressed preference that screening be undertaken by women doctors or nurses, every practice needs to ensure appropriate personnel are available. Some doctors are unwilling to delegate smear testing to trained nurses. One

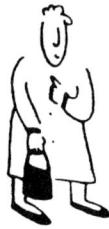

Why invite me?
All women between the ages of 20 and 64 are now being invited every five years

Isn't it just for young women?
No, in fact it is most important that women over 35 who have never had the test before should have one done

What if I'm past the change of life?
Even after the menopause women need to be tested regularly to make sure that the cervix is still healthy

Why me?

Why should I have the test?
There's nothing wrong with me.
The idea of the test is to find small changes that might cause problems later on, so that they can be dealt with before you get any symptoms

What if I've had a hysterectomy?
Some women who have had a hysterectomy still need to have a test. So ask your doctor what is right for you

What if I've had the test in the last five years?
If you think you are not due for another test check with your doctor or at the clinic

So are there any women who don't need a test?
All women would really benefit from having the test–even women who sometimes think they don't need the test any more such as widows and divorced women

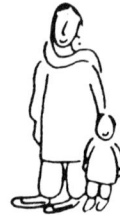

Do I need a test?

Fig. 24.6   Extract from the new edition of *You're invited* (Eardley et al 1988).

rationale is that doctors may screen for ovarian pathology by simultaneously performing a bimanual examination. However, there is no evidence that performing bimanual examinations on asymptomatic women will effectively identify preclinical ovarian carcinoma.

5. Doctors and nurses doing smears need feedback from the laboratory on the quality of the samples they obtain in relation to their peers. If performance is improved this will decrease the rate of false negative reports.

6. Cytology laboratories need computer systems to process information, and continuing quality assessment in order to minimize false negatives.

7. Family Health Service Authorities must agree nationally on the frequency with which women require surveillance because different policies cause confusion for patients and their doctors. To some extent, the system of 'targets' based on a 5-year time-scale addresses this issue.

8. Operating the call scheme has revealed the inadequacy of population registers. If FHSA registers are inaccurate and this inaccuracy leads to a poor response to screening, more radical solutions may be considered. In some Swedish counties each person is required to register a change of address with the parish in which they reside. This requirement is so interlocked with other government functions, including workers' compensation and health care, that compliance is virtually universal. With these registers, more than 90% of the eligible population have attended for cervical screening (Stenkvist et al 1984). To some, compulsory registration of change of address may seem to be excessively paternalistic.

Others may see it as a necessary prerequisite if screening is to be cost-effective. These issues need to be raised if screeners wish to create the political will to enable systems like those working in Sweden, to be introduced in the UK.

FOOTNOTE

Having considered the contributions of different disciplines to an understanding of cervical screening, the clinician returns to the patients.

1. Mrs Dodds, with postcoital bleeding, had never received an invitation for screening because she had moved house within the practice. On examination there was a hard lump on her cervix. She had invasive carcinoma.

2. When Mrs Afshar was invited for screening she was embarrassed about the prospect of a gynaecological examination. She came to see Dr Farnham as she felt it was more appropriate to have this done by another women.

3. Mrs Smart-Jones had mild dyskaryosis. Rather than wait for a repeat smear in 6 months she went to see a gynaecologist privately. She underwent colposcopy and laser treatment for CIN 2 and had a secondary haemorrhage.

4. Mrs Manson seemed to accept Dr Farnham's explanation that a cervical smear was not necessary. She said she was going back to America soon anyway.

REFERENCES

Anderson G H, Boyes D A, Benedet J L et al 1988 Organization and results of the cytology screening programme in British Columbia, 1955–85. British Medical Journal 296: 975–978

Beardow R, Oerton J, Victor C 1989 Evaluation of the cervical cytology screening programme in an inner city health district. British Medical Journal 299: 98–100

Beauchamp T L, Childress J F 1983 Principles of biomedical ethics, 2nd edn. Oxford University Press, New York

Britten N 1988 Personal view. British Medical Journal 296: 1191

BSCC Working Party on Terminology in Gynaecological Cytopathology 1986 Management of women with abnormal cervical smears. The Bulletin of the Royal College of Pathologists September No. 56: 1–2

Campion M J, Cuzick J, McCance D J, Singer A 1986 Progressive potential of mild cervical atypia: prospective cytological, colposcopic and virological study. Lancet ii: 237–240

Charney M C, Lewis P A 1987 Who is using cervical cancer screening services? Health Trends 19: 3–5

Chomet J 1987 Screening for cervical cancer: a new scope for general practitioners? Results of the first year of colposcopy in general practice. British Medical Journal 294. 1326 1328

Cook G A, Draper G J 1984 Trends in cervical cancer and carcinoma in situ in Great Britain. British Journal of Cancer 50: 367–374

Coulter A, Baldwin A 1987 Surveys of population coverage in cervical cancer screening in the Oxford region. Journal of the Royal College of General Practitioners 37: 441–443

Dixon P N, Morris A F 1974 A cervical cytology campaign using a computerized age-sex register. Journal of the Royal College of General Practitioners 24: 418–424

Duguid H L D 1986 Does mild atypia on a cervical smear warrant further investigation? Lancet ii: 1225

Eardley A, Alkind A, Spencer B et al 1988 Health education in a computer-managed cervical screening programme. Health Education Journal 47: 43–47

Eardley A, Elkind A K, Spencer B et al 1985 Attendance for cervical screening — whose problem? Social Science and Medicine 20: 955–962

Elkind A K, Haran D, Eardley A, Spencer B 1988 Reasons for non-attendance for computer-managed cervical screening: pilot interviews. Social Science and Medicine 27: 651–660

Ellman R, Chamberlain J 1984 Improving the effectiveness of cervical cancer screening. Journal of the Royal College of General Practitioners 34: 537–542

Evans D J D, Hudson E A, Brown C L et al 1986 Terminology in gynaecological cytopathology: report of the working party of the British Society for Clinical Cytology. Journal of Clinical Pathology 39: 933–944

Fox H 1987 Cervical smears: new terminology and new demands. British Medical Journal 294: 1307–1308

Giles J A, Hudson E, Crow J et al 1988 Colposcopic assessment of the accuracy of cervical cytology screening. British Medical Journal 296: 1099–1102

Havelock C, Edwards R, Cuzick J, Chamberlain J 1988 The organization of cervical screening in general practice. Journal of the Royal College of General Practitioners 38: 207–211

IARC working group on evaluation of cervical cancer screening programmes 1986 Screening for squamous cervical cancer: duration of low risk after negative results of cervical cytology and its implications for screening programmes. British Medical Journal 293: 656–664

Illich I 1976 Limits to medicine. Medical Nemesis: the expropriation of health. Penguin Books, Middlesex

Johnson I S, Milner P C, Todd 1987 An assessment of the effectiveness of cervical cytology screening in Sheffield. Community Medicine 9: 160–170

Laara E, Day N E, Hakama M 1987 Trends in mortality from cervical cancer in the Nordic countries: association with organized screening programmes. Lancet i: 1247–1249

La Vecchia C, Decavli A, Gentile A et al 1984 "Pap" smear and the risk of cervical neoplasia: quantitative estimates from a case-control study. Lancet ii: 779–782

McAvoy B R, Raza R 1988 Contraceptive service and cervical cytology. Health Trends 20: 14–17

Meadows P 1987 Study of the women overdue for a smear test in a general practice cervical screening programme. Journal of the Royal College of General Practitioners 37: 500–503

Nathoo V 1988 Investigation of non-responders at a cervical cancer screening clinic in Manchester. British Medical Journal 296: 1041–1042

Office of Population Census and Surveys 1985 Mortality statistics by cause: England and Wales 1984. HMSO, London

Office of Population Census and Surveys 1988 Cancer statistics registrations: England and Wales 1984. HMSO, London

Parkin D M, Moss S M 1986 An evaluation of screening policies for cervical cancer in England and Wales using a computer simulation model. Journal of Epidemiology and Community Health 40: 143–153

Pierce M, Lundy S, Palanisamy A et al 1989 Prospective randomized controlled trial of methods of call and recall for cervical cytology screening. British Medical Journal 298: 160–162

Posner T, Vessey M 1988 Prevention of cervical cancer: the patient's view. King's Fund Publishing Office, London

Pye M J 1988 Screening for cervical cancer: review of administrative arrangements. Journal of the Royal Society of Medicine 81: 82–83

Reelick N F, de Hues W F M, Shuurman J H 1984 Psychological side-effects of the mass screening on cervical cancer. Social Science and Medicine 18: 1089–1093

Ridsdale L L 1987 Cervical screening in general practice: call and recall. Journal of the Royal College of General Practitioners 37: 257–259

Roberts C J, Charney M C, Farrow S C 1985 How much can the NHS afford to spend to save a life or avoid a severe disability? Lancet i: 89–91

Robertson J H, Woodend B E, Crozier E H, Hutchinson J

1988 Risk of cervical cancer associated with mild dyskaryosis. British Medical Journal 297: 18–21

Sansom C D, Wakefield J, Yule R 1971 Trends in cytological screening in the Manchester area 1965–71. Community Medicine 126: 253–257

Scaife B 1972 Survey of cervical cytology in general practice. British Medical Journal 3: 200–202

Skrabenek P 1988 The physician's responsibility to the patient. Lancet i: 1155–1156

Spriggs A I, Boddington M M 1976 Protection by cervical smears. Lancet i: 143

Standing P, Mercer S 1984 Quinquennial cervical smears: every woman's right and every practitioner's responsibility. British Medical Journal 289: 883–886

Stenkvist B, Bergstrom R, Eklund G, Fox C 1984 Papanicolaou smear screening and cervical cancer: what can you expect? Journal of the American Medical Association 252: 1423–1426

Taylor P T, Andersen W A, Barber S R et al 1987 The screening papanicolaou smear: contribution of the endo-cervical brush. Obstetrics and Gynaecology 70: 734–737

Wilson A, Leeming A 1987 Cervical cytology screening: a comparison of two call systems. British Medical Journal 295: 181–182

Wilson J M G, Jungner G 1968 Principles and practice of screening for disease. WHO Public Health Paper, 34. World Health Organization, Geneva

Wolfendale M, Howe-Guest R, Usherwood M, Draper G 1987 Controlled trial of a new cervical spatula. British Medical Journal 294: 33–35

Woodman C B J, Yates M, Ward K et al 1989 Indicators of effective cytological sampling of the uterine cervix. Lancet ii: 88–90

The later years

25. Screening and surveillance of older people

Charles B Freer

INTRODUCTION

The belief that 'prevention is better than cure' makes eminently good sense and it is not surprising that it has widespread support in both professional and lay circles and is to be found regularly in party manifestos across the entire political spectrum. What is surprising and unlikely to be widely appreciated outside the medical profession is that, despite many decades of interest in preventive medicine, there remains deep controversy about its value (Lancet 1987).

Preventive care of older people provides an important illustration of the considerable problems in bridging the gap between attractive theory and effective practical implementation.

This chapter will describe the various surveillance strategies for the preventive and anticipatory care of older patients available to the primary care team; but this will be preceded by a detailed historical and theoretical review of the preventive care of older people, as this is likely to explain some of the very real difficulties in successfully achieving implementation and outcomes.

REVIEW OF THE LITERATURE

Modern interest in preventive care of older people dates from the pioneering Rutherglen screening experiment conducted by Anderson and Cowan (1955), which identified high levels of unreported problems among older people (see also Chapter 1). Since then a large number of papers have confirmed the existence of a high prevalence of previously unrecognized physical, social and psychological problems in the elderly population (Williamson et al 1964, Townsend and Wedderburn 1965, Thomas 1968, Hodes 1971, Williams et al 1972, Svanborg et al 1982). Only a small number of studies failed to find significant health problems not known to the general practitioner or other members of the team (Evans et al 1970, Irwin 1971, Freedman et al 1978).

This descriptive research was rapidly followed by studies of interventions to deal with problems detected at screening, several of which reported reduced prevalence (Lowther et al 1970, Pike 1976, Barber and Wallis 1978). A series of randomised controlled trials have also demonstrated benefits from the screening of older populations. Tulloch and Moore (1979) found that the study group had significantly shorter hospital admissions than the control group. Vetter et al (1984), who studied an urban and rural group, reported reduction in mortality in the former but no significant differences between the rural study and control group. A Danish study (Hendriksen et al 1984) found a reduction in mortality and significantly less hospitalization in their study group. An American randomised controlled study (Rubenstein et al 1984) has also reported a significant reduction in mortality and improved functional health status in the study group.

Despite all of this, geriatric screening has not become a prominent feature of primary care services in Britain, and one study of general practitioners in north west England found that only 10% of the study doctors had used any form of screening for their older patients (Williams 1983). The possible reasons for this will be discussed in the next section.

From about 1980, preventive care of older people has remained confined to a relatively small number of interested general practitioners, nurses, health visitors and other research workers, although two important changes in emphasis occured during this period. First, screening schedules concentrated more on the assessment of functional status and less on the detection of disease. Secondly, comprehensive universal screening of populations gave way to more selective and high-risk screening.

The most popular selective screening method has been a two-stage approach, whereby a large percentage of healthy older people are excluded from more detailed and time-consuming assessments by very brief but validated questionnaires in the first stage of the process. The range and practical details of these screening techniques will be described in detail later in this chapter.

The next development in this field was the response to some of the changes included in the UK Government's new contract with general practitioners, which took effect in 1990. Of particular relevance is that the enhanced capitation fee for patients aged 75 years or over requires them to be offered:

1. A home visit at once a year to see the home environment and to find out whether carers and relatives are available.
2. Social assessment (lifestyle, relationships).
3. Mobility assessment (walking, sitting, use of aids).
4. Mental assessment.
5. Assessment of the senses (hearing and vision).
6. Assessment of continence.
7. General functional assessment.
8. Review of medication
   (Department of Health and Welsh Office 1989).

The next section will examine some of the theory and arguments that underpin the profession's attitude to the preventive care of older people.

THEORETICAL AND PRACTICAL CONSIDERATIONS

To understand why geriatric screening and surveillance are not practiced more widely and why they remain controversial, it is necessary to review in detail some of the theoretical aspects of screening and the evidence available in the literature from the many studies published in the last 40 years.

Definitions

Over the past 40 years preventive care of older people has been more or less synonymous with geriatric screening. Like child screening, the literature on geriatric screening has from time to time reflected some confusion and inconsistency regarding terminology. In particular the definitions of screening and case-finding are not always clear. Traditional public health usage is based on the natural history of disease, with 'screening' used for diagnosis made at the asymptomatic stage and 'case-finding' for the identification of an established but undeclared problem. More recently, however, these terms have been used with reference to the organization of preventive care screening being doctor-initiated and case-finding occurring during a patient-initiated visit. (The latter is the usage

generally adopted in this book). Readers of the screening literature need to be aware of these different uses. 'Surveillance' is an all-embracing title for any strategy used to monitor the status of patients in a proactive fashion and 'anticipatory care' is a more recent term, which embodies both the proactive and predictive components of preventive care.

Principles of screening

Screening originates in the discipline of public health and traditionally has been used as a technique for the detection of hidden disease in an apparently healthy population. It was used to great effect in the 1950s when mass miniature radiography was used to tackle tuberculosis, and since then in the detection of carcinoma of the cervix and hypertension. It has not been possible to apply screening techniques to all diseases because there are a number of internationally agreed criteria that need to be satisfied before screening can be introduced with a reasonable expectation of success (Wilson 1966). One of the more important criteria is the need for an asymptomatic phase in the natural history of the disease when some abnormality or deviation from normal can be detected. Other criteria include the existence of cost-effective and acceptable screening techniques and the availability of effective treatment (see also Chapter 2).

In view of these criteria it is immediately obvious that the multidimensional screening of an entire age group, as opposed to screening for a well defined disease entity, is likely to meet considerable difficulties.

There are likely to be two types of hidden health needs in any population. The first are those hidden from the patient, i.e. asymptomatic disease — the basis of traditional public health screening. It is unlikely that this group of hidden needs accounts for major problems in the care of older people. The geriatric literature does not provide convincing evidence to suggest that asymptomatic deviations from normal lead to considerable amounts of preventable morbidity or mortality. The other group of hidden needs are those known to the patient but either hidden from or ignored by the doctor. The older person may not think that it is a legitimate or remediable problem, or may believe that it is to be expected in old age. The doctor may be equally guilty of ageism and assume that age and not, for example hypothyroidism or carcinoma of the colon, is the explanation of tiredness or constipation. Communication difficulties are greater in this age group and can add to the problem of reporting identified problems. This second group of hidden needs is likely to be considerably more important than the first group and, while screening programmes may contribute to better detection, better education of patients, relatives and doctors could be a more logical and efficient approach.

It is especially important for those outside general practice to avoid a reductionist view of primary care; demand-led care is not purely reactive. General practitioners are trained to use these opportunities for health promotion and anticipatory care. Efficient management of presented problems is also an important and frequently under-estimated form of preventive care.

Atypical characteristics of older populations

Any screening programme requires the establishment of normality, or at least some acceptable limits, on measured criteria. This can prove very difficult with older populations. Biochemical normality, for example, is likely to have been defined by studies of young healthy volunteers. In the case of diabetes this is likely to lead to an overestimate of cases unless age-correcting nomograms are used. Hypertension has, of course, proved very difficult to define and there is still no clear consensus on what levels of blood pressure in asymptomatic older people would benefit from treatment.

Experience with other screening programmes, such as child surveillance and carcinoma of the cervix, has found that poor attenders tend to be in the high risk groups. An interesting contrast has been found with older people. While many have predicted that those patients rarely seen by their doctors are likely to have problems and be in need of visiting, a series of British studies have all shown that, in the main, infrequently attending older people are likely to be fit and well (Williams 1984, Ebrahim et al 1984, Williams & Barley 1985). Concern for underconsulting has been a powerful force in preventive medicine but Ford and Taylor (1985) found little evidence of underconsulting in the older population. The presence of disease in older people is often less important than in younger age groups. Williams (1979) has described this as 'effective health', as many older people with medical problems nevertheless lead contented and fulfilling lives. This has led to the greater emphasis on the assessment of function rather than the detection of disease.

Cost-effectiveness and work-load

It is difficult to imagine that regular health surveillance of all older people would not yield some benefits, and earlier in this chapter reference was made to a number of randomised controlled studies that have demonstrated positive outcomes from geriatric screening.

However, only two such studies have been based in the UK (Tulloch and Moore 1979, Vetter et al 1984) and in the former the authors cautioned against generalisation because of the atypicality of the study practice. The other studies were done in the United States (Rubenstein et al 1984) and Denmark (Hendriksen et al 1984), which makes generalisation to the British situation even more precarious. Furthermore, the Danish study involved 4-monthly visits by nurses, a surveillance frequency quite unfeasible as a general policy in the UK.

The work-load implications of screening are vitally important and possibly the most telling argument against universal geriatric screening. Barber and Wallis (1982) estimated that to set up a full screening programme for those patients aged over 75 years in a Glasgow practice with a total population of 4000 would require 18 hours per week of health visitor time for the first year and 11 hours per week for subsequent years. In response to the Health Visitors Association joint statement with the British Geriatric Society on health visiting for older people (Health Visitors Association and British Geriatric Society 1986), Barley (1987) estimated that their proposals would require an additional 3000–6000 health visitors in the UK, a quite unrealistic target.

There are, in addition, possible ethical objections to the health screening of the elderly. First of all not all older people might want or welcome screening, and secondly the iatrogenic effects of the investigation and treatment of problems, some of which may be of dubious functional or prognostic significance, need to be carefully considered in any objective review of arguments for screening.

The evidence for the cost-effectiveness of screening is far from convincing, but perhaps financial considerations should not be the only criteria on which the provision of services should be based. It is likely that many older people would welcome an occasional check-up or reassurance about their health. Whether this means a formal screening or assessment is debatable, but perhaps the type of services and resources made available to older people should reflect the value society places on its senior citizens as much as, if not more than, whether it is a worthwhile investment.

Clearly the arguments about and the evidence for geriatric screening and surveillance are even more complex than those relating to, for example, hypertension and carcinoma of the cervix. It is also unlikely that any one strategy would suit every practice or practice team. In the final section of this chapter the range of practical approaches to the screening of older people will be considered.

PRACTICAL APPROACHES TO THE PREVENTIVE CARE OF OLDER PEOPLE

In the absence of any 'best buy' in terms of geriatric screening or surveillance, it seems reasonable for practices to choose methods compatible with their level of motivation and interest in the preventive care of the elderly and the resources and personnel available to them.

Universal and comprehensive screening

For those with a special interest in older people, the traditional approach of detailed screening on a regular basis, usually annually, is likely to be the most attractive option. The screening would take place in the patient's home, or at a special clinic, and a major part of it could be administered by a nurse or health visitor. The extent and content of the screening can be anything the practice team feel is appropriate, but there is a reasonable consensus in the literature for a functional orientation rather than a disease-based emphasis. A range of screening schedules have been used, including the detailed history and examination previously used by Williams (1979), the problem-based physical, social and psychological assessment, which has been validated by Barber and Wallis (1978) and the functional case-finding assessment used by Williamson (1987).

These assessments are available from the relevant authors but the reader should be aware that some of the early experiments with geriatric screening amount almost to mini-assessments (see Chapter 2) rather than brief screening schedules.

Arguments persist about when to initiate screening for the elderly. Seventy-five years is considered by many researchers to be the logical starting point because the yield of significant problems for the 65–74 year-old group does not justify including them in universal screening. But if preventive medicine is to be seen as an integral feature of primary care, it is probably necessary for prevention to be a continuous process with different protocols for different stages of the lifecycle, e.g. childhood, well-woman/man clinics, preretirement, etc.

For the majority of primary health care teams, however, screening of older people is unlikely to warrant full-scale, regular clinics, and for them the recent research interest in selective screening and brief approaches to geriatric screening will be of interest.

Selective screening

It is possible to identify individual patients at increased risk of health problems, e.g. those recently bereaved or discharged from hospital, but as yet it is not possible to use high-risk features to create subsets of elderly populations for selective screening, at least not with any degree of validity or reliability.

From about 1980 most of the groups interested in geriatric screening have used a particular selective approach, which has come to be known as two-stage screening. In the first stage a brief and rapid screening schedule is used to select those older patients thought to justify a more detailed assessment in the second stage. If the first stage could be done quickly and cheaply, leaving a relatively small number of patients requiring full assessment, this would have obvious work-load attractions.

Two-stage screening

Barber and his colleagues (1980) were the first to develop this approach and initially used a nine-item questionnaire, which was posted to all the patients to be screened (Table 25.1). All patients answering yes to one or more questions were referred for full second stage assessment. Early results were disappointing, as 80% of patients 'failed' stage one. Further analysis suggested that a major reason for this was the high percentage of false positive answers. This was remedied by a reduction in the number of questions included in the stage one questionnaire without any reduction in the case-finding efficiency of the instrument. Taylor and his colleagues (1983) found that by using questions 3, 5, 6 and 8 from Table 25.1, only 37% of the elderly would require follow-up for assessment. A meeting funded by the Chief Scientist's Office, which brought together many of the groups using the two-stage approach in Britain (Taylor & Buckley 1987), confirmed that many groups had developed an abbreviated version of Barber's initial questionnaire with many revised schedules omitting

Table 25.1 Postal screening questionnaire (from Barber et al 1980)

1. Do you live on your own?
2. Are you without a relative you could call on for help?
3. Do you depend on someone for help?
4. Are there many days when you are unable to have a hot meal?
5. Are you confined to your home through ill-health?
6. Is there anything about your health causing you concern or difficulty?
7. Do you have difficulty with vision?
8. Do you have difficulty with hearing?
9. Have you been in hospital during the past year?

questions 1, 2, 4 and 9. Anecdotal impressions suggested that question 6 had the highest predictive value.

Taylor and Buckley (1987) describe a range of geriatric screening schedules in some detail, but also list a number of practices and groups with contact addresses throughout the UK, any of whom would be able to provide more detailed practical information and an update on progress.

The two-stage, abbreviated approach appears to be the most popular approach at the time of writing, with a postal first stage being used in a number of practices. One variation of this has been the Edinburgh birthday card scheme (Porter 1987), where a brief questionnaire accompanies a birthday card. Initial experience suggested that this was very much appreciated by patients but there are some possible ethical objections based on the medicalisation of non-medical aspects of life, and perhaps raising health anxieties at a time when a person should be celebrating in a more positive way.

Other groups have organized volunteers to administer the first stage (Beales 1987, Carpenter and Demopoulos 1987) and in these projects the initial screening has used a modification of a shortened American questionnaire (Linn and Linn 1982). There is, however, an additional vehicle for two-stage screening based on the high contact rate between British general practitioners and their elderly patients.

Consultation-based screening of the elderly

On average, over 75-year-olds consult their general practitioner about 6.5 times per year (Office of Population Censuses and Survey 1984) and over 90% of this age group see their general practitioner at least once per year (Williams 1984, Freer 1985). There is therefore a valuable opportunity for screening to reach a significant percentage of older people by integrating it with routine care. This is even more feasible with the emergence of rapid, i.e. non-time-consuming), and validated first-stage screening schedules. Furthermore, concern about infrequent or non-attending older people has to a large extent been mitigated by the results of a number of studies showing that, in the main, these patients are fit and well (Ebrahim et al 1984, Williams 1984, Williams & Barley 1985). At worst, consultation-based screening would mean that only 10% of the elderly required contact by post or visiting. Pilot studies with a consultation-based system of screening have been encouraging and suggest that for some practices it may be a practical and efficient way to add a proactive

element to demand-led care, and thereby achieve comprehensive screening of the elderly patients in the practice (Freer 1987).

Self-screening

There is, in theory, one more approach to screening that is waiting to be tested — self-administration of stage one screening. There is certainly no reason why many patients could not review on a regular basis the questions in, for example, the abbreviated postal questionnaire and this would furthermore be in keeping with the increasingly popular notion that patients should be more involved in their own care.

CONCLUSION

We now have available a range of tested methods to organize screening and surveillance of older populations in primary care. It is something of a paradox, however, that the publication of this new edition comes in the wake of the introduction of a new general practitioner contract. Among a number of controversial new features is the requirement for general practitioners, or members of their team to offer to visit patients aged 75 years or over in their homes every year. This visit will involve an assessment of social status, mobility, mental state, hearing and vision, continence, functional status and medication. For this the general practitioner receives an enhanced capitation fee. The main criticism is that, as with the broader proposals in the National Health Service reforms, the ideas being introduced are untested. Yet screening and surveillance of older people, as discussed earlier, have received widespread research attention and results and experiences would offer no strong support for the method being forced on doctors by the revised contract. The latter fails to recognize that many older people are fit and well, are unlikely to be easily found at home and may, indeed, resent this intrusion. The inefficiency of annual home visiting of an age group, 90% of whom are seen at least once a year by their general practitioner, is difficult to justify. Worst of all, linked as it is to remuneration rather than the White Paper proposals on audit — which the medical profession welcomes and supports — screening of older people could be reduced to a delegated check-list procedure. The risk is that this would be completed to satisfy a contract and remunerative requirement, and not to promote genuine preventive and anticipatory care of older people.

This chapter has not been written for the 'enthusiast' but for all general practitioners, because if improvements are to occur in the anticipatory care of older people, all general practitioners — and not just those with a special interest — will need to be involved. It has been written in the belief that a genuine understanding of both the theoretical and practical implications of geriatric screening would assist practice teams to choose effective methods best suited to their practices.

Hopefully, changes currently occurring in UK general practice will allow for flexibility in the screening methods chosen, recognizing that variation in general practice is not only a reality but can be a strength.

REFERENCES

Anderson W F, Cowan N R 1955 A consultative health center for older people. Lancet ii: 239–240

Barber J H, Wallis J B 1978 The benefits to an elderly population of continuing geriatric assessment. Journal of the Royal College of General Practitioners 28: 428–433

Barber J H, Wallis J B 1982 The effects of a system of geriatric screening and assessment on general practice workloads. Health Bulletin 40: 125–132

Barber J H, Wallis J B, McKeating E 1980 A postal screening questionnaire in preventive geriatric care. Journal of the Royal College of General Practitioners 30: 49–51

Barley S 1987 An uncompromising report on health visiting for the elderly. British Medical Journal 194: 595–596

Beales D L 1987 The use of trained volunteers in a screening programme: an evaluative study. In: Taylor R C, Buckley E G (eds) Preventative care of the elderly: a review of current developments. Occasional Paper No. 35. Royal College of General Practitioners, London, p 4

Carpenter G I, Demopoulos G 1987 The use of a disability rating questionnaire in a case controlled screening surveillance programme. In: Taylor R C, Buckley E G (eds) Preventive care of the elderly: a review of current developments. Occasional Paper No. 35. Royal College of General Practitioners, London, p 11

Department of Health and Welsh Office 1989 General practice in the National Health Service: a new contract. Hmso, London

Ebrahim S, Hedley R, Sheldon M 1984 Low levels of ill health among elderly non-consulters in general practice. British Medical Journal 289: 1273–1275

Evans S M, Wilkes E, Dalrymple-Smith D 1970 Growing old: a country practice survey. Journal of the Royal College of General Practitioners 20: 278–284

Ford G G, Taylor R C 1985 The elderly as underconsulters: a critical reappraisal. Journal of the Royal College of General Practitioners 35: 244–247

Freedman G R, Charlewood J E, Dodds P A 1978 Screening of the aged in general practice. Journal of the Royal College of General Practitioners 28: 421–425

Freer C B 1985 Care of the elderly. Old myths. Lancet ii: 268–269

Freer C B 1987 Consultation-based screening of the elderly in general practice. A description and preliminary report. Journal of the Royal College of General Practitioners 37: 455–456

Health Visitors Association and British Geriatric Society 1986 Health visiting and the aged: a joint policy statement. Health Visitors Association, London

Hendriksen C, Lund E, Stromgard E 1984 Consequences of assessment and intervention among elderly people: a three year randomised controlled trial. British Medical Journal 289: 1522–1524

Hodes C 1971 Geriatric screening and care in group practice.

Journal of the Royal College of General Practitioners 31: 469–472

Irwin W G 1971 Geriatric practice in the health centre. Modern Geriatrics 1: 265–266

Lancet 1987 Primary health care: government's worthy word among the gloom (leading article). Lancet ii: 1307

Linn M W, Linn B S 1982 The rapid disability rating scale — 2. Journal of the American Geriatric Society 30: 378–382

Lowther C P, McLeod R D M, Williamson J 1970 Evaluation of early diagnostic services for the elderly. British Medical Journal 3: 275–277

Office of Population Censuses and Surveys 1984 Britain's Elderly Population Census Guide 1. OPCS, London

Pike L A 1976 Screening the elderly in general practice. Journal of the Royal College of General Practitioners 26: 698–703

Porter A D M 1987 The Edinburgh birthday card scheme. In: Taylor R C, Buckley E G (eds) Preventive care of the elderly: a review of current developments. Occasional Paper No. 35. Royal College of General Practitioners, London, p 22

Rubenstein L Z, Josephson K R, Wieland G D et al 1984 Effectiveness of a geriatric evaluation unit. A randomised controlled trial. New England Journal of Medicine 310: 1664–1670

Svanborg A, Bergstrom G, Mellstrom D 1982 Epidemiological studies on social and medical conditions of the elderly. World Health Organization (EURO reports and studies 62), Copenhagen

Taylor R C, Buckley E G (eds) 1987 Preventive care of the elderly: a review of current developments. Occasional Paper No. 35. Royal College of General Practitioners, London

Taylor R C, Ford G, Barber J H 1983 The elderly at risk. A critical review of problems and progress in screening and case finding. Age Concern research perspective monograph No 6, Mitcham, Surrey

Thomas P 1968 Experiences of two preventive clinics for the elderly. British Medical Journal 2: 357–360

Townsend P, Wedderburn D 1965 The aged in the welfare state. Occasional Papers on Social Administration No. 14. G. Bell, London

Tulloch A J, Moore V 1979 A randomised controlled trial of geriatric screening and surveillance in general practice. Journal of the Royal College of General Practitioners 29: 733–742

Vetter N J, Jones D E, Victor C R 1984 Effect on health visitors working with elderly patients in general practice: a randomised controlled trial. British Medical Journal 288: 369–372

Williams E I 1979 The care of the elderly in the community. Croom Helm, London

Williams E I 1983 The general practitioner and the disabled. The Journal of the Royal College of General Practitioners 33: 296–299

Williams E I 1984 Characteristics of patients over 75 not seen during one year in general practice. British Medical Journal 288: 119–121

Williams E S, Barley N H 1985 Old people not known to the general practitioner: low risk group. British Medical Journal 291: 251–254

Williams E I, Bennett F M, Nixon J V et al 1972 Sociomedical study of patients over 75 in general practice. British Medical Journal 2: 445–448

Williamson J 1987 Prevention, screening and case finding: an overview. In: Taylor R C, Buckley E G (eds) Preventive care of the elderly: a review of current developments. Occasional Paper No. 35. Royal College of General Practitioners, London, p 45

Williamson J, Stokoe I H, Gray S et al 1964 Old people at home. Their unreported needs. Lancet i: 1117–1120

Wilson J M G 1966 Some principles of early diagnosis and detection. In: Teeling-Smith G (ed) Surveillance and early diagnosis in general practice. Office of Health Economics, London

26. Sensory impairment in the elderly

Alastair J Tulloch

Because hearing and vision problems are common and often remediable causes of dysfunction and suffering, they should be important concerns of primary care. Untreated sensory deprivation also contributes to some forms of mental ill-health. (Health of the Elderly. Report of a WHO Expert Committee, 1989).

INTRODUCTION

In the search for higher standards of community care of the elderly it has become increasingly clear in recent years that the central task, and indeed ultimate objective of the care of this group is the promotion of function and independence so that they can lead the best life open to them in their chosen setting (usually their own homes) for as long as possible. To achieve this objective, high standards of diagnosis and management of disease must, as always, be the main line of attack but we cannot achieve optimal standards of care of older people unless the management of disease takes more account of its functional consequences than at present. Nowhere is this more obvious than in patients with sensory impairment, i.e. defective vision and hearing, particularly because, although each impairs social communication and integration, society reacts to the two impairments quite differently.

VISION

Society and the old person with impaired vision

Loss of vision is devastating because sight is central to almost everything we do and to the enjoyment of our environment. This problem is compounded by the incapacity of the blind to manage their own affairs entirely, an expression of their loss of autonomy. Thus, blindness is seen by society as the ultimate handicap and this is especially the case in the elderly, who are more likely to be suffering from other disabling medical and social disorders already. The blind or partially sighted person is the object of almost universal sympathy, compassion and support. It is easy to understand why, but the picture must be balanced by an appreciation that the blind person also is thought to develop a heightened perception and appreciation of sound and does not have to endure the terrible isolation of living in a silent world without the comfort of the human voice, like the deaf. This is not to underestimate the appalling problem of failing vision but simply to put it in context.

There are also a number of myths and misunderstandings about impaired vision in the elderly. First and foremost, society equates failing vision with the progressive loss of visual acuity, which is almost universal among people growing older and this, together with the fact that loss of vision is often gradual and progressive, leads the public to conclude, quite wrongly, that failing vision is simply the price of ageing. Of course impaired visual acuity is a measure of failing vision but the public takes too little account of the possible contribution of remediable conditions like cataract.

The visually impaired also tend to be seen, both by society and the caring professions, as an homogeneous group, which is not true in the elderly with their high rate of medical, functional and socioeconomic problems. Failing vision often magnifies these problems but it is not always the main disorder (Cullinan 1977).

Patients and their carers, formal and informal alike, also tend to be passive and pessimistic about deteriorating vision, often unaware that the cause is not infrequently remediable. As a result professional advice tends to be sought later than is desirable. Finally, the widely held belief that reading fine print strains the eyes and that subdued lights are restful in the case of old people is entirely without foundation.

These various misconceptions merely add to the burden of an old person whose eyesight is failing. As mentation and reflexes also tend to be impaired at this stage, it is easy to understand why elderly peoples' self-confidence, morale and self-esteem tend to be undermined, and why they are likely to dread the problem of failing eyesight.

Definition

There are at least 67 different definitions of 'blindness' around the world (Cullinan 1977) but it is generally agreed that total blindness is an inability to perceive light in either eye, while the WHO defines visual impairment as a Snellen Test Type distance visual acuity of 6/18 or less and classifies it as in Table 26.1.

Visual changes in old age are, of course, universal because hardening and decreased translucency of the crystalline lens, which comes with age (presbyopia), virtually always produces impaired visual acuity, although the rate of progress and the extent of the changes vary in different people. Lens opacities, glaucoma and macular degeneration, all more common in the elderly and threatening vision, further add to the burden. Decreased mobility of the iris tends to lead to a smaller pupil with less light reaching the retina. As a result, old people tend to find it difficult to adapt from bright light to dark surroundings and they are also more sensitive to glare. Tales of old people with perfect vision at all distances should be viewed with suspicion, although this phenomenon may be explained by some patients having a myopic eye used for near work and a 'normal' eye for everything else. Alternatively, one occasionally comes across a patient with a very small pupil and thus a large depth of field, which permits good distance and near vision.

Those old people who do consult their general practitioner may find them pessimistic on this subject and opthalmic surgeons, not fully briefed on the additional

disabilities, may have postponed operations (especially for cataract) inappropriately, although this is less likely now that impairment of quality of life is the indicator for cataract surgery.

Prevalence

Because of the wide differences in definition and methods of data collection it is impossible to provide firm figures on the prevalence of visual impairment. However Cullinan (1977) in a wide-ranging and thorough review of the subject came up with the following estimates:

1. The true prevalence of blindness, defined as WHO categories 2, 3, 4, 5 in the United Kingdom is about 190–220 per 100 000 of the total population.
2. 65–70% of the blind (and probably of the partially sighted) are over the age of 65 years. Between 65 and 74 the prevalence of blindness in the population rises to 550–600 per 100 000 and over the age of 75 it reaches at least 1500 per 100 000.

The General Household Survey 1986 also draws our attention to the fact that among people aged 65 or more with visual impairment, 22% wear glasses but still have difficulty in seeing (the figure for women is 26% and for men it is 16%), while over the age of 75 years the figure is 29% (women 33%, men 20%). This suggests that a significant minority of elderly people, particularly women over the age of 75, are overdue a visit to the optometrist, or have additional disorders affecting vision, some of which are certainly remediable.

Aetiology of visual impairment

The important causes of visual impairment are as follows:

Macular degeneration

This is the most important single cause of severe visual impairment. Jackson & Petrie (1969) reported a prevalence of 10.7%, although at this time macular degeneration was the cause in only 3.3% of the registered blind in Scotland.

Cataract

Firm figures for the prevalence of cataract are simply not available because of lack of population studies but it has been estimated that 50% of the population over 75 years have some form of cataract. Brennan and Knox (1975), reviewing the attendance at eye clinics, estimated the whole population prevalence as 59 per

Table 26.1 World Health Organization classification of blindness

WHO category	Maximum less than	Minimum equal to or better than
1	6/18	6/60
2	6/60	3/60
3	3/60 (or visual field < 10° or > 5°)	1/60 (finger counting at 1 metre)
4	1/60 (finger counting at 1 metre or visual field < 5°)	Light perception
5	No light perception	
9	Undetermined or unspecified	

100 000 for men and 99 per 100 000 for women. Most elderly people with cataracts who suffer from severe visual impairment also have some other eye disease, which leads to postponement of operation or makes the visual loss worse, e.g. macular degeneration.

Glaucoma

The prevalence of glaucoma was reported by Hollows & Graham (1966) as 840 per 100 000 in a population between 40 and 75 years of age and approximately 10% of people over the age of 70 years have glaucoma. Screening for glaucoma is discussed on page 260.

Diabetic retinopathy

The prevalence of this condition was reported by Sorsby (1972) as 6.4 per 100 000 for patients aged 60–69 and 10.3 per 100 000 for patients aged 70 years or more.

Archer (1985) estimates that 50% of those with proliferative retinopathy progress to blindness within 5 years, although with the advent of laser treatment this situation is clearly improving.

Shaw et al (1986), in a study of elderly hospital outpatients, reported new referral rates for the disorders:

1. Macular degeneration —12%
2. Cataracts — 25%
3. Glaucoma — 14%
4. Diabetic retinopathy — 4%

Other general disorders are associated with eye manifestations that may lead to preventable impairment of vision, e.g. hypertensive retinopathy. In other cases, e.g. the optic neuritis of multiple sclerosis, no treatment is as yet available, but its recognition may help to establish the diagnosis.

Screening for visual impairment

The benefits of a screening programme include:

1. Certain disorders, like cataract, can be corrected by surgery while others, like glaucoma, can be arrested in many cases.
2. The prescription of appropriate spectacles in patients with refraction errors can greatly improve visual acuity.
3. Better briefing of the patient about visual impairment, its implications and management and the services (see Appendix 1) and aids available to the patient.
4. Better education in the importance of bright lighting behind the patient's head, the use of low vision

aids and the absurdity of not reading in the interests of 'conserving' vision are all likely to offset the disability from impaired vision.

5. Detailed advice to carers, relatives and friends is also valuable in the handling of the visually impaired, e.g. introduction to the blind person each time and letting them take an arm rather than trying to steer them.
6. Organisation of a clear strategy, which the patient appreciates, for entering low doors, going upstairs, etc.
7. Making sure that trailing leads, curled up carpet edges, etc. are avoided to prevent falls.
8. Registration of the blind is most helpful and provides a variety of benefits (see Appendix 1).

Screening in practice

Questions are required to review the effect of impaired vision on day-to-day life as follows:

1. Do you have problems:
    a. reading the paper?
        i) ordinary newsprint?
        ii) even headlines?
    b. watching television?
    c. in other circumstances?
2. Does your impairment of vision:
    a. prevent you from getting around freely?
    b. lead to falls or other accidents?
    c. affect your day-to-day life significantly?
    d. make you feel depressed
        i) moderately?
        ii) severely?

Further assessment

Assessment of distant vision is made using the illuminated Snellen Test Type at a distance of 6 metres with a pin-hole. Assessment of near vision makes use of a standardised near test type chart.

Physical examination, including ophthalmoscopy and central visual field screening, should then be done to detect cataract, glaucoma and retinopathy.

In this process of screening, I see a most important role for the optometrist, with whom general practitioners must learn to work much more closely than in the past. They have more skill and experience in ophthalmoscopy than most family doctors, and this should be made available to patients during a screening programme. We should, therefore, be inviting optometrists to take part in such a programme, at least on an experimental basis. I recognise that there could be administrative problems, e.g. if one optometrist were seeing the patient of another, but these can be overcome. We must also try to ensure that optometrists are better briefed about relevant disorders, such as diabetes and hypertension, within the constraints of professional confidence, in the course of their ordinary work than at present.

When this screening is complete one has a clear profile of the patients' sensory status and a decision can be taken on the need for further investigation. In the event of hospital referral being necessary it is important for the consultant to be briefed about all the patient's previous medical history, as well as his/her health status, to aid the decision, e.g. in the case of cataract, on how soon to operate.

Finally, attention has been drawn to the fact that the abolition of routine free eye testing in April 1989 has led to a 30% fall in the number of people going to high street optometrists for eye examination (Rosenthal 1990). It is also believed that old people are deterred most, the very group in which macular degeneration and glaucoma — the two most usual causes of blindness — are most common.

Screening for glaucoma

The glaucomas can occur in all age groups and may even be congenital, but discussion of this subject seems most appropriately placed in a section devoted to the elderly, as it is in this age group in which most of the disability due to the condition occurs.

The following section concerns chronic, otherwise known as simple or open-angle glaucoma (as opposed to angle closure glaucoma). Simple glaucoma fulfils some of the prerequisites of a condition for which screening is justified: it is not uncommon, it produces significant disability and it has a prolonged presymptomatic phase when intervention is valuable. Furthermore, it is possible to define a population at special risk. However, screening for glaucoma is constrained by the need for a simple, reliable, sensitive and specific test.

Glaucoma — like toxaemia of pregnancy — has three cardinal features, more than one of which will usually be present. They are raised intraocular pressure (IOP), abnormalities of the optic disc (in particular increased cupping) and impairment of the visual fields. These have variously been used in screening.

Detection of glaucoma.

Intraocular pressure. Glaucoma screening has traditionally been based on measurement of intra-

ocular pressure with an applanation tonometer, as described by Pabalan & Weingeist (1985). However, tonometry has its limitations. Intraocular pressure resembles blood pressure in that it fluctuates throughout the day and is continuously distributed in the population, so that the choice of a cut-off point is a matter of judgement. Many authorities would favour a level of 21 mmHg, compared with a population mean of approximately 15.

Using applanation tonometry in the community setting, sensitivity figures of at best 50–70%, and specificity figures as low as 10–30% have been quoted (Shields 1985). Changing the cut-off point may lead to gains in one of these figures at the expense of the other.

While the low specificity figures indicate that a majority of patients with ocular hypertension do not currently have glaucoma, some will develop it later. Hitchins (1986) suggests that of patients with raised intraocular pressure, about 10% currently have glaucoma, while a further 10% will develop it within the next 10 years. Patients with ocular hypertension are therefore at the very least an at-risk group.

Applanation tonometers, such as the Schiotz, do not fulfil the requirement that a screening test should be simple and non-intrusive. They can cause discomfort, and carry a slight but significant risk of corneal abrasion and spread of infection. They must be used with a topical anaesthetic, which itself can cause sensitivity reactions. These problems have been partially overcome by the advent of non-contact tonometry (NCT), which can be used by relatively untrained staff without discomfort, although the equipment is not cheap.

Ophthalmoscopy. An increased cup:disc ratio is a hallmark of glaucoma. A ratio greater than 0.6 is usually taken as predictive.

It is sometimes advocated (Levi and Shwartz 1983) that ophthalmoscopy is a useful adjunct to, or indeed substitute for, tonometry. In a large Japanese study quoted by Shields (1987), involving 11 660 people, the yield of glaucoma with field loss was 0.49% (57 cases), using a combination of tonometry and ophthalmoscopy. Tonometry alone would have detected 28 cases, and ophthalmoscopy alone 39 cases. Some of the cases missed by tonometry had quite a significant degree of field loss.

On the other hand, ophthalmoscopy requires a high degree of expertise, and is particularly difficult in some elderly patients where a mydriatic has not been used.

Detection may be easier where the disease is unilateral, as asymmetry of intraocular pressures or of optic cups is likely to be significant.

Visual field measurement. The principal disability caused by simple glaucoma is restriction of the visual field. For this reason the most sensitive and specific technique for its detection is accurate visual field examination. However, this is often difficult — it requires a high degree of patient co-operation, a long attention span and a skilled operator with considerable time. A variety of manual and automatic procedures are now available for this purpose. Oculokinetic perimetry, as described by Damato (1985) has attracted much interest.

Population screening and selective screening. Fortunately, glaucoma is a condition in which certain risk factors can be identified. Family history is perhaps the best known. Hitchings (1986) reports a study of 1700 relatives of patients with glaucoma. In this group, covering all age groups, the prevalence of overt glaucoma was 2% (four times the population average), while 20% had physical signs placing them at risk of developing the condition. Other risk factors include increasing age, race, high myopia, vascular disease, long-term steroid treatment and diabetes mellitus.

While unselective population screening is unlikely to be feasible, there is a strong case for selective screening based on these risk groups. It is most important that all adult first degree relatives of patients with glaucoma be screened, particularly after the age of 40.

Screening by whom? If screening is to be carried out, who should do it? In general, screening is carried out in the community by optometrists. Where they have reason to suspect the condition, at least in the UK, they will advise the patient to attend his or her own general practitioner for onward hospital referral. However, it should be borne in mind that optometrists see a highly self-selected population — particularly since the introduction of charges for sight testing. Most will have coincidental visual symptoms, for example due to presbyopia, and some will have symptomatic glaucoma, which has advanced beyond the optimal stage for treatment.

While some general practitioners will be enthusiastic, skilled and equipped to carry out screening, they are likely in the foreseeable future to be a minority. For most, the main tool for the identification of glaucoma is a high index of suspicion, and a willingness to refer the relatives of patients affected by glaucoma, particularly if they also have other risk factors.

Further assessment. Patients in whom glaucoma is suspected will be referred to an ophthalmologist, where assessment will include a search for the cardinal manifestations mentioned previously, as well as slit-lamp examination to show the depth of the anterior chamber and look for evidence of synechiae.

Where a referral has been made and a patient has been confirmed to have glaucoma, life-long topical treatment is needed. For the patient with preglaucoma or ocular hypertension, long-term hospital follow-up has traditionally been the norm, although this is an area, like many others, with potential for general practitioner involvement.

HEARING

Old people with deafness in our society

Deafness is a disability which is increasingly prevalent with age and which, unlike blindness, is held in relatively low esteem by society. The deaf tend to find themselves regarded with impatience, often shouted at and treated as if they were stupid or backward. As a result, deafness carries a stigma and tends to make the patient feel a sense of shame. This, together with the view of older people that deafness is to be expected in old age, leads them to conceal the problem until it is quite severe and a major handicap. Relatives also tend to be pessimistic and passive about impairment of hearing which, as a result, they tend to collude in concealing, sometimes behaving as if they were vicariously ashamed of it. Even doctors are reported as sometimes, however unwittingly, leaving patients with the impression that deafness is often to be expected in old age and that little can be done for the deaf patient. Certainly there is a low rate of examination of the ears and poor standards of care when the ears are examined both in the UK and in the USA, although standards are higher in Denmark and Sweden. As a result, rates of referral for deafness are lower than might be expected. The availability of help is further impaired by long waits for out-patient care. Even in hospital, out-patient department briefing on the use of hearing aids is often poor and follow-up tends to be erratic. In addition, patients are not always advised that hearing aids are most helpful in face to face conversation and may be much less useful in a crowded room or noisy environment. It is scarcely surprising that poorly briefed patients, finding hearing aids ineffective in the above two settings, discard them as unsatisfactory. Even when they prove effective, older patients with reduced manual dexterity from, for example, arthritis or Parkinson's disease, may find the controls 'fiddly' due to poor design and, once again, the aid may be consigned to the drawer.

Thus, there are problems at all levels for patients whose hearing is failing, and they find society at the same time relatively unsympathetic and tending to afford their disability a relatively low priority. Yet to the patient it is a dreadful problem, leading to isolation, loneliness and loss of independence. It is hardly surprising that such patients feel neglected and are often unhappy and depressed, while some become suspicious and paranoid. The point is sometimes made that the deaf often seem more miserable, as a group, than those with the apparently greater disability of blindness. Society fails to understand the reason for this because we tend to underestimate the importance of the human voice in social contact and integration, which we take for granted in our day-to-day life, in addition to the other problems, listed above, which the deaf have to endure. Thus, a case can be made out for deafness being just as great, if not greater, a tragedy for the patient as blindness.

Certainly, there is much room for enlightenment in the attitude of society in general and professional carers in particular towards the problem of sensory impairment and especially deafness among older people. This would, at the very least, lead to patients seeking advice and help earlier than is often the case at present.

Definition of deafness

Defining deafness is not easy because hearing is impaired in many people as they grow older, yet only a minority of people could be described as deaf. However, a reasonable working definition of deafness suggested by Herbst and Humphrey (1981) was 'an average loss over the speech frequencies at 1 KHz, 2 KHz and 4 KHz of 35 decibels or more in the better ear'.

Prevalence

Approximately one-third of patients aged 65 years or more suffer from hearing loss 'which can have unfavourable social consequences' according to Fisch (1985). This figure was confirmed by the General Household Survey (GHS) (1986), men in this age group (35%) being more commonly affected than women (29%), probably due to the greater likelihood of them having worked in a noisy environment. The deafness, which may have been coming on gradually for many years, is more common in social class 5 (McAdam et al 1981).

The GHS (1986) also reported that only 1 in 3 of those with impaired hearing wore a hearing aid, and McAdam et al reported an even lower level of 1 in 5.

Aetiology

Presbycusis

Presbycusis is an impairment of hearing coming on with advancing years in the absence of pathological changes. It is a sensorineural loss, often relatively mild, which can range in severity from 10 to 50 dB.

However, disturbance of hearing in old age is not due simply to impaired sensitivity to sound. Other factors are involved, including abnormal appreciation of loudness (which can sometimes be increased), poor sound localisation, making it difficult sometimes for the patient to tell from which direction the sound is coming, and impaired capacity to interpret speech clearly, which is due to the fact that consonants, which project most information, generally tend to be in the higher frequencies in which hearing is most often lost, whether due to presbycusis or pathological changes. Finally, tinnitus and vertigo are each found in about one-third of patients aged 65 years or more and may compound the problems due to hearing loss.

Senescent changes

The main senescent changes in the auditory system are:

1. Thickening of the tympanic membrane.
2. Impaired articulation of the auditory ossicles.
3. Degenerative changes in the cochlea.
4. Nerve atrophy.
5. Degenerative changes in the basal nuclei and auditory cortex

Contributory factors

The most important contributory factor in impairment of hearing is environmental noise, followed by previous middle ear infection, vascular disease and trauma. Finally, earwax is common and easily remediable.

Screening for hearing impairment

Benefits of a screening programme

1. The deaf are recognised, understood and treated sympathetically with the nature and implications of the problem being carefully explained to the patient.
2. Consequently the cause of the deafness can be investigated and appropriate treatment instituted from as simple a measure as wax removal, which may greatly improve hearing, to the fitting of a hearing aid, careful briefing on its use and regular follow-up.
3. Education of the patient about deafness, its implications, its treatment and the aids and services available (see Appendix 2).
4. In appropriate cases training in lip reading.

5. Education of relatives about the problem and its implications, along with the need to be patient and supportive. Relatives should be advised to face the light, find the direction from which the patient hears best, look directly at him/her during conversation, speaking clearly and normally. They should be advised against mumbling, shouting, mouthing words unnaturally, smoking or putting their hands over their mouths.

Screening in practice

The advent, in 1990, of annual review visits to the over 75s has meant that an increasing number of patients have formal hearing assessment. However, as before, much of the screening will, in practice, be opportunistic.

First impressions are helpful in the ascertainment of hearing, although they can be deceptive. Our prime concern is to know how the patient functions day by day. Towards this end the patient should be asked:

1. Do you have difficulty in hearing:
   a. ordinary conversation?
   b. in a crowded room?
   c. on the telephone?
   d. the television?
   e. when the sound is loud and the hearing aid is turned up?
   f. in other conditions? (please detail)
2. Do you have difficulty in appreciating where sound comes from?
3. Does impaired hearing:
   a. affect your day-to-day life to any great extent? (please detail)
   b. cause you to feel at times that people are saying things about you that they do not want you to hear?

Further assessment needs to be carried out where there is doubt about a patient's hearing. This includes inspection of the ears for wax, Weber's test (which is particularly helpful in unilateral deafness) and Rinne's test, to distinguish between conductive and sensorineural deafness. The most objective information is provided by audiometry (see Fig. 18.5, p. 178), although the limitations of this technique should be recognised.

GENERAL

Failure of demand-led care in the identification of sensory impairment

Programmes of care involving screening of the elderly have been very common over the 35 years since Anderson and Cowan (1955) reported their classic Rutherglen Experiment — I was able to trace 45 done by doctors alone in the UK and nurses and health visitors have reported similar programmes of care. Yet I was unable to trace a single one in which identification of sensory impairment was reported as satisfactory.

The results of those programmes that did review recognition of sensory impairment can be summarised as follows:

1. Williamson et al (1964). These workers found that, in a population of 200 patients aged 65 years or more, 56 (28%) had slight or moderate visual defects and 17 showed severe visual impairment. Most of the former and three of the latter had been unrecognised by their family doctors. Thus, in the case of these three, the benefits of registration were not open to the patients.
2. Stokoe (1971) reviewed the same size of population and age group as Williamson et al (1964), finding that 43 patients (22%) had unrecognised visual defects and 46 (23%) hearing defects.
3. Sheard (1971). In a study of 462 patients aged over 70, Sheard reported 37 partially sighted (8%) and 17 blind (3.7%). Thirty-five of the partially sighted and 3 of the blind had not been registered and were thus not enjoying the benefit of this service. In addition, they were not well informed about services for the visually impaired at that time, i.e. they knew neither that the service was free nor that, if they were unfit to go to the optician, the optician would come to them. With regard to hearing, Sheard found that 137 people (30%) were 'unable to hear a forced whisper at conversational range'. Yet only 53 of them possessed hearing aids, not all of which were in use, although the author felt that many could have benefited from such an aid.
4. Tulloch & Moore (1979) reviewed a group of 145 patients aged 70 years or more and found unrecognised marked sensory impairment, i.e. at a level that materially affected their day-to-day life, in 9 patients — 2 with auditory and 7 with visual problems.
5. Barber & Wallis (1982). In screening a population of 97 patients aged 75 years or more, Barber & Wallis found 177 'new or deteriorating problems', 16 (9%) of them due to sensory impairment — 6 visual and 10 auditory.
6. McMurdo & Baines (1988) reported high levels of unreported visual problems among 50 patients aged 44–97 attending a geriatric day hospital — 32% had severe unsuspected visual impairment, more than half of which were remediable by cataract extraction.

7. Fenton et al (1975) found a large number of unrecognised visual handicaps among well-orientated patients in a typical geriatric ward. Thirty per cent of this group had their lot improved and some functioned as normal instead of nearly blind as a result of either surgery or the prescription of more appropriate spectacles.

These studies suggest that much sensory impairment in the community remains undiscovered and patients are not as well informed about available services as they could be — especially in relation to the use of hearing aids and registration of the partially sighted and blind.

DISCUSSION

The general result of identification and management of patients with sensory impairment is that they are less isolated and lonely. Wherever possible these disabilities are corrected and compensated so that patients are better integrated into their families and society. They can pursue their interests and recreations more easily, their mobility is improved and they are more likely to be able to remain independent in their chosen setting for longer. Institutional admission, which so many people fear, is likely to be postponed. Finally, associated disorders like anxiety, depression, confusion and paranoia (in the case of the deaf) and falls (in the case of the blind) may be mitigated.

Requirements for better maintenance of sensory function

Since the principal need is awareness of the importance of sensory impairment and its consequences to the patient, the first requirement is good education of the general public and of professional workers in this subject. Thus, myths and misunderstandings can be corrected, barriers of silence broken down and patients and their relatives encouraged to report these problems early. Some form of screening and continuing surveillance is also necessary to ensure not only that the disability is recognised early and appropriate treatment instituted, but that progress is kept under regular review and that patient and family education is fully maintained.

Early referral for specialist assessment is equally important and the consultant must be fully aware of the patient's other medical and social history before making a decision on, for example, the point at which cataract extraction should be undertaken. Careful follow-up should be ensured and, when patients default, the general practitioner should be informed so that one of the primary care team can visit to discover the reason for default.

To bring about such a programme as this calls for a basic change in the attitude both of the public and of the caring professions to sensory impairment, which is likely to take some time to come about. In the meantime, we must be prepared to be more active in seeking out these problems. This means supplementing demand-led care by screening and surveillance of higher risk groups, e.g. the old, diabetics, patients with a family history of glaucoma, cataract and otosclerosis and those who have worked in a noisy environment.

Screening in the elderly is a subject on which opinion is sharply divided, although the evidence from controlled studies is really unequivocal. There is no evidence that screening improves patient health, in the short-term at least, but screened patients are kept independent for significantly longer than unscreened matched groups, which is, after all, the ultimate objective of primary care of the elderly. This consistent finding in the three controlled trials that reviewed the effect of screening on institutional admission — Tulloch & Moore (1979), Hendriksen et al (1984), Rubenstein et al (1984) — seems to me to present an unanswerable case for the introduction of some form of screening for medical and paramedical problems likely to cause suffering and impair function. However, in so far as changes introduced in GP terms of service relate to the elderly under the new contract, they have clearly not been carefully thought through, are far too rigid and do not require the doctor undertaking the work to have special training. The two controlled trials which included costings — Hendriksen et al (1984) and Rubenstein et al (1984) — suggested that properly organised screening could also effect a cost saving by a reduction in prescribing and hospital 'bed days'.

The case for screening the elderly is therefore established and sensory impairment is a fertile field for this work given the problems described above. However, I would be opposed to screening for auditory and visual impairment in isolation. I believe it should be part of a carefully planned general screening programme. Between the ages of 65 and 74 this can be done at approximately 3-yearly intervals, and largely by the practice nurse, as suggested by Freer (1987), during routine care when the patient attends the surgery, with referral back to the general practitioner of the minority of patients with sensory impairment that affects day-to-day life to an extent not previously recognized. From the age of 75 years, and in a minority of high risk cases aged 65–74, patients should have a general review in a clinic in which assessments of hearing and sight are an important part, conducted by the doctor and practice nurse or health visitor. In some cases, especially in the very old, those with marked sensory impairment and in those with additional disabilities, it will be necessary to visit the patients to review the home environment.

Most, however, will be seen in the clinic where the equipment for review of sight and hearing is easily available.

CONCLUSION

There is well documented evidence of underdiagnosis of sensory impairment among the elderly. My impression is that this is attributable partly to the fact that doctors are sometimes unaware of the presence or severity of the problem — I have certainly been caught out in this connection myself. This is often due to under-reporting by the patients and their families but also to the rather passive attitude doctors adopt to sensory impairment in a system that remains largely demand-led. Thus, there is a need for a more active approach to these problems, coupled with much improved education of the general public, patients and their relatives.

This chapter has sought to document the problems of patients with sensory impairment and to establish the raison d'être of a more active programme of care of old people with sensory impairment and the means of achieving it.

APPENDIX 1

Services available for the registered partially sighted and blind

Financial

1. Extra DHSS allowance if already in receipt of income support.
2. Extra personal income tax allowance in some cases.
3. Lower TV licence fee (currently reduced by £1.25)
4. Concessionary train fares, which allow free travel to a sighted escort of a blind person going to a hospital appointment or job training. Also BR Disabled Person's railcard can be used for other concessions on rail travel.
5. Concessionary bus fares in some areas and help in some cases to get grants, e.g. for telephone rental.
6. Free postage on items sent under 'articles for the blind' label, e.g. Braille material, talking books and newspapers.
7. Rate relief under Rating (Disabled Persons) Act 1978.
8. Help with telephone installation charges and rental may be available.

9. Free permanent loan of radio and limited supply of batteries supplied by British Wireless for the Blind Fund.

Practical

1. Special equipment obtainable from the Royal National Institute for the Blind (RNIB) at concessionary rates, e.g. white stick, kitchen aids, adapted games, writing frames, etc. Special aids and equipment for work available on loan from the Manpower Services Commission.*
2. Radio or radio-cassette player provided free through Social Services (by Wireless for the Blind).
3. RNIB offers reduced rates on typewriters, tape recorders, electric razors, etc.*
4. Membership of RNIB talking book library and other cassette libraries and talking newspapers.*
5. Low vision aids can be prescribed by Hospital Eye Service.*
6. Parking concession under Orange Badge Scheme.
7. Personal reader service available in some areas.
8. Membership of organisations providing a variety of services for the blind.
   a. British Talking Book Service;
   b. RNIB providing braille library, tapes, transcriptions and recording services — also aids;
   c. free news publications.

Services

1. Visits from Mobility and Rehabilitation Officers to help advise on benefits and the best way to adapt to day-to-day problems and simply getting around.*
2. Visit from someone to teach Braille and touch typing.*
3. Blind Persons Resettlement Officer will advise in appropriate cases on retraining for a placement in work.*

In addition, the 'fares to work' scheme is available to the partially sighted and blind, with an additional disability allowance if unable to use public transport.

Both groups may be helped by local voluntary societies, which provide services like social activities, holidays, aids and limited financial assistance.

Finally, there is one problem with most of these concessions — the 'blind' person needs proof of identity, which does not come with registration. The doctor should therefore provide these patients with a letter certifying that they are registered blind.

---

* Services are also available to those registered partially sighted.

APPENDIX 2

Aids available to the hard of hearing:

1. Hearing aids — best supplied through the NHS with careful briefing and follow-up.
2. Telephone adaptations to make ringing and conversation more easily audible.
3. Doorbell conversion so that ringing gives way to flashing lights.
4. Ear trumpets, which look clumsy but still have a place in the elderly who dislike using ordinary hearing aids.
5. Use of hearing aid loop systems installed in communal rooms used by the elderly in institutional care.

REFERENCES

Anderson W F, Cowan N R 1955 A consultative centre for older people. Lancet ii: 239-240

Archer D B 1985 In: Phillips C (ed) Basic clinical ophthalmology. Pitman Publishing, London, pp 152-177

Barber J H, Wallis J B 1982 The effects of a system of geriatric screening and assessment on general practice workload. Health Bulletin 40/3: 125-132

Brennan M E, Knox E G 1975 The incidence of cataract and its clinical presentation. Community Health 7: 1

Cullinan T R 1977 The epidemiology of visual disability. Studies of visually disabled people in the community. Report No. 28. Health Services Research Unit, University of Kent

Damato B E 1985 Oculokinetic perimetry: a simple visual field test for use in the community. British Journal of Ophthalmology 69: 927-931

Fenton P J, Arnold R C, Wilkins P 1975 Evaluation of vision in slow stream wards. Age and Ageing 4: 3-48

Fisch L 1985 Special senses — the ageing auditory system. In: Brocklehurst J C (ed) Textbook of geriatric medicine, 3rd edn. Churchill Livingstone, Edinburgh

Freer C B 1987 Consultation-based screening of the elderly in general practice: a pilot study. Journal of the Royal College of General Practitioners 37: 455-456

General Household Survey 1986 The Office of Population Censuses and Surveys, Social Surveys Division. HMSO, London

Hendriksen C, Lund E, Stromgard E 1984 Consequences of assessment and intervention among elderly people: a three year randomised controlled trial. British Medical Journal 289: 1522-1524

Herbst K G, Humphrey C 1981 Prevalence of hearing impairment in the elderly living at home. Journal of the Royal College of General Practitioners 31: 155-160

Hitchings R A 1986 Screening for glaucoma. British Medical Journal 292: 505-506

Hollows F C , Graham D A 1966 The Ferndale Glaucoma Survey. In: Hunt L B (ed) Glaucoma. Churchill Livingstone, Edinburgh

Jackson C R S, Petrie E B 1969 Partial Sightedness. A Ross Foundation Report. W H Ross Foundation, Edinburgh

Levi L, Schwarz B 1983 Glaucoma screening in the health care setting. Survey of Ophthalmology 28: 164-174

McAdam D B, Siegerstetter J, Smith M C A 1981 Deafness in adults – screening in general practice. Journal of the Royal College of General Practitioners 31: 161-164

McMurdo M E T, Baines P S 1988 The detection of visual disability in the elderly. Health Bulletin 46/6: 327-329

Pabalan F J, Weingeist T A 1985 Glaucoma screening as part of the routine physical examination. What to look for and how to use the Schiotz tonometer. Postgraduate Medicine 77: 256-260

Rosenthal A R 1990 High street tests. Payments are deterring the elderly and blindness will increase. British Medical Journal 300: 695-696

Rubenstein L Z, Josephson K R, Wieland G D et al 1984 Effectiveness of a geriatric evaluation unit. A randomised controlled trial. New England Journal of Medicine 310: 1664-1670

Shaw D E, Gibson J M, Rosenthal A R 1986 A year in a general ophthalmic outpatient department in England. Archives of Ophthalmology 104: 1843-1846

Sheard A V 1971 Survey of the elderly in Scunthorpe. Public Health (London) 85: 208-218

Shields M B 1986 Glaucoma screening. In: Textbook of glaucoma. Williams & Wilkins, Baltimore, pp 132-136

Sorsby A 1972 The incidence and causes of blindness in England and Wales 1963-1968. DHSS Reports on Health and Medical Subjects No. 128. HMSO, London

Stokoe I H 1971 Care of the elderly. Update Plus 1: 677-684

Tulloch A J, Moore V 1979 A randomised controlled trial of geriatric screening and surveillance. Journal of the Royal College of General Practitioners 29: 733-742

Williamson J, Stokoe I H, Gray S et al 1964 Old people at home. Their unreported needs. Lancet i: 1117-1120

27. Problems of mobility in the elderly

Keith Thompson

INTRODUCTION

The process of ageing is slow and passes unnoticed by the individual, although clearly it is observed by others. Such slow change allows time for adaptation to take place, so that age is only experienced when one is faced with a challenge. Thus, at 25 one is too old to win the 100 metres free-style Olympic Gold Medal for swimming, at 30 too old to win the men's singles final at Wimbledon, at 35 a veteran footballer, and so on. By the age of 70 both the range and speed of physical performance have been reduced, so that most former activities have been abandoned, and more appropriate interests taken up.

The reasons for changed performance are infinitely complex and will not be discussed here. Nevertheless, we should remind ourselves that changes over time in the performances of different organ systems proceed at different rates. For example, whereas nerve conduction velocity diminishes by only 10% between the ages of 30 and 70, renal function, in contrast, falls by 50% over the same age span. These differences indicate clearly that each subject must be evaluated on a variety of performances. This will involve the assessor in having a rehabilitation profile scoring system to measure the degree of handicap and by which to measure progress considering not only the physical, but also the psychological and environmental contributions.

THE MUSCULOSKELETAL FAILURE SYNDROME

The musculoskeletal failure syndrome is one of the most common forms of disability in the elderly and consists of ambulation impairment due to minimal pathological lesions that effect muscles, nerves, joints and arteries which, taken together, may disable the patient, although no single system alone is sufficiently involved to constitute a primary disability.

Patients with minimal hypertrophic osteoarthritis or rheumatoid changes, often find it difficult to walk because knee and hip flexion deformity prevents normal standing, which requires an adequate degree of ankle dorsiflexion for the feet to be flat on the ground. Full extension of the knees and hips is required because, where a flexion deformity has developed, compensatory changes will occur at the other joints to maintain the centre of gravity. With flexed knees and extended hips the centre of gravity is thrown backwards, and compensation is provided by flexing the hips. If this position is maintained, a secondary flexion contracture takes place at the hips.

With the knees in full extension, the erect position is maintained with little quadriceps power because the locking home mechanism in the knee joint permits the erect position to be held with minimal corrective action by the quadriceps. But when the knees are flexed the quadriceps must be constantly active to prevent buckling, which produces fatigue with further flexion deformity, so that the greater the deformity the greater demand on the quadriceps, which becomes less and less able to support body weight.

Associated neurological conditions such as small strokes, or extrapyramidal lesions such as unsuspected parkinsonism may also contribute to musculoskeletal failure syndrome. The arterial circulation with mild ischaemic neuropathy, pain syndromes and loss of anterior horn cells may all be associated. Thus, in these patients, the deformity of the joints and the ambulation disability develop because of a combination of several mild pathological states, rather than from one major disorder. Such patients are often able to function well enough until some major illness occurs, when a period of bed rest augments the tendency toward the development of contractures and disuse atrophy of the muscles, and exaggerates negative psychological reactions. Recovery from the illness may result in a patient who was able to walk into hospital, but unable to walk out because of the musculoskeletal failure syndrome.

This syndrome is described not only because it is very common as a cause of mobility problems, but because it demonstrates the need to approach such problems from a wider aspect than the traditional medical method if we are to understand the individual's mobility problem.

ASSESSING MOBILITY PROBLEMS IN THE ELDERLY

Approach to the subject

The time-honoured disease-orientated approach of taking a thorough history, performing an exhaustive non-selective examination and obtaining appropriate laboratory and diagnostic tests is of value only if a single disease process explains the clinical picture, which is rarely the case in the elderly. A lot of data may be accumulated by the usual medical approach, yet one may have little understanding of a person's mobility status, because the clinical status is more than the sum of separate disease processes. Also, there is usually no consistent relationship between anatomical or biochemical abnormalities and physical signs.

The disease-orientated approach fails to recognise falling as a clinical entity in its own right. Falling is usually due to the accumulated effect of multiple chronic disabilities and is potentially preventable if the causative factors are recognised in individual patients. We should realise at the outset that concentration on diagnosing the disease for which little can be done can lead to underplaying symptoms or disabilities for which much can often be done.

We shall not consider how the gait or movement look, so much as concentrate on what the person can or cannot do. Every clinician has seen patients with abnormal gaits who manoeuvre safely and effectively. Also, it is more important to measure the effect of the environment than to analyse gait in an artificial setting. Thus, a patient with cardiac disease and painful arthritis may be unable to climb stairs to reach the toilet, but may manage quite well when rehoused in a ground-floor flat.

Nevertheless, it is important to be able to assess the ability to walk in older people, many of whom live alone. We need to note both the distance walked and the degree of mobility. A further note may also be added concerning the rate of walking in certain circumstances. Table 27.1 shows a simple grading system for mobility. It is, of course, necessary to assess the value of any aid and the way it is used. Sticks should be of the correct length, and be fitted with a ferrule. A stick for bearing weight should be stout and firm, not thin and whippy. When a walking stick is used because one leg is not functioning as it should, the stick should be held on the side of the better leg. A tripod may be too wide to be used on stairs.

The causes of immobility

There are many complex causes of immobility, which frequently interrelate. However, it may be useful to consider the commonly encountered physical and mental causes, bearing in mind that further consideration is always given to social circumstances and to interpersonal relationships (Fig 27.1).

Table 27.1 A simple grading system for mobility

Degree of mobility	Grading	Distance walked	Grading
Unable to walk	1	Unable to walk	1
Walks with help from 2 people	2	Walks less than 5 yards	2
Walks with help of 1 person	3	Walks 5–10 yards	3
Walks unsteadily with frame	4	Walks 10–100 yards	4
Walks steadily with frame	5	Walks more than 100 yards	5
Walks unsteadily with tripod	6		
Walks steadily with tripod	7		
Walks unsteadily with stick	8		
Walks steadily with stick	9		
Walks unsteadily without aid	10		
Walks steadily without aid	11		

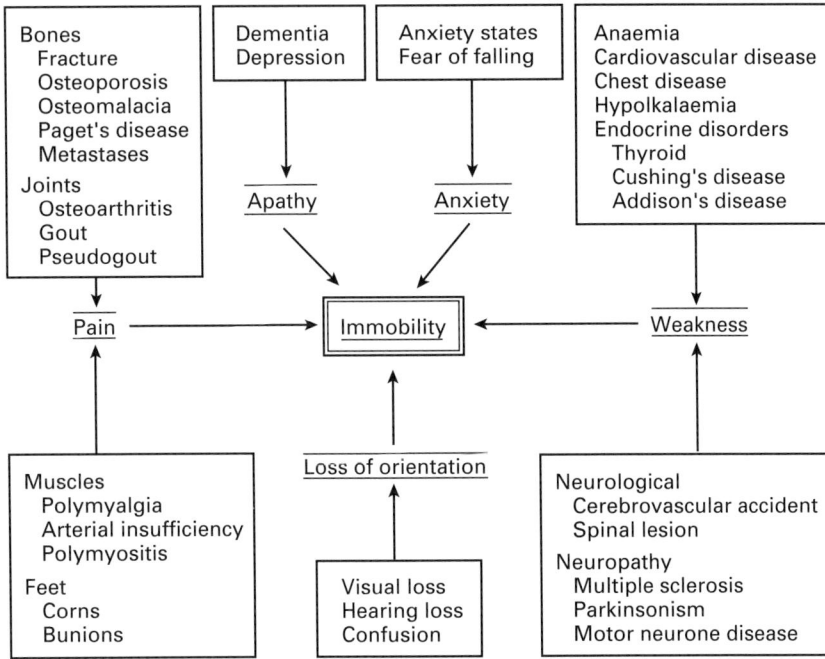

Fig. 27.1 Causes of reduced mobility.

The gait

Although there may be an opportunity to observe the way the patient enters the consulting room, this is not enough, but may only be suggestive where initial inspection raises doubts a more detailed assessment is in order. Table 27.2 sets out a method of analysing the walking pattern according to nine functions. This approach is preferable to applying terms such as 'festinant', which are often poorly defined by the one who uses them, although subjective attachment to them lingers on. The patient stands with the examiner at the end of an obstacle-free hallway. The examiner asks the patient to walk down the hallway at his/her usual pace and with the usual walking aid. The examiner observes one component of the gait at a time (as in a heart examination). For some components the examiner may walk behind the patient, for others, beside him/her. Several trips may be required to complete the examination.

The scheme provided here offers instructions to enable consistent observations between patients and to define the abnormality. Thus, for instance, in observing abnormal step symmetry, with the patient taking short steps on one side, with little lifting of the foot, one may be guided to the pain or weakness of the contralateral hip or leg necessitating decreased weight bearing. The physician is not, however, observing gait

to analyse every component meticulously, but to detect obvious problems that may be improved by therapeutic measures. It is important to remember that abnormal gait may be due either to neuromuscular or to musculoskeletal problems, but also represents a compensatory or adaptive manoeuvre to increase stability, and this is often seen in the slow short steps and flexed posture adopted by older patients. The examples given in Table 27.2 are meant to illustrate how the performance-orientated approach works, and to suggest that it is possible to approach a complex function such as mobility in a reliable and useful manner.

Balance and stability

Stability has been considered one of the four giants of geriatric medicine and is of cardinal importance because of the danger of falls. Therefore, when assessing an individual's mobility, attention must be paid to specific characteristics that may, in turn, influence balance, gait, awareness of the environment or desire to manoeuvre in the home. These matters are listed on Table 27.3 and include mental and emotional status, sensory functions, strength and coordination and such factors as neck and back flexibility and condition of the feet. Also associated with falling or decreased mobility of elderly persons are factors such

Table 27.2 Performance-orientated assessment of gait (from Tinetti 1986, reprinted with permission of the American Geriatric Society)

Components	Observation	
	Normal	Abnormal
Initiation of gait (patient asked to walk down hallway)	Begins walking immediately without observable hesitation, initiation of gait is single, smooth motion	Hesitates; multiple attempts; initiation of gait not a smooth motion
Step height (begin observing after first few steps: observe one foot, then the other	Swing foot completely clears floor but by no more than 2.5–5cm (1–2 in)	Swing foot is not completely raised off floor, or is raised too high (>2.5–5 cm (1–2 in))
Step length (observe distance between toe of stance foot and heel of swing foot; observe from side; do not judge first few or last few steps; observe one side at a time)	At least the length of individual's foot between the stance toe and swing heel (step length usually longer but foot length provides basis for observation)	Step length less than described under normal
Step symmetry (observe the middle part of the path not the first or last steps; observe from side; observe distance between heel of each swing foot and toe of each stance foot)	Step length same or nearly same on both sides for most step cycles	Step length varies between sides or patient advances with same foot with every step
Step continuity	Begins raising heel of one foot (toe off) as heel of other foot touches the floor (heel strike); no breaks or stops in stride; step lengths equal over most cycles	Places entire foot (heel and toe) on floor before beginning to raise other foot; or stops completely between steps; or step length varies over cycles
Path deviation (observe from behind; observe one foot over several strides; observe in relation to line on floor, e.g. tiles, if possible; difficult to assess if patient uses a walker	Foot follows close to straight line as patient advances	Foot deviates from side to side or toward one direction
Trunk stability (observe from behind; side-to-side motion of trunk may be a normal gait pattern, need to differentiate this from instability)	Trunk does not sway; knees or back are not flexed; arms are not abducted in effort to maintain stability	Any of preceding features present
Walk stance (observe from behind)	Feet should almost touch as one passes other	Feet apart with stepping
Turning while walking	No staggering, turning continuous with walking; and steps are continuous while turning	Staggers; stops before initiating turn; or steps are discontinuous

as postural hypotension, medication effects, and acute and chronic illnesses. It must be remembered that the risk of falling increases linearly with the number of abnormalities, therefore every successful intervention, no matter how seemingly insignificant, may reduce the chance of falling. Fear of falling will be indicated during examination by reluctance to attempt manoeuvres, a tendency to grab at objects or the adoption of a slow and studied pace. This decline in activity may change if asked to increase the pace, and this is an indication that overcoming this fear may be achieved by therapists.

Observing these everyday manoeuvres provides more useful information diagnostically, and prognostically, than indirect and non-specific tests such as the Rombergh test. It should also be made clear that when the nudge on the sternum is referred to, this should be performed firmly and gently, moving the patient through no more than 3–4 cm of space to test the self-righting reflexes. This may also be carried out laterally by nudging the shoulder from behind, with the patient's eyes open, then closed.

The tests are in some ways simple, even crude, and require no special apparatus. They can be performed with a high level of agreement by all members of a team. Pedants may object that they do not offer information about how the patient would perform on uneven ground. Nevertheless, by combining the various balance and gait observations, working hypotheses as to possible sources of problems can be formulated.

Stroke

Systematic evaluation of the motor capacity of patients with cerebrovascular disease is important for setting

Table 27.3   Performance-orientated evaluation of balance and gait (from Tinetti 1986)

Abnormal manoeuvre	Possible aetiologies*	Possible therapeutic or rehabilitative measures	Possible preventive or adaptive measures†
Difficulty arising from chair	Proximal muscle weakness (many causes) Arthritides (especially involving hip, knees) Parkinson's syndrome Hemi- or paraparesis Deconditioning	Treatment of specific disease states, e.g. steroids, L-dopa Hip and quadriceps exercises Transfer training	High, firm chair with arms Raised toilet seats Ejection chairs
Instability on first standing	Postural hypotension Cerebellar disease Multisensory deficits Lower extremity weakness or pain Foot pain leading to decreasing weight bearing	Treatment of specific diseases, e.g. adequate salt and fluid status, Florinef Hip and knee exercises Correct foot problems	Raise slowly Head of bed on blocks Supportive aid, e.g. walking aids
Instability with nudge on sternum	Parkinson's syndrome Back problems Normal pressure hydrocephalus peripheral neuropathy Deconditioning	Treatment of specific diseases, e.g. L-dopa, shunt Back exercises? Analgesia Balance exercises	Obstacle-free environment Appropriate walking aid (cane, walker) Night lights (more likely to fall if bump into object) Close observation with acute illness (high risk of falling) Avoid slippers Bright lights
Instability with eyes closed (stable with eyes open)	Multisensory deficits Decreasing proprioception, position sense, e.g. B12 deficiency, MS, etc.	Treatment of specific diseases, e.g. B12 Correct visual/hearing problems Remove cerumen Balance exercises Antiarthritic medication Cervical collar Neck exercises	
Instability on neck turning or extension	Cervical arthritis Cervical spondylosis Vertebro-basilar insufficiency		Avoid quick turns Turn body, not just head Store objects in home low enough to avoid need to look up
Instability on turning	Cerebellar disease Hemiparesis Visual field cut Decreasing proprioception Mild ataxia	Gait training Proprioceptive exercises	Appropriate walking aid Obstacle-free environment Properly fitting shoes
Unsafe on sitting down (misjudges distance or falls into chair)	Decreasing vision Proximal myopathies Apraxia	Treatment of specific diseases Coordination training Leg strengthening exercises	High, firm chairs with arms, in good repair Transfer training
Decreased step height and length-bilateral (there will often be a flexed posture with all of these conditions)	Parkinson's syndrome Pseudobulbar palsy Myelopathy (usually spastic gait) Normal pressure hydrocephalus Advanced Alzheimer's disease (frontal lobe gait) Compensation for decreasing vision or proprioception Fear of falling Habit	Treatment of specific diseases, e.g. L-dopa Correct vision Gait training (correct problems, suggest compensations)	Avoid loose rugs Good lighting Proper footwear (good fit, not too much friction or slip) Appropriate walking aid

* not an exhaustive list; †most not subjected to clinical trials, evidence for effectiveness is anecdotal

Table 27.4   The modified motor assessment chart according to Lindmark and Hamrin 1988

	Score 0–3				Score 0–3	

Part A: Ability to perform active movements

Upper extremity	P	NP	Lower extremity	P	NP
Sitting on the edge of the bed or on a chair			Supine, legs extended and resting on the bed		
1. Bring the hand to the mouth by bending the elbow and supinating the forearm and touch the lips with the fingers	...	...	1. Flexion of the hip and knee to more than 90 degrees flexion in both joints	...	...
2. Bring the hand to the back of the neck by abducting the shoulder, bending the elbow and pronating the forearm	...	...	2. Extension of the hip and knee from more than 90 degrees flexion in both joints	...	...
3. Flexion of the arm to 180 degrees with extended elbow	...	...	3. Abduction of the leg with the knee extended and the toes pointing towards the ceiling	...	...
4. Abduction of the arm to 180 degrees with extended elbow	...	...	4. Adduction of the leg with the knee extended and the toes pointing towards the ceiling	...	...
5. Bring the hand to the lateral side of the opposite knee by adduction and inward rotation of the arm, extension of the elbow and pronation of the forearm	...	...	Sitting on the edge of the bed or on a chair		
6. Supination of the forearm. For 1–2 p the elbow is flexed 90 degrees. For 3 p the elbow must be extended and the shoulder joint flexed about 45 degrees	...	...	5. Extension of the knee from 90 degrees flexion	...	...
7. Pronation of the forearm. For scoring see 6.	...	...	6. Flexion of the knee from full extension to more than 90 degrees flexion. The foot should be brought under the bed or the chair.	...	...
8. Bring the arm around the body and put the back of the hand against the waist	...	...	7. Dorsiflexion of the ankle. For 1-2 p the knee is flexed 90 degrees, for 3 p the knee is extended	...	...
Maximum score	24	+24	8. Plantar flexion of the ankle. For scoring see 7.	...	...
			9. One leg is brought across the other	...	...

Wrist			Standing with support		
For 1–2 p the elbow is supported, for 3 p the elbow is unsupported and extended			10. Flexion of the hip and knee to 90 degrees	...	...
1. Dorsiflexion	...	...	11. Extension of the hip backwards with extended knee	...	...
2. Palmar flexion	...	...	12. Standing on tiptoe	...	...
3. Circumduction	...	...			
Maximum score	9	+9	Maximum score, lower extremity	36	+36
			Maximum score, Part A	93	+93

Hand function			Part B: Ability to perform rapid movement changes		
1. Flexion of all fingers	...	...			
2. Extension of all fingers	...	...	Sitting on the edge of a bed or on a chair	P	NP
3. Opposition of the thumb against the tip of the second finger	...	...	1. Pro- and supination of forearm with the elbow flexed 90 degrees	...	...
4. Hook grasp. Hold around a stick with the metacarpophalangeal joints extended and the interphalangeal joints flexed	...	...	2. Flexion and extension of the elbow	...	...
5. Lateral grasp. A paper is held between the thumb and the lateral side of the second finger. The thumb must be extended and abducted	...	...	3. Extension and flexion of the knee	...	...
6. Pinch grasp. A pen is held between the thumb and second finger	...	...	4. Dorsi- and plantar, flexion of the ankle with the knee extended	...	...
7. Cylindrical grasp. A drinking glass is held with the thumb and the second finger opposing each other	...	...	Maximum score, Part B	12 +	12
8. Spherical grasp. A tennis ball is held with the fingers abducted and flexed around the ball	...	...	Maximum score, Part A + Part B	105	+105
Maximum score	24	+24	Maximum score, both sides together		210
Maximum score, upper extremity	57	+57			

	Score 0–3			Score 0–3	

Funtional capacity after stroke — motor assessment chart

Part C: Mobility	P	NP	Part D: Balance	P	NP
1. Supine to right lateral	...	...	1. Sitting without support	...	...
2. Supine to left lateral	...	...	2. Protective reactions — right side. The patient is blindfolded and pushed towards the right side	...	...
3. Supine to sitting upon on the edge of the bed	...	...			
4. Sitting on the edge of the bed to supine	...	...	3. Protective reactions — the left side. The patient, blind folded, is pushed towards the left side	...	...
5. Sitting to standing up	...	...			
6. Sitting down from standing up	...	...	4. Standing with support	...	...
7. Sitting with feet supported. Leaning forward and touching the feet	...	...	5. Standing without support	...	...
8. Walking score (0–6)	...	...	6. Standing on right leg	...	...
			7. Standing on left leg	...	...
Maximum score: Mobility = 21 and walking = 6	27	27	Maximum score	21	21

Footnotes to table

P, paretic side; NP, non-paretic side; p, points

Scoring

Mobility
0 = cannot perform the activity
1 = can perform the activity with much help
2 = can perform the activity with little help
3 = can perform the activity without help

Protective reactions
0 = no reactions
1 = only slight reactions
2 = clumsy or slow protective reactions
3 = normal reactions

Walking
0 = cannot walk
1 = a few steps with help of 2 persons
2 = can walk with the help of 1 person
3 = can walk with crutches, tetrapod, Moray
4 = can walk with one stick or crutch
5 = walks slowly or limps without aid
6 = walks at normal speed for his/her age

Standing with support
0 = cannot stand even with support
1 = can stand with strong support of 2 persons
2 = can stand with moderate support of one person
3 = can stand with only slight support of one hand

Standing without support
0 = cannot stand without support
1 = can stand without support for 10 sec
2 = can stand without support for 1 min
3 = can stand > 1 min while performing arm movements above shoulder level

Standing on one leg
0 = cannot stand on one leg
1 = can stand for a few sec
2 = can stand for longer than 5 sec
3 = can stand on one leg for > 10 sec

goals of rehabilitation, for therapeutic planning and for adjustment of treatment in accordance with the patient's recovery. An assessment chart with well defined numerical scores enables the physician to compare the patient's ability at different stages.

The mean age of patients suffering with stroke is 75 years, and of course patients of that age will frequently suffer from other motor disturbances. It is therefore advantageous to assess both sides, rather than just the hemiplegic side.

Selective movements, rather than power of different isolated muscle groups, should be assessed because the problem in these patients is a lack of motor control. These movements are chosen so that they reflect the patient's difficulties and possible progress as it follows a regular pattern. Disturbed balance, loss of sensation, pain and limited range of motion may also affect the motor function and impair the patient's ability to perform qualitatively well coordinated movements.

The functions investigated are the ability to perform active movements, rapid movement changes, gross mobility, walking, balance, sensation, passive range of motion, and pain. Table 27.4 may be helpful. Parts A and B of the table together give the motor function score, with a maximum of 105 points for each side of the body, and 210 points for the whole body. Part C is used for assessment of gross motor function and walking. Part D assesses seven activities concerning body balance.

The functional autonomy measurement system (SMAF)

This instrument, based on the WHO's classification of impairments, disabilities and handicaps, was developed for measuring the needs of the elderly and the handicapped (Table 27.5). It uses a 4-level measurement scale, and quantifies a subject's performance of 29 functions in 5 sectors of activity, but for each function the evaluator must also estimate available resources to compensate for any identified disability in order to estimate the handicap. The profile obtained is the basis for the prescription of home care or the allocation of chronic care beds. It takes an average of 42 minutes to administer but the reliability is not influenced by training, so that it is reliable for evaluators from different professions in the community, and the primary health care team.

The number of levels may be thought to be high, but this increases the sensitivity and avoids the centripetal result of choosing a mean level. The autonomy rating scale enables the evaluator to verify for each function how the patient's social and material

Table 27.5 List of items from the autonomy rating scale and their relation to the WHO's classification of disabilities

SMAF items	WHO's classification of disabilities	
	Section	Disabilities
Activities of daily living		
Eating	30	Personal
Bathing		dexterity
Dressing	60	
Grooming		
Urinary continence		
Faecal continence		
Using the bathroom		
Mobility		
Transfers	40	Locomotor
Walking inside		
Walking outside		
Putting on prosthesis or orthosis		
Moving around in a wheelchair		
Using the stairs		
Communication		
Seeing	20	Locomotor
Hearing		
Talking		
Mental functions		
Memory	10	Behaviour
Orientation		
Understanding		
Judgement		
Behaviour		
Instrumental activities of daily living		
Cleaning the house	50	Body disposition
Preparing meals		
Shopping		
Doing the laundry		
Using the 'phone		
Using public transport		
Taking medication		
Managing the budget		

Level 0 = complete autonomy
Level 1 = requires surveillance or stimulation
Level 2 = requires help
Level 3 = total dependence

resources compensate for disability. Thus, by weighing disabilities against resources the handicap rating can be scored, so that a score of minus 3 for being unable to use the stairs may be converted to zero once a stair lift has been installed. There is no absolute standard for disability measurement but this method has been found to be very effective in practice by providing the clinician with an evaluative tool that can be used for home care, for the allocation of chronic care beds, for setting care plans for health workers or for the management of services in community and institutional settings.

ASSESSMENT FOR MOBILITY ALLOWANCE

Claimants for the Assessment and Mobility Allowance must be aged between 5 and 75 years and the claim must be made before the 66th birthday. It is paid regardless of income, savings and National Insurance contributions and is a tax-free cash benefit designed to assist those unable or virtually unable to walk. It can be paid on top of other benefits, including Income Support, and can be the key to other services such as the Orange Badge Scheme and exemption from road tax.

The medical examination consists of answering questions concerning observation of the distance and terrain over which the claimant walked, the condition after the test, the gait, balance while walking, help or guidance needed, the speed of walking and how far the claimant would be able to walk out of doors without severe discomfort. Also considered are basic disorders giving rise to lack of ability to walk, the prognosis, and the patient's awareness of these facts.

The examination asks for height, weight, mode of arrival at the examination, attendance at hospital or training centre and the details of aids, appliances or artificial limbs. The examiner is required to take the pulse rate, blood pressure and perform a urine test for blood, sugar and albumen and to record the exact nature of any physical or mental abnormality, and its incidence. Newly introduced features include the assessment of the degree of hearing and eyesight loss insofar as they might relate to mobility. The examining doctor is then asked to give an opinion on walking ability using any prosthesis or orthosis.

Other social security benefits for which a disabled person may be eligible are:

1. Income Support;
2. Attendance Allowance;
3. Industrial Injuries Disablement Benefit;
4. Invalid Care Allowance;
5. Severe Disablement Allowance;
6. Crisis Loans;
7. Cold Weather Payment;
8. Social Fund.

REFERENCES

Lindmark B, Hamrin E 1988 Evaluation of functional capacity after stroke as a basis for active intervention. Scandinavian Journal of Rehabilitation Medicine 20: 103–109

Tinetti M 1986 Performance-orientated assessment of mobility problems in elderly patients. Journal of the American Geriatric Society 34: 119–126

28. Early detection and management of bladder and urological disorders

Peter Ellis

INTRODUCTION

The common urological disorders that affect elderly patients are incontinence of urine, urinary tract infections and prostatic disease; less common but also important is bladder neoplasm. While in some instances patients consult with symptoms, in others they do not.

Does the general practitioner have a role in screening patients in later years for bladder problems? Should the GP look for asymptomatic disease, seeking symptoms about which patients either are unconcerned or over which they have decided not to seek medical help?

GPs can try to identify disease early by their availability, clinical competence, skills in communication and attitude (features that, not surprisingly, were noted among the hallmarks of a good GP during assessment (Royal College of General Practitioners 1985)).

Of course, early detection of some conditions will be aided by screening in general practice.

Screening

Screening involves seeking out people with no overt symptoms of disease and asking them to undergo examination and tests to see whether the condition to be identified is present (DHSS 1976). Screening can be carried out opportunistically when the elderly patient presents to the GP or in specialised clinics run for the elderly. Each method has its advantages and a combination of both may be appropriate.

Opportunistic screening

Although possible in every general practice consultation (Stott & Davis 1979), opportunistic screening may sometimes be difficult for the doctor, for the patient and for the doctor–patient relationship (see Chapter 9). However, some people will not want to attend an organised 'elderly screening' session and, for such people, opportunistic screening is valuable.

Screening clinics

Where screening sessions are organised they may involve the GP or other member of the primary health care team, such as an attached health visitor or district nurse, or perhaps an employed practice nurse. Multiphasic screening has become popular, but scientific proof of benefit does not exist and such screening has not been shown to be cost-effective in the elderly. It also raises problems of resource allocation (Williamson et al 1987).

Complementary to screening for asymptomatic disease is the search for symptomatic disease already affecting the patient. Older people may fail to seek appropriate help and certainly some non-reporting exists (Williamson et al 1964). This appears to apply particularly to such conditions as chronic joint disease, foot problems and problems of the bladder (mainly prostatism and incontinence). Older people seem to consider that it is not worth bringing these problems to their GP's attention, perhaps because of little perceived prospect of benefit. There are claims that non-reporting is no longer significant but all practising clinicians must be aware that some disabilities come to light only at an advanced stage.

Surveillance of the elderly includes planned detection of established disability and detection of social problems. There are clearly problems deciding who will carry out these activities and also problems deciding how to share and pool any information gained with other primary care workers and client groups. It is also necessary to decide which group of old people are at risk. Postal questionnaires have been used as one method of identifying vulnerable groups (Barber et al 1980).

Primary and secondary care

The GP is the appropriate person to decide how far to investigate a particular symptom in an individual patient. The GP can be truly 'holistic' — thinking of the entire person and their relationship with the community — and needs to be aware of, receptive to, and certainly not dismissive of the patient's needs. GPs also need to know how secondary care resources match an individual's expectations.

Identification of disease, by whatever method, is important. Bladder disorders feature high, as shown in the studies of incontinence described later.

The management of bladder and urological disorders within primary care will depend on the expertise of the GP and the primary health care team. It will also depend on the resources available to the primary care worker. Furthermore, the interest and expertise of the secondary care services in the locality will influence when and how a referral is made.

Consideration of longer-term surveillance is important. Some hospital-based clinicians deal with long-term surveillance by tolerating tediously long out-patient clinics, with patients having to endure a long wait every 6 months or a year. Other secondary care clinicians arrange postal follow-up of patients and others discharge patients back to their GPs. This last option can be effective only if the standard of primary care is known to the secondary care clinicians, and if arrangements are made to ease re-referral when necessary.

INCONTINENCE

Prevalence

The most common bladder disorder in the later years is urinary incontinence, a condition in which involuntary loss of urine is a social or hygienic problem, and is objectively demonstrable (Hilton 1987). The actual prevalence of incontinence is difficult to define. A study by the Medical Research Council (Thomas et al 1980) showed a high prevalence of unrecognised incontinence, and it is thought that about 15% of elderly men and 20% of elderly women are sufferers.

Incontinence can result in rejection by carers and the prevalence among geriatric in-patients is higher than the average — 30–40% in some surveys (Scorgie 1983). Every general practice list will include around 15 elderly people at home with significant incontinence; fewer than 10% of these receive any specialist help (Ellis & McRoberts 1988). The majority of incontinence is unknown to the GP or the district nurse (Smith 1988a), partly because incontinence is a profound social handicap associated with shame and embarrassment.

Patients with stroke are a particular risk group and their rehabilitation is often constrained by incontinence (Currie 1986).

The GP, district nurse or health visitor visiting an elderly person at home should be alert to clues relating to incontinence — sheets being washed, chairs wet, smells lingering.

Assessment

Once a patient presents with incontinence, or is noted by screening or case-finding to be incontinent, the GP is often unsure how to proceed (Mandlestam 1983). It must be stressed that incontinence is a symptom (Ellis & McRoberts 1988) and should be investigated. However, the degree of investigation will vary with the patient, the practitioner and the clinical setting.

Traditionally, the symptoms of urinary incontinence are described by the terms stress, urge and continuous. Urodynamic assessment is sometimes advocated to allow more reliable diagnosis and appropriate treatment (Hilton 1987).

It is often useful for GPs to think of the causes of incontinence in terms of reversible, partially reversible and irreversible incontinence (Ellis 1985).

Reversible causes include environmental, mechanical, infective and iatrogenic causes, and reversible incontinence may also be caused by diuretics and illness (Table 28.1).

Partially reversible causes include sphincter weakness and detrusor instability.

Irreversible causes include dementia, postprostatectomy and neurogenic bladder.

Table 28.1   Reversible causes of incontinence

Environmental
   Positioning of toilet, stairs, warmth

Mechanical
   Faecal impaction, prostatic hypertrophy, bladder neck obstruction, urethral prolapse, mobility problems

Infective
   Urinary tract infections, toxic confusional state, vaginitis

Iatrogenic
   Diuretics, sedation, anticholinergic drugs

Diuresis
   Glycosuria, excess fluid intake

Illness
   Non-specific illness in the elderly

The initial assessment includes a detailed history, physical examination, urinalysis and the recording of the patient's toilet habits, using incontinence charts. It is important to assess the patient's mobility, dexterity, the toilet facilities and social circumstances. This assessment is ideally made by the GP and district nurse together, and in many health authorities the primary health care team can receive advice from a specialist nurse continence adviser.

The history needs to include fluid intake, alcohol consumption, drug history (especially sedatives, diuretics, anticholinergic and sympathomimetic drugs), the site of the toilet and problems getting there. Details of duration, onset and circumstances of incontinence are important. Stress incontinence is associated characteristically with coughing or sneezing. Nocturnal incontinence may be due to mobility problems.

A general examination should be performed. Incontinence may be precipitated in the vulnerable elderly person by medical, neurological, psychiatric, pelvic and environmental problems, as well as urological problems.

Examination needs to be made for a palpable bladder, as urinary retention due to prostatic hypertrophy or faecal impaction can lead to overflow incontinence. Rectal examination is necessary for assessment of prostatic and faecal impaction. Examination of the female external genitalia will show signs of vaginitis or urethral prolapse. Urinalysis must be performed to look for glycosuria and infection. If haematuria is found, consideration should be given to radiological investigation and to referral for cystoscopy.

The GP, district nurse and continence adviser should together assess the degree and cause of incontinence and should formulate a realistic management plan (Hilton 1987). Palliative measures, including personal hygiene, skin care and incontinence garments, are important.

Reversible causes of incontinence should be identified and treated appropriately. The partially reversible may be rather more difficult and may require specialised techniques. The referral pattern will depend on the interests of the primary and secondary care clinicians and their respective teams. Referral to secondary care may result in various investigations including urodynamics.

Urodynamic studies

Urodynamics should not be routine in the elderly but can be of use in appropriate cases (Scorgie, 1983).

Some clinicians advocate a simple regime of appropriate therapeutic trials. This would first exclude infection, also exclude vaginal, rectal and abdominal abnormality and exclude stress symptoms, and then would treat the patient as having an unstable bladder (Hilton & Stanton 1981). Where stress incontinence is the main complaint the patient is given pelvic floor exercises for a 3-5 month trial period. Intravaginal oestrogen can be used in postmenopausal women. In patients with mixed symptoms it may then be realistic to assume detrusor instability and give a therapeutic trial of an anticholinergic agent.

Some areas have keen, caring secondary care physicians who undertake urodynamic studies that allow the cause of incontinence to be more clearly defined (Mundy 1989) and this has led to improvements in treatment. Three main types of incontinence are identified by urodynamic studies:

1. Extra-sphincteric causes, e.g. vesicovaginal fistula.
2. Non-neuropathic causes — including stress and urge incontinence, reduced awareness, postprostatectomy, and hypnotic drugs.
3. Neuropathic causes, as in diabetes and parkinsonism.

Stress and urge incontinence are common in clinical practice. Stress incontinence is usually due to sphincteric weakness but urge incontinence can be due to a motor urge — detrusor instability — or sensory urgency due to urinary tract infection, bladder stone and other causes. Stress incontinence is best treated by pelvic floor exercises but there is the possibility of surgical treatment, and oestrogens can be helpful for atrophic vaginitis/urethritis.

Urge incontinence can be treated with anticholinergic drugs, e.g. propantheline or terodiline. Flavoxate is a smooth muscle relaxant and is sometimes of use. Prostaglandin synthetase inhibitors such as flurbiprofen are sometimes beneficial and calcium antagonists have been used.

Irreversible incontinence

A number of patients remain incontinent and the primary health care team can help make things more manageable. Regular toileting, perhaps on a 2-hourly daytime basis, with late night and early morning toileting, is sometimes helpful. Incontinence that still persists can be managed by appliances to enable the patients to live with dignity. There is a range of appliances and they should be chosen with an individual in mind. Absorption garments, collection devices and catheters all need to be considered. Attention must be given to the person's capabilities and the type of incontinence.

Absorption garments, such as pads and pants, are available for men and women (Smith, 1988b). Special sheets are available, and there may be a local Incontinence Service. Collection devices, such as condom drainage systems, can be suitable for some male patients. For both male and female, an indwelling catheter will sometimes be appropriate (Belfield 1988). However, the hazards of ascending infection should be borne in mind — this problem can be largely avoided in selected patients by recourse to intermittent self-catheterization.

Certainly, the majority of women reporting incontinence can be diagnosed by a GP and improved by appropriate intervention (Jolleys 1989).

URINARY TRACT INFECTIONS

Many elderly patients present with symptoms of dysuria and frequency. Some have nocturia or haematuria. The incidence of nocturia rises with age and women over 70 normally have to void at night (Cardozo 1986). Infection may be associated with residual urine in the bladder. This may be associated with prostatism in men, but it can be easy to miss a large residual urine on clinical examination in an elderly lady. Urine must be tested for sugar and examined for infection — stick testing for nitrites and leucocytes, if positive, may indicate the need for laboratory culture. Haematuria should probably be examined further, as should sterile pyuria if this is genuine and not due to previous antibiotic use or to contamination of urine samples. Urinary tract infection also needs to be considered in elderly patients presenting with a toxic confusional state, or if any elderly person 'goes off' non-specifically.

Infection, if shown to be present in a urine sample, by whatever criteria (Lipsky et al 1987), should be treated appropriately, although there are no clear guidelines about the necessary length of treatment.

Some would advocate that men with urinary tract infection should be investigated because urological abnormalities are likely to be present. Treatment for 2 weeks may be necessary in men (Gower 1989).

Repeated urinary tract infection may be a reason for referral to an interested secondary care urologist or geriatrician. Sometimes medication, such as regular long-term prophylactic antibiotics may be appropriate for symptomatic repeated urinary tract infection. There is usually no need for long-term surveillance in secondary care.

Prevalence of *asymptomatic* bacteriuria increases with age, approaching 1 in 4 in men over the age of 70, and is even more common in patients living in institutions (Gower 1989). Predisposing factors include prostatic hypertrophy, urinary tract instrumentation and catheterisation, dementia and concurrent infections, such as pneumonia. Routine antimicrobial treatment, short or long-term, is not justified in patients with asymptomatic bacteriuria.

Whilst maintaining an awareness of the possibility of urinary tract infections in an elderly person, there would seem to be no reason for screening the well-elderly for infection of the urinary tract.

PROSTATISM

Whilst prostatic hypertrophy can cause incontinence and be associated with urinary infection, the majority of elderly male patients seeing a urologist have prostatism.

The patient will again have come to see his GP with symptoms, or the early symptoms of prostatism will have been picked up during planned or opportunistic screening. The GP will then take a history and perform an examination, which should include the bladder, genitalia and the rectum. Some patients will be investigated further in primary care before referral to a urologist for assessment. Unfortunately, some further investigations, e.g. X-ray examination carried out at the request of GP, will prove to be a waste of time and money (Bransby-Zachary & Sutherland 1989). Patient investigation is an important part of the work of a GP (Kelly & Barber 1988), but there is a likelihood of duplication and X-rays are sometimes not available when the patient is seen at an out-patient clinic.

The timing of referral will depend on the doctor, the patient, the symptoms and hospital policy. Various treatment options are now possible, but operative transurethral resection is probably the best method of managing patients who need treatment for benign prostatic hypertrophy (Chisholm 1989).

BLADDER CANCER

The average GP can expect to see one new bladder tumour every 3 years. The great majority of such tumours are transitional cell carcinomas, and most present with haematuria. Before macroscopic haematuria occurs, there is a phase of microscopic haematuria, during which testing of urine with dipsticks may lead to a diagnosis.

Groups at particular risk are workers in certain occupations — particularly those who have been in contact with aniline dyes and certain other substances. The surveillance of these groups is covered by statute, and may include regular cytological urine examination.

Bladder tumours in the general population are almost confined to the elderly. Is there a case for routine screening of this group?

In a study by Britton et al (1989), 578 patients aged 60–85 had their urine tested for blood using dipsticks. Of these, 132 (23%) were positive and 87 of these were investigated. 45 (52%) of those investigated had urological abnormalities, although only four had tumours. The predictive value of a positive test was therefore a very disappointing 0.03. Although the study provides no evidence as to sensitivity, it should be remembered that haematuria may be intermittent.

Routine dipstick testing is a blunt instrument, and would generate a large number of patients requiring further investigation — probably in the form of flexible cystoscopy. Furthermore, although bladder tumours are amenable to treatment, there seems at present to be little evidence that detection at the stage of microscopic haematuria results in increased survival, beyond the expected lead-time effect (Plail 1990).

Although it is, of course, essential to follow up any finding of microscopic haematuria made on routine testing, the arguments for population screening at present appear less than compelling.

SUMMARY

GPs have an important role in the early detection of incontinence and other urological disorders in patients of later years and they can certainly make a welcome contribution to the well-being of these patients. Every primary care worker needs to have a positive and caring attitude enabling problems to be discovered and managed appropriately.

REFERENCES

Barber J H, Willis J B, McKeating E 1980 A postal screening questionnaire in preventive geriatric care. Journal of the Royal College of General Practitioners 30:49

Belfield P W 1988 Urinary catheters. British Medical Journal 296: 836–837

Bransby-Zachary M A P, Sutherland G R 1989 Unnecessary X-ray examinations. British Medical Journal 298: 1294

Britton J P, Dowell A C, Whelan P 1989 Dipstick haematuria and bladder cancer in men over 60: results of a community study. British Medical Journal 299: 1010–1012

Cardozo L 1986 Urinary frequency and urgency. British Medical Journal 293: 1419–1923

Chisholm G D 1989 Benign prostatic hyperplasia: the best treatment. British Medical Journal 299: 215–216

Currie C T 1986 Urinary incontinence after stroke. British Medical Journal 293: 1322–1323

DHSS 1976 Prevention and health: everybody's business. HMSO, London

Ellis P 1985 Urinary incontinence in the elderly. The Physician 4: 525–526

Ellis P McRoberts A 1988 Management of urinary incontinence by the primary health care team. Update 36: 2521–2525

Gower P E 1989 Urinary tract infection in men. British Medical Journal 298: 1595–1596

Hilton P, Stanton S L 1981 Algorithmic method for assessing urinary incontinence in elderly women. British Medical Journal 282: 940–942

Hilton P 1987 Urinary incontinence in women. British Medical Journal 295: 426–432

Jolleys J V 1989 Diagnosis and management of female urinary incontinence in general practice. Journal of the Royal College of General Practitioners 39: 277–279

Kelly M H, Barber J H 1988 Use of laboratory services and communication of results to patients in an urban practice: an audit. Journal of the Royal College of General Practitioners 38: 64–66

Lipsky B A, Ireton F C, Fiton S D et al 1987 Diagnosis of bacteriuria in men: specimen collection and culture interpretation. Journal of Infectious Diseases 155: 847–54

Mandlestam D A 1983 Aids for the incontinent. Update 27: 1107–1114

Mundy A R 1989 Incontinence. Update 969–976

Plail R 1990 Detecting bladder cancer. British Medical Journal 301: 567–568

Royal College of General Practitioners, 1985 Report from General Practice 23, What sort of doctor? Royal College of General Practitioners, London

Scorgie R 1983 Incontinence. The Physician. November: 344–346

Smith N K G 1988a Continence advisory services in England. Health Trends 20: 22–23

Smith N 1988b Aids for urinary incontinence. British Medical Journal 296: 772–773

Stott N C H, Davis R H 1979 The exceptional potential in each primary care consultation. Journal of the Royal College of General Practitioners 29: 201–205

Thomas T M, Plymat K, Blannin J, Meade T W 1980 Prevalence of urinary incontinence. British Medical Journal 281: 1242–45

Williamson J, Stokoe I H Gray S et al 1964 Old people at home: their unreported needs. Lancet i: 1117–20

Williamson J, Smith R G, Burley L E 1987 Primary care of the elderly: a practical approach. John Wright, Bristol

29. Gastrointestinal disorders

Roger Jones

INTRODUCTION

Disorders of the gastrointestinal tract account for 8–10% of consultations with general practitioners; about half of these consultations are due to digestive disorders related to the upper gastrointestinal tract, with most of the remainder being due to disturbances in large bowel function. Although the majority of patients presenting in general practice will turn out to have relatively minor and self-limiting conditions, inflammatory and neoplastic disease still have major implications for morbidity and mortality. Peptic ulceration and its complications, for example, account for about 10% of acute hospital admissions and gastrointestinal haemorrhage carries a mortality rate of approximately 10%. The socio-economic consequences of uncomplicated peptic ulcer disease are also considerable. Colorectal cancer is responsible for almost 20 000 deaths each year and is the second most common cause of death from cancer in the UK. Gastric cancer is common, with over 12 000 registrations annually in England alone. The majority of gastric cancers occur in the age range 65–79 years and the incidence of colorectal cancer also increases sharply with age. It is because of this distribution that this Chapter falls into the section of the book dealing mainly with the elderly, although it should be emphasized that much of what follows is also applicable to younger age groups.

The investigation and treatment of gastrointestinal disorders in general practice also have substantial resource consequences. The technology used to provide imaging of the upper and lower gastrointestinal tract is expensive, as are the widely prescribed ulcer-healing agents used to treat peptic ulcer disease.

Although the natural history and epidemiology of many important gastrointestinal conditions are becoming clearer, causative agents and risk factors associated with the development of inflammatory and neoplastic disorders of the gut are still being sought. This means that preventive strategies for many of these conditions

are difficult to establish. Similarly, appropriate and acceptable screening techniques for many of these conditions are, with a number of important exceptions, not yet available.

However, the present state of knowledge does enable us to identify certain groups in whom clinical suspicion of the presence of serious organic gastrointestinal disease should be heightened and others in whom screening and secondary and tertiary prevention are appropriate.

OESOPHAGEAL DISORDERS

The oesophagus is emerging as an important organ in terms of the spectrum of digestive disorders encountered in general practice. Peptic oesophagitis is the most common endoscopic abnormality recorded in patients referred for investigation (Jones 1986), while motility disturbances of the oesophagus are an important cause of non-cardiac chest pain, so that specialised oesophageal laboratories are being established in which manometry and pH measurements can be performed. Although relatively rare, carcinoma of the oesophagus remains an important disorder, although one generally diagnosed only when advanced disease produces troublesome symptoms.

Benign oesophageal conditions

Reflux of gastric and duodenal contents, including bile, into the oesophagus produces inflammation, ulceration and eventual fibrosis and stricture formation. The precise nature of the lower oesophageal sphincter mechanism remains controversial; significant reflux can occur without the presence of a hiatus hernia and significant symptoms are often accompanied by relatively normal endoscopic appearances. Under these circumstances, oesophageal biopsy and pH and manometric studies are frequently required to confirm the diagnosis. There is little scope for screening or primary prevention for peptic oesophagitis, although once the condition has been diagnosed, prevention of complications becomes important. Appropriate dietary advice, encouragement of weight loss and instructions concerning posture at mealtimes and at rest are of importance. Although patients with typical reflux symptoms, which respond adequately to conventional acid-suppressing therapy, may not require early investigation, those with persistent or recurrent symptoms, and certainly patients in whom there is any suspicion of dysphagia, merit endoscopic evaluation with a view to identifying severe oesophageal damage, leading to fibrosis and stricture formation.

An important complication of gastro-oesophageal reflux disease is the development of the so-called Barrett's oesophagus, in which part of the oesophagus becomes lined with columnar epithelium. This may be found at endoscopy in as many as 16% of patients with established reflux oesophagitis and a small proportion of these patients, between 8 and 15%, will go on to develop adenocarcinoma. The presence of dysplasia in oesophageal biopsies in columnar epithelium is an indication for endoscopic surveillance, although the workload implications of these recommendations are considerable. It has been calculated, for example, that with yearly endoscopy, 77 examinations would be required to detect one adenocarcinoma. However, this approach has the potential advantage that cancers might be detected at the presymptomatic stage, when surgery is more likely to be curative. Recent work suggests that DNA analysis using flow cytometry may offer hope of more reliable predictability of malignant change in columnar epithelium in the oesophagus (Atkinson 1989).

Cancer of the oesophagus

Mortality from oesophageal cancer appears to be rising, with registrations increasing by 2% per annum during the last decade. There are almost 4000 cases of the disease each year in the UK, which means that in a practice of 2500, one new case is likely to be seen every 4 years. The incidence increases sharply with age and is almost twice as great in men as in women. A number of risk factors for oesophageal cancer have been identified. In western countries the major risk factors are cigarette smoking, which increases the risk by a factor of at least two, and alcohol consumption, which is responsible for the excess incidence of oesophageal cancer in Northern France. In other, non-European, populations oesophageal cancer is much more common and more specific risk factors seem to

be at work. For example, in the South African homeland state of Transkei, cancer of the oesophagus accounts for up to 20% of all adult deaths. The disease is also common on the shores of the Caspian Sea in northern Iran and in the Henan and Shanxi provinces of China. A factor linking the high incidence of oesophageal cancer is these areas seems to be a diet rich in cereal and poor in fresh fruit and vegetables, with deficiencies in riboflavin and vitamins A and C. There also appear to be trace element deficiencies in the soil of these areas, particularly of zinc and molybdenum. The Xhosa people in the Transkei ferment the dietary maize to make Xhosa beer, which contains a high concentration of nitrosamines. These substances are also present in high levels in Xhosa tobacco, which is absorbed not only by smoking but also by the local habit of swallowing the hot juices, injonga, from the stems of tobacco pipes (Sagar 1989).

For the general practitioner working in the UK, modification of alcohol and smoking habits appears to offer the only realistic scope for prevention; patients with gastro-oesophageal reflux disease who also have these additional risk factors should be regarded as a group at particular risk of developing oesophageal cancer. In the regions of China where the incidence of the disease is particularly high, brush biopsy endoscopic techniques have been introduced to attempt early diagnosis.

PEPTIC ULCERATION

Dyspeptic complaints are extremely common, both in the community and in general practitioners' surgeries. The 6-month period prevalence of significant dyspepsia in the general population is about 40% and approximately one-quarter of these patients will seek medical advice for their symptoms (Jones 1989). General practitioners are faced with real difficulties in making decisions about investigating patients with dyspepsia, because only a small proportion of all dyspeptic patterns seen in general practice will turn out to have organic lesions of the stomach and duodenum to account for their symptoms, with the remainder having so-called non-ulcer dyspepsia, in many cases related to dysmotility of the gastro-intestinal tract. Studies performed in endoscopy and radiology departments have, however, yielded guidelines, which should enable us to divide dyspeptic patients into those at low risk of having organic disease and those at relatively high risk and requiring early investigation. Patients' age is the most important factor, with peptic ulceration and cancer being uncommon under the age of 50.

Male sex and smoking add to the likelihood of the presence of peptic ulcer disease, as does a previous history of peptic ulceration. Clinical features are surprisingly unhelpful, both in determining the presence of ulceration or, indeed, its site. Although night pain is a fairly strong predictive factor for the presence of duodenal ulceration, the correlation between clinical diagnosis and endoscopic diagnosis is surprisingly poor, so that patients with risk factors require investigation to establish the site and nature of the predicted lesion (Heatley & Rathbone 1987, Colin-Jones 1988, Williams et al 1988).

Gastric and duodenal ulcer are both common conditions throughout Europe, with duodenal ulcer being consistently two to three times more common. However, the epidemiology of these conditions has been constantly changing over the last 100 years. At the end of the nineteenth century gastric ulcer was the predominant peptic lesion in Britain and at this time was mainly a disease of young women. The prevalence of duodenal ulcer disease began to increase at about the time of the First World War and over the last 50 years it has become much more common than gastric ulcer in most areas. It seems that duodenal ulcer disease reached a peak in the 1950s and, long before the introduction of histamine(H$_2$) receptor antagonists, its prevalence began to decline slowly.

Changes have also occurred in the complication rates of peptic ulcer disease; perforation rates in men have fallen substantially and bleeding has replaced perforation as the major complication. Perhaps the most important change of all has been the emergence of elderly women taking non-steroidal anti-inflammatory agents as the group at particular risk of the complications of peptic ulceration (Walt et al 1986). The prescribing rate for these drugs in older women is quite alarming, with prescriptions now approaching 1400 scripts per 1000 women per year. The complication rate in terms of number of prescriptions written for the whole population is rather low – about one in every 3000 prescriptions for women over 60 and one in 20 000 prescriptions for those under 60 — but because over 24 million prescriptions for NSAIDs are written every year, the size of the problem is considerable. As well as evidence from hospital admission studies, there are also suggestions that sudden death due to gastrointestinal haemorrhage in elderly people may also be linked to NSAID ingestion.

Prevalence and mortality rates for peptic ulcers are higher in smokers than in non-smokers and both types of ulcer have a raised incidence in patients of blood group O and in non-secretors. There also seems to be a link between peptic ulcer disease and coffee intake and a recent study suggests that the temperature at which caffeine-containing beverages are taken may be important, with peptic ulcer patients preferring significantly hotter drinks that normal controls (Pearson & McCloy 1989). Education about the harmful effects of smoking is at present likely to offer the only major preventive strategy, but an awareness of the dangers of non-steroidal anti-inflammatory prescribing, particularly in older women, is of great importance.

Early detection and treatment of peptic ulcer disease might be achieved by earlier investigation of appropriate patients; providing open access to upper gastrointestinal endoscopy may be one way of doing this. There is evidence that such diagnostic services are used effectively by general practitioners (Jones 1985) although their impact on morbidity and mortality remains uncertain.

CANCER OF THE STOMACH

Gastric cancer is now the second most common cause of cancer death in males in the United Kingdom and the fourth in women, after breast, colon and bronchus. Age is an important determinant, with 60% of cases occurring in the age range 65–79 years. There is also a marked social class gradient in gastric cancer incidence, with the standardised mortality rate in social class 5 being three times that in social class 1; this is a probable explanation for the geographical variations in cancer rates observed, with high rates in the north of England and in Wales. Gastric cancer is responsible for 10% of all cancer deaths in the United Kingdom. Three new cases will be seen in a list of 2500 patients every 4 years. A number of risk factors have now been identified, with a unifying hypothesis being that dietary nitrate, which is converted to nitrite by bacterial action, leads to the production of nitrosamines which, as in oesophageal cancer, are carcinogenic. The incidence of the disease is particularly high in areas where rich nitrate deposits occur in the soil, which may explain the high incidence in some South American countries. A similar association with the nitrate content of drinking water has also been demonstrated. The chemical preservation of food also involves the use of nitrates and the high incidence of gastric cancer in Japan, in which pickled and cured food is widely consumed, is probably linked to this. A recent decline in incidence rates in western countries may be partly explained by the use of refrigeration rather than chemical methods of food preservation. Case control studies suggest that the consumption of fresh vegetables and milk may protect against gastric cancer, possibly by inhibition of the conversion of nitrites to nitrosamines. There is also a four-fold increase in the risk of gastric cancer in achlorhydric conditions, such as atrophic gastritis and pernicious anaemia, and in patients who have had partial gastrectomies for duodenal ulcer. The absence of gastric acid encourages nitrosamine production from ingested nitrate. Early fears that H_2 receptor antagonists, by producing profound suppression of gastric acid secretion, might contribute to this process, have subsequently been shown to be unfounded (Colin-Jones et al 1988). Other risk factors exist, including cigarette smoking and red wine consumption. The disease is also more common in coal miners and in workers in the metal and rubber industries.

The clinical course of gastric cancer remains depressing. In a recent review of gastric cancers treated over a 25-year period, from 1957 to 1981, 79% of patients presented with stage 4 disease and less than 1% were found to have stage 1 disease at presentation (Allum et al 1989). The resulting curative resection rate was only 21%, with high operative mortality rates. Overall, age-adjusted 5-year survival was only 5%; 5-year survival for stage 1, 2 and 3 disease was 72%, 32% and 10% respectively.

Prevention and early detection of gastric cancer in the UK remain elusive goals. Changes in food preservation and diet seem to have had some impact on the incidence of the disease, but the use of chemical fertilisers containing nitrate is unlikely to change for the foreseeable future. Although patients with achlorhydric states are at greater risk of malignant change, there is no agreement about appropriate screening or surveillance strategies for them.

The poor prognosis, linked to presentation at a late histopathological stage, of gastric cancer in the UK has led to suggestions that dyspeptic patients should receive much earlier investigation in the hope of detecting early disease. This recommendation is based partly on experience in Japan, where gastric cancers affect 10% of men. In this population, early diagnosis using endoscopic screening and gastrocamera techniques, has resulted in the discovery of substantial numbers of early gastric cancers, confined to the submucosa. Cure rates of up to 90% have been reported in these patients. There is a real question, however, about whether the natural history of gastric cancer is the same in the UK as it is in Japan. Very few early gastric cancers are discovered, even opportunistically, at the time of investigation for other indications; a substantial increase in the number of dyspeptic patients submitted to endoscopy would create an unsustainable workload on gastroenterology units and the pick-up rate of early, curative lesions remains a subject for speculation.

COLORECTAL CANCER

In 1983, there were 24 000 recorded new cases of large bowel cancer in the UK, making it the second most common cancer in men, after carcinoma of the lung, and the second most common in women after cancer of the breast. Colorectal cancer accounts for 15% of all cancers detected in western Europe and North America. More than two cases will occur annually in a list of 2500 patients. The highest incidence of the disease is found in the USA and although most western countries have a high incidence, the disease is uncommon in Japan, Asia, Africa and in most of South America. The 5 year survival rate remains low, at about 30%, although this is directly linked to the histopathological stage of the cancer at the time of treatment. The incidence of the disease increases sharply with age and is marginally higher in women until the age of 60 years, but a little higher in men thereafter. The incidence of the disease in migrants coming from countries with a low disease incidence changes very rapidly, faster than for any cancer other than that of the skin.

There is growing evidence that diet is the most important exogenous factor in the aetiology of bowel cancer and that other factors such as genetic disposition are of relatively minor importance. The disease is one of developed societies and most epidemiological work has demonstrated a clear link between large bowel cancer and a diet with a high beef and fat intake. One possibility is that fat intake stimulates the release of bile acids, which are subsequently converted to carcinogens. Other research also suggests that dietary fibre protects against colon cancer and in British studies fibre pentose correlates more closely with regional cancer incidence than any other constituent of fibre. It seems likely that both fibre and beef are intimately involved in the development of colorectal cancer, with one being protective and the other causal.

A number of pathological conditions are associated with an increased risk of colonic cancer. The most important of these is familial polyposis, which has a prevalence of about one in 10 000. It is inherited as an autosomal dominant with 80% penetrance and gives rise to malignant change by the age of 60 years in almost all of those affected. Other colonic polyps also possess a potential for malignant change, particularly when greater than 2 cm in diameter. Ulcerative colitis is another premalignant condition, particularly when it has been present for over 10 years. The excess risk in ulcerative colitis is probably about ten-fold and neoplasms may arise in proximal areas of the colon unaffected by colitis.

Although cancer of the rectum has many similarities to colon cancer, there are sufficient epidemiological differences between the two that they may be considered as distinct conditions. The highest incidence is, inexplicably, found in Denmark. At all ages rectal cancer is more common in men than in women and, unlike colonic cancer, which is more frequent in the higher social classes, no social class differences have been noted for rectal cancer. The dietary risk factors for colon cancer have also been implicated in rectal cancer, although the associations are weaker. Alcohol consumption in the form of beer has been implicated in a number of studies, as well as ulcerative colitis, Crohn's disease and rectal polyps, which are regarded as premalignant conditions for carcinoma of the rectum; pelvic irradiation for cervical and testicular cancer has also been identified as a risk factor.

Prevention of colorectal cancer has to be considered under the three headings of modifying risk factors, early recognition and early detection (screening).

Dietary risk factors

Although a clear link with the affluent diets of western countries has been demonstrated, it seems unlikely that, without a major change in our eating habits, substantial changes in disease incidence can be effected at present. The protective effect of fibre offers one opportunity for education, although the consumption of beef remains an integral part of the western diet.

Early recognition

In practice this means an awareness of the abnormal signs and symptoms in patients that should raise a suspicion of colorectal cancer. These are altered bowel habit, rectal bleeding, lower abdominal pain, the rectal passage of mucus, weight loss and the development of iron deficiency anaemia.

Patient education is of potential importance here, although no studies are available to confirm its efficacy. Early investigation by general practitioners of patients with these symptoms is crucial but current evidence suggests that too few patients seen in general practice are adequately examined when they present with these suspicious symptoms. A recent study from St Mark's hospital, London, has caused concern because it was shown that less than half the patients

sent to a rectal clinic had even had a rectal examination (Springall & Todd 1989). A substantial number of rectal cancers are palpable on digital rectal examination and over half of all colorectal cancers can be identified at sigmoidoscopy. One salutary observation is that between 10 and 20% of patients eventually diagnosed as having colonic cancer had received treatment for 'piles' from their general practitioner in the 2 years preceding diagnosis.

Adequate investigative facilities need to be provided at the primary care level for the investigation of patients presenting with symptoms suggestive of colorectal cancer. In practice, this means the use of proctoscopy and sigmoidoscopy in general practitioners' surgeries and the provision of open access not only to barium enema examination but to colonoscopy for these patients. In a recent evaluation of an open access colonoscopy service in Southampton, the diagnostic yield of significant lesions was found to be 57%, with 25% of patients referred having neoplasia, a higher figure than that detected in the open access, double contrast barium enema service during the same period (Tate & Royle 1988). Although the workload implications of providing open access to colonoscopy are considerable, the evidence at present suggests that general practitioners are able to use this service effectively and efficiently.

Screening

The evidence and arguments to support population screening for colorectal cancer are becoming compelling. The rationale for screening asymptomatic patients hinges largely on the fact that prognosis is related to the extent of tumour spread at the time of diagnosis and that earlier diagnosis of symptomless disease is likely to offer the best hope of reducing mortality. Also, as most colorectal cancers arise from benign adenomas, it may be possible to prevent the development of cancer by the earlier detection and removal of these premalignant lesions.

The method used to detect the presence of colorectal neoplasia is faecal occult blood testing, and most studies have now concluded that guaiac testing is the most appropriate method to use. A small sample from two parts of the stool is smeared on to three slides of a guaiac-impregnated filter paper over three consecutive days and the slide is developed with hydrogen peroxide. The presence of haemoglobin, indicating bleeding from a colorectal lesion, is shown by a blue coloration. As an instrument for detecting occult blood, the guaiac test has a sensitivity variously reported as lying between 40 and 80% and a specificity as high as

97 to 99%, meaning that while the false positive rate is only about 2% there may be many more false negative results. These figures are not altered in patients taking non-steroidal anti-inflammatory agents. More recently, immunological tests with even greater sensitivity have been introduced. Another approach to improving the acceptability of faecal occult blood testing has been a system in which an impregnated tissue, which changes colour in the presence of occult blood, is dropped into the lavatory after defaecation. Unfortunately, the specificity and sensitivity of this test compare unfavourably with the more established guaiac methods.

Two studies in the United Kingdom have suggested that this approach to the early detection of colorectal neoplasia is acceptable and effective, although the effect of screening on mortality from colorectal cancer remains to be evaluated.

In Southampton, Nicholls et al (1986) carried out a randomised trial of compliance with screening for colorectal cancer using the Haemoccult guaiac test. Screening was offered to over 17 000 people and the overall compliance rate was 42%. A variety of methods of invitation to screening were devised by the participating general practices. Either a letter and the test were sent to the patient or a letter with an appointment to attend the surgery was sent or, during a routine consultation, the general practitioner invited patients to participate. Some patients received educational booklets about bowel disorders and screening. Compliance was significantly altered by the method of invitation, although the educational booklet did not have an impact. Compliance was highest (57%) in the group that was offered the Haemoccult test during a routine consultation. In this group the compliance rate achieved by individual general practitioners ranged from 26 to 82%. Compliance was significantly higher in the older (55–70) age group and in households in which two or more people were offered screening.

In this study, 1% of the patients screened had a positive test and 38% of the positive patients who were subsequently investigated proved to have neoplastic disease. The yield in this study was 1.2 cancers and 1.2 benign adenomas greater than 1 cm in diameter per 1000 people screened. This relatively low yield was probably due to the fact that people between 40 and 70 years were screened, rather than an older age group.

In a larger study in Nottingham, Hardcastle et al (1989) have sent faecal occult blood tests to over 50 000 people between the ages of 50 and 74 years identified from the lists of general practitioners. The faecal occult blood test packs were sent with an explanatory letter from the general practitioner concerned. Initial tests were carried out without dietary restrictions and patients with an initial positive test were asked to repeat the test over a 6-day period, excluding red meat and vegetables high in peroxidase from their diets. Subjects with a second positive test were then submitted to full investigation by endoscopy. Subjects with a negative second test after dietary restriction were asked to repeat the faecal occult blood tests, again with dietary restriction, after 3 months. Those with a positive test at this stage were also investigated.

In this study, 2.3% of patients had positive tests and 63 cancers (52% of which were at Duke's stage A) and 376 adenomas were identified, giving rates of 2.3 cancers per 1000 patients accepting the test and 8 adenomas per 1000 patients screened. Although Nicholls had found that the general practitioners' offer of opportunistic screening at consultation provided the highest level of compliance, the compliance rate in Hardcastle's study, of over 50%, is encouraging. In other studies in Sweden and Denmark, compliance rates of 66% and 67%, respectively, were achieved although in one of these personal telephone calls were used in addition to reminder letters.

These results suggest that faecal occult blood testing is an effective and acceptable means of screening for asymptomatic colorectal neoplasia. There is evidence from Hardcastle's study that lesions are discovered at a significantly earlier histopathological stage in the screened population than in a control group. However, recommendations for the institution of a national screening programme for colorectal cancer cannot be made until the impact on mortality of these screening approaches has been established. It is, nonetheless, important to remember that the death rate from colorectal cancer is ten times that from cervical cancer, for which a screening programme has been in existence for many years.

Endoscopic surveillance

Although faecal occult blood testing is likely to be the correct approach for screening asymptomatic patients, endoscopic surveillance is appropriate for patients at particularly high risk of developing new or recurrent lower bowel malignancy. In particular, this means that patients with familial polyposis, those with longstanding ulcerative colitis and patients who have had successful resections of colonic cancer should be examined. At present the recommendations for patients in the first two groups are that annual colonoscopies should be performed, but the guidelines for follow-up of colorectal cancer survivors are less clear. In particular, it is important that patients who have had ulcerative colitis for over 10 years are followed up, even if they have predominantly distal disease, because adenocarcinomas can arise de novo in the proximal colon. In practice, this means that an average district general hospital will perform 12 colonoscopies per 100 000 of population annually (Jones et al 1988). The likely cost for each carcinoma detected in this way is approximately £6000.

DIVERTICULAR DISEASE

This condition is a very common incidental finding at barium enema and at autopsy throughout the western world, although the clinical features of diverticular disease are extremely variable and an unknown but probably large proportion of people with this condition are asymptomatic. The link between diverticular disease and fibre intake is very strong, so that the disease appears in Africans and Asians who have adopted western eating habits or who were reared in the west on a fibre-deficient diet; these changes are accompanied by a rise in bowel transit times and a fall in stool weight. The prevalence of the condition in the UK increases linearly with age, without sex differences. It is responsible for substantial morbidity, although it is a rare cause of death.

The link between diverticular disease and dietary fibre offers the only feasible means of preventing the disorder and of forestalling complications in patients with established disease.

LIVER AND BILIARY DISORDERS

Liver disease

Although liver disease is uncommon in general practice, a number of groups at particular risk of hepatic damage can be identified, so that prevention and screening do have some place. Two-thirds of cases of hepatic cirrhosis in Britain are due to alcohol abuse, with the risk of developing liver damage directly related to the amount of alcohol consumed and to the length of heavy drinking. Although there is wide variation in susceptibility to alcohol, women have a systematically greater likelihood of liver damage than men. Deaths from cirrhosis are rising and have increased by one-quarter during the last decade. Although there has been a considerable increase in the prevalence of cirrhosis in young men under 25, the peak mortality continues to be in the age group 50–60 years, with a peak about a decade earlier in women. There are clear social class and occupational links, with the highest mortality in social class one and the highest incidence

of cirrhosis in occupations associated with the liquor trade or with a traditionally high alcohol intake.

Patients falling into these groups, or in whom excess alcohol consumption is suspected for any other reason, merit particular attention in terms of lifestyle modification and surveillance for the development of hepatic damage (see also Chapter 34).

Primary liver cancer is extremely rare and in 90% of cases is liver cell carcinoma (hepatoma). There are 800 cases annually in the UK and, although rare in the young, the incidence rises sharply with age and is twice as common in men as in women. Hepatomata are extremely common in the black population of central and southern Africa, in south-east Asia, Japan and eastern Europe. The major risk factor in developing countries appears to be contamination of food with aflatoxin, which is a toxin produced by the fungus *Aspergillus flavus*. In developed countries the major risk factors for hepatoma are hepatic cirrhosis of all kinds, and chronic hepatitis B virus infection, with the geography of hepatoma in Europe closely following that of the hepatitis B carrier state.

The link with chronic hepatitis B infection in western societies offers scope for prevention, by means of providing immunisation against hepatitis B for those at increased risk.

Gallstones

The prevalence of gallstones reported in autopsy studies is extremely variable, ranging from 5% in Portugal to 44% in Malmo, Sweden. Some of this variation is due to the occurrence of two distinct types of gallstones — unpigmented cholesterol stones and pigmented stones, containing bilirubin. There seem to have been changes in the relative proportion of these stones, with a recent increase in the incidence of cholesterol stones. The prevalence of gallstones is high in northern Europe and North America and much lower in tropical areas. Gallstones are two to three times more common in women than in men and the incidence and prevalence increase with age. Although the frequency of gallstones found in autopsy studies in defined populations does not seem to have changed, there has been a steady rise in the number of cholecystectomies performed in recent decades.

The association between gallstone formation and diet is rather weak but there is a strong association between obesity and symptomatic gallstones, and even moderate overweight may significantly increase the risk of gallstone formation (Maclure et al 1989). In this study specific dietary links were not made, except for the interesting finding that an average alcohol intake of over 5 g daily was associated with a 40% reduction in risk of symptomatic gallstones among non-obese women.

Dietary measures to prevent obesity should be adopted; in obese female patients in particular, it is worth bearing in mind the possibility that gallstones, rather than acid-related disorders, may be responsible for upper abdominal digestive complaints.

CONCLUSIONS

Available evidence suggests that lifestyle influences represent the most important risk factors for the development of a wide spectrum of gastrointestinal disease, although this statement may simply reflect limitations in the scope of studies so far performed. Specific agents and deficiency states have been identified in only a small number of these disorders, so that the opportunities for prevention and screening are limited; major changes in western eating and recreational habits are unlikely to occur in the foreseeable future.

Perhaps the most important condition for which screening and surveillance are appropriate is colorectal cancer, in which the arguments for population screening are strong and likely to outweigh those related to some current, established screening programmes. Although the best way of delivering population screening for colorectal cancer to the population remains to be established, there is good evidence that general practitioners play an important role, at least in co-operation with hospital services, by helping to identify patients in at-risk groups and possibly by actually providing the screening facilities at primary care level.

Beyond this, general practitioners are now well-placed to detect gastrointestinal lesions at an early stage because of good access to investigative facilities. Open access to barium studies is generally fairly widely available and almost one-third of hospitals are now offering open access to upper gastrointestinal endoscopy for general practitioners. Open access to colonoscopy and to fibre-optic sigmoidoscopy is also developing and this trend is likely to increase in the future despite the increased workload for gastroenterology units. An awareness of some of the groups at risk of developing inflammatory, peptic and neoplastic gastrointestinal disease is important in making wise choices about the use of these investigations, particularly during a time of shrinking resources for health care.

REFERENCES

Allum A W H, Powell D J, McConkey C C, Fielding J W L 1989 Gastric Cancer: a 25 year review. British Journal of Surgery 76: 535–540

Atkinson M 1989 Barrett's oesophagus — to screen or not to screen? Gut 30: 2–5

Colin-Jones D G, Langman M J S, Lawson D H, Vessey M P 1988 Cimetidine and gastric cancer: preliminary report from post-marketing surveillance study. British Medical Journal 285: 1311

Colin-Jones D G 1988 Management of dyspepsia: report of a working party. Lancet i: 576–579

Hardcastle J D, Thomas W M, Chamberlain J et al 1989 Randomised, controlled trial of faecal occult blood screening for colorectal cancer. Lancet i: 1160–1164

Heatley R V, Rathbone B J 1987 Dyspepsia: a dilemma for doctors? Lancet ii: 779–781

Jones H W, Grogono J, Hoare A M 1988 Surveillance in ulcerative colitis: burdens and benefits. Gut 29: 325–331

Jones R 1985 Open access endoscopy. British Medical Journal 291: 424–426

Jones R 1986 Open access endoscopy — a view from general practice. Journal of the Royal College of General Practitioners 36: 6–8

Jones R 1989 Dyspeptic symptoms in the community. Gut 30: 893–898

Maclure K, Hayes K C, Colditz G A et al 1989 Weight, diet and the risk of symptomatic gallstones in middle-aged women. New England Journal of Medicine 321: 563–569

Nicholls S, Koch E, Lallemand R C et at 1986 Randomised trial of compliance with screening for colorectal cancer. British Medical Journal 293: 107–110

Pearson R C, McCloy R F 1989 Preference for hot drinks associated with peptic disease. Gut 30: 1201–1205

Sagar P M 1989 Aetiology of cancer of the oesophagus: geographical studies in the footsteps of Marco Polo and beyond. Gut 30: 561–564

Springall R G, Todd I P 1989 General practitioner referral of patients with lower gastrointestinal symptoms. Journal of the Royal Society of Medicine 81: 87–88

Tate J J, Royle G T 1988 Open access colonoscopy for suspected colonic neoplasia. Gut 29: 1322–1325

Walt R P, Katchinkski B, Logan R et al 1986 Rising frequency of ulcer perforation in elderly people in the United Kingdom. Lancet i: 489–492

Williams B, Luckas M, Ellingham J H M et al 1988 Do young patients with dyspepsia need investigation? Lancet ii: 1349–1351

30. Deficiency disorders in older people

E Graham Buckley

INTRODUCTION

Deficiency disorders are a miscellaneous group of conditions unified only by the concept of a person lacking an essential element. Everyone accepts dietary deficiency in folates, which leads to macrocytic anaemia as a deficiency disorder, but the book *Sans everything: a case to answer* (Robb 1967) appropriately makes the point that deficiencies in respect and care have a profound impact on the health and well-being of older people in institutional care. Thus, deficiency disorders in the elderly, as in other age groups, range from the deficiency of a particular molecule, such as vitamin B12, to the deficiency of a basic human need, such as warmth. This chapter looks at just a few of the deficiency disorders that affect older people.

A selective approach to screening and surveillance for deficiency disorders is sensible. This approach is supported by findings such as those of the South-East London Study Group (Holland et al 1977). The development of automatic machines capable of carrying out multiple biochemical and haematological tests led to early enthusiasm in North America for screening whole populations, a practice termed 'multiphasic screening'. In the South-East London study, middle-aged men who were screened in this way were no better off at a subsequent assessment that the control group of men who had not been screened.

Similarly, Murray & Young (1970) found no correlation between multiphasic screening of people aged 65 years and their subsequent cause of death. A non-selective approach to screening for deficiency disorders that are revealed in biochemical and haematological tests is therefore unlikely to be useful. Anticipatory care is not a mechanistic exercise — it should be a thoughtful and integral part of clinical medicine, tailored to the needs of individual patients. However, there are tests that can sensibly be carried out on the whole population. Screening for phenylketonuria in infants is one of the few screening tests

that meet Wilson's criteria of screening (Wilson 1966). As yet, no screening tests for older people meet these criteria.

OLD PEOPLE

In affluent western countries, the people most likely to suffer deficiency disorders are the elderly. Chronic illness, multiple medication, poor mobility and poor nutrition contribute to produce this state of affairs. For the majority, the deficiency is subclinical and symptoms may be difficult to disentangle from those caused by underlying disease. Studies that have sought to establish the prevalence of deficiency disorders in the elderly have proved difficult to interpret because of lack of established normal biochemical values in older people. Nevertheless, it is clear that older people, both in institutional care and in the community, are at risk of nutritional deficiencies. Ironically, it is older people in hospital who are most at risk. A fixed menu, which may have low nutritional value to start with, may not appeal to an older person and the intake of both calories and nutrients may be low. In the community, old men living alone may subsist on tea, alcohol and cigarettes, and teaching men to cook may be one of the best preventive measures against deficiency disorders, as well as striking a blow for social equality between the sexes. However, for many older men living alone, the meals on wheels service can make a major impact on the problem.

The dietary guidelines for older people are similar to those for younger age groups: a mixed diet so that all nutrients are present, calorie intake adjusted to energy expenditure, fat and sugar content kept to a minimum, and as much fibre as possible in the form of wholegrain bread and fruit. However, energy needs decrease in old age. On average the calorie intake at the age of 70 years is 33% less than at the age of 20 years. In contrast to energy needs, nutrient requirements do not diminish with age (Chernhott & Lipschitz 1988). The deficiency disorders that are particularly likely to affect older people are deficiencies in their environment and total energy deficiency (particularly in the form of protein calorie malnutrition, resulting in hypothermia, tiredness, mental confusion and weight loss), potassium deficiency due to diuretic therapy and bone problems due to osteoporosis and osteomalacia. These latter conditions will be considered first.

OSTEOPOROSIS

Osteoporosis is usually considered along with specific deficiency disorders, such as osteomalacia, although its cause is uncertain. Fractures of osteoporotic femurs are a major cause of morbidity and mortality in older women. People are living longer and the age-specific incidence of fractures has increased; the reason for this is not known. Fractures of the neck of the femur have almost doubled in incidence in the past 30 years for all age groups (Boyce Vessey 1985).

Loss of bone mass is a normal part of the ageing process. Bone mass begins to decrease around the age of 40 and, in advanced old age, the skeleton shrinks by 30%. Osteoporosis is said to exist when bone density is much less than expected for the subject's age. Although the condition may arise from chronic gastrointestinal and endocrine disorders, in most cases there is no obvious cause. Screening for the disorder is difficult because of the lack of simple reliable tests.

In the past, epidemiological studies used the ratio of the area of cortical bone to the total bone area in a metacarpal bone as the marker for osteoporosis. This was of limited value as a research technique and impractical as a screening instrument.

Routine biochemical tests are normal in people with osteoporosis. Single and dual photon absorptiometry and quantitative computerised tomography now allow accurate measurement of bone mass. These tests are not appropriate for routine screening but are being used in research projects to predict the groups of people most at risk of osteoporosis and to monitor the effect of different treatments (see also p. 220).

Established osteoporosis is difficult to treat and prevention is the best approach. Previous fracture (possibly due to osteoporosis), early menopause, lean build, white or Asian race and high alcohol intake have been identified as important risk factors. Corticosteroid therapy, rheumatoid arthritis, chronic liver disease, thyrotoxicosis and the endocrine disorders directly leading to bone loss, such as primary hyperthyroidism, may lead to secondary osteoporosis.

The diet of middle-aged and older people is frequently deficient in calcium and providing calcium supplements in moderate amounts in staple foods would appear to be a sensible preventive measure for all people. However, there is a poor correlation between osteoporosis and calcium intake. This is because the intake of calcium does not directly determine the net balance of calcium in the body. For 40 years, bread and flour in the UK were fortified with calcium and there is no evidence that, as a result, the bones of older people in this country are less brittle than those of old people in other countries.

However, a 14-year longitudinal study showed that those men and women aged 50 and over who were taking more than 765 mg dietary calcium per day had a 60% lower rate of hip fracture than those taking less (Holbrook et al 1988). In established osteoporosis, calcium in pharmacological quantities (1.5–2.5 g/day) has been shown to decrease the number of subsequent fractures (Riggs et al 1982). There is no agreed quantity of daily calcium that can be recommended to older people, but supplements of 800 mg/day for women and 400 mg/day for men are reasonable. Skimmed milk contains 700 mg of calcium per pint. Exercise in the form of 30 minutes walking, jogging or dancing has been shown to reduce bone loss in postmenopausal women (Chow et al 1987) and this form of prevention is desirable on many counts.

Oestrogens have been shown unequivocally to delay loss of bone mass in postmenopausal women. Indeed, it is the only form of treatment that prevents the rapid bone loss than occurs soon after menopause (Horsman et al 1977). Hormone replacement therapy should be considered in women with menopause or oöphorectomy before the age of 45 years. Cyclic progestogens should be given to women with a uterus to minimise the risk of endometrial carcinoma. The optimum length of treatment is uncertain but should probably be at least 5 years and possibly 10 years, if significant long-term benefit is to be achieved. Vitamin D has no role in the management of osteoporosis although research assessing the effect of its metabolites on bone loss in patients with established osteoporosis continues. More promising are the findings of research into the effect of diphosphonates on steroid-induced osteoporosis (Reid et al 1988). Etidronate is the diphosphonate being advocated for prevention of primary osteoporosis.

Calicitonin could theoretically be beneficial in the prevention and treatment of osteoporosis because of its inhibition of osteoclast activity in bone resorption. However, it must be given by injection and can cause hypercalcaemia.

Anabolic steroids have been shown to increase bone mass in women with established osteoporosis (Chestnut et al 1983) but it remains uncertain whether they decrease the risk of fractures. The adverse effects of anabolic steroids make them unsuitable as preventive agents.

OSTEOMALACIA

The diet of older people may be seriously deficient in vitamin D as well as calcium. Older people who are particularly at risk of developing osteomalacia are those who are confined indoors and those suffering chronic illnesses that affect calcium metabolism and diminish the appetite (Dunnigan et al 1986, Toss & Sorbo 1986).

Early recognition of osteomalacia is important. The clinical features are bone pain and weakness of the proximal muscles. Fractures of the softened bones can occur. The proximal muscle weakness may simulate paraplegia and cause difficulty when rising from a chair. Once suspected, diagnosis using biochemical and X-ray tests is relatively straightforward. A raised serum alkaline phosphatase of bony origin occurs in Paget's disease and after fractures but the combination of this finding with a low serum level of calcium and/or phosphate should confirm the diagnosis. Pseudofractures of the scapula or femur noted by radiologists are sometimes the way in which the diagnosis is made. Serum levels of 25-hydroxy vitamin D can be measured in some laboratories but are not routinely available. The definitive diagnosis is made by histological examination of a bone biopsy, but this is only rarely necessary.

The recommended daily intake of vitamin D is 2.5 µg. It has been suggested that the housebound and institutionalised elderly should receive a weekly supplement equivalent to a daily dose of 10 µg. However, giving pharmacological doses of vitamin D to older people is hazardous. Perhaps because of a reduction in vitamin D binding protein, hypercalcaemia may be produced in this age group by relatively moderate doses of the vitamin. Osteomalacia can be prevented by ensuring that the staple foods have a high vitamin D content. For example, margarine, but not butter, has added vitamin D in the UK. Equally beneficial effects have been demonstrated, although admittedly in the warm environment of Aukland, New Zealand, as a result of 30 minutes of daily exposure to sunshine (Reid et al 1986).

HYPOTHERMIA

Like other deficiency disorders, the aetiology of hypothermia in the elderly is often multifactorial.

Identified risk factors include serious chronic diseases, e.g. arthritis, previous strokes and diabetes; a history of falls or unsteadiness; malnourishment or known poor housing; use of sedatives and/or hypnotics; alcohol abuse; senile dementia; a need to get up at night, e.g. nocturia or insomnia; severe immobility and social isolation. Taken individually these risk factors are present in a large proportion of the old elderly, especially those over the age of 85. In this age group temperature regulation is impaired in the sense that old people cannot maintain body temperature as well as younger people when exposed to cold environments.

Hypothermia as the direct cause of death is relatively rarely recorded. The true extent of hypothermia and the effect of cold weather on older people can be assessed from the overall seasonal mortality figures in the UK. These show a yearly mortality of around 40 000 related to cold weather. This discrepancy may be due to underrecognition by doctors that hypothermia may have contributed to the development of conditions such as pneumonia. However, Harris (1986a,b) has shown that the prevalence of conditions such as arthritis and depression show seasonal variations and not all the excess mortality seen in the winter in the country may be due to cold. Other countries in Northern Europe show less excess mortality in the winter than the UK. This is a good advertisement for central heating and Scandinavian triple glazing.

Slakes (1988) investigated the circumstances surrounding the deaths of people in Barnsley who were identified as dying from hypothermia. He found that the average age was 74 years. One-third of the deaths could be linked to housing and heating problems (sometimes the heating was adequate but not used even though there was no serious financial hardship). In just under one-third of the deaths, mental illness was a major contributing factor. A sad but typical scenario was for an elderly person to wander away from home, hospital or nursing home and later be found dead.

Otty and Roland (1987) attempted to introduce a programme in general practice to prevent hypothermia. They inspected the records of patients aged over 75 years in one general practice. Those with two or more of the risk factors listed about were visited early in the winter and advised how hypothermia could be prevented. They were revisited during very cold weather to see if any changes had been made. Although some improvements in heating arrangements had been made, the median temperature in houses without central heating was 10°C below World Health Organization recommended temperatures. Even with media publicity and visits from carers and doctors, 17 out of 24 elderly people studied continued to live in an environment in which they were at risk of developing hypothermia.

Screening for the risk factors for hypothermia in general practice is not difficult. The great difficulty lies in persuading older people that they are at risk and in changing the environment in which they live. Housing policies and changes in the methods of supervising old people with dementia are likely to have more impact on the mortality statistics for hypothermia than individual action by general practitioners, whose main clinical responsibility as doctors lies in the recognition of mild cases of hypothermia. Patients themselves will not complain of the problem, which creeps up on them without overt symptoms until major illnesses, such as pneumonia, occur.

IATROGENIC DEFICIENCY DISORDERS

Medicines taken by older people can cause specific deficiencies, as in potassium depletion due to diuretic therapy or protein calorie malnutrition due to the toxic effects of drugs such as digoxin. Older people frequently need to take multiple medications and often add analgaesics and laxatives to prescribed drugs. There is a clear need for efficient monitoring of the effects of medicine taking in the elderly.

COMMENT

A major problem in screening and surveillance for deficiency disorders lies in the non-specific symptoms associated with mild deficiencies and the problems encountered in trying to define the normal ranges of body constituents. This is particularly true for the elderly and many studies that have been reported to show a high prevalence of deficiency disorders in this age group may have used inappropriate end-points in separating normal from deficient subjects. Excessive consumption of vitamin tablets constitutes a health hazard; excessive dietary calcium and vitamin D leads to hypercalcaemia and renal calculi; high intake of pyridoxine and vitamin A can cause neurological problems, including ataxia and headaches. For some vitamins, particularly vitamin D, the difference between a therapeutic and a toxic dose is small and in our enthusiasm to correct deficiencies we should not create problems due to excessive treatment.

REFERENCES

Boyce Vessey M 1985 Rising incidence of fracture of the proximal femur. Lancet 150–151
Chernhoff R, Lipschitz D A 1988 Nutrition and ageing. In: Shils M E, Young V R (eds) Modern nutrition in health and disease, 7th edn. Lea and Febinger, Philadelphia
Chestnut C H et al 1983 In: Dixon A, Russel R, Stone T (eds) Osteoporosis, a multidisciplinary problem. Academic Press, London
Chow R, Harrison J E, Notarius C 1987 Effect of two randomised exercise programmes on bone mass of healthy postmenopausal women. British Medical Journal 295: 1441–1444
Dunnigan M G et al 1986 Prevention of vitamin D deficiency in the elderly. Scottish Medical Journal 31: 144–149
Harris C M 1986a Further observations on seasonal variation. 1. Osteoarthritis. Journal of the Royal College of General Practitioners 36: 316–318
Harris C M 1986b Further observations on seasonal variation. 2. Depression. Journal of the Royal College of General Practitioners 36: 319–321
Holbrook T L, Barrett-Connor E, Wingard D L 1988 Dietary calcium and risk of hip fracture. 14-year prospective study. Lancet ii: 1046–1049
Holland W W, Crease A L, D'Souza M F et al 1977 A controlled trial of multiphasic screening in middle age: results of the South East London screening study. International Journal of Epidemiology 6: 357–363
Horsman A, Gallagher J C, Simpson M, Nordin B E C 1977

Prospective trial of oestrogen and calcium in post menopausal women. British Medical Journal 789–792
Murray T S, Young R E 1977 Correlation of causes of death with multiple screening in a geriatric population. Update 15.11: 1103–1107
Otty C J, Roland M L 1987 Hypothermia in the elderly: scope for prevention. British Medical Journal 295: 419–420
Reid I R, Gallagher D J A, Bosworth J 1986 Against vitamin D deficiency in the elderly by regular sunlight exposure. Age and Ageing 15: 35–40
Reid I R et al 1988 Prevention of steroid-induced osteoporosis with (3-amino-1-hydroxypropylidine)-1,1-bisphosphonate (APD). Lancet i: 143–146
Riggs B L, Seeman E, Hodgson S F et al 1982 Effect of the fluoride/calcium regimen on vertebral fracture occurring in postmenopausal osteoporosis. New England Journal of Medicine 306: 446–450
Robb B 1967 Sans everything: a case to answer. Nelson, London
Slates D N 1988 Death from hypothermia: are current views or causative factors well founded? British Medical Journal i: 1643–1644
Toss G, Sorbo B 1986 Serum concentrations of 25 hydroxy vitamin D and vitamin D-binding protein in elderly people. Acta Medica Scandinavica 220: 273–277
Wilson J M G 1966 Some principles of early diagnosis and detection. In: Teeling-Smith G (ed) Surveillance and early diagnosis in general practice. Office of Health Economics, London

FURTHER READING

Passmore R, Eastwood M A 1986 Human nutrition and
  dietetics. Churchill Livingstone, Edinburgh
Truswell A S 1986 ABC of nutrition. British Medical Journal
Publications, London
Shils M E, Young V R 1988 Modern nutrition in health and
  disease. Lea & Febinger, Philadelphia

31. Depression and dementia

Sanjeebit J Jachuck

Depression and dementia are common clinical problems among the elderly. The number of patients with these clinical conditions is set to increase as the number of people aged 75 and over will rise by 20%, and those over 85 by 50%, by the end of the century. Increasing age was reported to be associated with impairment in mental function (Jachuck et al 1986) and consequent loss of independence (Kay 1989), sometimes necessitating a shift of care to institutions. There will, therefore, be an increasing need for provision of appropriate care for the elderly infirm. It has been estimated that the need for institutional care for those above 85 years of age will increase more than 10 times faster than for the 65–74 age group (Clarke et al 1979). It is not surprising that increasing emphasis is being placed on this issue.

Loss of job, change in house and environment, death of spouse and close associates, loss of income and loss of support through movement of children and other carers usually accompany the ageing process. It may also be associated with gradual decline in vision, hearing, mobility and continence. It is reported that approximately 60% of disabled people are above 65 years of age (Royal College of Physicians 1986). Such disability can lead to progressive dependency, insecurity, change in personality and motivation, disharmony with relatives and social isolation, which in turn contribute to psychiatric illness (Miller 1985, Kay 1989).

Extracranial, as well as intracranial, vascular diseases often cause deterioration of mental function (Sourander & Sourander 1977). The pathophysiology was thought to be decreased cardiac output, increased cerebrovascular resistance or hypotension resulting in disseminated cerebral infarction. In my own practice, a study of 378 individuals above 70 years of age revealed that 129 (34%) had recorded clinical evidence of cardiovascular, cerebrovascular or peripheral vascular disease (Table 31.1). Impaired mental function was seen more commonly in those elderly people with vascular disease. Depending on the degree of decompensation, vascular disease manifests as transient cerebrovascular ischaemia and ischaemia affecting heart and limbs. Patients with such disability may also have depressive illness.

One of the unmet needs of stroke survivors is the failure to recognise impaired mental function (Folstein et al 1977, Fiebel et al 1979). Stroke affects approximately 500 out of every 100 000 individuals living in Britain (Wade et al 1985) and accounts for their psychiatric symptoms (Folstein et al 1977, House 1987). Not all patients with cerebral infarction manifest organic brain syndrome and it has been shown that a small stroke in a 'silent' area of the brain may not produce a sudden change in intellect, personality or character (Fisher 1968). Mental illness following

Table 31.1 Details of vascular disease affecting heart, brain and extremities in 378 elderly patients

Disease	Male (%) (n = 120)	Female (%) (n = 258)	Total (%)
Ischaemic heart disease	19 (15.8)	56 (21.7)	75 (19.8)
Cerebrovascular disease	9 (7.5)	16 (6.2)	25 (6.6)
Peripheral vascular disease	3 (2.5)	4 (1.5)	7 (1.8)
Combination of the above	9 (7.5)	13 (5.0)	22 (5.8)
Total	40 (33.3)	89 (34.5)	129 (34.1)

stroke is directly due to haemodynamic changes and may also arise indirectly through functional disability (Holbrook 1982, House 1987). The age-specific incidence and prevalence of such multi-infarct disorders in the elderly community has not been well documented (Henderson & Kay 1984).

The increased incidence of morbid conditions seen in elderly individuals is also associated with increased use of prescribed and non-prescribed medication. Drugs used in the elderly may affect mental function by reducing cerebral perfusion, causing sedation and blocking neurotransmitters.

The structure and function of the brain change with age. Age-related cell deaths are rather selective: as well as reduction in weight and volume of the brain there is substantial neurological loss in the cerebral cortex (Tomlinson 1980). The histological changes and changes in neuropharmacology are associated with reduction in presynaptic markers leading to functional decline (Rossor 1985).

Depression and dementia are separate entities but both these conditions can be associated with affective disorder and memory impairment (Thielman & Blazer 1987). In a study by Kahn and associates (1975), which evaluated self-reporting of memory complaints in 153 patients with depression and organic brain syndromes, 25% were found to have no memory problem, and the severity of memory complaint was associated with the severity of depression. Studies by Folstein & McHugh (1978) and by Kazzniak et al (1981) suggested that depression is common in patients with dementia, but this has been denied by Cavanaugh & Wettson (1983), who suggest that apparent cognitive deficit in depressed patients was due to unreliable assessment methods. The cognitive deficit observed in a group of depressed elderly was found to be more common in those with a history of electroconvulsive therapy (Thielman & Blazer 1987). There is a need for further studies to improve our understanding of this subject.

In reviewing this complex subject, it is important to understand the pathophysiology of the ageing process and the associated clinical, social and psychological problems that directly or indirectly contribute to the condition. The two clinical conditions, depression and dementia, also need to be clearly outlined for proper evaluation.

DEPRESSION

Depression is more common in the elderly than during early life (Herrington 1983) and twice as common as dementia (Patterson & Crone 1986). Although depressed people consult their general practitioners more often, they cannot be relied upon to report their symptoms to their doctors (Henderson & Kay 1984). Williamson and colleagues (1964) studied elderly individuals belonging to three general practices and reported that 16 out of 21 cases of depressive illness were not known to their general practitioner. It is possible that not all patients with the clinical condition are recognised by the general practitioner (Goldberg & Blackwell 1970). A study by MacDonald (1986), on the other hand, suggested that general practitioners do recognise the condition, but tend not to refer or treat with medication.

The need for a proper epidemiological study was stressed in the Second National Morbidity Survey (Dunn 1983) and there have been some attempts to evaluate the prevalence of depression in the elderly in this country (Henderson & Kay 1984, Maule et al 1984, Bond 1987, Copeland et al 1987, Jack et al 1988). Freeling and associates (1985) had reported that the incidence of depression diagnosed by the general practitioner was 31.4 in 1000 in 1970–71. Subsequently, a review of the Third National Morbidity Survey by Smeaton (1989) reported a decline of 35% in the general practitioners' recording of mental illness compared to that observed 10 years previously. The decline was attributed to the different recording system and changes in attitude to recording of the illness.

It is not easy to make an accurate description of the prevalence of depression in the elderly community because changes in sleep patterns and decline in physical ability are associated with the ageing process, and there are more than 25 rating scales in common use to detect the disorder (Gallagher 1987). Kay and colleagues (1964) initiated a study in which they reported a prevalence of depression of 10% in the elderly in Newcastle upon Tyne. MacDonald (1986) reported depression in 19% of elderly men and 37% of elderly women in a study carried out in London. The reported diagnosis of depression in a random sample of population in Edinburgh was 3.7% of men and 6.6% of women (Maule et al 1984). Copeland & colleagues (1987) studied a sample of 1070 in Liverpool and reported 11.3% as having depressive illness. A study carried out in my own practice in Newcastle upon Tyne (Jack et al 1988) revealed 15% of elderly men and 18% of elderly women to be depressed. Studies in the USA and Canada report the prevalence of depression among the elderly to be between 13 and 65% (Blazer & Williams 1980, Gurland et al 1980, Patterson & Crone 1986). Lower rates of depressive illness in the community have been reported in Iceland, Sweden and (West) Germany (Eastwood & Corbin 1985).

Depression is one of the affective disorders that is associated with physical incapacity, loneliness, poverty and acute realisation of poor outlook for future life (Blazer & Williams 1980, Herrington 1983). Those affected tend to manifest with apathy, blue mood, sadness, tearfulness, emptiness, sleep disturbances, preoccupation with somatic complaints and loss of interest and pleasure (Blazer & Williams 1980, Gurland et al 1983, Hanley & Baikie 1984). Depression is more commonly seen in those who have experienced severe life events and social difficulties (Murphy 1982). Social difficulties are encountered when individuals are deprived of the company of their spouse, children and friends, either through physical loss or through their personal inability to maintain contact. In a study of elderly bereaved, Heyman & Giauturo (1973) found that 25% of women were still depressed 21 months after losing their spouse. Women seemed to be affected more by death than men (Linn et al 1980). Progressive loss of finance, security and purpose in life leads to an anxiety state and depression. Lack of activities tends to affect the men more (Hale 1982). Increasing vandalism and physical assault on the elderly infirm have added further stress to their life in recent years.

Progressive increase in physical illness is a major contributory factor for the depressive state (Murphy 1982). Murphy reported that the risk of depression increased from 25% with one contributing risk factor, to 80% when associated with health problems and major social difficulties. The most common illness contributing to depression is stroke. The prevalence of depression a week after a stroke is reported to be 22–27% (Robinson et al 1983, House 1987) but with time it declines. Depression is more common in those with left hemisphere damage, particularly in those patients with involvement of the anterior hemisphere and aphasia (House 1987). Other intracranial conditions responsible for depression are cerebral tumour, head injury, Parkinson's disease (Strub 1985, Gotham et al 1986) and myocardial infarction (Hanley & Baikie 1984). Depression is also associated with loss of vision, painful joint movements, sexual difficulties and many physical disabilities (House 1987), which threaten the independence of the individual.

Millard (1983) stated: 'no matter what is done a third get better, a third stay the same and a third get worse'. Despite the self-limiting course, depression seen in general practice can be severe (Burton & Freeling 1982). All general practitioners need to be aware of the difficulties experienced by the patients and by the carers so that efforts can be made to provide appropriate cure, care and comfort for the patients. This should enable us to dispel the criticism made by Johnson (1973) when he stated: 'patients with depressive illness do not receive the best treatment in general practice'. In fact, general practitioners are most suitably placed to detect the affective disorders early because 95% of the elderly consult them (Grey 1987). If general practitioners do not assume this responsibility of early detection and care, an intolerable burden will be imposed on the hospital services, and inappropriate community care for the elderly with psychiatric disorders will be perpetuated (Jack et al 1988).

Psychiatric assessment requires more consultation time than is conventionally offered in general practice. Not only do most elderly individuals see their general practitioners regularly (Williams 1984, Clarke et al 1984), but the general practitioners are aware of their social difficulties (Hooper 1988), contrary to the claim made by Williamson and colleagues (1964). In practice, general practitioners encounter three types of patients in whom affective disorders are seen:

1 Known depressives — these include younger patients who are depressed and enter old age.
2 Occult depressives — these elderly are depressed but either not diagnosed or not receiving treatment.
3 Potential depressives — those elderly who are at high risk of developing depressive illness.

In a Swiss study (Ciompi 1969) the severity of depression did not change in patients with early onset of depressive illness when they entered old age. A subsequent follow-up study by Post (1972) revealed a greater recurrence of depression in later life in this group of patients. Such relapses may remain undetected (Sadavoy 1981) if an appropriate surveillance plan is not instituted. It is therefore important for all general practitioners to be aware of their depressive patients when they enter old age. It is not difficult to identify those patients receiving regular treatment because most general practitioners have a system for assessing repeat prescriptions; introduction of computerisation will certainly facilitate detection. However, it is not easy to identify those patients who have completed treatment before entering old age or those who have never received medication unless the practitioners maintain a morbidity register for their patients.

In view of the reported high prevalence of the illness in the elderly community, efforts should be made to identify those elderly who are clinically or subclinically depressed so that a plan of care can be organised to promote their quality of life. It is important to detect the illness early because such late onset depression carries a reasonable prognosis (Roth 1955, Cole 1983) and in this group planned care influences the outcome (Baldwin 1988).

The term 'potential depressives' describes a group of elderly who have clinical or social conditions that predispose to depressive manifestation. Stressful life events, loss of spouse, stroke, myocardial infarction, Parkinson's disease, loss of vision and other conditions have already been mentioned. Depression is also common in those who enter residential care. Mann and colleagues (1984) described significant depressive symptoms in 40% of elderly residents in London local authority homes.

'Recurrent brief depression' is a recently described disorder, which manifests with short episodes of major depression and carries a risk of deliberate self-harm over 10 years in 13% of patients (Baldwin 1989). Baldwin reported that the World Health Organization and the American Psychiatric Association intend to use this new term in their classification scheme. This is an interesting diagnosis, as it will account for some of the differences in the reported prevalence of depression in the literature and will contribute to the solution of difficulties encountered in assessing and managing such patients.

Use of a short, reliable, easily-administered questionnaire is the most effective method of identifying those elderly individuals with depressive symptoms. Those in whom the questionnaire reveals psychiatric symptoms are called psychiatric 'cases' (Bond 1987, Goldberg & Bridges 1987, Jack et al 1988), as not all of them suffer from clinical depressive disorders. Therefore, it is necessary to establish the clinical diagnosis by proper psychiatric assessment. To the best of my knowledge there is no published long-term follow-up study of those psychiatric 'cases' who do not suffer from a clinical depressive disorder, and this would constitute an interesting research exercise in the future.

The commonly used questionnaires to detect depression in the elderly are the Hamilton Self-Rating (HSR), the Schedule for Affective Disorders and Schizophrenia (SADS), the Diagnostic Interview Schedule (DIS), the Beck Depression Inventory (BDI), the Mood Assessment Scale (MAS), the Zung Self-Rating Depression Scale (SDS) and the Geriatric Depression Scale (GDS). Blazer and Williams (1980) used the Duke-Oars methodology (OARS 1978) in their study in USA but it is complicated and inappropriate for use in general practice (Jachuck & Mulcahy 1987). GDS and BDI were used in my own practice study (Jachuck 1988). Both these questionnaires were easy to administer and the outcome was useful. I would recommend BDI as a good screening questionnaire as it is reliable in detecting depression and it is sufficiently sensitive to identify a patient's distress (Gallagher 1987). If all clinicians used a standardised

screening method it would be possible to produce a comprehensive account of the subject.

A comprehensive clinical assessment is an important method of excluding contributing causes with their somatic symptoms and establishing the correct diagnosis of affective disorder. Freeman and associates (1985) and Alexopoulos (1989) describe transient neurological abnormalities, such as left hemiparesis with increased deep tendon reflexes and extensor plantar reflexes, associated with depressive episodes. I have never encountered such clinical manifestation in any of my elderly patients with depressive illness who do not have an organic neurological disorder. It is necessary to record the morbidity pattern and the associated functional disability because they play a significant role in contributing to depression. The three major determinants of depression in the elderly were considered to be disease, disability and dependance (Gurland et al 1983).

Laboratory investigations are used primarily to support the clinical diagnosis. Increased mortality in depressed patients with associated ventricular enlargement has been reported (Jacoby et al 1981) but I do not consider it justifiable to screen all depressive patients for this. To differentiate dementia from depression, the dexamethasone suppression test, average evoked response test and event related potential test have been suggested (Thielman and Blazer 1987) but such tests are not easily accessible to most general practitioners and very few patients warrant them.

DEMENTIA

Dementia is a syndrome of intellectual dysfunction manifesting with progressive impairment in performance related to memory, orientation, communication and certain cortical functions of comprehension, calculation and solving problems (Fozard 1985; Copeland 1987, Gurland et al 1987, Kendrick 1987). It is often described as organic brain syndrome and cognitive dysfunction. Confusional states may be seen in patients with dementia but not all those with confusional state suffer from dementia. Clinicians should be precise about the terminology to promote our understanding and management.

There are two principal types of dementia — primary and secondary. Primary dementia, the most common type, is associated with cerebral degenerative changes for which no obvious cause has yet been established. Secondary dementia is associated with certain known pathological conditions, which affect the brain directly or indirectly through structural changes

Table 31.2 Causes of dementia

Primary	Secondary
Alzheimer's disease	Multi-infarct dementia
Pick's disease	Cerebrovascular insufficiency
Creutzfeldt–Jakob disease	Depressive disorders
Huntington's disease	Metabolic disease, e.g. myxoedema
Parkinson's disease	Infection
	Drug-induced
	Alcohol-induced
	Hydrocephalus (normal pressure)
	Intracranial space-occupying lesion
	Subcortical
	Haematological, e.g. pernicious anaemia

Table 31.3 Commonly prescribed drugs that cause cognitive disorders

Analgesics
  Dextropropoxyphene
  Salicylates
  Opiates
Cardiovascular
  Clonidine
  Digitalis
  Methyldopa
  Nitrates
  Propranolol
Gastrointestinal
  Cimetidine
Central nervous system
  Barbiturates
  Carbamazepine
  Diazepam
  Levodopa
  Phenytoin
Psychotropic
  Benzodiazepines
  Lithium
  Monoamine oxidase inhibitors
Steroids
  Corticosteroids

and impaired circulation or neurotransmission. This form of dementia is of considerable interest to clinicians because in some instances the condition is amenable to appropriate and timely intervention.

Primary dementia is a characteristic pathological condition commonly represented by Alzheimer's type of disease, which accounts for in excess of 50% of those suffering from dementia (Neshkes & Jarvik 1985). Matsuyama & Jarvik (1982) reported that up to 11% of siblings of affected cases are at risk of suffering from the disease. Autosomal dominant inheritance has been postulated as the genetic deficit in some cases (Neshkes & Jarvik 1985). Huntington's disease is also an autosomal dominant familial disease, which is characterised by choreiform movements although cognitive dysfunction may be an early manifestation in this disease. This condition is discussed in greater detail in Chapter 10. The Alzheimer type of dementia is also commonly seen in association with Parkinson's disease. Onset of dementia is rather late in this clinical condition. Pick's disease and Creutzfeldt–Jakob disease are two very rare forms of primary dementia. Pick's disease usually presents as personality disorder and dementia is a late manifestation in Creutzfeldt–Jakob disease (Table 31.2).

Secondary dementia is commonly seen in multi-infarct dementia. The incidence varies from 8–29% of all dementias (Neshkes & Jarvik 1985). Legh-Smith and colleagues (1986) reported impairment in mental function in 20–25% of patients within a year following a stroke. It is claimed that such impairment in mental function is encountered when vascular insufficiency affects 50–100 ml of cortical or subcortical areas (Roth 1978). Other conditions that may be responsible for secondary dementia include myxoedema, pernicious anaemia and occult neoplasm.

Iatrogenic dementia may constitute the most common type of treatable secondary dementia. The prescribing rate is high in the elderly. In my own study (Jachuck 1988) of 455 individuals over 70 years of age in a group practice, 361 were receiving prescriptions for medication at the time of my evaluation. The drugs commonly implicated in impaired mental function are shown in Table 31.3.

Diseases causing secondary dementia usually affect cortical function through hypoxia, electrolyte imbalance, vascular insufficiency, hormonal changes, toxic changes, interference with neurotransmitters or through changes in intracranial pressure. With increasing research in this field, more and more causes are being added to the list. Recent studies implicate high serum aluminium in patients undergoing renal dialysis as the cause of impairment of mental function (Altmann et al 1989) but this supposed association needs further scientific investigation.

Not all older people suffer from dementia. In fact, in excess of 95% of the older people who live in the community do not (Clarke et al 1984, Jachuck et al 1986). The reported prevalence of dementia in elderly individuals living in the community varied between 1% and 10% (Clarke et al 1984, Jachuck et al 1986). A study in Newcastle upon Tyne by Kay and colleagues (1964) reported a rate of 13% in the community. The prevalence of the condition in a group of hospitalised patients in the same city was found to be 27.8% (Evans et al 1979). In a study carried out in my own practice in Newcastle upon Tyne (Jachuck et al 1986), using identical screening methods to the hospital study (Evans et al 1979) severe mental impairment was observed in only 0.8% of patients. A study by Clarke and associates (1986) in Melton Mowbray reported that 1.6% of individuals over 75 years of age and living in the community suffered from dementia. The figures quoted so far refer only to severe cognitive impairment representing almost end-stage cognitive function. In an average general practice with a list of 2500, it is estimated that there will be 40 patients with dementia, and 20 of these will be severely affected (Mohanaruban & Sastry 1989). Ineichen (1987) has predicted a tripling in the prevalence of dementia by the year 2000.

Early detection

Progressive decline in cognitive performance is reported in all elderly individuals and it is claimed to affect people even before 60 years of age (Gilleard 1984). Despite such a decline, individuals are capable of leading an independent life in the community, provided that the deficit is not too severe and the rate of decline is not accelerated by certain factors (Pearce 1984). It is difficult for individuals to remain in the community without support when their cognitive impairment reaches a critical point through physiological ageing or as a result of pathological conditions. It is therefore important to record the rate of decline in cognitive performance, as well as to search for those who have cognitive deficit sufficiently severe to impair independent existence.

In clinical practice it is not easy to detect the early changes, which are often mistaken for the physiological ageing process (Kendrick 1987). To identify early changes it is suggested (Heston & White 1983, Jachuck et al 1986) that efforts should be made to assess cognitive performance at regular intervals when monitoring the mental function of the elderly individual. This will document the rate of normal decline, identify factors accelerating the rate of decline and detect the 10–15% patients who are amenable to treatment (Pearce 1984). Such information would strengthen our claim for adequate and appropriate resources to pro-

vide the necessary support and service for the needy. Investment in resources for early detection would facilitate research in the field of aetiology, pathology, assessment and management. Research in this field is sparse (Henderson & Kay 1984) and emphasis has been placed (World Health Organization 1986, Heston & White 1983) on the need to identify the small group of patients with severe mental impairment who are incapable of maintaining themselves in the community and who make heavy demands on their carers, the health service and society (Pearce 1984). The reported factors contributing to pathological acceleration of such a decline are:

1 Degenerative changes associated with ageing.
2 Increased incidence of morbidity and its treatment.
3 Functional disability.
4 Social difficulties.

The assessment of patients with dementia is not easy. In general practice, they usually present to clinicians through their inability to maintain an independent life or because of their carers' inability to support them in the community. Incontinence of urine and faeces is an important manifestation of patients with severe dementia. Isaacs and Walkey (1964) observed that 80% of those who were doubly incontinent had organic brain syndrome. This can manifest in a variety of forms, such as wandering aimlessly, accidents, fractured femur, non-compliance to medication, failure to pay bills and poor hygiene in the house. In my experience such a presentation represents a fairly advanced state of dementia and any intervention tends not to alter the course significantly. Reviewing the management of such demented elderly in the community, Bergmann et al (1978) reported that 70% of the patients were either dead or in institutional care within 12 months of diagnosis. Some patients with moderate dementia are brought to the attention of their practitioners when the cognitive deficit is further enhanced by certain infective, metabolic or cerebrovascular conditions.

To detect dementia early, the aim of assessment should be to identify deterioration of cognitive performance suggestive of impaired mental function and then to identify a cause for such deficit by clinical and other assessment. Increased awareness of the condition and factors that contribute to it will enhance early detection. The most important manifestation that commonly receives attention is memory loss (Kendrick 1987).

It is of great practical value to design a simple screening device that is sufficiently sensitive to detect the deficit early (Beaumont 1982). Those interested in this field have made attempts to perfect questionnaires which identify impaired mental function and which could be correlated with characteristic pathological changes. Since the study by Blessed and colleagues (1968) several screening methods have been used to achieve the objective but no universally accepted standardised technique or diagnostic criteria have been agreed upon as yet (Copeland 1987). Copeland and colleagues (1986) have produced a very powerful assessment tool, AGECAT, a computerised program to standardise diagnosis, but as yet it has not been adapted to clinical practice. I adopted a simple 13-point questionnaire, previously used in hospital (Evans et al 1979) to screen elderly people in general practice (Jachuck et al 1986). The questionnaire was well accepted by all the elderly and easily administered by a member of the primary health care team. A high score (11) indicated normal mental function and those who scored less than 3 were found to have severe mental impairment. It is a two-stage questionnaire, in which the primary care team refers these elderly people with lower scores for specialist assessment. It also offers the opportunity to undertake reappraisal of each individual and to evaluate serial changes for longitudinal studies in the community. Clarke and colleagues (1986) used a similar, easily administered assessment method, Clifton Assessment Procedures for the Elderly (CAPE) (Pattie & Gilleard 1979). CAPE has a fixed cut-off point to decide between normal and abnormal mental function. It does not identify those who have moderately impaired mental function, unlike the procedure used by Evans and colleagues (1979). In the questionnaire assessment, low scores correlate well with the diagnosis of dementia but loss of specificity and increase in false positives are observed with high scores (Kay 1989). In general practice, it is necessary to have a relatively simple questionnaire, which can be used by all members of the primary care team who are in regular contact with the elderly. Such a questionnaire could form part of the annual review of over 75s, which is now part of a general practitioner's terms of service.

All patients in whom preliminary screening raises suspicions of dementia should be fully assessed clinically and by appropriate laboratory investigations. This is necessary not only to confirm the diagnosis but also to identify contributing causes and to enable a positive plan for long-term management to be made. The clinical assessment is to identify the manifestations and contributing causes. Examination should cover the central nervous system, cardiovascular and endocrine systems, respiratory function and nutritional state, and should seek evidence of neoplasm. Such an assessment is also used to compile a complete morbid-

Table 31.4 Laboratory investigations in dementia

Neurological investigations
  Electroencephalography
  Scan
  Ventriculography

Other investigations
  Haemoglobin
  Serum electrolytes
  Liver function tests
  Thyroid studies
  Chest X-ray
  Electrocardiograph

ity pattern, to quantify the associated functional disability and to produce an appropriate plan of care for the patient and support for the carers.

The laboratory investigations are usually designed to exclude secondary causes of dementia, but results of some of the investigations may also support the primary diagnosis of dementia. Table 31.4 shows a set of investigations from which clinicians may wish to choose. Finally, the GP is likely to be involved at the patient's death. An increase in autopsy will significantly increase histological confirmation of the disease and factors contributing to it (Black & Jachuck, 1984).

CONCLUSION

The information pertaining to mental illness in the elderly community is rather sketchy. To accommodate the rising demand for care of the elderly community, it is imperative that proper priority is given to establish the magnitude of the problem by introducing a simple screening programme that can identify those in need of special assessment. Such a screening programme will be less effective if it is not supported by information relating to the associated morbid conditions, medication prescribed and functional assessment (Jachuck 1989) for each individual. Facilities and resources should be made available to maintain such a screening and surveillance programme, and to produce a standardised data base of good quality information upon which to plan future development of management, education and research.

To develop an effective, efficient and economical service to benefit elderly people, an appropriate framework should be introduced in primary care practice. It should be based on quality information with which to select patients who would benefit from scientific and technological advances. Without such infrastructure it would be impossible to apply clinical, biochemical, radiological and pathological techniques to their fullest advantage.

REFERENCES

Alexopoulos G S 1989 Late life depression and neurological brain disease. International Journal of Geriatric Psychiatry 4: 187–190

Altmann P, Dhanesha U, Hamon C 1989 Disturbance of cerebral function by aluminium in haemodialysis patients without overt aluminium toxicity. Lancet i: 7–11

Baldwin D 1989 Recurrent brief depression. British Medical Journal 299: 413–414

Baldwin R 1988 Depression in later life. A fresh challenge to an old problem. In: Murphy E, Parker S W (eds) Current approaches to affective disorders in the elderly. Duphar Laboratories Ltd. Publication, Southampton, pp 18–27

Beaumont G 1982 Dementia and general practice. Psychiatry in Practice 1: 5

Bergmann K, Foster E M, Justice A W, Mathews V 1978 Management of the demented elderly patients in the community. British Journal of Psychiatry 132: 441–449

Black D, Jachuck S J 1984 Death certification in general practice: review of records. British Medical Journal 288: 1127–1129

Blazer D, Williams C D 1980 Epidemiology of dysphoria and depression in an elderly population. American Journal of Psychiatry 137: 439–444

Blessed G, Tomlinson B E, Roth M 1968 The association between quantitative measures of dementia and of senile changes in the cerebral grey matter of elderly subjects. British Journal of Psychiatry 114: 797–811

Bond J 1987 Psychiatric illness in later life. A study of prevalence in a Scottish population. International Journal of Geriatric Psychiatry 2: 39–57

Burton R H, Freeling P 1982 How GPs manage depressive illness. Journal of the Royal College of General Practitioners 32: 558–561

Cavanaugh S V A, Wettson R 1983 The relationship between severity of depression, cognitive dysfunction and age in medical inpatients. American Journal of Psychiatry 140: 495–496

Ciompi L 1969 Follow-up studies on the evaluation of former neurotic and depressive states in old age. Journal of Geriatric Psychiatry 3: 90–106

Clarke M, Lowry R, Clarke S 1986 Cognitive impairment in the elderly — a community survey. Age and Ageing 15: 278–284

Clarke M, Clarke S, Odell A, Jagger C 1984 The elderly at home: health and social status. Health Trends 16: 3–7

Clarke M, Hughes A O, Dodd K J et al 1979 The elderly in residential care: pattern of disability. Health Trends 11: 17–20

Cole M G 1983 Age of onset and course of primary depressive illness in the elderly. Canadian Journal of Psychiatry 28: 102–104

Copeland J R M 1987 The diagnosis of dementia in old age. In: Pitt B (ed) Dementia: medicine in old age. Churchill Livingstone, Edinburgh, pp 52–68

Copeland J R M, Dewey M E, Wood N et al 1987 Range of mental illness among the elderly in the community. Prevalence in Liverpool using GMS — AGECAT package. British Journal of Psychiatry 150: 815–823

Copeland J R M, Dewey M E, Griffiths-Jones H M 1986 Computerised psychiatric diagnostic system and case nomenclature for elderly subjects: GMS and AGECAT. Psychological Medicine 16: 89–100

Dunn G 1983 Preliminary communication; longitudial records of anxiety and depression in general practice: the second national morbidity survey. Psychological Medicine 13: 897–906

Eastwood R, Corbin S 1985 Epidemiology of mental disorders in old age. In: Recent advances in psychogeriatrics, vol 1. Airie T (ed) Churchill Livingstone, Edinburgh, pp 17–32

Evans J G, Prudham D, Wandless I 1979 A prospective study of fracture of the proximal femur: factors predisposing to survival. Age and Ageing 8: 246–250

Fiebel J H, Berk S, Joynt R J 1979 The unmet needs of stroke survivors. Neurology 29: 592

Fisher C M, 1968 Dementia in cerebral vascular disease. In: Toole J F, Siekert R G, Whisnant J P (eds) Cerebral vascular diseases, 6th conference. Grune and Stratton, New York

Folstein M F, McHugh P R 1978 Dementia syndrome of depression. In: Katzman R, Terry R D, Bick K L (eds) Alzheimer's disease: senile dementia and related disorders. Raven Press, New York

Folstein M F, Maiberger R, McHugh P R 1977 Mood disorder as a specific complication of stroke. Journal of Neurology, Neurosurgery and Psychiatry 40: 1018–1022

Fozard J L 1985 Psychology of aging — normal and pathological age differences in memory. In: Brocklehurst J C (ed) Textbook of geriatric medicine and gerontology, 3rd edn. Churchill Livingstone, Edinburgh 122–144

Freeling P, Ros B M, Paykel E S et al 1985 Unrecognised depression in general practice. British Medical Journal 290: 1880–1883

Freeman R C, Galaburda A M, Cabal R D et al 1985, The neurology of depression. Cognitive and behavioural deficits with focal bindings in depression and resolution after electroconvulsive therapy. Archives of Neurology 42: 289–291

Gallagher D 1987 Assessing the affects in the elderly. Clinics in Geriatric Medicine 3(1): 65–85 W B Saunders Company, Philadelphia

Gilleard C J 1984 Assessment of cognitive impairment in the elderly: a review. In: Hanley I, Hodge J (eds) Psychological approaches to the care of the elderly. Croom Helm, London

Goldberg D, Bridges K 1987 Screening for psychiatric illness in general practice: the general practitioner versus the screening questionnaire. Journal of the Royal College of General Practitioners 37: 15–18

Goldberg D, Blackwell B 1970 Psychiatric illness in general practice: A detailed study using a new method of case identification. British Medical Journal 1: 439–443

Gotham A M, Brown R G, Marsden C D 1986 Depression in Parkinson's disease: a quantitative and qualitative analysis. Journal of Neurology, Neurosurgery and Psychiatry 49: 381–389

Grey D P 1987 Preventive care of the elderly. Journal of the Royal College of General Practitioners 37: 98

Gurland B J, Dean L, Cross P, Golden R 1980 The epidemiology of depression and dementia in the elderly: the use of multiple indicators of these conditions. In: Cole J, Barrett J E (eds) Psychopathology in the aged. Raven Press, New York, pp 37–60

Gurland B, Copeland J, Kuriansky J et al 1983 The mind and mood of aging. Croom Helm, New York

Gurland B J, Cote L J, Cross P S, Tonner J A 1987 The

assessment of cognitive function in the elderly. Clinics in Geriatric Medicine 3(1) 53–63

Hale D 1982 Correlates of depression in the elderly; sex differences and similarities. Journal of Clinical Psychology 38: 253–257

Hanley I, Baikie E 1984 Understanding and treating depression in the elderly. In: Psychological approaches to the care of the elderly. Hanley I, and Hodge J (eds) Croom Helm, London

Henderson A S, Kay D W K 1984 The epidemiology of mental disorders in the aged. Handbook of studies on psychiatry and old age. Elsevier Science, Amsterdam, pp 53–88

Herrington R N 1983 Antidepressant drugs and the elderly. In: Caird F I, Evans J G Advanced geriatric medicine, 3rd edn. Pitman Books Ltd, London pp 105–118

Heston L L, White J A 1983 Dementia. Freeman, New York

Heyman D K, Gianturo D T 1973 Long term adaptation by the elderly to bereavement. Journal of Gerontology 28: 259–262

Holbrook M 1982 Stroke and social and emotional outcome. Journal of the Royal College of Physicians (Lond) 16: 100–104

Hooper J 1988 Case finding in the elderly: does the primary care team already know enough? British Medical Journal 297: 1450–1452

House A 1987 Depression after stroke. British Medical Journal 294: 76–78

Ineichen B 1987 Measuring the rising tide: how many dementia cases will there be in 2001? British Journal of Psychiatry 150: 193–200

Isaacs B, Walkey F A 1964 A survey of incontinence in elderly hospital patients. Gerontology 6: 367–376

Jachuck S J 1989 Caring for the elderly. The Royal College of General Practitioners Members' Reference Book. Royal College of General Practitioners, London, pp 375–378

Jachuck S J 1988 Evaluation of the need in care of the elderly in a general practice. Medical Research Centre, Newcastle upon Tyne

Jachuck S J, Mulcahy J R 1987 Minimum data set necessary to promote the care of the elderly in general practice. Journal of the Royal College of General Practitioners 37: 207–209

Jachuck S J, Stobo S A, Sahgal A 1986 Evaluation of the mental function of the elderly in a general practice. Journal of the Royal College of General Practitioners 36: 123–124

Jack M A, Stobo S A, Scott L A et al 1988 Prevalence of depression in general practice patients over 75 years of age. Journal of the Royal College of General Practitioners 38: 20–21

Jacoby R J, Levy R, Bird J M 1981 Computed tomography and the outcome of affective disorder: a follow-up study of elderly depressives. British Journal of Psychiatry 139: 288–292

Johnson D A W 1973 Treatment of depression in general practice. British Medical Journal 2: 1061–1064

Kahn R L, Zarit S H, Hilbert H M, Niederehe G 1975 Memory compliant and impairment in the aged: the effect of depression and altered brain function. Archives of General Psychiatry 32: 1569–1573

Kay D W K 1989 Ageing of the population: measuring the need for care. Age & Ageing 18: 73–76

Kay D W K, Beamish P, Roth M 1964 Old age mental

disorders in Newcastle upon Tyne. British Journal of Psychiatry 110: 146–158

Kazzniak A W, Wilson R S, Lazarus et al 1981 Memory and depression in dementia. Presented at the Ninth Annual Meeting of the Neuropsychological Society, February 4–7th, Atlanta, Georgia

Kendrick D C 1987 Psychological assessment. In: Pitt B (ed) Dementia: medicine in old age. Churchill Livingstone, Edinburgh, pp 69–89

Legh-Smith J, Wade D T, Langton-Hewer R 1986 Service for stroke patients one year after stroke. Journal of Epidemiological Community Health 40: 161–165

Linn M W, Hunter K, Harris R 1980 Symptoms of depression and recent life events in the community elderly. Journal of Clinical Psychology 36: 675–682

MacDonald A J D 1986 Do general practitioners 'miss' depression in elderly patients? British Medical Journal 292: 1365–1367

Mann A, Graham N, Ashby D 1984 Psychiatric illness in residential homes for the elderly: a survey in one London borough. Age and Ageing 13: 257–265

Matsuyama S S, Jarvik L F 1982 Genetics: what the practitioner needs to know. Generations 7: 19–21

Maule M M, Milne J S, Williamson J 1984 Mental illness and physical health in older people. Age and Ageing 13: 349–356

Millard P H 1983 Depression in old age. British Medical Journal 287: 375–376

Miller A 1985 A study of dependency of elderly patients in wards using different methods of nursing care. Age & Ageing 14: 132–138

Mohanaruban K, Sastry B S D 1989 Assessment and diagnosis of dementia. Geriatric Medicine 19: 81–84

Murphy E 1982 Social origins of depression in old age. British Journal of Psychiatry 141: 135–142

Neshkes R E, Jarvik L F 1985 The central nervous system — dementia and delerium in old age. In: Brocklehurst J C, Textbook of geriatric medicine and gerontology, 3rd edn. Churchill Livingstone, Edinburgh pp 309–327

OARS methodology 1978 Multidimensional functional assessment: the OARS methodology, 2nd edn. Duke University Centre for the study of Aging and Human Development, North Carolina

Patterson L J, Crone P 1986 Depression in the elderly patients. Update 32: 580–590

Pattie A H, Gilleard C J 1979 Manual of the Clifton assessment procedures for the elderly (CAPE). Hodder and Stoughton Educational, Sevenoaks

Pearce J M S 1984 Dementing illness. In: Pearce J M B (ed) Dementia: a clinical approach. Blackwell Scientific Publications, London, pp 1–11

Post F 1972 The management and nature of depressive illness in late life: a follow through study. British Journal of Psychiatry 121: 393–404

Robinson R G, Starr L B, Kubos K L, Price T R 1983 A two year longitudinal study of post stroke mood disorder: findings during the initial examination. Stroke 14: 736–741

Rossor M N 1985 The central nervous system — neuro-chemistry of the aging brain and dementia. In: Brocklehurst J C (ed) Textbook of geriatric medicine and gerontology. Churchill Livingstone, Edinburgh, pp 284–308

Roth M 1978 Epidemiological studies. In: Katzman R, Terry R D, Bick K L (eds) Alzheimer's disease: senile dementia and related disorders. Aging, vol 7. Raven Press, New York

Roth M 1955 The natural history of mental disorder in old age. Journal of Mental Science 101: 281–301

Royal College of Physicians Report 1986 Physical disability in 1986 and beyond. Journal of the Royal College of Physicians (Lond) 18: 128–131

Sadavoy J 1981 Psychogeriatric care in the general hospital. Canadian Journal of Psychiatry 26: 334–336

Smeaton N C 1989 Episodes of mental illness in general practice: results from the Third National Morbidity survey. Health Trends 21: 21–31

Sourander L, Sourander P 1977 Organic brain syndrome and circulatory disorders in old age. In: Wheatley D (ed) Stress and heart. Raven Press, New York.

Strub R L 1985 Mental disorders in brain disease. In: Vinken P J, Bruyen G W (eds) Handbook of clinical neurology, vol 2, (46). Elsevier, New York, 413–442

Thielman S B, Blazer D G 1987 Depression and dementia. In: Pitt B (ed) Dementia: medicine in old age. Churchill Livingstone, Edinburgh, pp 251–264

Tomlinson B E 1980 The structural and quantitative aspects of dementia. In: Roberts P J (ed) Biochemistry of dementia. John Wiley, Chichester, p 15

Wade D T, Hewer L J, Skilbeck C E, David R M 1985 Stroke: a critical approach to diagnosis, treatment and management. Chapman and Hall, London

Williams E I 1984 Characteristics of patients over 75 not seen during one year in general practice. British Medical Journal 288: 119–121

Williamson J, Stokoe I H, Gary S et al 1964 Old people at home: their unreported needs. Lancet i: 1117–1120

World Health Organization 1986 Dementia in later life: research and action: report of a WHO scientific group in senile dementia. Technical Report Series 730. World Health Organization, Geneva

FURTHER READING

Post F, Shulman K 1985 New views on old age affective disorders. In: Arie T (ed) Recent advances in psychogeriatrics, vol 1. Churchill Livingstone, Edinburgh, pp 119–140

Williams I 1979 Mental illness in old age. The care of the elderly in the community. Croom Helm, London, pp 163–173

Lifestyle and health

32. Health promotion and primary care

Simon Smail

By 1990, the primary health care system of all Member States should provide a wide range of health-promotive, curative, rehabilitative and supportive services to meet the basic health needs of the population and give special attention to high-risk, vulnerable and underserved individuals and families.

(Target 28, World Health Organization 1985)

The notion that primary care services should be involved in preventive activity dates back many years; in the United Kingdom, both the Peckham experiment (Pearce and Crocker 1944) and the Dawson Report (Ministry of Health 1920) foreshadowed the emphasis on preventive care that was later to be incorporated as a key element in the NHS Act of 1946. Nevertheless, since 1946 the reality has been that preventive care in the NHS has never received more than a very small per-centage of overall resources. During the 1980s, a rise in consumerism and an increased emphasis in socio-medical research on lay concepts of health and illness both led to a re-examination of models of preventive medicine and health education. The concept of health promotion as proposed by the World Health Organization European Region (WHO 1984) does not fit easily with traditional models either of health education or of preventive medicine.

The roots of the health promotion movement lie in an appreciation of the fundamental determinants of health, whereas traditional health education as practised both in primary care and elsewhere derives almost entirely from a biomedical framework and the questionable assumption that simple educational techniques can have a major influence on health outcomes.

The purpose of this chapter is to examine the relationship between current concepts of health promotion and primary care, with particular reference to the role that primary health care professionals, particularly doctors and nurses, may play in promoting health.

THE CHALLENGE OF 'HEALTH FOR ALL'

During the late 1970s and throughout the 1980s, the World Health Organization played an important role as a catalyst in reviewing and re-examining the fundamental basis of health, the determinants of health, and in particular the role of primary health care in achieving health. Whilst the phrase 'health promotion' has become increasingly used by primary care practitioners, the background concepts may still be unfamiliar to many. The position statements and declarations published by the WHO summarise many of these concepts and advance the case for a broadly based model of health promotion.

The Alma-Ata declaration

An international conference on primary health care was held in 1978 in Alma-Ata in the Soviet Republic of Kazakstan (WHO 1978). The conference agreed an important declaration, which has since formed the basis for much discussion about the role of primary health care.

First, the declaration stated that health is a fundamental human right, which can be achieved only if certain prerequisites are acknowledged. These include a reduction in inequalities between developed and developing countries by sustained economic and social development and world peace.

The declaration reaffirmed the principle that people have the right and duty to participate individually and collectively in the planning and implementation of their health care. Governments, however, have a responsibility in providing adequate health and social measures; the declaration proposed that a main social target for governments should be 'the attainment of all peoples by the year 2000 of a level of health that will lead to a socially and economically productive life.'

The Alma-Ata declaration also affirmed that primary health care is the key to attaining this target. However, the definition of primary health care drawn by the conference is somewhat wider than that usually understood by practitioners within the United Kingdom:

Primary Health Care is essential health care based on practical, scientifically sound and socially acceptable methods and technology made universally accessible to individuals and families in the community through their full participation and at a cost that the community and country can afford... It is the first level of contact of individuals, the family and community with the national health system... and constitutes the first elements of a continuing health care process. Primary health care... is based on the application of relevant results of social, biomedical and health service research and public-health experience; addresses the main health problems of the community, providing promotive, preventive, curative and rehabilitative services accordingly; involves in addition to the health sector all related sectors and aspects of national and community development, in particular agriculture, animal husbandry, food, industry, education, housing, public works, communications and other aspects; relies at local and referral levels on health workers including physicians, nurses, midwives, auxiliaries and community workers.

The conference called on all governments to collaborate in introducing and maintaining primary health care in accordance with the spirit and content of the declaration.

By 1981, WHO Geneva had coordinated many of the important themes in the Alma-Ata declaration and published their *Global strategy for health for all by the year 2000* (WHO 1981). A new programme of work was introduced to achieve progress on the challenging new agenda.

Targets for health for all

The European Office of WHO published a series of 38 specific targets for the European region in order to achieve progress towards the overall goal first proposed at Alma-Ata (WHO 1985).

There are targets for health improvement (targets 1–12), targets aimed at improving lifestyles (targets 13–17), targets aimed at improving the environment (targets 18–25) and targets for setting up appropriate care, particularly emphasising the importance of primary health care (targets 26–31). The remaining targets concern health research and support for the development of appropriate programmes of work. The philosophy of this document draws strongly on the principles expressed in the Alma-Ata declaration, but emphasises the contribution of many different sectors to achieving health and, in particular, charges governments with the responsibility for developing policies, support and resources for promotion of healthy lifestyles. Emphasis is also given to the need for various sectors involved in the promotion of health to work together to maximise the potential of individual inputs ('inter-sectoral collaboration').

So far as primary health care is concerned, yet again its fundamental importance is emphasised, and indeed its role in coordinating efforts to achieve health for all: '... all member states should have mechanisms by which the services provided by all sectors are co-ordinated at the community level in a primary health care system' (Target 30).

The Ottawa charter for health promotion

The concepts of health promotion were further developed at a WHO conference in Ottawa in 1987 (WHO 1987).

A definition of health promotion was adopted by the Ottawa conference: 'Health promotion is the process of enabling people to increase control over and thereby improve their health'. Rather than focusing on professional roles, health promotion is seen as focusing principally on the community, involving not just the health sector but individuals and the wider community. Health promotion seeks to empower individuals and the community to achieve change. The philosophy echos that of the WHO Targets document (1985): 'Health for all will be achieved by people themselves. A well informed and actively participating community is the key element for the attainment of the common goal'.

The Ottawa charter defined the fundamental conditions and resources for health — peace, shelter, education, food, income, a stable ecosystem, sustainable resources, social justice and equity. Five major areas of action were then defined for health promotion action:

Build healthy public policy

Health should be on the agenda of policy makers in all sectors and at all levels, directing them to be aware of the health consequences of their decisions and to accept their responsibilities for health.

Create supportive environments

The impact of environments on health must be recognised. Systematic assessment of a rapidly changing environment — particularly in areas of technology, work, energy production and urbanisation — is essential and must be followed by action to ensure positive benefits to the health of the public.

Strengthen community action

Effective community action involves setting priorities, making decisions, planning strategies and implementing them to achieve better health. At the heart of this process is the empowerment of communities.

Develop personal skills

Health promotion supports personal and social development by the provision of information, education for health and by the enhancement of life skills. By so doing it increases the options available to people to exercise more control over their own health and over their environments and to make choices conducive to health. Settings for this activity include school, home, work and the community, with action through education, professional, commercial and voluntary bodies.

Reorient health services

The role of the health sector must move increasingly in a health promotion direction, beyond its responsibilities for providing clinical and curative services. Health services need to embrace an expanded mandate, which is sensitive and respects cultural needs. This mandate should support the needs for individuals and communities for healthier life and open channels between the health sector and broader social, political, economic and physical environment components. Reorienting health services also requires stronger attention to health research as well as changes in professional education and training.

The Ottawa charter suggested three key skills for achieving health promotion action — advocacy for health, enabling all people to achieve their fullest health potential and mediating between differing interests in society for the pursuit of health.

In 1988, a follow-up conference on the methodology for achieving health through healthy public policy was held at Adelaide, South Australia (WHO 1988). The recommendations of this conference emphasised the issue of public accountability for health, and four key action areas for policy development — the health of women, food and nutrition policy, tobacco and alcohol policy and creating supportive environments.

KEY ISSUES IN HEALTH PROMOTION

Many commentators have found difficulty in coming to terms with the concept of health promotion. As Green and Raeburn (1988) have pointed out, practitioners may latch onto one or more of the strategies or individual concepts and ignore others. For some people, the visionary language employed and the almost unachievable Utopia suggested by the prerequisites of world peace, equity etc., act as a barrier to any real consideration of the practical issues involved in health promotion.

Perhaps the most important issue to grasp in considering health promotion is the breadth of the concepts involved. Health promotion is clearly not the same as preventive medicine, nor is it a modern equivalent of health education, although both are important components. Unfortunately, the terminology has been confused in the United Kingdom by a variety of usages. For example, the UK government (Department of Health 1989) has referred in the new contract for general practitioners to 'health promotion clinics' when they apparently mean the provision of preventive medical services and one-to-one health education.

Some authors (for example Tannahill 1988) interpret health promotion as three overlapping spheres of activity — health education, disease prevention and health protection (including legislation for health). Yet such a model neglects, to a degree, the community focus of the health promotion movement, and does not sufficiently address some of the key issues in health promotion.

The concept of 'lifestyle'

Any discussion of health promotion will inevitably involve consideration of lifestyle. However, it is important that lifestyle is carefully defined; it is not the same as health behaviour. Lifestyle has to be seen as a general way of living based on the interplay between living conditions in the wide sense, and individual patterns of behaviour as determined by sociocultural factors and personal characteristics (Nutbeam 1986). In their critique of health promotion and the Ottawa charter, Green and Raeburn (1988) emphasise the need to take an ecological perspective: 'Health is the product of the continuous interaction and interdependence of the individual and his or her ecosphere: that is the family, community, culture, societal structure and physical environment. Characteristic modes of interacting over time constitute a lifestyle'.

Individual versus collective responsibility

The Ottawa charter emphasises both individual and collective aspects of responsibility. On the one hand governments, professional bodies and institutionalised systems of care have their responsibilities towards policy development and supporting health environments. On the other hand a primary objective in health promotion is also to empower individuals to take control over their own health, and to assist them in adopting appropriate health behaviours.

Some practitioners, commentators and politicians may emphasise one of these two approaches to the almost total exclusion of the other, but there is no dichotomy between the two and they must be seen as complementary. To argue for one approach only at the expense of the other leads to a dangerous and potentially sterile argument.

In a debate in the House of Commons in 1987 (Hansard 1987) the then Minister of Health said:

'surely people should accept responsibility at least in some part for their own health whatever their income. There is a real divide between those who know that their health is in their hands and can do something about it and those who do not and will not. Both groups are present throughout the country. The Government cannot compel people to be healthy, but they can help, and we are determined to do so.'

In the same debate, contributors from other parts of the political spectrum emphasised the importance of improving the environment and dealing with poverty and homelessness. Mr Sam Galbraith pithily summarised such approaches: 'To get people to co-operate we should not blame them. We should take them along with our ideas and make facilities available.'

There is a real danger in any health promotion programme of 'victim blaming': the belief that responsibility for health and health problems is placed chiefly if not exclusively with the individual, neglecting the influence of social, economic and physical environments and the constraints on healthy lifestyle imposed by these factors (Nutbeam 1986).

An unthinking application of traditional approaches to the provision of health information can very readily lead to victim blaming. Many patients just do not believe that basic self-care practices are relevant to their health; attempts at health education may be misinterpreted by the individual, who fails to understand how any change in practices could improve his or her health.

Empowerment

Health promotion involves a movement away from institutional control and high technology towards control of health by the community and people. Empowerment implies valuing the unique contribution that individuals and communities can make, and endeavouring to contribute to and build on this contribution (WHO 1987).

There are a number of different approaches to empowerment, although essentially they can be analysed according to the framework of the Ottawa charter. Perhaps one of the most important areas is that of community action, with its emphasis on self-help groups, community projects and neighbourhood and community development.

The provision of health skills will almost inevitably involve initiatives from the health care sector. Yet lay leaders (natural community leaders or voluntary workers) may also prove effective in demonstrating health skills and in influencing others (Puska et al 1986). Lay leaders can also effectively diffuse innovations in social or health behaviour throughout the community: the theory behind this activity has been reviewed by Rogers (1983).

The ethics of health promotion

Moving from a 'controlling' preventive medicine approach (which can be viewed as a beneficent approach) towards a community-based focus implies a shift in emphasis towards valuing the autonomy of the individual. Yet there are a variety of ethical dilemmas and implications for practitioners. For example, the style of information provision must respect the autonomy of the individual rather than adopting a coercive approach. The relationship between health and the environment constitutes another area of difficulty in ethical terms. The risks of industrial practices in terms of damage to health have often not been quantified, nor indeed is there any consensus on the difficult issues of the balance between financial returns and productivity of industrial processes on the one hand and the health impacts on the environment or workforce. There is an increasing need for a 'health promotion ethic' (Gillon 1987, Manciaux et al 1987).

IMPLICATIONS FOR PRIMARY CARE

The concept of Primary Health Care accepted in the United Kingdom is generally taken to include the activities of the Primary Health Care Team, i.e. doctors, health visitors, district nurses and midwives (Standing Medical Advisory Committee 1981). Although this definition is narrower than that proposed by the Alma-Ata declaration, the reality is that such services are the core services of primary health care in the UK and, as such, have a major contribution to make to the pursuit of the philosophies embodied in the 'Health for All' approach.

Preventive care in British general practice

The role of UK general practitioners in preventive care and health education has tended to develop according to traditional models, often linked to local programmes of preventive care organised by community physicians. The emphasis has been on disease prevention (immunisation programmes, family planning services, antenatal care) and secondary prevention (screening programmes). In concept, these services are based on a medical model of preventive care rather than on a patient-oriented perspective (Calnan 1988, Hart 1988).

The Royal College of General Practitioners' influential reports on prevention (RCGP 1983, 1984) developed the theme of the provision of preventive services through general practice, emphasising for example the importance of ascertaining patients' risk factors for coronary heart disease.

New approaches for primary care professionals

The essential shift of emphasis for primary health care professionals in responding to the challenge of 'Health for All' is an expectation that they will: 'concentrate on the commitment to fostering self-reliance and social action of an intersectoral nature, and on people-oriented health technology which meets the needs of people whilst giving appropriate consideration to the needs that are recognised epidemiologically as demanding urgent attention' (WHO 1983). In essence this implies a shift away from process-oriented health technology to a people/community-oriented perspective. Primary care practitioners in a sense perhaps need to remember their roots: as part of a service within and for the community. It is necessary to develop a better understanding of what can be called the 'health culture' of the community and to work with individuals and groups to enable community members to play a greater part in planning and developing the health care programme.

Public expectations

There is ample evidence that the public expect their primary care practitioners to be interested in health issues as distinct from illness. Wallace et al (1987) found that patients are concerned about their lifestyle and would welcome relevant counselling. Coulter (1987) found in a survey of Oxford residents that 44% would welcome advice on a 'healthier lifestyle'. (It is interesting to note in this paper that many respondents, particularly those in the lower social classes, specifically mentioned environmental issues — unemployment, low income, pollution and housing — as important factors in determining health).

In attempting to respond to such expressed needs, primary health care professionals should have a sensitivity for the potential difference between their patients' views of health needs and their own, professional view of 'needs'. There will be an area of dialogue between the two extremes, which should provide a basis for negotiation. Rather than concentrating on an isolated behaviour (such as smoking), the trend in health education practice should be to examine the general lifestyle of the individual and, crucially, the barriers that exist to adopting any new proposed behaviour. Action in reducing barriers may be vastly more effective than concentrating on an individual behaviour approach. Ensuring that a young unmarried mother has all the social security benefits to which she is entitled may be much more beneficial in helping her to feed her family a more nutritious diet than any amount of education about the nutritional value of unfamiliar foodstuffs.

Styles of communication

Once primary health care professionals have accepted the underlying philosophy of health promotion, it follows that the style of communication between practitioner and patient must value the patient's perspective. This implies not only respecting the individual's autonomy but also, crucially, attempting to understand the beliefs and motivations of the individual so far as these may be relevant to health behaviour. Health behaviour research has sought to address these problems. Such research covers a number of different behavioural science disciplines including anthropology, sociology and social psychology. Each of these sciences brings a particular perspective to the issues, and to the untrained observer there may be a confusion of themes, theories and methodologies (Stacey 1988). Nevertheless, from such research it is perfectly clear that the simplistic notion of a professional giving straightforward 'advice' in a didactic fashion to individuals or groups can rarely be expected to achieve any major impact on health or lifestyles, although such activity may well have a place in a panoply of other action.

One of the themes that is often quoted in discussions of health behaviour is the 'health belief model' developed by Rosenstock (1966) and Becker et al (1977). Put at its simplest, this model suggests that health behaviour is determined by peoples' perception of their own susceptibility to a specific disorder, their perception of how serious the disorder is and whether or not they view the proposed health behaviour or health action as a viable option in their own terms. Factors that might modify a health decision could include the general health motivation of the individual and any cues or other triggers that tip the balance of decision one way or another, such as the advice of a health professional.

Whilst it may help professionals to understand some aspects of health behaviour, it is clear from subsequent research that the health belief model can explain only a relatively small part of health behaviour (Morgan et al 1985). The model was developed in the context of an investigation into the use of preventive services, and does not specifically address more fundamental issues of the origins of basic self-care practices or daily health habits. The work of Pill and Stott (1985, 1986, 1987) has shown that positive health practices (which involve day-to-day lifestyle choices) and procedures (which involve health professionals and services) are nevertheless to some extent linked. They also define an index, the 'Salience of Lifestyle Index', which is a measure of the extent to which the women in their studies believe that lifestyle choices are relevant for health status. This index was a powerful predictor of health practice performance.

Pill and Stott also demonstrated that a large proportion of a working class population of women are fatalistic about their health. Only one in three recognised the relevance of day-to-day behaviour for their health status. Positive health maintenance was an unfamiliar concept, although food and nutrition were the most widely known factors, followed by exercise and physical activity, sleep, rest and relaxation. They concluded that when discussing health behaviour with individuals, primary care professionals should understand that any approach to stereotyping individuals can be counterproductive in the one-to-one consultation.

The importance of self-care practices in health promotion has also been investigated by Dean (1989) who reported on self-care practices of a large population sample in Denmark. Over half of this sample did not report any deliberately undertaken health protective behaviour. However, some interesting correlates emerged. Active health protection behaviour was more common amongst women than men yet social support was less important for health maintenance forms of self-care than had been expected. Health promotion behaviour was conceived quite narrowly by the bulk of the population.

Dean concludes that there may be an excessive focus in health education practice on a few individual health behaviours, to the neglect of other factors such as action to protect the environment.

Many health information programmes operate as though personal behaviour is a simple matter of informed choice

rather than of complex processes involving opportunities for choosing healthy ways of living combined with personal strength and resources for making health enhancing choices. The evidence from the investigation indicates that the socioeconomic situation exerts more influence on self-care behaviour than health attitudes and knowledge.

Communication with patients should therefore recognise not only that individuals may be fatalistic in respect of the impact of health behaviour on their health, but also that the health environment is a legitimate topic for discussion with patients. Empowerment implies helping individuals and groups to influence their own health environment. Practitioners could therefore examine with patients the various barriers to the achievement of better health and help patients to overcome such barriers, rather than concentrating entirely on one or two health behaviours in isolation.

The place of screening/anticipatory care

Much of the emphasis in preventive care during the 1970s and 1980s was on developing screening services. The rapid development of such services has often been questioned (Bayliss 1981), and indeed controlled trials of multiphasic screening have sometimes yielded negative results (Olsen et al 1976)(see also Chapter 1). Yet there are well formulated criteria for judging whether or not screening services are likely to reduce morbidity and mortality (Wilson 1965), and many programmes of screening, described elsewhere in this book, have now been instituted. Anderson (1983) found that the majority of the population (78%) now expect a screening service and many (22% of a sample of 836) reported undergoing a preventive check-up.

However, the problems of screening programmes must be acknowledged. There is a danger that screening services may develop into a technique for removing personal responsibility for health from the individual and placing it with the institution or authority that organises screening. Patients may be seduced into a feeling that 'everything will be all right' if they have a multiphasic check-up, even if their health practices continue to be damaging.

Some screening programmes have been found to generate considerable psychological distress (Posner and Vessey 1988, Marteau 1989). Stoate (1989) found a significant increase in psychological disorder amongst patients 3 months after attending a general practice screening clinic for coronary heart disease (see also Chapter 4).

Screening programmes can undoubtedly identify patients with significant medical disorders (Fullard et al 1987), but the programmes should be run in a way that acknowledges the principles already discussed. It would seem that individual screening programmes consisting simply of one test, or of identifying one behaviour or risk factor, are most likely to prove upsetting for patients. Pre- and post-test counselling by skilled primary care practitioners must be considered an essential prerequisite for any such programme, whether the test is a simple blood pressure or cholesterol measurement or a more complicated test such as mammography. Simply identifying risk factors within a patient population is of little intrinsic value unless carefully followed through with advice and, where necessary, treatment. Advice about health behaviour must be based on a thorough understanding of the individual's background, health habits and self-care perspectives. A patient's own primary care practitioners (doctors or nurses) are in a unique position to provide sensitive screening programmes and advice. They are also able to follow up patients who have been identified in screening programmes to reassess risk factors at regular intervals.

There has also been much debate in the UK concerning the merits of different approaches to the organisation of primary care screening programmes (Stott 1983). Some practitioners favour specific programmes organised as a separate part of service provision, whilst others favour the provision of screening and health advice during the consultation (Stott and Davis 1979) (see also Chapter 9). Organised screening programmes may, however, fail to reach the people who have the highest risks. Stott and Pill (1988) found that high risk patients, with poorer self-care practices, were less likely than lower risk patients to attend a general practitioner's surgery following an invitation for a health check concentrating on cardiac risk factors. Both they and other authors (Smail 1982, Fowler 1985a, b) point out that as 65% of people see their GP every year, and around 90% every 5 years, opportunistic advice during routine consultations may be preferable. Another study (Pill et al 1989) found that over 48% of a cohort of 130 women remembered being given general health advice during a routine general practice consultation over a 5-year period.

Community involvement

A number of authors, particularly Calnan (1988), have pointed out that both organised screening and opportunistic health advice during consultations may be conceived as placing an undue burden on individuals to accept responsibility for their own health (victim blaming). Screening programmes are generally instituted to

detect those patients at highest risk from specific diseases or to detect presymptomatic disease. This approach to prevention is known as the 'high-risk' approach. However, primary care practitioners are in a unique position to integrate such an approach with the 'low-risk', or population, approach to prevention. Essentially this will entail a more community-oriented programme of activities for the primary health care team. Such a programme of activity can be seen as an important adjunct to the use of opportunistic health education and prevention within the consultation.

Should primary care practitioners not become more heavily involved in alternative health promotion strategies other than screening and 'health advice'? They have a potentially strong role in advocacy for health, both at the local level, and, collectively, at the national level. Similarly, they may at times be in a position to mediate to improve the health environment. Health visitors in the UK and public health nurses in other countries, e.g. Canada and Finland, have at times become involved in a variety of community initiatives for health. The various professional members of the primary health care team may each have particular roles in working more actively with the community. One admirable example from British general practice involved community action by a group of practitioners to promote the provision of exercise facilities for the benefit of the local community (Campbell et al 1985). However, many general practitioners and nurses are inexperienced in such activity and may feel that their place is in the surgery, behind their desks. As a first step towards becoming involved in community initiatives, any practice can investigate the local provision of lay care groups and health interest groups, and learn to use them more effectively. Similarly, the philosophy of intersectoral collaboration is important. Other sectors that are important in community terms include not only the voluntary sector but also education, the churches, industry, occupational health, housing and the leisure and amenity services of local authorities. It must, however, be acknowledged that active cooperation with other sectors may at times be handicapped by lack of a shared goal and lack of resources for implementing joint programmes of work.

Primary care practitioners also have an important role to play in 'agenda setting' for the local community. Doctors and nurses act as powerful role models in the community and many consider that they have a personal obligation to follow appropriate health behaviours, reinforcing their role as advocates for health. A number of general practitioners also act as a resource for the local media sources, providing information and advice for newspapers and radio programmes (Smail

1983, 1985). Such activities can raise the profile of health issues, although ultimately personal advice from a health professional may be more successful in influencing individual health behaviour. Local media may be an important avenue for raising the profile of issues concerning the local health environment.

ORGANISING PRIMARY CARE FOR HEALTH PROMOTION

Several authors have suggested that a new breed of general practitioner is needed to provide community-oriented care. Mant and Anderson (1985) suggested that there should be integration of general practice and community medicine, whilst Hart (1988) suggests that a 'new kind of doctor' is needed. He proposed a number of possible scenarios, including a much closer link between community physicians and general practitioners, with an enhanced role in health promotion for nurses attached to group practices, or alternatively a fully salaried service for general practitioners.

The Community Nursing Review for Wales (Welsh Office 1987) suggested an enhanced structure for practice teams, with clearly defined goals and a commitment to developing work with the community.

New management structures are being brought into place in UK primary care at the time of writing. However, the scientific basis for some of the services demanded of general practitioners by the 1990 contract have been challenged. Morrell (1991) has pointed out that the general philosophy of the new contract ignores much earlier research, especially in relation to screening services.

Policies for health promotion action are needed, but these should take into account the principles of 'Health for All'. Primary care teams must never be seen as isolated units responsible or accountable for the health status of the population they serve. Such an approach is a denial of the responsibilities of other sectors for health, as well as a reflection of a missed opportunity for real progress in developing a central coordinating role for primary care teams. Although emphasis has been placed on achievement of targets for screening and immunisation, there are real moral and ethical dangers in developing an approach that is orientated towards such centrally determined process targets (such as recording of blood pressure levels or other risk factors) rather than an approach oriented towards more fundamental health goals and based on sensitivity to patients' beliefs, needs and perceptions.

Training for health promotion

A recent survey of European medical schools demonstrated that the medical teachers in only 3 countries were 'very familiar' with the Alma-Ata declaration, although the medical schools in 11 out of 26 countries emphasised the responsibilities of the community in participating in decisions about their own health (Walton 1985). The development of teaching of general practice throughout Europe is also patchy. Nevertheless, Walton found some reasons for satisfaction in that attitudes have clearly been changing very rapidly; but further progress 'will only result from a major reorientation in medical education'.

It will be difficult for medical schools, and particularly departments of primary care, to teach about health promotion unless a clear lead is given by governments. It will also be essential for schools to have access to, and to be involved in, active health promotion projects that can be used as a base for teaching. In Wales, the 'Heartbeat Wales' programme (Smail and Parish 1989) has formed the basis for new developments in postgraduate education, with the foundation of an academic Institute of Health Promotion; core funding is provided by the Health Promotion Authority for Wales.

CONCLUSION

Primary care practitioners must accept that they have a central role to play in changing the lifestyle of individuals, families and populations. However, they must also realise that the determinants of lifestyle include not just health behaviour, but also societal and environmental factors. To influence lifestyles, practitioners should bear in mind environmental barriers to the adoption of better lifestyles and seek to modify them directly by using new methods of health promotion action, or by empowering individuals to address the barriers for themselves. Health promotion through primary care therefore involves a broad range of activities, best carried out by a team of professionals with a variety of different skills. The skills for community development, of advocacy, mediating and enabling may be new to practitioners. In particular, skills for intersectoral working may need to be developed.

A shift in emphasis is needed away from the technology of process-oriented preventive medicine towards a renewed understanding of the way that patients and communities behave and an understanding of the manifold influences upon such behaviour.

REFERENCES

Anderson R M 1983 Public attitudes to and experience of medical check ups. Community Medicine 5: 11–20

Baylis R I S 1981 The medical check-up. British Medical Journal 283: 631–634

Becker M H, Haefner D P, Kasl S V et al 1977 Selected psychological models and correlates of individual health-related behaviours. Medical Care 15(5): Suppl 27–46

Calnan M 1988 Examining the general practitioner's role in health education: a critical review. Family Practice 5(3): 217–223

Campbell M J, Brown D, Waters W E 1985 Can general practitioners influence exercise habits? Controlled trial. British Medical Journal 290: 1044–1046

Coulter A 1987 Lifestyle and social class: implications for primary care. Journal of the Royal College of General Practitioners 37: 533–536

Dean K 1989 Self-care components of lifestyles: The importance of gender, attitudes and the social situation. Social Science and Medicine 29(2): 137–152

Department of Health 1989 General Practice in the National Health Service: A new contract. Department of Health, London

Fowler G 1985(a) Health education in general practice. Health Education Journal 44(1): 44–45

Fowler G 1985(b) Health education in general practice: giving advice. Health Education Journal 44(2): 103–104

Fullard E, Fowler G, Gray M 1987 Promoting prevention in primary care: controlled trial of low technology, low cost approach. British Medical Journal 294: 1080–1082

Gillon R 1987 Health education and health promotion. Journal of Medical Ethics 13: 3–4

Green L W, Raeburn J M 1988 Health Promotion. What is it? What will it become? Health Promotion 3(2): 151–159

Hart J T 1988 A new kind of doctor. Merlin Press, London

Hansard 1987 Parliamentary Debates 23 October 1987; House of Commons Official Report 120(29): 1026–1094

Manciaux M, Pissaro B, Zucman E 1987 Ethics and health promotion. Health Promotion 2(1): 1–3

Mant D, Anderson P 1985 Community General Practitioner. Lancet ii: 1114–1117

Marteau T M 1989 Psychological costs of screening. British Medical Journal 299: 527

Ministry of Health 1920 Interim report on the future provision of Medical and Allied Services (Dawson Report) Cmnd 693, HMSO, London

Morgan M, Calnan M, Manning N 1985 Sociological approaches to health and medicine. Routledge, London

Morrell D C 1991 Role of research in development of organization and structure of general practice. British Medical Journal 302: 1313–1316

Nutbeam D 1986 Health promotion glossary. Health Promotion 1(1):113–127

Olsen D M, Kane R L, Proctor H 1976 A controlled trial of multiphasic screening. New England Journal of Medicine 294(17): 925–930

Pearce I H, Crocker L H 1944 The Peckham experiment: a study in the living structure of society. George Allen and Unwin, London

Pill R, Stott N C H 1985 Preventive procedures and practices among working class women: new data and fresh insights. Social Science and Medicine 21: 975–983

Pill R, Stott N C H 1986 Looking after themselves: health protective behaviour among British working class women. Health Education Research 1: 111–119

Pill R M, Stott N C H 1987 The stereotype of 'working-class fatalism' and the challenge for primary care health promotion. Health Education Research 2(2): 105–114

Pill R M, Jones-Elwyn G, Stott N C H 1989 Opportunistic health promotion: quantity or quality? Journal of the Royal College of General Practitioners 39: 196–200

Posner T, Vessey M 1988 Prevention of cancer: the patient's view. King Edward's Hospital Fund for London, London

Puska P, Koskela K, McAlister A et al 1986 Use of lay opinion leaders to promote diffusion of health innovations in a community programme. Lessons learned from the North Karelia project. Bulletin of the World Health Organization 64(3): 437–446

RCGP 1983 Promoting prevention. Occasional Paper 22. Royal College of General Practitioners, London

RCGP 1984 Combined reports on prevention. Reports from General Practice Nos 18–21. Royal College of General Practitioners, London

Rogers E 1983 Diffusion of innovations. The Free Press, Macmillan Publishers, London

Rosenstock I 1966 Why people use health services. Millbank Memorial Fund Quarterly 44: 54–127

Smail S A 1982 Opportunities for prevention: the consultation. British Medical Journal 284: 1092–1093

Smail S A 1983 Doctor on the air. Practitioner 227: 1839–1845

Smail S A 1985 Medicine and the media. Journal of the Royal College of General Practitioners 35: 363–366

Smail S A, Parish R 1989 Heartbeat Wales — a community programme. Practitioner 233: 343–347

Stacey M 1988 In: Anderson R, Davies J K, Kickbusch I et al (eds) Health behaviour research and health promotion. Oxford Medical Publications, Oxford, pp 270–279

Standing Medical Advisory Committee 1981 The primary care team. HMSO, London

Stoate H G 1989 Can health screening damage your health? Journal of the Royal College of General Practitioners 39: 193–195

Stott N C H 1983 Primary health care. Springer-Verlag, Berlin

Stott N C H, Davis R H 1979 The exceptional potential in each primary care consultation. Journal of the Royal College of General Practitioners 29: 201–205

Stott N C H, Pill R M 1988 Health checks in general practice.University of Wales College of Medicine, Cardiff

Tannahill A 1988 Health promotion and public health: a model in action. Community Medicine 10(1): 48–51

Wallace P G, Brennan P J, Haines A P 1987 Are general practitioners doing enough to promote healthy lifestyles? Findings of the Medical Research Council's general practice research framework study on lifestyle and health. British Medical Journal 294: 940–942

Walton H J 1985 Primary health care in European medical education: a survey. Medical Education 19: 167–188

Welsh Office 1987 Nursing in the community — A team approach for Wales. Report of the review of Community Nursing in Wales. Welsh Office, Cardiff

WHO 1978 Primary health care. Report of the Internal Conference on primary health care. Alma-Ata, USSR,

6–12 September 1978. "Health for All" series No. 1. World Health Organization, Geneva

WHO 1981 Global strategy for health for all by the year 2000. "Health for All" series, No. 3. World Health Organization, Geneva

WHO 1983 New approaches to health education in primary health care. Technical Report Series 690. World Health Organization, Geneva

WHO 1984 Health promotion: A discussion document on the concepts and principles. World Health Organization, Copenhagen

WHO 1985 Targets for health for all. WHO Regional Office for Europe, Copenhagen

WHO 1987 Ottawa charter for health promotion. Health Promotion 1(4): iii–v

WHO 1988 The Adelaide recommendations: healthy public policy. Health Promotion 3(2): 183–186

Wilson J M G 1965 Some principles of early diagnosis and detection. In: Teeling Smith G (ed) Surveillance and early diagnosis in general practice. Office of Home Economics Press, London, pp 5–10

33. Disorders of diet, eating and weight

Peter Campion   Elizabeth M E Poskitt

NUTRITION AND HEALTH

Imbalance between dietary intake and nutritional requirements, due either to nutrient deficiency or excess, may result in ill health. Gross food deficiencies lead to protein energy malnutrition or starvation, or

Table 33.1   Groups at risk from diet-related diseases

Disorder	Group(s) at risk
Obesity	Those with family history of obesity Children of single parents; single children Low social class Sedentary occupation Physical handicap
Eating disorders	Females aged 12–35 Overweight
Protein calorie malnutrition	Chronic illness Prolonged hospitalisation Extreme social deprivation Psychological eating disorder Total vegetarian diets 'Eccentric' diets (macrobiotic, fruitarian) Confused, impoverished, elderly
Vitamin C deficiency	Confused, impoverished, elderly Edentate Chronically sick Prolonged hospitalisation Extreme social deprivation
Vitamin D deficiency	Anticonvulsant or steroid treatment Asian or middle-east origin Lack of sunlight: housebound Elderly
Iron deficiency	Premature babies Those on vegetarian diets All children Premenopausal women
Vitamin B deficiencies	Alcoholics Total vegetarians

anorexia nervosa. Inadequate intake of trace substances or 'micronutrients' leads to vitamin and mineral deficiencies, such as rickets and dietary anaemias. Simple obesity is the result of an excess of energy intake over requirements, while dental caries can be considered as the result of both a deficiency of a micronutrient, fluoride, and an excess intake of dietary sugar.

Screening the population for dietary 'deviance' may seem attractive but is impractical for several reasons. The assessment of dietary intake is never very reliable, particularly when carried out in a clinical setting. Dietary intakes vary from day to day and recorded intakes, especially of micronutrients, are inaccurate over short periods. Population dietary needs are expressed through 'Dietary reference-values' (Department of Health 1991) but these represent safe levels for whole populations rather than guidelines on minimal requirements for individuals, which vary widely.

If it is assumed that some dietary patterns may contribute to future morbidity, and that risks can be reduced if diets are modified, it becomes important to identify those groups at increased risk of developing diet-related diseases. Routine enquiries about diet may identify individuals likely to be at risk from nutritional deficiency, excess, or imbalance, and screening procedures may then be applied to them.

Table 33.1 lists at-risk groups for those diet-related diseases common in the UK. Many nutritional problems common in some parts of the world are not seen in the UK, except in association with other underlying illness. The remainder of this chapter therefore focuses on conditions of sufficient frequency in the UK to make the presymptomatic screening of whole populations worthwhile — obesity, anorexia and bulimia, vitamin D deficiency and iron deficiency.

OBESITY

Obesity is defined as an excess of body fat. Excess fat is usually associated with increased lean body mass but there are no clinically practical methods of measuring lean and fat body mass separately and accurately. Garrow (1988) showed that, independent of height, body weight rises by 1.27 kg for every 1 kg fat gained: 75% of excess weight is fat. Even so, weight alone cannot be used as a measure of fatness, as height is a major determinant of total body weight. To overcome this problem various indices relating weight to height have been developed to assess obesity. The Body Mass Index (BMI) or Quetelet index:

$$\frac{\text{weight (kg)}}{\text{height (m}^2)}$$

is widely used, although it invokes no direct measurement of body fat. It is simple to determine and provides a reasonable measure of relative fatness in adults. Garrow (1988) has classified obesity in terms of the BMI as follows:

Underweight	< 20
Grade 0	20 – 24.9
Grade I	25 – 29.9
Grade II	30 – 40
Grade III	> 40

BMI is not a useful indicator when used alone as an estimate of fatness in children because the relationship of weight to height varies with age. A more suitable index (Cole 1979) relates the BMI of the index child to the BMI of a theoretical child of the same age and with weight and height on the 50th centile for age. A slide rule has been developed to simplify estimation of this percentage expected BMI and is available from Castlemead Publications, 12 Little Mundells, Welwyn Garden City, Hertfordshire, AL7 1EW. Alternatively, a visual comparison of the relative positions of height and weight on standard growth charts (Tanner et al 1966) gives a rough estimate of the extent of overweight where applicable.

Both BMI and percentage expected BMI indices are only indirect estimations of fatness and should be used circumspectly, particularly when considering individuals at the extremes of height, or those with unusual physical activity levels (greater or less than normal) in whom the relation of fat to lean tissue is likely to be abnormal. The thickness of subcutaneous fat layers can be measured directly by using skinfold callipers but these are less practical and are imprecise if used by the inexperienced (see Garrow 1988, p 39 for details).

Health implications of obesity

Individuals with Grade III obesity (BMI > 40) have significantly greater risk for morbidity and mortality than those of normal weight. BMI > 40 is equivalent to a weight of 130 kg (20 stones) in an individual of 179 cm (5 feet 10 inches) or > 90 kg (14 stones) for someone of only 151 cm (5 feet). Most individuals with this degree of obesity recognise they are overweight and are often anxious to lose weight. The role of health professionals is to consider what intervention can be applied. Some reduction in weight, even if not achieving ideal body weight, is likely to result in reduced morbidity and enhanced well being.

Cardiovascular morbidity and mortality rise significantly as BMI rises above 30 — Grade II obesity (Tuomilehto et al 1987). As other cardiovascular risk factors, such as elevated blood lipids and hypertension, are also commonly associated with overweight, the extent to which overweight itself directly influences risk is widely questioned (Jarrett 1986, Keys 1986). Nevertheless, this degree of obesity remains a threat to health for at least some individuals (Dawes 1984). As these individuals do not necessarily recognise they have weight problems, screening by weight and height measurement and calculation of BMI, will expose otherwise unrecognised health risks.

Grade I obesity (BMI 25–30) appears to have very little association with illness in the absence of other adverse factors such as diabetes mellitus, hyper-

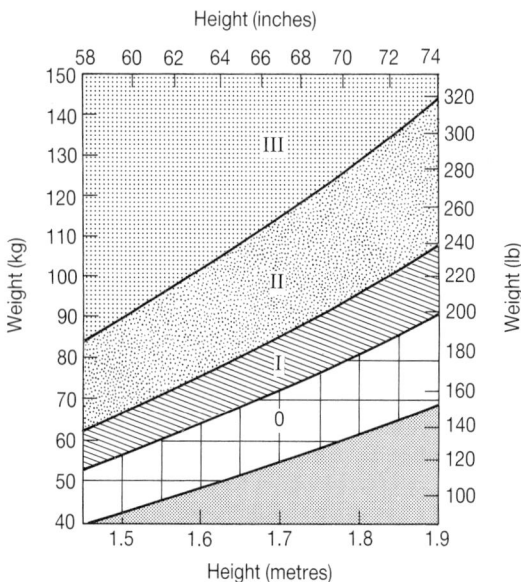

Fig. 33.1   Relation of weight to height defining desirable range (0), and grades I, II and III obesity, marked by boundaries W/H^2=25-29.9, 30-40, and over 40 respectively (from Garrow 1988).

lipidaemia or hypertension. Does this BMI represent a risk factor for more severe obesity and thus a risk to health? Braddon et al (1986) followed a cohort of over 5000 individuals born in 1946 for over 30 years and concluded that obesity frequently appears in young adults and increases in severity with time. Thus there is an argument for identifying milder degrees of obesity in young adults in the hope of preventing the development of more severe obesity.

Other anthropometric indices: waist/hip and waist/thigh circumference ratios

Recently it has been recognised that fat distribution, independent of the extent of obesity, may be an important risk factor and a better predictor of cardiovascular problems than the degree of overweight alone. Cardiovascular disease is more strongly associated with central or abdominal fat than with more peripherally deposited fat (Kissebah et al 1982, Lapidus et al 1984, Seiden et al 1989). Estimations of waist:hip circumference ratios reflect the distribution of fat between abdominal and subcutaneous sites and may have a place in screening (Ashwell et al 1985). Further studies of correlations between body fat distribution and morbidity suggest that the waist:mid-thigh circumference ratio may give even better correlations between anthropometric measurements and clinical problems (Mueller et al 1987).

The Bogalusa studies in the USA demonstrated that truncal obesity in children is associated with high levels of very low density lipoprotein and low density lipoprotein-bound cholesterol, decreased high density lipoprotein-bound cholesterol and decreased apolipoprotein A_1. These are lipid profiles associated with increased risk of cardiovascular problems in later life (Freedman et al 1989).

Body image

Actual weight and perceived weight are not the same. Brodie & Slade (1988) distinguish between body dissatisfaction, which is associated with fatness, and body image inaccuracy, which is not associated with fatness, but is related to the eating disorders, anorexia nervosa and bulimia (see below). Thus, patients who present to their doctor complaining of their weight should be assessed psychologically as well as anthropometrically to avoid the potentially disastrous mistake of exacerbating an eating disorder by inappropriately discussing dieting in a vulnerable individual.

Can obesity be treated?

An important criterion for any screening procedure is that the condition should be amenable to treatment. Garrow (1988) proposed that an explanation for the reluctance of many doctors to recognise obesity as a problem may be the widespread but erroneous view that it is untreatable! The evidence on treatment has been reviewed by Cohen (1985) and Garrow (1988), and can perhaps be summarised in the one word 'perseverance', applied to both patients and physicians. There is no magic cure, the laws of thermodynamics are inviolable, weight loss takes time and relapse prevention must be part of any treatment strategy.

Coupar and Kennedy (1980), clinical psychologist and general practitioner respectively, showed the moderate but measurable effectiveness of small group therapy in a general practice setting, using conventional dietary education and behaviour therapy. After 10 months, 7 of their original 16 obese patients had maintained a loss of at least 5% of body weight. Such weight losses are depressing if compared with the total amount of excess fat but any weight loss is likely to be associated with improved self-image, improved exercise capacity and some reduction in cardiovascular health risks. The fact that return to ideal body weight is probably an unrealistic goal is no contraindication to attempting some weight reduction and should not deter the doctor from recommending weight reduction.

Screening for obesity in general practice

There is no evidence that routine recording of height and weight in healthy individuals does harm and, because established obesity is so difficult to treat (Pacy et al 1987), there is a case for general practitioners 'screening' for obesity by documenting changes in patients' BMI over time (Frame 1986), perhaps at 3-yearly intervals. This could coincide with the currently recommended 3-yearly check of cervical cytology in women. Review of all adults not seen in the preceding 3 years became part of the contractual duties of general practitioners in the UK in 1990 (DOH 1989), and the recording of data that allow the BMI to be calculated is stipulated as part of this review.

EATING DISORDERS

The diagnostic criteria for eating disorders defined in DSM-III-R (American Psychiatric Association 1987, Fairburn 1987, 1990) are as follows:

Anorexia nervosa

1. Intense fear of becoming obese, which does not diminish as weight loss progresses.
2. Disturbance of body image, e.g. claiming to 'feel fat' even when emaciated.
3. Weight loss of at least 25% of original body weight or, if under 18 years of age, > 25% weight loss from original body weight combined with projected weight gain expected from growth charts.
4. Refusal to maintain body weight over a minimal normal weight for age and height.
5. No known physical illness that would account for the weight loss.

Bulimia

1. Recurrent episodes of binge eating (rapid consumption of a large amount of food in a discrete period of time, usually less than 2 hours).
2. At least three of the following:
   a. consumption of high-calorie, easily ingested food during a binge;
   b. inconspicuous eating during a binge;
   c. termination of such episodes by abdominal pain, sleep, social interruption, or self-induced vomiting;
   d. repeated attempts to lose weight by severely restricted diets, self-induced vomiting, or use of catharctics or diuretics;
   e frequent weight fluctuations greater than 10 pounds (4.5kg) due to alternating binges and fasts.
3. Awareness that the eating pattern is abnormal and fear of not being able to stop eating voluntarily.
4. Depressed mood and self-deprecating thought following eating binges.
5. The bulimic episodes are not due to anorexia nervosa or any known physical disorder.
6. Persistent over-concern with body weight and shape.

For each condition, a corresponding 'partial syndrome' is defined by the presence of all criteria except those relating to weight.

Prevalence

A recent British survey from four general practices in South London (King 1989) screened consecutive attenders aged between 16 and 35: 186 males and 534 females. The screening test was the widely used Eating Attitudes Test (EAT) (Garner et al 1982). High scorers and a sample of low scorers were interviewed using two research interview schedules. The figure for prevalence of full eating disorder was $1.1 \pm 1.0\%$, while for all forms (full and partial anorexia and bulimia) it was $3.9 \pm 1\%$. In addition to identifying 7 cases of bulimia nervosa and 15 cases of partial bulimia or anorexia, the remaining high scorers on the EAT were classified as obsessional dieters (13), normal dieters (23), obese (3) and disturbed (4). In another British survey (Johnson-Sabine et al 1988) 1.8% of a sample of 1000 unselected London schoolgirls aged 14-16 showed evidence of either full or partial eating disorder.

Whitaker et al (1989), using the EAT with a large population of American schoolchildren, reported point prevalences for anorexia and bulimia (DSM-III criteria) of 0.2 and 1.2%, respectively, in girls and 0.4% for bulimia in boys. No boy showed the full syndrome of anorexia nervosa. Point prevalences for the partial anorexia and bulimia syndromes, i.e. not fulfilling the weight criteria, were 7.6% and 1.2% in girls and 0.6% and 0.4% in boys, respectively. True prevalences would have been higher because children in hospital for management of eating disorders were not included in the survey. As bulimic behaviour represents a threat to health, the authors argue that screening for this form of eating disorder is as important as screening for the better known anorexia.

Slade (1982) developed a model of the aetiology of eating disorders, which proposed the two 'setting conditions' of general dissatisfaction with life and self, and perfectionist tendencies, which together generated a 'need for total bodily control', and in the presence of successful dieting led to anorexia nervosa. Slade & Dewey (1986) have subsequently developed a screening questionnaire, the 'SCANS', which has been shown to discriminate between patients with eating disorders and normal controls, in five dimensions — general dissatisfaction, perfectionism, social and personal anxiety and weight control — patients with eating disorders scoring higher than controls on all scales. These authors argue that, as many studies have shown that the best predictor of outcome is the duration of the eating disorder before the start of treatment (the shorter the better), early intervention is likely to prove worthwhile. Disorders of short duration may well include more of those likely to resolve spontaneously so the effects of early intervention have yet to be proved.

Implications for general practice

Computerised self-administered tests are being developed (King 1989), which will assess the risk of developing an eating disorder in populations of schoolchildren, or other groups of adolescents such as college students, or occupational groups. The outcome of such testing remains to be seen, but it seems likely that general practitioners need to become more aware of the significance of abnormal eating behaviour and attitudes. King (1989) gave information to general practitioners on half the patients with high EAT scores to assess the effect on the GP's practice. Only one of these patients with a high EAT score was referred for specialist care, and none for whom information was not given to the GP. Several patients were referred, at their own request, to a dietitian. There is a danger that general practitioners misunderstand the symptoms of eating disorders and respond in terms of dietary advice, thus colluding with patients whose real problems are not dietary, but those of self-image, self-satisfaction, and relationships with their environment.

IRON DEFICIENCY

Iron deficiency in children is common and important (Illingworth 1986). It is a consequence of the high iron requirements of rapidly growing children, the low bioavailability of iron in many foods, the low iron content of many children's diets and the effect of frequent infections on appetite and absorption. Premature and small-for-date infants, because of lower total body iron at birth and rapid growth, are particularly at risk, especially once birth weights have doubled and iron stores in the tissues and the high haemoglobin of the neonate have been utilised (Poskitt 1988).

The inclusion of tests for iron deficiency in programmes of routine child surveillance in general practice showed the prevalence of iron deficiency (defined by haemoglobin < 10.5 g/dl and mean corpuscular volume < 75 fl) as 16% (James et al 1988) and 17% (Grant 1990), respectively. Serum ferritin < 10 μg/litre was regarded as confirmation of iron deficiency. Iron deficiency was three times more common in non-Caucasian children than in Caucasians (25% compared with 8%) and slightly more common in those below than those above the 10th centile weight for age (James et al 1988).

Hall (1989), in the report of a joint working party on child health surveillance, gives more details of haematological criteria for the diagnosis of iron deficiency but does not recommend universal screening until more research has been done. There is some evidence that iron deficiency retards physical and mental development (Illingworth 1986) and that these changes can be reversed by treatment with oral iron (Aukett et al 1986, Pollitt et al 1986). Screening preschool children for iron deficiency anaemia seems justifiable and, as the studies

by James et al (1988) and Grant (1990) included 650 children, screening seems both feasible and acceptable as well.

VITAMIN D DEFICIENCY

Deficiency of vitamin D in childhood causes rickets, classically presenting in neonates, infants, young toddlers and adolescents, especially those whose families originate from the Indian subcontinent (Arneil and Barltrop 1978). A large scale survey in Glasgow (Goel et al 1976) found that 12% of children of Asian origin showed evidence of florid, minimal or healing rickets. More recently, public health strategies and adaptation to a more British way of life by Asian communities have reduced the incidence of rickets in this vulnerable group (Dunnigan et al 1981). However, children with vegetarian diets and those with lack of sunlight exposure remain at risk. In one survey 17% of a group of children from Rastafarian families who followed total vegetarian diets showed evidence of rickets (James et al 1985).

Accurate diagnosis of the presence or absence of mild rickets is not easy, particularly as summer sunshine may initiate spontaneous cure and confuse biochemical and radiological findings. Useful investigations are serum calcium, phosphate and alkaline phosphatase, coupled with X-rays of wrists and knees (Goel et al 1976). Elevated alkaline phosphatase with calcium and phosphate which are low, or at the lower limit of normal suggests active rickets, but alkaline phosphatase may be elevated in a number of situations, including early in the adolescent growth spurt, and thus results must also be interpreted with clinical and radiological information. Screening even high risk populations for rickets is probably unnecessary provided effective health education is available to families of high risk groups. It needs to be remembered that rickets can be a problem for dark skinned children, those on vegetarian diets and those infants changed on to whole cow's milk early and not given supplementary vitamin D.

Vitamin D and the elderly

The report of the DHSS Working Party on the Fortification of Foods with Vitamin D (1980) stressed the importance of osteomalacia due to inadequate vitamin D ingestion or production by the elderly. Prevalence may be about 2–5% of the elderly population (Campbell et al 1984). It has been suggested that osteomalacia in this age group may contribute to the risk of fracture of the femoral neck and other bone and muscle problems. Levels of the main circulating metabolite of vitamin D (25-hydroxy vitamin D) are significantly lower in the elderly than in younger people and levels are lower in elderly women than men; values show smaller summertime rises than in younger people. The elderly probably expose less skin to the summer sun and have smaller intakes of vitamin D because of lower total food intakes. They fail to build up adequate stores of vitamin D in summer to maintain 25-hydroxy vitamin D levels above those at which osteomalacia develops (< 5 ng/ml) throughout the winter (Lawson et al 1979). Problems are most likely in those over 75 years. Screening for vitamin D deficiency by enquiries about clinical symptoms such as bone pain, muscle weakness, difficulty going up and down stairs (common symptoms in all the very old!) and further assessment by measurement of calcium, phosphate and alkaline phosphatase when there is concern, are therefore important, (see also Chapter 30).

INDIVIDUALS WITH RESTRICTIVE DIETARY PRACTICES

There appear to be increasing numbers of individuals adopting vegetarian or more restricted diets in Britain for either religious, moral or ethical reasons or because these diets are perceived as enhancing health. Lacto-ovo-vegetarian diets present few problems except in the very young (Nutrition Standing Committee of the British Paediatric Association 1988) and the very old, but total vegetarian (vegan) diets can lead to calcium, riboflavin and vitamin B12 deficiency. All vegetarian diets, but particularly total vegetarian diets given to young children, risk inadequate intakes of many nutri-ents, including protein and energy (Nutrition Standing Committee of the British Paediatric Association 1988). More restrictive diets than vegan diets, e.g. fruitarian, macrobiotic, should be discouraged.

It is likely that some of those voluntarily pursuing strict vegetarian diets will not welcome routine screening for deficiency problems. Nevertheless, regular growth monitoring is essential so that families can be advised if the children's growth appears to be less than expected because of their diet. In adults, occasional monitoring of weight and clinical checking for evidence of anaemia, with dietary advice or investigation where indicated, would seem the most appropriate form of surveillance. Those following strict total vegetarian diets should be advised to seek nutritional and dietary advice from reliable informed sources such as the Vegan Society.

CONCLUSION

Screening for dietary disorders is not a precise procedure because the boundaries between normal and abnormal are often ill-defined and both excessive and inadequate intakes can be causes for concern. Perhaps the most useful activity is the measurement of height and weight as part of the clinical evaluation of both individuals and groups. Amongst groups it is those at the extremes of age, those more or less dependent on others for their nutrition (children, confused elderly, handicapped and bedridden), and those pursuing extreme lifestyles, who are most at risk of nutritional complications.

REFERENCES

American Psychiatric Association 1987 Diagnostic and statistical manual of mental disorders, 3rd edn, revised (DSM-III-R). American Psychiatric Association, Washington DC

Arneil C, Barltrop D 1978 Nutrition and nutritional disorders. In: Forfar J O and Arneil G C (eds) Textbook of paediatrics. Churchill Livingstone, Edinburgh, p 1119–1128

Ashwell M, Cole T J, Dixon A K 1985 Obesity: new insight into the anthropometric classification of fat distribution shown by computed tomography. British Medical Journal 290: 1692–1694

Aukett M A, Parks Y A, Scott P H, Wharton B A 1986 Treatment with iron increases weight gain and psychomotor development. Archives of Disease in Childhood 61: 849–857

Braddon F E M, Rodgers B, Wadsworth M E J, Davies J M C 1986 Onset of obesity in a 36 year birth cohort study. British Medical Journal 293: 299–303

Brodie D A, Slade P D 1988 The relationship between body-image and body-fat in adult women. Psychological Medicine 18: 623–631

Campbell G A, Kemm J R, Hosking D J, Boyd R V 1984 How common is osteomalacia in the elderly? Lancet ii: 386–388

Cohen J 1985 Obesity: a review. Journal of the Royal College of General Practitioners 35: 435–441

Cole T J 1979 A method of assessing age and standardised weight for height in children seen cross sectionally. Annuals of Human Biology 6: 249–268

Coupar A M, Kennedy T 1980 Running a weight control group: experiences of a psychologist and a general practitioner. Journal of the Royal College of General Practitioners 30: 41–48

Dawes M G 1984 Obesity in a Somerset town: prevalence and relationship to morbidity. Journal of the Royal College of General Practitioners 34: 328–330

Department of Health 1989 Terms of service for doctors in general practice. Department of Health, London

Department of Health 1991 Dietary reference values for food energy and nutrients for the United Kingdom. Report on Health and Social Subjects No 41, HMSO, London

Department of Health and Social Security 1980 Rickets and

Osteomalacia. Report on Health and Social Subjects No. 19, HMSO, London

Dunnigan M G, McIntosh W B, Sutherland G R et al 1981 A policy for the prevention of Asian rickets in Britain: an assessment of the Glasgow rickets campaign. British Medical Journal 282: 357–360

Fairburn C 1987 Eating disorders. Medicine International 2: 1846–1850

Fairburn C 1990 Bulimia nervosa. British Medical Journal 300: 485–487

Frame P S 1986 A critical review of adult health maintenance: Part 4 Prevention of metabolic, behavioural, and miscellaneous conditions. Journal of Family Practice 23: 29–39

Freedman D S, Srinavasan S K, Harsha D W et al 1989 Relation of body fat patterning to lipid and lipoprotein concentrations in children and adolescents. The Bogalusa Heart Study. American Journal of Clinical Nutrition 50: 930–939

Garner D M, Olmstead M P, Bohr Y, Garfinkel P E 1982 The eating attitudes test: psychometric features and clinical correlates. Psychological Medicine 12: 871–878

Garrow J S 1988 Obesity and related diseases. Churchill Livingstone, Edinburgh

Goel K M, Logan R W, Arneil G C et al 1976 Florid and subclinical rickets among immigrant children in Glasgow. Lancet i: 1141–1145

Grant 1990 Prevalence of iron deficiency in rural pre-school children in Northern Ireland. British Journal of General Practice 40: 112–113

Hall D M B (ed) 1989 Health for all children. Oxford University Press, Oxford

Illingworth R S 1986 Anaemia and child health surveillance. Archives of Disease in Childhood 61: 1151–1152

James J A, Clark C, Ward P S 1985 Screening Rastafarian children for nutritional rickets. British Medical Journal 290: 899–900

James J, Evans J, Male P et al 1988 Iron deficiency in inner city pre-school children: development of a general practice screening programme. Journal of the Royal College of General Practitioners 38: 250–252

Jarrett R J 1986 Is there an ideal body weight? British Medical Journal 293: 493–495

Johnson-Sabine E, Wood K, Patton G et al 1988 Abnormal eating attitudes in London schoolgirls — a prospective epidemiological study: factors associated with abnormal response on screening questionnaires. Psychological Medicine 18: 615–622

Keys A 1986 Is there an ideal body weight? British Medical Journal 293: 1023–1024

King M B 1989 Eating disorders in a general practice population. Prevalence, characteristics and follow-up at 12 to 18 months. Psychological Medicine Monograph Supplement 14. Cambridge University Press, Cambridge

Kissebah A H, Vydelingum N, Murray R et al 1982 Relation of body fat distribution to metabolic complication of obesity. Journal of Clinical Endocrinology and Metabolism 54: 254–260

Lapidus L, Bengtson C, Larsson B et al 1984 Distribution of adipose tissue and risk of cardiovascular disease and death: a 12 year follow up of participants in the population study of women in Gothenberg, Sweden. British Medical Journal 289: 1257–1261

Lawson D E M, Paul A A, Black A E et al 1979 Relative contribution of diet and sunlight to vitamin D status in the elderly. British Medical Journal 2: 303–305

Mueller W H, Wear M L, Harris C L et al 1987 Body circumferences as alternatives to skinfold measurement of body fat distribution in Mexican Americans. International Journal of Obesity II: 309–318

Nutrition Standing Committee of the British Paediatric Association 1988 Vegetarian weaning. Archives of Disease in Childhood 63: 1286–1292

Pacy P J, Webster J D, Pearson M, Garrow J S 1987 A cross-sectional cost/benefit audit in a hospital obesity clinic. Human Nutrition: Applied Nutrition 41a: 38–46

Pollitt E, Saco-Pollitt C, Liebel R L, Viteri F E 1986 Iron deficiency and behavioural development in infants and schoolchildren. American Journal of Clinical Nutrition 43: 555–565

Poskitt E M E 1988 Practical paediatric nutrition. Butterworths, London, p 117

Slade P D 1982 Towards a functional analysis of anorexia nervosa and bulimia nervosa. British Journal of Clinical Psychology 21: 771–775

Slade P D, Dewey M E 1986 Development and preliminary validation of SCANS: a screening test for identifying individuals at risk of developing anorexia nervosa and bulimia nervosa. International Journal of Eating Disorders 517–538

Seiden J C, Cigolini M, Duerenberg P et al 1989 Fat distribution, androgens and metabolism in non-obese women. American Journal of Clinical Nutrition 50: 269–273

Tanner J M, Whitehouse R H, Takaishi M 1966 Standards for birth to maturity for height, weight, height velocity and weight velocity in British children in 1985. Archives of Disease in Childhood 41: 454–471

Tuomilehto J, Salonen J, Martin B et al 1987 Body weight and risk of myocardial infarction and death in the adult population of eastern Finland. British Medical Journal 295: 623–627

Whitaker A, Davies M, Shaffer D et al 1989 The struggle to be thin: a survey of anorexic and bulimic symptoms in a non-referred adolescent population. Psychological Medicine 19: 143–163

34. Screening for patients with excessive alcohol consumption

Paul Wallace

INTRODUCTION

Alcohol consumption in the United Kingdom has more than doubled in the last 40 years and is continuing to increase (Central Statistical Office 1986). Somewhere in the region of 65% of the adult population now consume alcohol regularly and, on average, each person drinks the equivalent of nine pints of beer weekly (Wilson 1980, Office of Health Economics 1981). Excessive alcohol consumption can have adverse effects on an individual's psychological and physical health as well as on his or her social well-being, with both acute and chronic effects. Acute intoxication may lead to accidents and acts of violence and crime, while regular heavy drinking has a variety of serious psychological and social consequences and is responsible for a range of physical harms including raised blood pressure, increased risk of strokes and certain forms of cancer, gastritis and peptic ulceration, brain damage and liver cirrhosis. A number of studies point to alcohol as a principal factor in the illness of up to 30% of patients admitted to hospital (Williams et al 1978, Jariwalla et al 1979), and there is little doubt that alcohol is, as the report of the Royal College of Physicians put it, 'a great and growing evil' (Royal College of Physicians 1987). Recent estimates put the number of individuals drinking to excess at 7 million, with 1.5 million drinking at 'dangerous levels' and between 25 000 and 40 000 dying annually as a result of their alcohol consumption (Royal College of General Practitioners 1986).

In general practice, detection and intervention strategies for alcohol-related problems have evolved rapidly in recent years, and much of this is due to a change in diagnostic classifications.

For much of the first half of this century, problems resulting from alcohol use were regarded as complications of a single disease, 'alcoholism', which was considered to have a predominantly genetic basis and a predictable natural history. This concept was particularly favoured in North America and spawned a number of treatment programmes, including Alcoholics Anonymous. An alternative approach was developed by Edwards and Gross, who formulated the concept of the 'alcohol dependence syndrome' (Edwards & Gross 1976), a psychobiological state characterised by a cycle of dependence, which included the reorientation of life around alcohol, an awareness of a compulsion to drink and drinking to avoid the discomfort of withdrawal. A distinction was made between this syndrome and the broad spectrum of problems resulting from harmful drinking (the 'alcohol-related disabilities' (Edwards et al 1977)) but both were considered to exist within a continuum of severity rather than as distinct disease entities. From this, it was but a short step to the formulation of the terms 'hazardous' and 'excessive' drinking, and now weekly alcohol consumption is as widely accepted as a 'risk factor' as serum cholesterol levels for coronary heart disease and blood pressure values for cerebrovascular disease: the greater the quantity of alcohol consumed, the greater the risk to the individual. Excessive alcohol consumption may be defined as the consumption of alcohol at levels where psychological, social and physical sequelae are likely to occur, and the definition of safe, hazardous and dangerous levels is designed to aid in quantifying the level of risk. There has been considerable debate around what constitutes 'safe' levels of drinking, but since 1986 the Royal Colleges of Physicians, Psychiatrists and General Practitioners have all come forward with the same recommendations (Table 34.1).

Table 34.1 Levels of risk for alcohol consumption

	Level of risk (units/week)		
	Low	Intermediate	High
Men	< 20	20–50	> 50
Women	< 15	15–35	> 35

The role of surveillance and screening for alcohol problems in general practice has been profoundly modified by the evolution of the definitions described above. While it is still vital for the GP to be vigilant for the 'hidden alcoholics', described so elegantly by Wilkins (Wilkins 1974), the principal task has now become the detection of the much larger number of individuals at risk because of their excessive drinking. This is intrinsically attractive, both because it provides the GP with an alternative to the difficult and often unrewarding task of working exclusively with patients with full-blown alcohol dependence and because it opens up new possibilities in the ever more popular and important field of prevention. Furthermore, the large number of people drinking to excess are actually responsible for a greater contribution to the overall public health problems of alcohol than the relatively few people with alcohol dependence.

SCREENING AND SURVEILLANCE

Do surveillance and early intervention programmes work? The evidence from a number of studies has indicated that this approach can be effective. Heavy drinkers frequently want to cut down on their drinking and when treatment is available they come forward for help (Plant et al 1979, Cust 1980). A study using a minimal intervention method in general practice (the DRAMS scheme — Drinking Reasonably And Moderately with Self-control), demonstrated that at 6 months follow-up, general practitioners' advice was effective in reducing the alcohol consumption of heavy drinkers (Heather et al 1987). In the MRC Study on Lifestyle and Health — a multicentre, randomised controlled trial to determine the effectiveness of advice from the general practitioner to heavy drinkers to cut down their alcohol consumption — patients in the treatment group were interviewed by their general practitioner and received advice and information about how to reduce their consumption. Follow-up was within 1 month and again at 4, 7 and 10 months. These patients reduced their consumption on average by 18 units/week, compared with only 8 units/week in the controls (Wallace et al 1988). The proportion of men with excessive consumption at interview dropped by 44% in the treatment group compared with 26% in the control group, and the mean value of gamma glutamyl transpeptidase (GGT) had fallen significantly in the treated men at 1 year. Similar, although less marked results, were obtained in the case of women, and for both sexes a reduction in both consumption and GGT was evidenced in proportion to the number of general practitioner interventions. The results indicate that, at a conservative estimate, advice from general practitioners in the United Kingdom could reduce to moderate levels the alcohol consumption of some 250 000 men and 67 500 women currently drinking to excess each year.

Further evidence for the effectiveness of early intervention comes from a Scottish study involving the counselling of heavy drinkers on medical wards. The patients given counselling showed significant improvements compared with the controls (Chick et al 1985). Finally, in a study in Sweden involving the identification of and intervention in heavy drinking in middle-aged men (Kristenson et al 1983), the GGT values in both groups were significantly decreased, but there were differences between the two groups with regard to sick absenteeism, hospitalisation and mortality. Compared with the control group the treatment group showed a significant reduction (80%) in sick absence at 4-year follow-up, a reduction of 60% in hospital days at 5-year follow-up and a 50% reduction in mortality at 6-year follow-up. The intervention programme, which included repeated encouragement to lower overall alcohol consumption and biofeedback information in the form of GGT measurements, was effective in preventing medicosocial consequences of heavy drinking.

Given the evidence that early intervention is effective, what strategies are available in general practice for surveillance or screening? The shift in emphasis to primary prevention by intervention in 'at-risk' drinkers has required a critical reappraisal of the methods used in detection as well as of the intervention process itself. Clinical skills used as part of the consultation should naturally still be employed. Traditionally, laboratory tests have been used, often surreptitiously, to confirm clinical suspicion of alcohol dependence. These tests are certainly useful in some cases, but their performance in surveillance programmes is generally poor. More recently, questionnaires and structured questioning have been shown to be at least as effective as the other methods.

Clinical indicators

Some patients are particularly likely to be heavy drinkers. These include those with high blood pressure and those who are overweight. Other associated factors are a history of recurrent injuries or accidents, non-specific gastrointestinal complaints, marital problems or a history of absenteeism and anxiety, depression or insomnia. Further risk factors for heavy drinking include certain occupations (journalists, businessmen and those working in the catering trade), a strong family history of drinking and early signs of harm, such as abnormal liver function tests. General practitioners are expert at physical assessment in the surgery and as a minimum, a check should be made on pulse and blood pressure, on the liver for tenderness or enlargement, on the hands for tremor or sweating and on the breath for smell of alcohol.

Liver function tests

Liver function tests (GGT, ALT and alkaline phosphatase) can be extremely helpful in detecting patients with advanced alcohol-related disease. They appear to act largely as indicators of hepatocellular damage and may be raised in up to 85% of 'alcoholics' (Rosalki & Rau 1974). However, they also have a rather high false positive rate (up to 25%), which limits their usefulness in screening, even for these patients. Elevated GGT levels may be associated with pregnancy, obesity, diseases of the liver and biliary tract and the use of pharmacologically active agents, notably anti-epileptics and warfarin. The rise of the enzyme in the serum is primarily due to hepatic enzyme induction. There is a quantitative relationship between GGT levels and the quantity of alcohol consumed (Shaper et al 1985). Increased GGT activity in the serum can be observed after a few weeks of alcohol intake and, following reduction in drinking, serum GGT levels fall rapidly, returning to normal levels within 2–4 weeks. The sensitivity in detecting patients with alcohol dependence may be as high as 90%, but in relation to heavy drinking, it is very much lower — about 30% (Baxter et al 1980). This seriously limits the usefulness of the test for screening purposes. However, raised levels almost certainly precede liver damage and the test can be useful in monitoring abstinence or large scale reductions in consumption.

Mean corpuscular volume

Mean corpuscular volume (MCV) has been reported to be raised in as many as 90% of alcoholics (Wu et al 1974), probably as a result of interference with the developing red cell membrane. It appears that this is not the direct result of nutritional deficiency, because the effect is reversed when alcohol is withdrawn. The proportion of heavy drinkers who have an MCV over 98 femtolitres ranges somewhere between 15 and 30% and the false positive rate is between 4 and 6%. MCV is an unreliable indicator of heavy drinking.

Complex laboratory tests

A number of more complex tests are available. For example, excessive alcohol consumption is associated with an increase in the ratio of plasma transferrin pI 5.7 to total transferrin. In one study, the sensitivity of this assay was 100% and the specificity 97% (Vesterberg et al 1984) but this involved alcohol dependents. A recent study on carbohydrate-deficient transferrin showed it to be more effective in detecting 'self-confessed alcoholics' than the standard biological markers, with a 91% sensitivity and 98.8% specificity (Kapur et al 1989). However, although the authors suggest that it may be an important advance in the detection of alcohol abuse, there appears to be no evidence about its performance in detecting patients with lower levels of excessive alcohol consumption. These assays are not generally available in the clinical setting, presumably because of their high cost, and this is a major limitation to their usefulness in screening and surveillance programmes.

Combined laboratory tests

Results of laboratory tests may be combined to increase the sensitivity and specificity of the assessment. In one study, a combination of GGT and MCV results led to the identification of 91% of 'alcoholics' whereas only 72% were correctly identified by GGT alone and 78% by MCV alone (Clark et al 1983, Chan et al 1987). However, there has been insufficient work carried out on the application of these principles to the identification of excessive drinkers in the general population to allow confident advocacy of such combinations for general use.

Thus, the armamentarium of laboratory tests available to detect heavy drinkers has serious limitations, and this may in part explain why so many heavy drinkers are unidentified by their general practitioners.

Alcohol meters

Alcohol meters measure the breath ethanol concentration and are essentially the same as those used by the police in roadside checks. They are relatively inexpensive. The one major study of their use in general practice (Wiseman et al 1982) found that 3.5% of patients aged over 15 years gave a positive result. Of the 35 patients with positive readings, 11 were not previously thought to have a problem related to alcohol. Breath and blood alcohol measurement can be useful, particularly if positive readings are obtained on samples taken during a morning surgery. However, as alcohol is eliminated from the body within hours and many heavy drinkers who are not dependent on alcohol will abstain from drinking before attending surgery, this method lacks sensitivity.

Questionnaires and interviews

There has recently been increasing interest in the use of simple questionnaires and face-to-face questioning in the assessment of alcohol consumption. Many doctors are cautious about asking direct questions about alcohol, perhaps believing that their relationships with their patients will be harmed. In fact it appears that the majority of patients perceive questioning about alcohol consumption and other areas of lifestyle as a legitimate topic for enquiry by their general practitioner (Wallace & Haines 1984). More importantly, it is widely believed that, if asked, patients will lie about their alcohol consumption or evade the issue. A number of studies have now shown that most patients in general practice will provide a sufficiently truthful account of their consumption to give a reasonably accurate indication of their risk (Poikalainen 1985, Wallace & Haines 1985). Questioning about alcohol consumption is also important because it can make patients aware of the importance of placing alcohol on the health agenda. Systematic measurement using a questionnaire is more useful than just asking a patient 'How much do you drink?', to which the responses are likely to be a vague 'not very much', or 'I'm only a social drinker', or 'a fair bit at weekends'. A simple quantity frequency scale in which patients are asked how often they usually drink and how much is drunk on each drinking occasion is an easy and systematic method of questioning. Calculation of weekly consumption is then a question of simple multiplication. Such a method has been shown to be reliable and, furthermore, patients are generally willing to respond. This appears to be particularly true for general lifestyle questionnaires, such as the Health Survey Questionnaire, where questions about smoking, exercise, dieting and weight are included with those about alcohol. The use of such a questionnaire may be particularly helpful in identifying heavy drinkers and one study demonstrated a 5 fold increase in the numbers of such patients known to their general practitioners as a result of using this method (Wallace & Haines 1985).

Questionnaires may also be used for identifying individuals suffering psychosocial consequences because of their drinking. Of the numerous questionnaires available the MAST (Michigan Alcohol Screening Test) and the CAGE have been used most widely. The MAST questionnaire takes about 15 minutes to complete in its full length (25-question) form, and rather less in the shortened (10-question) form. In its original study using a cut-off score of 6 and above, the brief MAST identified all of 60 'alcoholics' and gave a false positive rate of 7 out of 62 non-alcoholics (Pokorny et

al 1972). It has subsequently been tested extensively in such patients and has performed consistently well, although rather less is known about its effectiveness in detecting excessive drinkers. The CAGE questionnaire consists of four questions:

1. Have you ever felt you should Cut down on your drinking?
2. Have people Annoyed you by criticising your drinking?
3. Have you ever felt bad or Guilty about your drinking?
4. Have you ever had a drink first thing in the morning to steady your nerves or get rid of a hang-over (Eye-opener)?

This questionnaire was originally validated in a population of known alcoholics; 81% answered positively to two or more of the questions, compared with 11% of non-alcoholics (Mayfield et al 1974). Although it has performed well in clinic settings, in general practice and community settings the CAGE questionnaire has failed to detect approximately half those individuals who are known to be at risk (Saunders & Kershaw 1980). However, it has the great advantage of being short and thus quick to administer and, when used in a modified form, including questions on smoking, exercise and weight (Wallace & Haines 1985) it was found to be 78% sensitive and 98% specific in detecting men with excessive consumption, although it appeared to perform rather less well with women.

The World Health Organization has recently developed a core screening instrument for screening persons with early signs of alcohol-related problems. The maximum possible score is 40. Using a cut-off point of a score of 10 in community settings the instrument accurately identified 80% of individuals at risk because of their drinking. The instrument had a false positive rate of 11%. A positive finding had a predictive value of 60% and a negative finding a predictive value of 95% (Saunders & Aasland 1987).

SURVEILLANCE AND SCREENING IN PRACTICE

In the light of the above evidence on screening methods, what strategies for early detection should be adopted? Each practice will wish to make its own decision about this and there are no absolute recommendations to be made. However, there seems little point in relying on laboratory tests or breath alcohol meters for surveillance when simple questionnaires are at least as effective and are cheaper and more acceptable to patients. Given the exceptional potential for opportunistic screening in general practice, this approach would appear to be more attractive than actively calling up patients as part of a screening programme. The practice will have to decide which instrument to adopt, but a simple quantity–frequency scale, with or without the addition of the CAGE or MAST questions, would be highly suitable. Information about patients' consumption can be obtained and recorded at various stages of their contact with the surgery. An ideal time to distribute the questionnaire is at registration, when many practices already seek clinical and social data; the 1990 GP contract requires such registration checks to be carried out. Receptionists may be asked to put copies of a questionnaire into the notes of patients as they attend for surgery so that they can then be handed a copy to complete when they check in at the desk for their appointment. A supply of questionnaires may be kept in the doctor's surgery or nurse's room to be given to the patient during the consultation. Coupled with routine questioning about alcohol consumption as part of the consultation, this method of opportunistic surveillance should allow the practice to detect the majority of its patients who are at risk because of their drinking. Provided that the programme is maintained, each patient's records can be updated regularly, say at every fifth consultation or every 2 years, whichever comes first.

Responding to the surveillance programme

Again, each practice will need to develop its own plans for assessing and managing the problems that arise form the use of alcohol.

The following guide for action is graded according to the patient's level of alcohol consumption.

Review

The large majority of any practice population will consist of people who drink less than 15 units (women) or 20 units (men) weekly and show no extra vulnerability, as shown in Table 34.2. The general practitioner should record the present level of consumption, discuss any concerns about drinking which the patient may have, provide simple information, such as the booklet *That's the Limit* (Health Education Authority 1986) and arrange for review after, say, 5 years or whenever any significant change occurs in the patient's life, e.g. pregnancy or bereavement. Some of those who have low consumption but high vulnerability will suffer form transient conditions and alcohol should be kept on the agenda for any consultations for those conditions. Review should be arranged after, say, 3 years.

Table 34.2   Expected numbers of patients in drinking categories

Classification of risk	Units	Expected numbers (Practice total = 2000)
Low	Women < 15	700
	Men < 20	500
Intermediate	Women 15–35	75
	Men 21–50	250
High	Women > 35	25
	Men > 50	50

Minimal intervention

Women who normally drink between 15 and 35 units/week and men drinking 20–50 units/week should be given advice and information about the risks they are taking and encouragement and help in reducing consumption. They should be offered review in, say, a year. Those drinking the same amount but who are more vulnerable should be assessed for existing harms in social, psychological and physical terms, advised about reducing consumption and supported in that endeavour, whether by the doctor or another team member.

Men drinking between 20 and 35 units a week should be kept under careful review, as should women drinking between 15 and 21 units per week. In the case of people aged under 18 or over 64, lower levels may be appropriate. For pregnant women much lower levels may be appropriate because of risk to the baby, e.g. 1 or 2 units once or twice a week. Of course it is acceptable to decide on different limits for specific patients. It is often helpful to follow a fairly standard sequence; whether the patient believes that alcohol is affecting his or her health and/or life. Make a note of the patient's drinking habits: weekly consumption/type of drink/regular heavy drinking days. Fill in a drinks diary recording consumption for the previous 7 days, starting with the previous day and work backwards.

Recall is assisted by asking about morning, lunchtime and evening of each day. Indicate the patient's position on the histogram (Fig. 34.1). This will correct beliefs about the 'normality' of the patient's own consumption or that of his/her peers. Mention the risks of increased drinking, such as accidents and injuries, anxiety and depression, weight problems, sexual difficulties, stomach upsets, difficulties in sleeping, liver disease, raised blood pressure, headaches and hangovers. Detail the potential benefits of reduced drinking, such as financial savings, safer driving, improved concentration at work, improved general health and any factors specific to individual patients.

Histogram

Distribution of units consumed weekly by men
England and Wales

Distribution of units consumed weekly by women
England and Wales

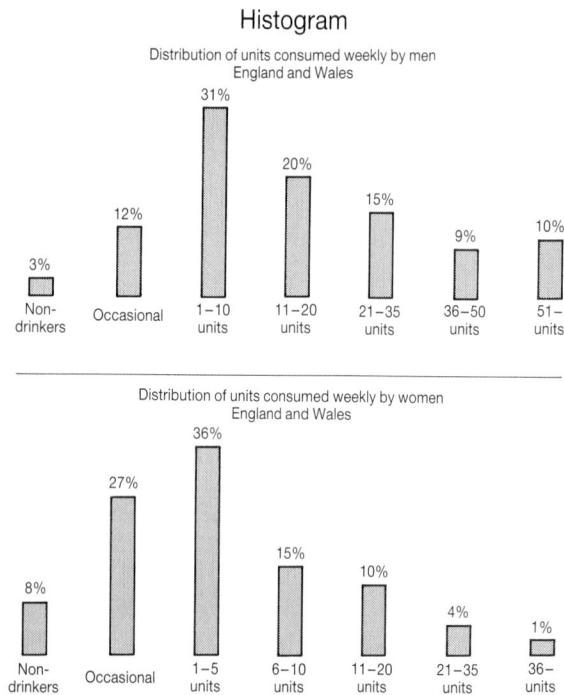

Fig. 34.1   Histogram showing drinking habits. (Each unit of alcohol costs approx. £1 at 1991 prices.)

Give firm but friendly advice to cut down. Bearing in mind individual circumstances, it is suggested that in general men are advised not to drink more than 20 units per week and women not to drink more than 15 units per week. Give the patient an information booklet such as *That's the Limit* (Health Education Authority 1986) or the *Cut down on your Drinking* leaflet (Health Education Authority and Alcohol Concern, 1987, Fig. 34.2) and arrange a follow-up appointment within the next 2–4 weeks. Explain that you will be asking about the patient's alcohol consumption at future attendances at surgery. Note the interview and the date in the patient's notes or on the computer. You may also wish to attach a sticker inside or outside the notes to remind you to check on patients' consumption at their next consultation.

Intensive intervention and referral

Women consuming above 35 units or men consuming above 50 units weekly will require fuller assessment, with advice, support and regular follow-up. Full assessment may take some time and it is sometimes helpful to divide it into several sessions. Together with the patient, complete a 7-day drink diary for the week prior to consultation. You can help in the recall by working backwards one day at a time and asking about the day in components: morning/lunchtime/evening. Try to gauge the patient's views about his/her levels of consumption and find out whether he/she has considered cutting down. As always in medical assessment, the past history is vital. It is essential to discover when heavy drinking started, events that were linked at the time, accounts of any bouts of heavier drinking, including the days before and after. Try to find out what the patient felt and thought at the time and obtain information about previous attempts to cut down or abstain as well as the events surrounding relapse. It may also be helpful to find out about the attitudes and behaviour of those close to the patient and obtain a brief summary of the patient's early life and upbringing, particularly a family history of heavy drinking. Regular consultations may be necessary to continue assessment and monitoring of the patient's drinking, but fundamentally the same approach to intervention can be adopted as detailed above. Unless there is evidence of alcohol dependence, there is no requirement for the patient to stop drinking altogether, although sometimes it may become apparent that this is the most appropriate policy (some experts would not necessarily advise abstinence even in the presence of obvious dependence). A drinking diary will help both the patient and the doctor/nurse to monitor drinking between consultations, and clear instructions should be given as to how this should be completed.

The majority of heavy drinkers and patients with alcohol problems can be helped by support from members of the primary care team and their own families. However, there are some whose problems are more severe or who lack a supportive environment who may need referring on to a specialist agency. When a referral is made it is important to maintain your relationship with the patient and give a further appointment to discuss what took place. Without this continuing contact, the referral may feel like a rejection. Many areas have local councils on alcohol, voluntary agencies whose responsibilities include co-ordinating available services and which provide counselling and advice for heavy drinkers and their families. Addresses of local counselling services may be found in the telephone directory, or alternatively Alcohol Concern publishes a directory of national and local services. Alcoholics Anonymous provides a supportive self-help group. It asks members to acknowledge that they are 'alcoholic' and that abstinence is the only way to recovery. Al-Anon and Al-Teen provide support for the spouses and teenage children of problem drinkers. Addresses are in the telephone directory.

Only under exceptional circumstances will detoxification be required, and it is advisable in these cases to

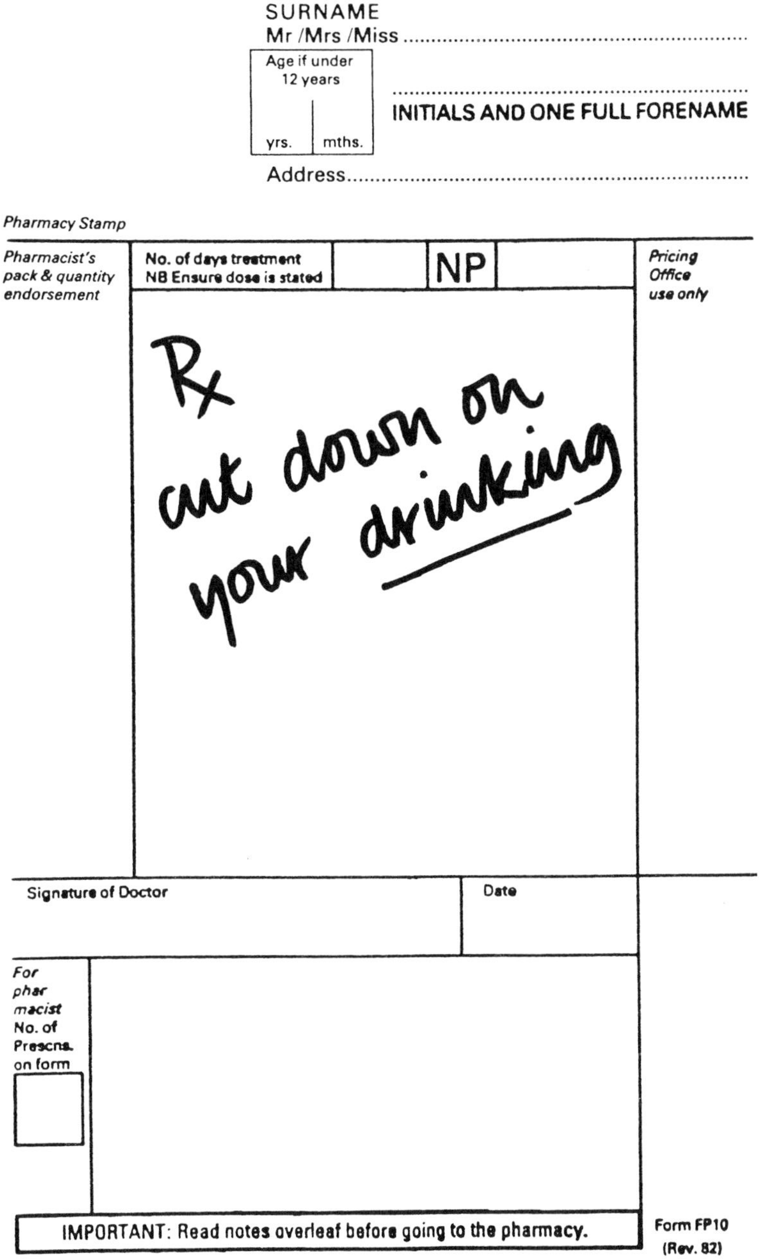

SURNAME
Mr /Mrs /Miss ....

| Age if under 12 years | |
| yrs. | mths. |

....
INITIALS AND ONE FULL FORENAME

Address..

Pharmacy Stamp

| Pharmacist's pack & quantity endorsement | No. of days treatment NB Ensure dose is stated | **NP** | Pricing Office use only |

Rx
cut down on
your drinking

| Signature of Doctor | Date |

| For pharmacist No. of Prescns. on form | |

IMPORTANT: Read notes overleaf before going to the pharmacy.   Form FP10 (Rev. 82)

Fig. 34.2 *Cut down on your drinking* (Health Education Authority and Alcohol Concern 1987).

seek the assistance of a consultant with a special interest in alcohol or a community alcohol team. Community alcohol teams (CATs) are multidisciplinary groups, often involving social workers, probation officers, psychiatric nurses, counsellors, psychologists and others, who are often attached to, or at least have close links with, alcohol treatment units.

Alcohol treatment units are usually associated with psychiatric units, have facilities for detoxification and offer a range of approaches to treatment.

In all cases where patients are referred on to other agencies, it is vital to demonstrate an ongoing interest in the welfare of the patient and to offer regular follow-up.

REFERENCES

Baxter S, Fink R, Leader A R, Rosalki S B 1980 Laboratory tests of excessive consumption evaluated in general practice. Alcohol and Alcoholism 15: 164–166

Central Statistical Office 1986 Social Trends 16. HMSO, London

Chan A W K, Welte J W, Whitney R B 1987 Identification of young adult alcoholics by blood chemistry. Alcohol 4: 175–179

Chick J, Lloyd G, Crombie E 1985 Counselling problem drinkers in medical wards. British Medical Journal 290: 965–7

Clark P M, Holder R, Mullet M 1983 Sensitivity and specificity of laboratory tests for alcohol abuse. Alcohol and Alcoholism 18: 261–269

Cust G 1980 Health education about alcohol in the Tyne Tees area. In: Aspects of Alcohol and Drug Dependence

Edwards G, Gross M M 1976 Alcohol dependence: provisional description of a clinical syndrome. British Medical Journal 1: 1058–1061

Edwards G, Gross M M, Keller M et al (eds) 1977 Alcohol related disabilities. WHO Offset Publications No. 32. WHO, Geneva

Health Education Authority 1986 That's the limit. Health Education Authority, London

Health Education Authority and Alcohol Concern 1987 Cut down on your drinking (pack) Health Education Authority, London

Heather N, Campion P D, Neville R G, McCabe D 1987 Evaluation of a controlled drinking minimal intervention scheme (The DRAMS Scheme) in general practice. Journal of the Royal College of General Practitioners 37: 358–363

Jariwalla A G, Adams P H, Hore B D 1979 Alcohol and acute medical admissions to hospital. Health Trends 11: 95–7

Kapur A, Wild G, Mulford A, Triger D R 1989 Carbohydrate deficient transferrin — a marker for alcohol abuse. British Medical Journal 299: 427–431

Kristenson H, Ohlin H, Hulten–Nosslin M B et al 1983 Identification and intervention of heavy drinking in middle-aged men; results and follow-up of 24–60 months of long-term study with randomised controls. Alcoholism, Clinical and Experimental Research 7: 203–9

Mayfield D, McLeod G, Hall P 1974 The CAGE questionnaire; validation of a new alcoholism screening instrument. American Journal of Psychiatry 131(10): 1121–1123

Office of Health Economics 1981 Alcohol: reducing the harm. White Crescent, Luton

Plant M A, Piries F, Kreitman N 1979 Evaluation of the Scottish Health Education Unit's 1976 campaign on alcoholism. Social Psychiatry 14: 11–24

Poikalainen K 1985 Underestimation of recalled alcohol intake in relation to actual consumption. British Journal of Addiction 80: 215–6

Pokorny A D, Miller B A, Kaplan H B 1972 The brief MAST: a shortened version of the Michigan Alcoholism Screening Test. American Journal of Psychiatry 129: 342–345

Rosalki S B, Rau D 1974 Serum gamma glutamyl transpeptidase activity in alcoholism. Clinica Chimica Acta 39: 41–47

Royal College of General Practitioners 1986 Alcohol — a balanced view. Report from General Practice No. 24. RCGP, London

Royal College of Physicians 1987 A great and growing evil: the medical consequences of alcohol abuse. Tavistock, London

Saunders W M, Kershaw P W 1980 Screening tests for alcoholism — findings from a community study. British Journal of Addition 75: 37–41

Saunders J B, Aasland O G 1987 WHO collaborative project of identification and treatment of persons with harmful alcohol consumption. Report on phase 1: development of a screening instrument. WHO, Geneva

Shaper A G, Pocock S J, Ashby D et al 1985 Biochemical and haematological response to alcohol intake. Annals of Clinical Biochemistry 22: 50–61

Vesterberg O, Petren S, Schmidt D 1984 Increased concentrations of a transferrin variant after alcohol abuse. Clinica Chimica Acta 141: 33–39

Wallace P G, Haines A P 1984 General practitioner and health promotion; what patients think. British Medical Journal 289: 534–536

Wallace P G, Haines A P 1985 Use of a questionnaire in general practice to increase the recognition of patients with excessive alcohol consumption. British Medical Journal 290: 1949–1953

Wallace P G, Cutler S and Haines A P 1988 Randomised controlled trial of general practitioner intervention in patients with excessive alcohol consumption: findings of the MRC's general practice research framework study on lifestyle and health. British Medical Journal 297: 663–668

Wilson P 1980 Drinking in England and Wales. HMSO, London

Williams A T, Burns F H, Morey S 1978 Prevalence of alcoholism in a Sydney teaching hospital. Medical Journal of Australia 2: 608–611

Wilkins R H 1974 The hidden alcoholic in general practice: a method of detection. Paul Elek, London

Wiseman S M, Thompson P V, Barnett J M et al 1982 Use of an alcohol meter to detect problem drinkers. British Medical Journal 285: 1089–1090

Wu A, Chanerin I, Levi A J 1974 Macrocytosis of chronic alcoholism. Lancet i: 829–830

35. Drug abuse

D M Thomson   J R Robertson

INTRODUCTION

The increased numbers of individuals who have inject-ed drugs over the last two decades have given rise to the need for services from a range of agencies. A crisis of funding and confidence in the mid-1980s among designated drug dependency units allowed the devel-opment of a wider range of services including volun-tary and non-statutory agencies. It also allowed prima-ry care to define a role for itself in the range of require-ments expressed by illegal drug takers. Primary care has therefore become an acknowledged focus for engaging new or recent drug takers, particularly in an attempt to prevent the spread of infectious diseases such as hepatitis B and AIDS.

TRENDS

Trends in drugs of abuse and patterns of drug taking have also influenced policy and therapy options. The high availability of heroin throughout the UK in the early 1980s has given way to a wider variety of street drugs of abuse including cocaine, amphetamine and 'designer' drugs. In addition, the enthusiasm for sub-stitute prescribing by the medical profession has encour-aged the abuse of several prescribed drugs. Agents such as buprenorphine; benzodiazepines, e.g. diazepam, temazepam, triazolam; dipipanone and barbiturates all continue to be abused by injection, sometimes in preference to the more conventional drugs of abuse but more com-monly as a substitute in the absence of heroin or cocaine.

THE OBJECTIVES OF SCREENING AND SURVEILLANCE

The ultimate purpose of intervention in drug usage must be to help the patient achieve a drug-free lifestyle by early detection and effective management. For many patients with established physical and psychological depen-dence a rapid transition to complete abstinence is not possible and lesser, more achievable objectives must be set in the medium term. The failure of several national policies on drug abuse control, together with the arrival of HIV infection, have forced considerable change in priorities in dealing with drug abuse. Thus it has become clear that, for example, the rational man-agement of chaotic drug misusers with a lifestyle adapted to obtaining and using drugs, with drug habits that sustain substantial health risks for both themselves and their families, may be to help them to achieve stable, low-risk drug usage through education, coun-selling and support. The problems caused by and asso-ciated with drug abuse are, at least, as important as the abuse itself.

THE NATURE OF DRUG ABUSE

Although the physical dependence induced by a wide range of mood-altering drugs is of considerable impor-tance in sustaining drug abuse, purely pharmacological concepts of abuse are unlikely to be a successful basis for management. The nature of abuse in any one indi-vidual is likely to be the result of the interplay of a wide range of influences — of the personality, relationships and social supports of the individual, of the availability and acceptability of drugs of misuse within his/her sub-culture and of the restrictions placed on these drugs by society as a whole.

Throughout history mankind has always sought and used psychotropic agents and equivocated over their control. Alcohol and tobacco usage are constrained by taxation. In contrast, benzodiazepine tranquillisers are controlled through prescription. Yet the major mor-bidity and mortality associated with alcohol, tobacco and tranquillisers considerably outweigh those associated with 'street drugs' in modern society. Ambivalence about the 'medicalisation' of drug abuse management is understandable, although erroneous. That society as a whole, or the medical profession in particular, should display hypocrisy is less acceptable.

Medicine must take a lead in identifying current problems and proposing solutions. Individual practitioners must accept a personal responsibility to contributing to this initiative.

RECOGNISING THE PROBLEM

The patient

There is no 'typical' drug misuser. Although there are clear associations between emotional/social deprivation and a predisposition to drug usage this link is neither sufficiently strong nor has sufficient specificity to be a helpful means of identification. Types of usage range from the experimenting school adolescent, the recreational/intermittent user, the regular 'stable' user to the chaotic polydrug user (contact with whom may have prejudiced the attitudes of general practitioners). Drug users are, in short, a heterogenous group.

The symptoms

The importance and severity of physical withdrawal symptoms tend to be overemphasised in presentation, diagnosis and management. The 'drive' to use drugs in an abuse pattern is of psychological origin and is sustained more often by the social framework and lifestyle of the user than by physical withdrawal symptoms. The principal objective in management is to provoke lifestyle changes and to prevent sustained relapse into psychological and physical dependency. Even high-dose long-term heroin abusers, with whom physical withdrawal is most clearly associated, often have prolonged periods of abstinence, either voluntarily or due to supply problems.

The drug

Although generalisations may be made about the psychopharmacological effects of the drugs of abuse (Table 35.1) there are dangers in this approach because (i) the range of drugs is expanding rapidly; (ii) many drug users will employ a mixture of drugs, including alcohol; (iii) with the varying availability of drugs each user may have an inconsistent drug taking pattern. Users are less likely to present when they have achieved their 'target' effect and more likely to present with toxicity, physical withdrawal or with a powerful anxiety about maintaining their supplies.

Most general practitioners will be familiar with the wide range of symptom strategies employed by drug users (deceit, aggression, profoundly expressed desires to 'kick' the habit and tearful pleading). Not all will have devised appropriate strategies to expose, control and amend these approaches nor have found it possible to establish a relationship that holds the potential for positive therapeutic activity.

The clinical signs

Other than the behavioural traits, there are few clinical signs of abuse. Severely dependent users will show evidence of self-neglect. The pinpoint pupils of opiate users are characteristic even in those who have high tolerance levels. Sweating may be profuse in opiate withdrawal and amphetamine toxicity. Persistent nasal sniffing may be observed in opiate withdrawal. Tachycardia, hypertension and cardiac arrythmias may be noted in amphetamine users. Repeated use of cocaine produces a chronic rhinitis and occasionally a perforated nasal septum. Those who abuse volatile solvents may

Table 35.1 Drugs of abuse: general psychotropic effects

	Target effects	Toxicity	Withdrawal effects
CNS depressants Opiates Sedatives Cannabis	Relaxation Euphoria	Drowsiness Respiratory depression Coma Death	Anxiety Insomnia Sweating Muscle cramps Confusion Psychosis
CNS stimulants Amphetamines Cocaine	Assertiveness Self-confidence	Irritability Suspiciousness Restlessness	Lethargy Depression
Perception-altering drugs Hallucinogens Volatile solvents	Euphoria Abnormal sensory perceptions	Recklessness Aggression	

present with a characteristic rash around the nose and mouth although this may be transient; their clothes may retain some of the characteristic odour of the solvents. Signs of past and present skin ulceration, abscesses, thrombophlebitis and evidence of arterial damage are suggestive of intravenous misuse.

USEFUL CLINICAL HABITS

There is no substitute for a high index of suspicion in the detection of drug misuse. Even when it is not possible to establish the diagnosis it is entirely reasonable to record this suspicion to trigger further enquiry at a later date whether by that doctor, by a partner, a trainee or the practice nurse. Confirmed abuse should be recorded in the records of not only that patient but in the records of spouses, cohabitees, sexual partners and children. Practice receptionists often detect the characteristic consulting patterns of previously unknown drug users and should be encouraged to relay their suspicions to the doctor. Observe the user's friends who patiently wait outside the surgery premises. Beware the self-admitted user; the non-dependent patient may simply be acting as a supplier to a friend or as a street dealer. Many prescribed drugs have a small but important potential for abuse, e.g. salbutamol, cyclizine and anti-depressants, and may be unwittingly supplied in quantities in excess of needs. Beware too, the atypical supplier — those elderly who supplement their meagre old age pension by selling their hypnotics and analgesics, or families of users who have succumbed to persuasion or coercion. Drug users with whom the doctor has established a good relationship may often provide information on other patients in the practice, often out of genuine concern for a friend who is running excessive risks. Check clinical information where possible with hospitals, previous GPs and any available drug abuse circulars. The local pharmacist may well have clear suspicion of drug users who have succeeded in registering with more than one GP often under a series of assumed names. Generally avoid prescribing at the first consultation but offer constructive help for the future. Place your own safety and that of your staff first and, if necessary, give in to important physical threats. Keep your prescription pads and drugs well guarded. Write prescriptions with amounts in numbers and figures and with a total number of supply days. Give only short supplies of drugs and do so ideally only by contract which excludes negotiation. Consider writing the prescription before the consultation begins, using the consulting time for information-giving, advice and counselling; hand over the prescription only as the final act in the consultation.

ASSESSING THE SEVERITY OF DRUG ABUSE

The social context

Although drug use is not confined to one end of the social spectrum there is no doubt that the contemporary drug problem is largely concentrated in inner city populations. Drug users tend to be adolescents or young adults who are unemployed or in temporary employment, have few academic attainments and have limited prospects for self-advancement. Crime and imprisonment are a feature in many studies of drug problems. However, the relationships between social disorganisation and drug use are complex and there is characteristic disruption and confusion in any family or social group associated with a drug user. Although this occurs across the social spectrum, it may be more easily contained and disguised within families with strong financial and emotional resources.

An early indication of the severity of drug use may be the effect on social and family harmony. The family may indeed be the initiators of requests for help for the drug user. There is also an obvious need for support for the family and relatives; a role for which the family doctor is ideally suited.

Physical and psychiatric aspects of ill health

The most common mode of presentation of a drug problem to the general practitioner is the occurrence of physical health problems. The incidence of injection site abscesses, thromboses or local trauma to GP or Accident Units is a clear guide to the scale of intravenous drug abuse in a community. Similarly the incidence of these problems in any one individual provides an indication of the degree of 'unhealthy' drug misuse and a fair index of risk. In contrast, behavioural and emotional disorders, commonly resulting from stimulant or depressant drugs other than heroin, are increasingly being recognised within primary care.

Infectious diseases are a common clinical expression of drug use, acute bacterial endocarditis, septicaemia and hepatitis B being among the most common. Slowly developing AIDS may present in a multiplicity of manners, most importantly as the acute diagnostic illness of *Pneumocystis carinii* pneumonia.

HIV infection and AIDS

The HIV status of the present or past intravenous drug user is the highest indicator of risk. The full expression of HIV in drug users is not yet apparent and experience is accordingly limited. Our knowledge both of the disease and its management is undergoing rapid change. Subsequent upon the important development of the HIV antibody test in 1985, the availability of laboratory tests for beta 2 microglobulin and CD4 lymphocyte counts has enabled early diagnosis and staging of the disease process.

The availability of zidovudine therapy has made it increasingly important to draw those infected into early contact with medical care, as will the availability of prophylactic antibodies for the management of opportunistic infection. There is a need for education of those infected or at risk of infection to combat heterosexual spread — the mode of transmission that is likely to affect the largest population. The potential for, and the responsibility of general practitioners towards, early diagnosis and intervention is clear (see also pp. 345–348).

WHAT HAPPENS TO DRUG MISUSERS?

There is no easy answer to this question. Of all drug abuse opiate use has been most studied. Long-term studies have emphasised that opiate misuse must be regarded as a chronic relapsing problem associated with, at one extreme, an increased mortality rate due to suicide, accidental overdosage, infection and criminal activity/association and, at the opposite extreme, a small but important minority who 'mature' out of drug usage, often spontaneously. The policies of 'damage-limitation' or 'harm-reduction' in the drug users, their friends or family must therefore play an important part in plans for long-term support.

TREATMENT

The broadening of interest in drug misuse, which has occurred as a result of HIV infection, has led to the recognition of the need for and the development of many resources for support and treatment of drug users. In addition the increased range of drugs of misuse have widened our horizons as to what we may contribute to the individual or to the community.

1. Provision of a service open enough to attract adolescents with problems or drug users with anxieties is an early but fundamental step. This is often associated with a rapid uptake of services.
2. Provision of sterile injecting equipment, substitute drug prescribing and supported 'healthy' drug usage may be controversial but are showing increasing signs of being worthwhile.
3. Liaison with non-statutory agencies is a useful adjunct to coping with an increasing problem. Other than advantages for patients/clients, such liaison may provide important interprofessional support.

4. Association with local treatment centres and specialist facilities is mandatory. Referrals must be selective, appropriate and targeted to the prevailing local problem.
5. It is easy to become dissatisfied with the outcome of intervention because relapse is common. Long-term survival in chronic drug usage is good in the absence of AIDS, violence or suicide. Accordingly, an expectation of the need for long-term support rather than cure is both realistic and professionally satisfying.

The consultation and control

It is important to establish an appropriate relationship with a drug misuser. The context of general practice is substantially different from that of, for example, a community support group where formalised relationships may be unhelpful. The general practitioner has to work within the disadvantage of being a point of access to legal drugs. The two extremes of either being a 'soft touch' for users or of maintaining a 'never prescribe under any circumstances' policy (which may do much to protect doctor and practice but little to combat the tide of abuse and its attendant risks to society) have little to commend them. The principal challenge to the doctor is to remove by whatever means the supply of drugs as being the principal item on the patient's consultation agenda. Drug users have medical needs other than those deriving from their drug habits. Appropriate control is therefore an important issue in preliminary assessment and in follow-up. Control may often be best established where care is shared between the GP and a community resource, e.g. a specialist community drug service.

Counselling

There are several distinct aspects of 'counselling' that deserve emphasis: (i) information concerning the nature of drug misuse and its attendant risks; (ii) advice, tailored to the needs of that individual, in respect of reduction regimes, 'healthy' drug usage, sexual behaviour and social relationships; (iii) true counselling wherein the doctor, avoiding giving proscriptive advice, helps the patient to explore the complex issues of personal emotions and relationships that are inevitably associated with drug misuse, and supports the patient along a predictably uneven progress towards control or abstinence.

PREGNANCY, CHILDREN AND FAMILIES

Drug abuse has a wide variety of effects on sexual activity. Chronic opiate usage is associated with decreased sexual drive and with amenorrhoea. In contrast, the high-risk lifestyle of chronic drug users is displayed consistently in their unwillingness, despite counselling, to employ 'safer' sexual activities. The twin risks of unwanted pregnancy and infection (HIV and hepatitis B) are therefore of considerable importance to users, their consorts(s) and their children, present or prospective. Remember hepatitis B immunisation. Many consorts of chronic drug users are surprisingly not themselves users and effective counselling may be most appropriately directed towards them.

The most powerful source of support, whether established or potential, for drug users in the community may be their families — who in turn may need considerable support from, amongst others, the family doctor.

CHECKLIST

Confronted by a complex and difficult problem often presented by patients whose behaviour does not conform to the social norms, it is easy to choose a management pathway that avoids rather than confronts the problem. It is, however, possible to adopt a positive and constructive approach to drug misuse through the areas

defined in the general practitioner checklist (Table 35.2).

Table 35.2 General practitioner checklist for drug abuse

Objective	Possible benefit
Early contact Hepatitis B vaccine Substitute prescribing Supply sterile equipment Education re dangers of septic equipment	Prevention of infection with HIV and hepatitis B through ignorance or lack of equipment
Contraceptive advice	Prevent unwanted pregnancy
Liaison with agencies	Appropriate support to GP, patient and family
Provide general medical services	Detection and management of non-drug related problems
Educate family/partners	Prevent heterosexual spread
Family therapy Continuous care	Provide support through crises
Notify drug addiction agency	National audit size of drug misuse problem

FURTHER READING

Banks A, Waller T A N 1988 Drug misuse. A practical handbook for GPs. Blackwell, Oxford
Ghodse H 1989 Drugs and addictive behaviour. A guide to treatment. Blackwell, Oxford
Robertson R 1987 Heroin, AIDS and society. Hodder and Stoughton, London

36. The sexually transmitted diseases

Ian Redhead

The purposes of screening for sexually transmitted diseases is to attempt to remove potential transmitters from an infectious pool and to treat infected persons prior to complications. If inexpensive and valid tests are available, screening has great appeal as a method to attempt to control the spread of these diseases.

THE SIZE OF THE PROBLEM

According to the returns made to the World Health Organization, approximately 200 million new cases of gonorrhoea and 40 million new cases of syphilis are notified each year. New cases of other sexually transmitted diseases, especially non-specific genital infection, occur in untold numbers. In the last decade vast numbers of people have been infected with the HIV viruses, especially in the African Continent (N'Gally & Ryder 1988) and increasingly throughout the world. Sexually transmitted diseases constitute a pandemic possibly without precedent.

In the UK, consultants in charge of clinics for sexually transmitted diseases are required to make quarterly returns to the Chief Medical Officer. This requirement was set down in the Venereal Disease Regulations of 1916, which also provided for the establishment of a free and confidential service for the treatment of sexually transmitted diseases (STD) under the auspices of local authorities. This duty was undertaken by the National Health Service at the time of its establishment in 1948. At that time, the medical profession, including many doctors working in the field of STD, considered that modern antibiotics had the measure of these diseases and it seemed that the need for the special clinics to manage them was fast diminishing. However, the incidence of new cases began to rise. In 1960 the number of new cases attending clinics in England and Wales was 120 000. By 1977 it was 400 000 and in 1986 it was 645 000. By 1987 the number of new cases seen was 620 000 (DHSS 1989), a fall of 25 000 on that in 1986 and a decrease of 4%.

Although relatively small, this was the first time since 1962 that the number of new cases had declined. Preliminary figures for the first quarter of 1988 suggested a further slight decline and, in 1987, there were falls in the number of new cases of most conditions compared with 1986. The decline was particularly marked in gonorrhoea — there were nearly 40% fewer cases of gonorrhoea in 1987 than in 1986. This could be due to changes in sexual behaviour following the publicity about AIDS/HIV, especially in homosexual men. There is little evidence of a change in sexual practices in the heterosexual male.

Figure 36.1 illustrates the trend and conditions seen over 10 years and its main components. New cases of syphilis and gonorrhoea accounted for only 4% of new cases, as compared with 16% in 1977. New cases of non-specific genital infection (NSGI), which includes chlamydia, non-specific urethritis, proctitis and cervicitis, decreased by 5500 (17%) in 1987 compared with 1986. Nevertheless, NSGI still accounted for 20% of new cases and remained the most commonly recorded condition.

Candidiasis and trichomoniasis were more commonly seen in women and accounted for 20% of female conditions seen. Both were declining in frequency, as was herpes simplex in both sexes. The decline in cases of candidiasis seen in genitourinary medicine (GUM) clinics could be the result of general practitioners diagnosing and treating this disease in their practices. Although candidiasis is recognised as an STD it is not necessarily so, and in most instances it is not.

The wart virus is one of the few conditions that showed an increase between 1986 and 1987 and currently this disease is of epidemic proportions. This condition is of particular interest and concern because of the possible link with cervical cancer, and it is especially common in the younger age groups. Other conditions not classified as sexually transmitted diseases are seen at clinics and these may not require treatment or may need referral elsewhere, most frequently to the

341

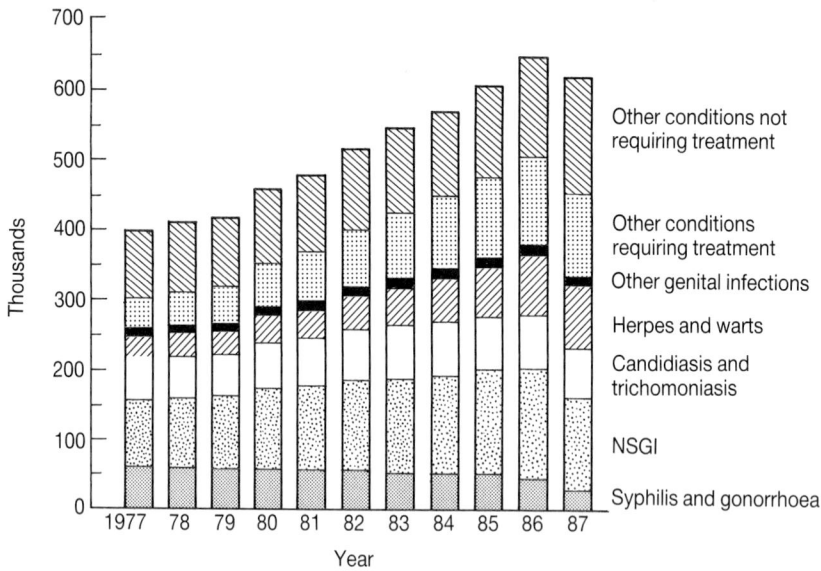

Fig. 36.1   New cases seen at NHS genitourinary medicine clinics in England (1977-87) (reproduced with the permission of the Department of Health Statistics and Research Division).

dermatologist or gynaecologist. In 1987 there were 288 000 such cases, more than double the number in 1977. Conditions not requiring treatment increased from 143 000 in 1986 to 168 000 in 1987, an increase of 18%. This category includes those coming for HIV testing, who were concerned about an infection mainly as a result of the HIV/AIDS publicity campaign. One-quarter of all cases seen in GUM clinics came under the category of 'other conditions not requiring treatment' and amongst these are the so-called 'worried well', anxious about HIV or AIDS.

The number of cases of HIV infection are not recorded in the figures up to 1987. Such cases are included under 'other conditions requiring / not requiring treatment' as appropriate. However, HIV and AIDS are distinguished in the new document on which consultants in GUM clinics have to record the new cases seen, although HIV and AIDS cases frequently do not present at genitourinary medicine clinics but are diagnosed as a result of manifestations such as chest infections and skin conditions.

The statistics discussed do not provide the real total of cases of STD that occur. It is estimated that about 10% of patients suffering from STD are treated in the private sector and a few by their own NHS general practitioner without referral to a clinic. No doubt large numbers of patients suffering from candidiasis are treated by their general practitioner but how many of these cases have been confirmed microbiologically is not known.

SCREENING FOR STD — GENERAL CONSIDERATIONS

In the planning of the screening programme the application of the principles and practice of screening for disease listed by Wilson & Jugner (1968) should be considered. More sophisticated postulates have been advocated since 1968 (Hudson et al 1988) but the simplicity of the original paper makes it highly acceptable in the context of general practice. The principles are listed in Tables 2.2 and 2.3.

Relating these principles to individual sexually transmitted diseases, gonorrhoea and syphilis would fulfil the criteria except that their incidence in this country is declining, so that they accounted for only 4% of the total new cases attending GUM clinics in 1987. A screening programme for syphilis in pregnant women is undertaken nationally in antenatal clinics. This will be discussed later.

Non-specific genital infection (NSGI) represented 20% of new cases attending clinics in 1987 and *Chlamydia trachomatis* was thought to be responsible for about half that total. Some of the increase in NSGI may have been due to the recording of epidemiological treatment, that is the treatment of contacts exposed to infection, which is widely practised. However, the steep rise in the laboratory diagnosis of genital *Chlamydia trachomatis* suggests that this represents a real increase in the disease. Chlamydia infection is associated with pelvic inflammatory disease, which is increasing, and also with consequent ectopic pregnancy, which resulted in 3000 hospital discharges and deaths in 1967, rising to 4600 in 1985 (CDSC 1989). It is a common cause of infertility.

Screening programmes for trichomoniasis and candidiasis do not fulfil the criteria as described above. Nevertheless, the development of new, simple tests designed for the rapid diagnosis of these conditions are being evaluated (Carney 1989). It is a fact that trichomoniasis frequently masks underlying gonorrhoea and, after treatment of the former, tests for neisserial infection should be undertaken.

Mass screening for herpes simplex is not indicated, nor is screening for pubic lice, scabies and the tropical venereal diseases. Sexually transmitted hepatitis B is of high incidence in homosexual men and screening for this disease is indicated in this high risk group. A vaccine is highly effective.

The incidence of wart virus infection is increasing and, although as a disease it does not fulfil the criteria for a screening programme, it is important that the partners of males with genital warts should be investigated because of the suspected relationship between this virus and cervical cancer, especially in younger women (British Cooperative Clinical Group 1987).

ROLE OF THE GENERAL PRACTITIONER

Apart from the opportunistic diagnosis of STD in patients with symptoms and signs such as urethral discharge and dysuria in men, vaginal discharge and dysuria in women, genital warts and other obvious pointers, screening for sexually transmitted disease generally is not undertaken in general practice (M P Vessey, personal communication). This fact is the result of the limited place of the general practitioner in the diagnosis and management of STD. A large proportion of patients attending GUM clinics self-refer and prefer not to present themselves to their personal doctor with symptoms that they suspect could have been the result of a sexual encounter. In taking a history from such a patient the general practitioner requires extreme tact and discretion, whereas the doctor in the clinic can be more direct. In addition, specialists in genitourinary medicine prefer patients to attend the clinic for diagnosis and management, having at their disposal full diagnostic and therapeutic facilities. GUM clinics have the service of a health adviser, one of whose major tasks is to follow up the contacts of patients and persuade them to have appropriate treatment. Contact tracing in general practice is more difficult because so frequently the

sexual partner of a patient has a different general practitioner.

Taking into account these considerations the question must be asked, has the general practitioner any part to play in screening and surveillance in STD? Formal screening, in the sense of calling in patients for routine testing, e.g. for NSGI, is not practical and is contraindicated. There are, nevertheless, three major fields in which the GP can play a part. These are screening for chlamydia infection, blood testing of pregnant women and cervical cytological screening. The problem of screening for HIV/AIDS will be discussed later.

CHLAMYDIA TRACHOMATIS INFECTION

About 40–50% of the cases of non-specific genital infection seen at GUM clinics in the UK and the USA are caused by *Chlamydia trachomatis*. It was estimated that over 4 million persons aquire chlamydia infection each year in the United States (Judson 1985). In England and Wales, returns from GUM clinics in 1987 reported approximately 65 000 cases of chlamydia genital infection (DHSS 1989). This must be a gross underestimate of the real total of chlamydia infection. Alexander (1988) stated that as a group genitourinary physicians in the UK cannot accurately diagnose chlamydia in the bulk of the patients attending their clinics because of a lack of laboratory facilities for diagnosing this infection. General practitioners are at an even greater disadvantage. Only a small minority of laboratories throughout the country give open access to general practitioners for diagnosis of chlamydia.

The frequently symptomless nature of chlamydia infection in both sexes can be misleading. In particular the inadequate follow-up by gynaecologists and general practitioners of the male partners of women with pelvic inflammatory disease ensures that a large number of cases of the infection go undetected. Infection with chlamydia in women is serious. It is frequently symptomless, and if there are symptoms, they are usually minimal (Ayra et al 1981). The first suggestion that the patient has had a previous chlamydia infection may be when she presents with infertility. Even in those with symptoms, the clinical presentation may give little indication of the extent and severity of the inflammation found at laparoscopy (Lancet 1986).

Chlamydia infection is more common in persons under 25, especially adolescents (Report of US Preventive Services Task Force 1989). Other risk factors for chlamydia in asymptomatic persons include multiple sexual partners, a new partner in the previous 2 months and a partner with a chlamydia infection.

It has been estimated that between 2 and 37% of mothers will have a chlamydia infection during pregnancy, with higher rates in younger patients and in the lower socio-economic groups (Hardy et al 1984, Wood et al 1984). Amongst those newborn at risk it has been estimated that 33–50% get conjunctivitis and 10–20% get pneumonitis (Lancet 1986).

The screening tests

The most sensitive and specific test for chlamydia infection is direct culture. It has the disadvantages of expense, limited availability and problems of transport and storage. It is therefore unacceptable for screening. Recent technological developments have made available tests that are less expensive and have less complicated transport and storage requirements. One of these is the direct monoclonal antibody test (Micro Trak, Syva) and is reported to be comparable with the traditional culture method in sensitivity and specificity (Longhurst et al 1987). Another is the enzyme linked immunoassay (ELISA), which does not require the special laboratory equipment and skilled technicians required by Micro Trak, although its sensitivity and specificity for chlamydia infection is uncertain (Report of US Preventive Services Task Force 1989). However, a note of caution should be introduced in regard to the new antigen detection chlamydia tests as they have only been evaluated properly in high prevalence populations and not in those at low risk (P E Munday, personal communication).

Effectiveness of early detection

Early detection of chlamydia infection in asymptomatic persons permits the early initiation of antibiotic treatment and the prevention of complications. Few controlled trials have been performed but it is believed that occult infection,which may result in serious complications, accounts for a large proportion of chlamydia infections (up to 80% in women and 10–20% in men). Over 95% of such infections can be cured by a 14-day course of an appropriate antibiotic. Treatment failures are usually the result of not treating the sexual partner or of non-compliance by the patient. Chlamydia screening in pregnant women reduces the incidence of neonatal infection by the treatment of positives with erythromycin (Schachter et al 1986).

Screening for chlamydia using direct antigen testing is considered to be cost-effective in the high risk groups, such as those attending GUM clinics and the younger age groups, including those attending family planning clinics (Nettleman & Jones 1988, Trachtenberg et al

1988). The absence of proper evaluation of the effectiveness of direct antigen tests in low risk groups has made an assessment of cost-effectiveness impossible.

The role of the general practitioner

From the evidence above it can be seen that there is a reservoir of chlamydia infection lying hidden within each general practice. Persons the general practitioner should consider screening for chlamydia (utilising swabs for microscopy and culture from the urethra in the male and cervix in the female) are:

1. The younger age groups considered at high risk attending for family planning.
2. Women who are known to have multiple sexual partners.
3. Women with other STD, e.g. genital warts.
4. Pregnant women less than 20 years of age, unmarried, known to have had multiple sexual partners or with a past history of sexually transmitted disease.
5. Women suffering from clinical pelvic inflammatory disease.
6. The sexual partners of women suffering from pelvic inflammatory disease (PID).

Knowledge of the infecting organism would improve the management of PID but what is of paramount importance is to prescribe an antibiotic regimen effective against chlamydia and other likely pathogens and pursue the sexual partners enthusiastically.

In addition to these high risk categories, opportunistic screening should be performed on those in the sexually active years who complain of sometimes relatively minor symptoms which, at the outset, do not suggest a diagnosis of STD. These include women with frequency and dysuria suggestive of a urinary tract infection but who have a normal midstream urine specimen or just mild pyuria and no growth on culture; women with unexplained abdominal pain without the clinical signs of pelvic inflammatory disease (Munday et al 1986); and men with frequency and dysuria with no urethral discharge. These men should be assumed to be suffering from STD, possibly chlamydia, unless proved otherwise by laboratory testing.

A negative chlamydia culture does not exclude the possibility of chlamydia infection and in suspicious cases repeated testing should be performed or referral to a clinic considered. The decreasing incidence of gonorrhoea should not deter a search for neisserial infection. Swabs for microscopy and culture from the urethra in the male, from the rectum in homosexuals and from the cervix and urethra in females, should be

Table 36.1   Reported AIDS, UK. By exposure category

	Cases reported to CDSC and CD(Scotland)U up to end November 1990					
	Male		Female		Total	
Exposure category	Cases	(Deaths)	Cases	(Deaths)	Cases	(Deaths)
Homosexual/bisexual male	3152	(1748)	–	(–)	3152	(1748)
Injecting drug user (IDU)	120	(49)	37	(20)	157	(69)
Homosexual/bisexual male and IDU	59	(32)	–	(–)	59	(32)
Haemophiliac	223	(152)	3	(2)	226	(154)
Blood/components recipient						
Abroad	13	(9)	24	(14)	37	(23)
UK	16	(13)	13	(9)	29	(22)
Heterosexual contact						
Partner(s) with above risk factors	11	(6)	22	(13)	33	(19)
Others[1]						
known exposure abroad[2]	136	(68)	60	(23)	196	(91)
no evidence of exposure abroad	13	(5)	12	(4)	25	(9)
Child of at risk/infected parent	13	(5)	20	(10)	33	(15)
Other/undetermined	37	(27)	4	(2)	41	(29)
Totals	3793	(2114)	195	(97)	3988	(2211)

[1] Partner(s) not known to have above risk factor(s)
[2] Includes persons, without other identified risks, from, or who have lived in, WHO transmission pattern II countries

taken. Clinical differentiation between chlamydia and neisserial infection is impossible.

The place of general practitioners as contact tracers can be underestimated (Owen et al 1988). It is true that many of the sexual contacts of their patients frequently have another general practitioner but at the heart of contact tracing is the provision of information to patients about their infection. They must be told how chlamydia infection is frequently silent and they must know about the long-term consequences of this silent disease. Repeated badgering at successive consultations might persuade the patient to drive his/her sexual partner to the clinic for investigation and treatment.

HIV AND AIDS

The incidence of HIV and AIDS in the UK

The first reported case of acquired immune deficiency syndrome (AIDS) was diagnosed in 1979. The cumulative total of cases reported on 30 November 1990 was 3988 (Table 36.1). Of these, 3152 were homosexual/bisexual men, 157 were intravenous drug abusers and 226 were haemophiliac. The incidence of AIDS amongst heterosexuals has remained low. Table 36.2 shows the geographical distribution of patients diag-

Table 36.2   Reported AIDS, UK. By country and region of report

Cumulative cases and deaths reported to CDSC and CD(Scotland)U up to end November 1990		
Country	Cumulative total	Deaths
England		
Northern	82	46
Yorkshire	101	63
Trent	76	41
East Anglia	41	30
NW Thames	1601	788
NE Thames	680	386
SE Thames	444	266
SW Thames	141	100
Wessex	93	60
Oxford	82	48
South Western	75	50
West Midlands	91	53
Mersey	51	36
North Western	156	91
Channel Islands	4	4
Wales	59	41
Northern Ireland	20	17
Scotland	191	91
Total (UK)	3988	2211

Table 36.3   Reported HIV-1 antibody-positive persons. Cumulative reports to end September 1990

Exposure category	Male	Female	Unknown	Total
Homosexual/bisexual male	7738	–	–	7738
Injecting drug user (IDU)	1306	615	32	1953
Homosexual/bisexual male and IDU	151	–	–	151
Haemophiliac	1208	7	1	1216
Blood/components recipient	68	61	2	131
Heterosexual contact Partner(s) with above risk factor(s)	20	151	1	172
Others* known exposure abroad[†]	336	223	9	568
no evidence of exposure abroad	29	26	2	57
undetermined	157	167	.	324
Child of at risk/infected parent	80	81	34	195
Multiple risks	14	4	–	18
Other/undetermined	1821	237	142	2200
Total	12 928	1572	223	14 723

* Partner(s) not known to have above risk factor(s).
† Includes persons, without other identified risks, from, or who have lived in, transmission pattern II countries.

nosed as having AIDS: it should be interpreted with caution because many of the patients ascribed to the London regions have been referred or migrated there.

In September 1990 the cumulative UK total of HIV-1 antibody positive persons was 14 723 (Table 36.3). Just under half of these were homosexual/bisexual males, 1953 were injecting drug abusers and 1216 were haemophiliac. Notwithstanding the substantial number coded as 'undetermined', the advance of HIV disease into the heterosexual population has been slower than expected.

In its conclusions and recommendations, the Cox Report (Department of Health 1988) said: 'the uncertainties of the epidemic are such that there is a wide range of plausible predictions of the numbers of new cases of AIDS. ...If a single figure is demanded we give 3600 as the recommended basis for planning for 1992'.

Over the following 10–15 years the report predicted that there would be 16 000–40 000 new cases of AIDS amongst those already HIV antibody-positive. The report commented that the increase in the monthly figures had been less rapid than expected but added that it would be a gross error to regard the lower predictions as grounds for complacency. The degree of uncertainty in the forecasts could only be reduced by more precise information about the current level of seroprevalence.

Screening and surveillance

When the principles and practice of screening for disease (Wilson & Jugner 1968) are considered relating to HIV infection, a fundamental principle does not apply; there is no medical treatment that will eliminate the virus nor is there a vaccine. However, treatment that has been shown to delay progression and to combat many of the opportunistic infections that occur is available and early diagnosis can prolong life and help protect potential sexual partners. It is for these reasons that screening for HIV infection is justified.

As a legal prerequisite in all cases the patient's consent is required to obtain blood and to perform an HIV antibody test. Pretest counselling as to the consequences of such a test proving positive must be performed, thus allowing the patient to accept or decline.

Patients found to be HIV positive present a complex situation. There are important social, economic and other personal consequences for the individual concerned. Confidentiality is of crucial importance when HIV infection or AIDS has been diagnosed. Any difficulties concerning confidentiality will usually be overcome if doctors are prepared to discuss openly and honestly with the patient the implications to others of condition.

The case for anonymous screening for HIV infection is made in the summary of recommendations in the

Cox Report: 'Urgent consideration should be given to methodological, ethical and legal issues associated with ascertaining seroprevalence more accurately via anonymous/blind testing on a national scale'. Such a screen would facilitate future planning required to cope with the epidemic.

Anonymous free testing for HIV infection in Sweden was reported by Herlitz and Brorsson (1989). One-quarter of the population of that country in the age groups 16–44 years had been tested over a 3-year period, resulting in a positive rate of 0.4%. This could be useful in health planning but the campaign had been financially extremely expensive. In England the Public Health Laboratory Service Working Group (1989) reported a study of the prevalence of HIV antibody in high and low risk groups. Anonymous testing of 34 222 subjects took place between October 1986 and December 1987. The incidence of HIV was significantly higher in the high risk groups – homosexual and bisexual men and intravenous drug users. Heterosexual spread of infection was evidently confined to subjects whose partner had an identifiable risk. The continuing complacency evident in the heterosexual male is likely to change this picture as time goes on.

Ethical arguments against anonymous screening have been voiced from several quarters in the UK, including the British Medical Association (Lancet 1988). It had misgivings including the obvious fact that anonymous screening would not provide an opportunity for identifying and counselling HIV seropositive individuals. The Association saw this objection not as an argument against anonymous testing but as one for making voluntary testing more widely available. The Royal College of General Practitioners considered that testing without the informed consent of the patient would be an infringement of the rights of the individual (RCGP Working Party 1988).

Screening in high risk groups has been advocated. Quinn et al (1988) advocated that all patients attending STD clinics should be screened. Loveday et al (1989) believed that there was a need for aggressive education for heterosexual men about HIV and AIDS and Curtis et al (1989) proposed the screening of intravenous drug abusers.

The case for mass HIV screening is being fiercely debated, especially in the United States. Rhame & Maki (1989) advocated HIV testing for all US adults below the age of 60 years, regardless of history. Wider testing would benefit not only society but also the carrier of the virus, for whom appropriate treatment of opportunistic disease could be prescribed. Smith (1989) summed up a body of opinion that challenges a patient's right to confidentiality in certain circumstances and cited the risks to surgeons from infected patients. The extreme view was taken by Seale at a conference of the London Medical Group (1989) who urged the introduction of routine and universal testing to combat AIDS: 'The decision to test should be taken by society and the individual must submit for the benefit of all individuals whether he likes it or not — as is the case with payment of taxes'.

The role of the general practitioner

The current controversy that surrounds the problem of screening for HIV infection makes an assessment of the role of the general practitioner exceedingly difficult. In instances the GP may know of patients in the practice who are at high risk, such as homosexual or bisexual men and intravenous drug abusers. However, there will be others who are also in these high-risk groups. Many an experienced general practitioner has been astonished to find that a male patient, known to them for many years, is homosexual or bisexual, and to miss a diagnosis of HIV infection can have serious consequences (Norell 1986).The refusal of many of those infected with HIV to allow the information to be given to their general practitioner can result in the doctor working at a serious disadvantage, and not only at a personal risk but at a risk to practice staff and to the patient him or herself.

In certain cases, testing for HIV infection is being requested and performed for political or other reasons. In these instances the principles of screening as defined in this chapter are void. Several countries insist on an HIV antibody test before allowing a person to enter. Some insurance companies require this test before providing insurance cover and, as the epidemic progresses, it seems certain that more companies will insist upon more testing. Insurance companies can also create a problem by placing a loading on the premiums of those individuals who admit to having had an HIV test. Occasionally, certain employers also require the test. Full pretest and post-test counselling is required in all these cases. This procedure is extremely time-consuming and could add considerably to the heavy workload of the general practitioner.

The role of the general practitioner in screening and surveillance for HIV infection is likely to be radically altered following a placebo controlled multicentre clinical trial supported by the United States National Institute of Allergy and Infectious Diseases (NIAID). Zidovudine (Retrovir), when given to persons with early AIDS-related complex (ARC), appears significantly to slow the progress to AIDS. The announcement made by NIAID (Wellcome Foundation 1989) stated that: 'significantly fewer persons receiving zidovudine progressed to advanced ARC or AIDS. This finding could extend treatment to an estimated 1 or 200 000 persons in the United States'. The report emphasised how critical it was that persons at risk from HIV infection be tested and seek prompt medical care. Early intervention was considered important in HIV infection and zidovudine was well tolerated in persons with early ARC.

If time confirms the beneficial effects of this drug in the early stages of HIV infection then it seems inevitable that a more positive screening programme can be anticipated in the UK, and it is likely that the general practitioner could play a major role in this programme. The impact on the National Health Service could be profound. Not only would the Government be required to fund the treatment and management of many more persons suffering from HIV infection, but support would be necessary to provide counselling facilities for the vastly increased number of persons who would submit to HIV testing.

BLOOD TESTING IN PREGNANCY

Antenatal screening for syphilis

Syphilis is rare in the UK, having fallen from a total of 3964 in 1975 to 2203 in 1986 (CDSC 1989). This fall can be almost certainly attributed to a substantial decrease of the disease in homosexuals. In the United States a rise in infectious syphilis has been reported in young heterosexuals and a similar trend has been observed in the UK, especially amongst young people.

In such circumstances, antenatal screening for syphilis must continue (Clay 1989). Screening has played a crucial part in the decline of the disease and is cost-effective if performed in the first trimester. As women become pregnant the serological tests performed constitute a massive screening programme not only of women but indirectly of men.

The results of treatment of the disease in early pregnancy are excellent both for the mother and for the fetus. Results of treatment later in pregnancy have as yet not been determined but the impression is that they are disappointing. Screening as early as possible in pregnancy is therefore essential. In higher risk groups it would be wise to repeat serological testing, but to perform such tests routinely is not cost-effective.

The antenatal testing for syphilis has been a highly effective compaign. It was summed up succinctly by Clay (1989): 'as in the case of AIDS, if prevention is done properly then precisely nothing happens'. Pride

should be taken in an achievement that had been quietly and laboriously attained (see also Chapter 11).

Antenatal testing for HIV

Routine testing for HIV in pregnancy is not being performed at the present time. However, Howard et al (1989) studied the transmission of HIV by heterosexual contact with reference to antenatal screening in an area with a very high prevalence of HIV infection within the local community. The results of the survey indicated increasing heterosexual spread of HIV infection. With one exception the 12 pregnant women found to be HIV antibody positive during the survey were in known high risk groups. Of the men seen in the genitourinary medicine clinic during the same period the majority, 22 out of a total of 32, were intravenous drug abusers. The authors concluded that if the present trend continued, more women will become infected, often unaware that they were at risk, and this would not be detected unless HIV testing was offered to all pregnant women and widely accepted. Decisions on local policy should be based on the available estimates of prevalence of HIV infection in that community.

Recent surveys in the United States have suggested that a significant minority of pregnant women infected with HIV did not belong to a high risk group and would therefore go undetected by current voluntary screening programmes (American Family Physician 1988). It was considered that it may be just a matter of time before HIV testing would become a routine part of prenatal screening in the United States.

One benefit of HIV screening in the antenatal clinic is that it allows pregnant women the opportunity to consider the possibility of termination. It is considered that about 30-50% of the offspring will be infected. The risk to the mother is difficult to quantify. Initial reports showed a high mortality from AIDS (Scott et al 1985) but later work (Mok et al 1987) was more reassuring. Howard and co-workers suggested that other benefits of HIV screening would include the counselling of patients about the advisability of future pregnancies and universal HIV testing in pregnancy would also serve to reassure midwives. It seems inevitable that the general practitioner will have to face the problem of antenatal screening for HIV within the next few years, initially in the areas of high risk but, in the long term, probably elsewhere.

CERVICAL CYTOLOGY

The role of the cytologist in screening for sexually transmitted disease is confined to the field of genital warts. Infection by the human papilloma virus (HPV) is one of the few conditions that has shown an increase in incidence in recent years. The association between this virus and carcinoma of the cervix has been recognised and it is therefore important to take measures to deal with this threat.

Ismail et al (1989) reported that experienced histopathologists showed considerable interobserver variability in grading intraepithelial neoplasia. Their conclusion was that the interpretation of cervical biopsies was very subjective. However, having accepted variations in interpretation various changes are recognised under the microscope with HPV. All male partner should be examined for the presence of genital warts and if present these should be treated and condoms used at least until the warts have disappeared.

Tait et al (1988) reported that although HPV was the most important sexually transmitted agent associated with cervical intraepithelial neoplasia (CIN), HPV was present in most patients with false negative and false positive cytology results in a series of 632 patients attending a clinic for STD. Thirteen out of 51 cases biopsied at colposcopy had false negative cytology results. The conclusion was that colposcopy as well as cervical cytology must be available for certain STD clinic patients. This gave an added incentive for the general practitioner to consider referring women with genital warts to the GUM clinic for colposcopy.

Richardson and Lyon (1981) reported a study of condom use in cases of CIN in the United States. In all cases the disease was biopsy proven. The 286 patients in whom child-bearing function was to be preserved were instructed to use a condom throughout intercourse as soon as a diagnosis of CIN was confirmed. Some patients had active surgical treatment but 139 were treated with condom use only. Of these, 136 showed complete regression within 6 months or more. No patients showed progression of the disease whilst using the condom and all grades of CIN proved to be reversible. The authors concluded that a mechanical barrier at intercourse should be recommended in any programme for the conservative treatment of CIN. In interpreting the results of this interesting paper it would be wise to take into account the considerable interobserver variability described by Ismail and his colleagues. Despite an exhaustive search, no studies similar to that of Richardson and Lyon have been found in the literature.

The ethical implications of repeating such a trial are considerable and even prohibitive. However, it would seem reasonable to examine in a closely controlled trial the effect of condom use on cases recognised to have cytological evidence of wart virus changes or early dyskaryosis.

Cytologists have no role to play in screening for herpes, although they will occasionally note multinucleated giant cells, which are suggestive of herpes but are not a reliable guide. Evidence of trichomonal infection or monilia may be noted but this observation is not really of value in screening for these conditions.

CONCLUSION

The evidence suggests that although the general practitioner has a small role to play in the screening and surveillance of sexually transmitted disease, it is a significant one. If the question was to be asked what tasks should be given priority, then three are suggested:

1. The screening for chlamydia infection in male sexual partners of women suffering from pelvic inflammatory disease. The vast majority of these infectious but symptomless men are most unlikely to attend a clinic for genitourinary medicine.
2. The screening of all the sexual partners of men or women suffering from genital warts.
3. An awareness that the HIV/AIDS epidemic is making slow but relentless inroads into the heterosexual population and, as a consequence, GPs should be prepared to counsel and offer testing to patients whom they suspect could be infected.

REFERENCES

Alexander I 1988 Letter. British Medical Journal 297: 791
American Family Physician 1988 Editorial: HIV screening in pregnancy 37(4): 93–96
Ayra O P, Mallinson H, Goddard A D 1981 Epidemiological and clinical correlates of chlamydia infection of the cervix. British Journal of Venereal Disease 57:118–124
British Cooperative Clinical Group 1987 Cervical cytology screening in sexually transmitted diseases clinics in the United Kingdom. Genito Urinary Medicine 63:40–43
Carney J A 1989 Rapid tests for the diagnosis of vaginal candida and trichomonas infection. Labmedica April/May 31–38

Clay J 1989 Antenatal screening for syphilis must continue. Leading article British Medical Journal 299:409–410
Communicable Disease Surveillance Centre Public Health Laboratory Service 1989 Sexually transmitted disease:1985–6. Genito Urinary Medicine 65: 117–121
Curtis J L, Crummy F C, Baker S N et al 1989 HIV screening and counselling for intravenous drug abuse patients, staff and patient attitudes. Journal of the American Medical Association 261(2): 258–262
Department of Health and Social Security 1989 Returns from departments of genito urinary medicine. Department of Health, London

Department of Health and Welsh Office 1988 Short term prediction of HIV infection and AIDS in England and Wales. Report of a working group. Chairman Cox, D. HMSO, London

Handsfield H H, Jasman L L, Robert P Z 1986 Criteria for selective screening for chlamydia trachomatis infection in women attending Family Planning Clinics. Journal of the American Medical Association 255(13): 1730–1734

Hardy P H, Hardy J B, Nell E E et al 1984 Prevalence of six sexually transmitted disease agents among pregnant inner city adolescents and pregnancy outcome. Lancet ii: 333–337

Herlitz C, Brorsson B 1989 HIV testing in 25 cent of Swedish population aged 16–44. Lancet ii: 386–387

Howard L C, Hawkins D A, Marwood R et al 1989 Transmission of human immuno deficiency virus by heterosexual contact with reference to antenatal screening. British Journal of Obstetrics and Gynaecology 96: 135–139

Hudson T W, Rheinhart M A, Rose S D et al 1988 Clinical preventative medicine. Little, Brown & Co, Boston/Toronto

Ismail S M, Colclough A B, Dinnen J S et al 1989 Observer variation in histopathological diagnosis and grading of cervical intraepithelial neoplasia. British Medical Journal 298:707–710

Judson F N, 1985 The incidence of chlamydia infection in the United States. Journal of Reproductive Medicine 30: 269–272

Lancet 1988 Notes and news. Lancet ii: 582

Lancet 1986 Leading Article. Chlamydia in women: a case for more action. Lancet i: 892–894

London Medical Group 1989 Report of 26th Annual Conference 1989. Bulletin of Institute of Medical Ethics 43: 19–20

Longhurst H J, Flower N, Thomas B J et al 1987 A simple method for the detection of chlamydia trachomatis infections in general practice. Journal of the Royal College of General Practitioners 37: 255–256

Loveday C, Pomeroy L, Weller I V D et al 1989 Human immuno deficiency viruses in patients attending a sexually transmitted disease clinic in London 1982–87. British Medical Journal 298:419–421

Mok J Q, Giaguinto C, Derossi A et al 1987 Infants born to mothers seropositive for human immuno deficiency virus. Preliminary findings from a Multicentre European Group. Lancet i: 1164–1168

Munday P E, Thomas B J, Taylor-Robinson D 1986 The Micro Trak Test for rapid detection of chlamydiae in diagnosing and managing women with abdominal pain. Genito Urinary Medicine 62: 15–16

Nettleman M D, Jones R B 1988 Cost effectiveness of screening for women at moderate risk for genital infections caused by chlamydia trachomatis. Journal of American

Medical Association 260(2): 207–213

N'Gally B, Ryder R W 1988 Epidemiology of HIV infection in Africa. Journal of Immune Deficiency Syndromes 1: 551–558

Norell J S 1986 In aid of doctors suffering from complaints about AIDS. British Medical Journal 293: 1213–1215

Owen P, Munro J, West R 1988 Letter. British Medical Journal 297: 1269

Public Health Laboratory Service Working Group 1989 Prevalence of HIV antibody in high and low risk groups in England. British Medical Journal 298: 422–3

Quinn T C, Glasser D, Cannon R D et al 1988 Human immuno deficiency virus infection among patients attending clinics for sexually transmitted diseases. New England Journal of Medicine 318(4): 197–202

Report of US Preventive Services Task Force 1989 Guide to clinical preventive services. Screening for chlamydia infection p 99–101 (in press)

Rhame F, Maki D 1989 The case for wider testing for HIV infection. New England Journal of Medicine 320: 1248–1254

Richardson A C, Lyon J B 1981 The effect of condom use on squamous cell cervical intraepithelial neoplasia. American Journal of Obstetrics and Gynaecology 140: 909–913

Royal College of General Practitioners Working Party 1988 Human immuno deficiency virus infection and acquired immune deficiency syndrome in general practice. Journal of Royal College of General Practitioners 38: 219–225

Scott G B, Fischl M A, Klimas N et al 1985 Mothers of infants with acquired immuno deficiency sydrome. Evidence for both symptomatic and asymptomatic carriers. Journal of American Medical Association 253: 363–366

Schachter J, Sweet R L, Grossman M et al 1986 Experience with routine use of erythromycin for chlamydia infections in pregnancy. New England Journal of Medicine 314: 276

Smith S 1989 Aids test polarises debate on surgery safety and privacy. New Scientist 13(5): 37

Tait I A, Alawattegama A B, Rees E 1988 Screening for cervical dysplasia in departments of genito urinary medicine. Genito Urinary Medicine 64: 255–8

Trachtenberg A I, Washington A E, Halldorson S 1988 A cost based decision analysis for chlamydia screening in California Family Planning Clinics. Obstetrics and Gynaecology 71: 101–108

Wellcome Foundation 1989 New data on the use of zidovudine in early ARC. Letter to Consultants in GUM in UK. The Wellcome Foundation Ltd, Cheshire

Wilson J M G, Jugner G 1968 Principles and practice of screening for disease. Public Health Paper No.34. World Health Organization, Geneva

Wood P L, Hobson D, Rees E 1984 Genital infections with chlamydia trachomatis attending an antenatal clinic. British Journal of Obstetrics and Gynaecology 91: 1171–76

37. The family and its problems

Peter Tomson

INTRODUCTION

Working with families is probably less amenable to the protocol of screening considered in this book than other subjects but may nevertheless be rewarding. The recognition of certain characteristics within a family or its members can be a pointer to both present and future troubles and may allow useful preventive work and anticipatory care to take place.

First we need to decide what is meant by the term 'family'. It is a central word in our vocabulary but we may not always know what we mean by it. Various attempts have been made to define it: 'the family is a significant group of intimates with a history and a future' (Ransome & Vandervoort 1973). 'The family may be also be defined as a group of adult partners with or without children and single parents with children. These people function in a setting where there is a sense of home and they have an agreement to establish nurturing relationships' (Smilkstein 1975).

There is little research on healthy families and what there is may only apply to white families in the USA (Textor 1989). If a 'healthy' family cannot be defined, then neither can a 'sick' family, but in reality all families will have more and less healthy parts and times. However, there are various circumstances in which there is a greater likelihood of sickness occurring in either the individual or the family. It is these that I wish to explore.

'The family is the patient' is a provocative statement (Marinker 1976). In general practice we are used to focusing on the individual, although we may, and perhaps should, always think of the individual in the context of his/her family. This chapter will consider both the effect of the family on an individual's illness and the effect of that illness on the family. Serious or chronic illness in a family member can lead to problems in the family as a whole; it can also put other members at risk of becoming sick. On the other hand, a family that appears to be 'sick' may not actually contain any members that are overtly 'sick'. It is deliberate that no distinction has been made between physical, psychological and behavioural disturbances because there is very little research linking individual or family trauma to specific outcomes.

The likelihood of illness in the family will depend, as in an individual, on the balance between the strengths and weaknesses of the family and the stresses to which it is subjected.

The first half of the chapter will describe the various family circumstances that increase or decrease the risks of problems and the second half will look at ways in which these ideas may be used in general practice.

RISK FACTORS

Genetics

This is not the chapter to elaborate on this theme but it might be helpful to remember that whatever the likelihood of a person developing a condition that is known to exist in the family, the fear of developing it may be a source of continuing anxiety and behaviour. We could also remember the interaction between the genetic and the environmental in almost all conditions, of which schizophrenia is a good example (Tarrier 1989) (see also Chapter 10).

Family structure

There is a presumption that intact nuclear families are less vulnerable to dysfunction than disrupted or reconstituted families.

A girl whose mother dies before she reaches the age of 12 is known to be at risk of depression in later life (Brown & Harris 1978). A period of separation from parental and particularly maternal care in infancy or childhood can have deleterious effects, particularly if there is inadequate substitute parental care. Initially this may manifest itself as a cognitive delay, while in later life boys may develop behavioural problems and girls depressive tendencies (Rutter 1972). However, short periods of well managed separation may actually strengthen the ego and prepare the person for the difficulties of adult life.

Single parent families are often financially poorer than intact ones and there is some evidence that they present more illness to the general practitioner (Jennings & Sheldon 1985). Remarried or reconstituted families often have difficulties coping with their children — the mythology of the wicked stepmother may well have some basis in reality.

Three-generational households may offer support for the parents but in our current culture may provide opportunities for inappropriate alliances and rivalries. Many incidents of sexual abuse are perpetrated by men, other than the natural fathers, who live in the household or have easy access to the victim. This may include stepfathers.

The family life cycle

Families have life cycles just as individuals do (Medalie 1979) (Fig. 37.1). At any one time in the family life cycle various tasks need to be achieved if 'health' is to be maintained and development sustained. At these periods the family may be in a state of crisis, with the implication that there are opportunities for both growth and disaster. For example, around the birth of the first child the parents may need to accomplish the following changes, amongst others:

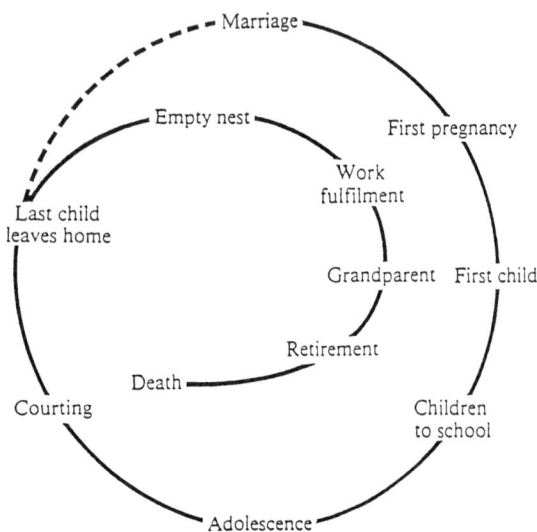

Fig. 37.1 The family life cycle (from Tomson 1983).

1. Acceptance of the loss of independence both socially and economically, especially for the mother.
2. Definition of their roles as parents.
3. Recreation of their sexual life, perhaps with contraception for the first time.
4. Re-evaluation of their economic status.
5. Coping with the increased interest of the grandparents.
6. Rejoining the social community as parents.

If these adaptations are not successfully accomplished they may be at risk of:

1. Maternal depression.
2. Father opting out or going to the pub (Lawrence 1915).
3. Separation.
4. Poor parenting and child abuse.
5. Recurrent sickness in the child.

It requires only imagination and common sense to create the tasks and risks of the other life cycle stages. By remembering the family life cycle, general practitioners should be able to provide anticipatory guidance and counselling.

Unexpected crises and life events

There is now much evidence connecting life events to ill health and death in individuals (Rahe & Holmes 1967). Similarly, in a prospective study of life events in New Zealand, Beautrais et al (1982) found an association between life events and attendance of children to the medical services for a variety of ailments. The hierarchy of stressful events is headed by losses but also includes illness, conflict, deprivation and change. Loss embraces not only death but divorce, separation, losing a limb and getting the sack, with loss of status and self-esteem.

Top of the list of stressful events is death, and no doctor can fail to be aware of the effect of death on the surviving relatives. Van Eijk et al (1988) found that there was an increase of minor illness among relatives after an expected death, and of more serious illness after a sudden one. We may not always be aware of the long-term effects of some deaths, particularly if the process of grieving has not been successfully accomplished. If a grandparent dies at the same time as a baby is born, the parent is both grieving and celebrating at the same time and this may disrupt early parenting. Similarly, if one twin dies and the other lives, the parents are having to cope with conflicting emotions at the same time.

Acute serious illness in one member may lead to increased reporting of serious illness in other family members, depending on the coping skills of the family (Van Eijk 1985).

In families with a chronically sick or disabled person there is a strong probability of one of the carers also becoming ill. Having a handicapped child (Romans-Clarkson et al 1986), a mother with bulimia (Stein & Fairburn 1989), a relative with a stroke (Carnwath & Johnson 1987), a mentally infirm person to cope with (Gilleard et al 1984), asthma (Davis 1977) or indeed even someone with an acute illness in the family (Johnson et al 1985) have all been shown to be associated with increased morbidity, usually psychiatric.

In many conditions not only is the rest of the family affected but the family itself may be involved in the aetiology or the maintenance of the condition. This leads to the idea that including the family in consultations may be helpful in resolving the problem. Obvious examples are behavioural problems, especially the abuse of alcohol (Orford 1987, Lanier 1984), depression (Widmer et al 1980), anxiety, somatoform symptoms particularly headaches, chronic fatigue, high attendance rates at surgery, compliance difficulties and psychosomatic conditions.

Children at risk may be identified from certain factors in the family history. Such factors include:

1. Being born after another child has died or after an abortion or stillbirth.
2. Being born after a time of subfertility.
3. Being born at a time of crisis in the family; death of a family member, moving house, serious illness and unexpected unemployment.
4. Having a chronically sick parent or sibling.
5. Being born after a difficult pregnancy or labour.
6. Being unwanted or the wrong sex.

The larger system or the external world does, of course, have a profound effect on the family system. Poverty, inadequate housing, poor education, unemployment and bad medical facilities are obvious examples.

Family functioning

There have been many attempts to assess family functioning and perhaps the best researched for the purpose of general practice is that of McMasters (Epstein et al 1978). It incorporates assessing the family's problem-solving abilities, communications, roles, affective responsiveness, affective involvement and behaviour control.

A simpler and perhaps more useful framework for assessing family function contains only two dimensions, adaptability and cohesiveness (Fig. 37.2). Families that are rigid in the face of stress are more likely to develop

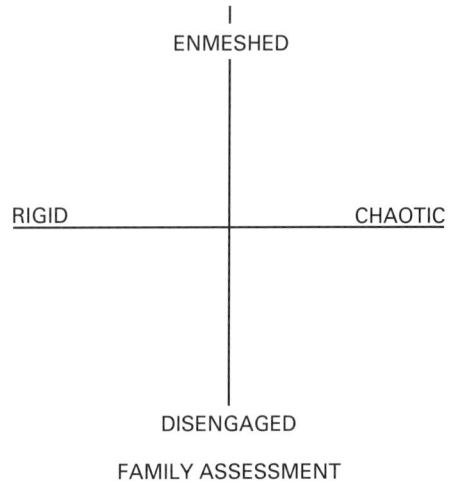

Fig. 37.2   Family assessment.

either family or individual distress. To cope adequately with any stress demands flexibility of roles, the ability to communicate and appropriate emotional interaction. Conversely, families who have no guidelines and wander haphazardly from the path are also likely to become sick or drift apart.

Cohesion in some families is so close that members think for each other, speak for each other and share emotions but may be unable to discuss or resolve conflicts. They are 'inside each others' skins' and often overprotective. Such families can present as nice, happy people but the degree of rigidity may be restrictive. If the ethos of not quarrelling prevails so the only escape route is into illness, such families are thought to develop psychosomatic disorders (Minuchin 1974, Wirsching and Stierlin 1985).

At the other end of the scale families are described as chaotic. They seem to care little for each other, go their own way and they may quarrel violently. These families are more at risk of behavioural problems, including involvement with the law, substance abuse, etc. Most families will be at times close and at others distant, sometimes inflexible and sometimes malleable, it is only the extremes that are vulnerable.

While it is probable that dysfunction in the other areas of interaction are important and predictive of family health, they are difficult to assess and do not seem applicable to surveillance or screening without some experience of family therapy. Those interested in pursuing the ideas about problem-solving, communication, affect and behaviour control are referred to Epstein et al (1978) and to Christie-Seeley (1984).

Abuse, both sexual and physical, recurs in successive generations. At some time, perhaps antenatally, mothers and fathers could be asked about their own childhood experiences.

Huygen (1988) has shown that maternal grandparents with nervous disorders predict frequent new periods of illness among the grandchildren, so this area may also be worth anticipating.

Data Base

NAME			FORENAME		DATE

DATE OF BIRTH		RELIGION	

COUNTRY OF ORIGIN		TEL. NO.	

Single☐ Married☐ Divorced☐ Remarried☐ Separated☐ Widowed☐

FAMILY HISTORY

		ALIVE		IF DEAD	
	FIRST NAME	YEAR OF BIRTH	ANY SERIOUS ILLNESS	CAUSE OF DEATH	AGE AT DEATH
MOTHER					
FATHER					
BROTHERS 1					
BROTHERS 2					
BROTHERS 3					
SISTERS 1					
SISTERS 2					
SISTERS 3					
HUSBAND/ WIFE					
CHILDREN 1					
CHILDREN 2					
CHILDREN 3					
CHILDREN 4					
CHILDREN 5					
CHILDREN 6					P.T.O.

Fig. 37.3   Family database.

Protective factors

SCREEM is an acronym for Social, Culture, Religious, Economic, Educational and Medical resources (Smilkstein 1975). Having a confiding relationship seems to be protective against physical disorder (Medalie 1976) and against depression (Brown and Harris 1978). The relationship is most often with a spouse but need not be so to be helpful; social networks also have a protective action. Berkman & Syme (1979), in a sample of 6928 adults, showed that people without social ties had an increased risk of death, while Henderson et al (1978) found an inverse relationship between social bonds and neurotic symptoms. In a general practice study, religious allegiance has been found to be associated with a lower number of symptoms of all kinds (Hannay 1980). Beale & Nethercott (1988) in Calne, Wiltshire have shown the deleterious effects of unemployment and the threat of unemployment on family health.

The role of the primary care team

It is not the objective of this book to introduce a lot more 'shoulds' into practice but there is some implication of expectancy in the use of the word 'could'. The themes of this book are screening, surveillance and case-finding. In the field of detecting family problems I would like to suggest a further option: taking a history of the family either from an individual member of the family or preferably from the whole family. This latter idea has been used in the USA (Gropper et al 1987) but not in the UK as far as I know.

The past history of a family is fixed and although it will need updating with time, most of it needs to be ascertained only once. How accurate and how complete it is will depend on the method and skill of the clinician and the memory and attitude of the story teller. Like any history it is not just a matter of fact but also

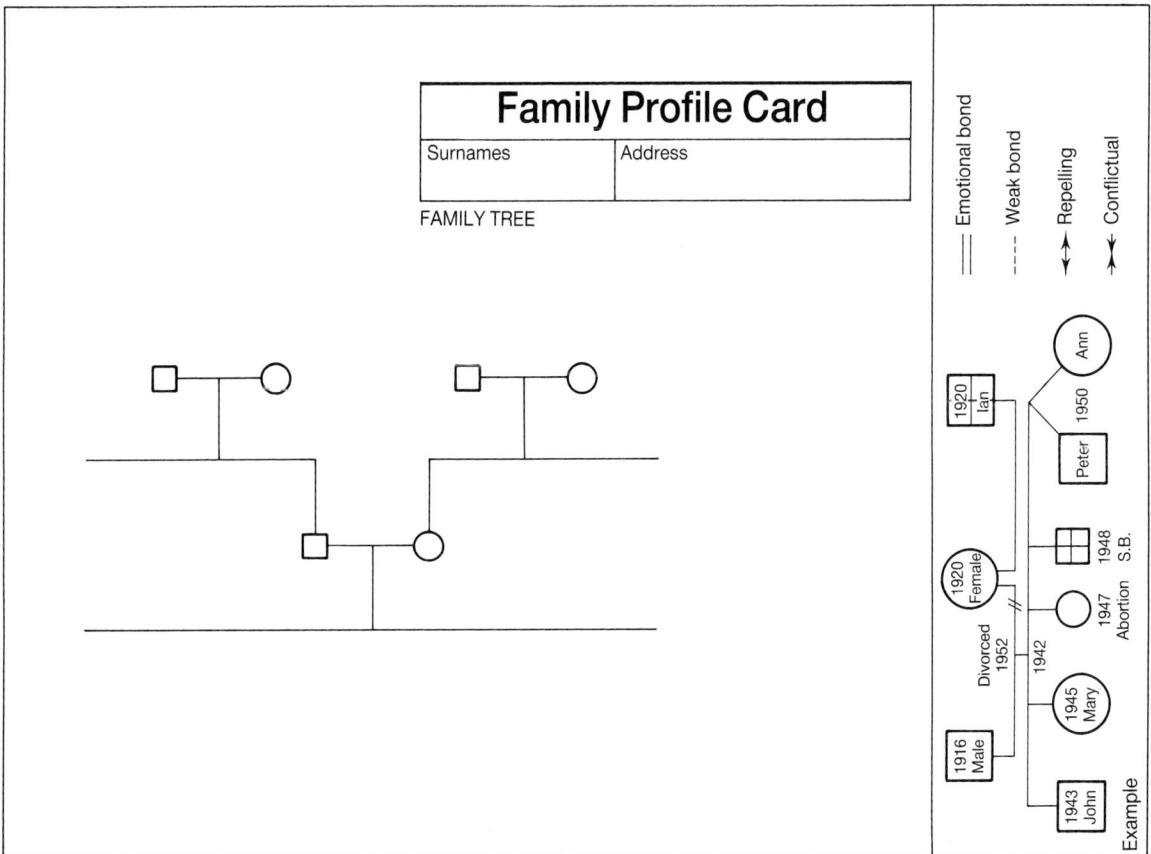

Fig. 37.4 Family profile card.

of interpretation. If both partners of a marriage are asked to relate the family history each will give a picture which varies in some aspects. Nevertheless, the basic family tree is fairly reliable. Later in the chapter I will outline a way of taking a family history — the genogram — which produces much useful information.

A basic family history can be taken by giving newly registered patients or old patients, if suitably introduced, a questionnaire about their general health containing a section about their family history (Murray et al 1974) (Fig. 37.3). This section should include, as a minimum, information about the dates of all births and deaths of three generations, the causes of death and major illnesses, abortions and stillbirths. These data become much more meaningful if they are translated into a family tree; an activity that has been done by a secretary with very little extra training (Tomson et al 1986). It can then be recorded on each person's records, which is time-consuming and creates difficulties in keeping it up to date, or it can be detailed on a family record card (Fig. 37.4) (Tomson 1986 et al). In our practice these cards are kept separately and are made available to the doctors at all consultations, together with the ordinary record cards or folders. Thus, at every consultation the family structure is visible and can be updated. The cards we have designed also have space on the inside for information about the health of the individual members of the family that are registered with the practice (Fig. 37.5). (The database card (patient questionnaire) and the family record card can obtained from General Practice Supplies, 314 St Albans Rd, Watford, Herts, WD2 5PD.)

Whether the family history is ascertained by questionnaire or by face to face contact it could be validated and discussed by the clinician of first contact, who might be the nurse, health visitor or doctor. In the course of this discussion an opportunity could be made to ask about the childhood experiences of the parents with specific questions about sexual and physical abuse.

The family health tree provides information about the genetics, the family life cycle, the structure of the family, repetitive patterns of illness and some of the unexpected crises that the family has suffered (Prince-Embury 1984). It does not provide any information about family dynamics or support.

If I were redesigning the cards I would incorporate the simple question 'How many people do you have that you can readily count on for real help in times of trouble or difficulty, such as to baby-sit, watch over pets, take you

Forename (and surname if different) & Relationship	D of B	D of D	Current Problems	Past History	Family Dynamics	Occupations	EXTENDED FAMILY			
							Problems	Cause of Death	D of B	D of D
F						....	F	....		
						....	M			
M						....	F	....		
						....	M			
						....				
						....				
						....				
						....				
						....				
						....				
						....				

Fig. 37.5 Family record card.

```
┌─────────────────────────────────────────────────────────────────────┐
│                     Family Interview Questionnaire                    │
├─────────────────────────────────────────────────────────────────────┤
│                                                                       │
│  Family Life Cycle                                                    │
│    (I)*  1.  How many are there in the family?                        │
│    (I)   2.  Who lives at home?                                       │
│    (A)   3.  In what phase of the family life cycle is this family?   │
│    (I)   4.  What problems does this raise for them presently?        │
│    (I)   5   What major problems has this family had in the past      │
│              (inquire about death, separation, major physical or      │
│              mental illness, financial crisis, etc)?                  │
│    (I)   6.  Does this family feel these problems were dealt with      │
│              satisfactorily?                                          │
│                                                                       │
│  Family Process or Psychosocial Interior                             │
│    (I)   1.  Who are the major decision makers in the family?         │
│    (I)   2.  Who can each person talk to most easily?                 │
│    (I)   3.  What are the family members' expectations of each other? │
│              Are these expectations being acheived? (Are they         │
│              realistic?)                                              │
│    (I)   4.  How does each member of this family get attention?       │
│    (A)   5.  How much tolerance for individual difference and         │
│              self-expression is there in the family?                  │
│                                                                       │
│  Social Milieu                                                        │
│    (I)   1.  How much contact do you have with relatives? Are they    │
│              helpful? Do they create problems?                        │
│    (I)   2.  Do the family members have many friends in their         │
│              neighbourhood? To what groups or clubs do family         │
│              members belong?                                          │
│    (I)   3.  What sort of community resources has the family used?    │
│              Would they use them again?                               │
│    (I)   4.  What is the educational level and status of the parents  │
│              of the family?                                           │
│                                                                       │
├─────────────────────────────────────────────────────────────────────┤
│         *I—Inquire                                                     │
│          A—Assess                                                     │
└─────────────────────────────────────────────────────────────────────┘
```

Fig. 37.6 Family interview questionnaire (from Arbogast 1978).

to hospital or shops or help you if you are sick?' Blake & McKay (1986), in the USA, showed that adults responding 0-1 had a higher risk of morbidity than patients who had 2 or more possible helpers. This single question was as predictive as a 12-item questionnaire.

Arbogast et al (1978) have described a 15-item questionnaire that they have used to attempt to ascertain the family health (Fig. 37.6). This was found to be helpful but did not elicit enough about the internal dynamics of the family. It has not been used as a screening tool as far as I know, but it does give an idea of the range of questions that might need to be asked when assessing a family.

The genogram

The genogram (Lieberman 1979, McGoldrick & Gerson 1986, Markus et al 1989) is a family tree that includes family dynamics, illness, health hazards,

occupations and other data that seem important. It is also a way of taking a family history with a patient or with a whole family that includes not only the family tree and physical illnesses but begins to look at the meaning of the events to the family and at the interpersonal dynamics.

It is created *with* the individuals or members of the family and is not *extracted* from them. It starts with a fairly simple family tree of three generations but the doctor also asks about the meaning and implications of the history and its effect on the relationships within the family. I think that it is a technique that *could* be learnt by all primary health care workers with benefit. Like et al (1988) describe an approach to interpreting the data.

Rogers & Durkin (1984), in a semi-controlled screening project of 72 newly registered patients, found that the genogram elicited psychosocial problems in 60% of patients, compared with none referred for counselling among the controls who had a standard history taken. The genogram took 20 minutes to complete and 98% of the patients felt that it improved the doctor-patient relationship. A later study (Rogers & Cohn 1987), using a self-administered genogram, again found that more information was discovered but that it did not lead to more counselling-type activity by the physicians. It seems that personal contact is more helpful than questionnaires in this situation.

In their day-to-day consultations, doctors and other members of the primary care team will be alerted to family problems by the illnesses presented (see p. 353).

Formal screening

In 1978 Smilkstein devised the family APGAR, a self-administered tool for assessing family dysfunction. It consists of five questions eliciting information about Adaptation, Partnership, Growth, Affection and Resolve (Fig. 37.7). It has been used to screen new patients (Hilliard et al 1986), routinely attending patients (Mengel 1987) and newly registering adolescents (Shapiro et al 1987). In all examples it detected family distress. It would thus seem that the test is capable of identifying family and psychosocial problems. It fulfils some criteria of good screening in that the problems to be identified are common, it is a cheap, easy to administer and non-invasive screening device, but we have no evidence about its sensitivity or specificity, nor do we have any researched evidence about its effectiveness in helping patients or families.

An antenatal prospective study using the family APGAR and FACES (the Family Adaptability and Cohesion Evaluation Scales (Olsen et al 1978)) demonstrated an ability to predict low birth weight (Ramsay et al 1986). Whether these instruments are used or not, the antenatal period is a useful time for assessing the possibility of poor parental bonding with the infant and future child abuse. Clues include the mother's own experience of childhood, single parents, unsupported families, isolation, alcoholism, economic poverty and marital dysfunction, all of which *could* be inquired about.

Postnatal depression

There is evidence that postnatal depression is under-diagnosed. Playfair & Gowers (1981) showed that 24.3% of their population had three or more depressive symptoms at 3 months postnatally and Kumar & Robson (1978) also found 24% of primigravidae in their study to have a depressive neurosis. Not only is postnatal depression a very distressing illness but it is known

to have deleterious effects on the child's development (Cogill et al 1986). Ancill et al (1986) tackled this by antenatal use of the Hamilton depression rating scale, adapted for self-rating and administered by a microcomputer. They found that there was a significant correlation between antenatal scores and the development of postnatal depression. The Edinburgh postnatal depression scale (Cox et al 1987) has only 10 questions and positive scores correlate well with clinical depression. I think the Edinburgh postnatal depression scale *could* be given to all postnatal patients at their postnatal visit by the doctor or midwife.

The family life cycle

We have discussed the importance of assessing the family antenatally and postnatally but assessment at other stages can also be useful. Farmer & Markus (1986) describe assessing family influences on the development of psychological problems in teenagers. Doctors do not often have the opportunity to counsel engaged couples, but should the chance arise it might be helpful to do a genogram with the couple. Similarly Caplan (1986) describes the importance of counselling families in the throes of separation to mitigate the distress to the children.

Bereavement has effects not only on the bereft spouse but also on the children and this is a priority time to help the family, perhaps with a family counselling session (Ersrtling & Devlin 1989).

Clues to family problems

There are various presentations that suggest that family dynamics may be involved in the maintenance of an individual's symptoms. I would be alerted by recurrent non-specific symptoms, overutilisation of the practice by the family, poor compliance in chronic illness, behavioural disorders, lifestyle diseases, depressions and chronic headaches. Using the APGAR can help to reveal to the family that there was a family problem and the genogram might help to confirm this and to suggest areas of difficulty that could be worked on.

Management

This chapter so far has discussed ways of identifying problems in families or the individuals in them. One very important criterion for successful screening is that there is a satisfactory treatment. In patients presenting with symptoms Comley (1973) showed that family therapy done by family physicians decreased the number of visits to the doctor, increased patient satisfaction and

The following questions have been designed to help us better understand you and your family. You should feel free to ask questions about any item in the questionnaire.

The space for comments should be used when you wish to give additional information or if you wish to discuss the way the question is applied to your family. Please try to answer all questions.

Family is defined as the individual(s) with whom you usually live. If you live alone, your "family" consists of persons with whom you now have the strongest emotional ties.

For each question, check only one box

	Almost always	Some of the time	Hardly ever
I am satisfied that I can turn to my family for help when something is troubling me.	☐	☐	☐

Comments: _____

| I am satisfied with the way my family talks over things with me and shares problems with me. | ☐ | ☐ | ☐ |

Comments: _____

| I am satisfied that my family accepts and supports my wishes to take on new activities or directions. | ☐ | ☐ | ☐ |

Comments: _____

| I am satisfied with the way my family expresses affection and responds to my emotions, such as anger, sorrow and love. | ☐ | ☐ | ☐ |

Comments: _____

| I am satisfied with the way my family and I share time together. | ☐ | ☐ | ☐ |

Comments: _____

Scoring: The patient checks one of three choices, which are scored as follows: "Almost always" (2 points), "Some of the time" (1 point) or "Hardly ever" (0). The scores for each of the five questions are then totaled. A score of 7 to 10 suggests a highly functional family; a score of 4 to 6 suggests a moderately dysfunctional family; a score of 0 to 3 suggests a severely dysfunctional family. We think that a low family score more accurately reflects a high level of current dissatisfaction in one family member than unmistakable evidence of severe family dysfunction. The latter diagnosis will require more evidence about the family system.

[According to which member of the family is being interviewed, the physician may substitute for the word "family" either "spouse," "significant other," "parent," or "children".]

Fig. 37.7 Family APGAR questionnaire (from Smilkstein 1978).

improved family relationships. Huygen (1978), in Holland, also found a diminution of patient attendance after simple family therapy in general practice. Doherty & Baird (1983) have described a method of counselling families that is applicable to general practice and Ersrtling & Devlin (1989) write about the single session family interview.

Counselling and individual therapy have also been shown to be effective (Trepka & Griffiths 1987, Kolvin et al 1988). There is no consensus about who should be doing the counselling. The teaching of counselling techniques to undergraduates and doctors has been neglected and experiences in training may actually undermine any natural skills they have (Rowland et al 1989). The same comment may apply to health visitors and nurses. There is, as always, a possibility of side-effects or even adverse effects from psychotherapy (Furman & Ahola 1989).

As yet there is no defined place for psychologists or trained counsellors in the primary care team (Gray 1988). It is interesting that, in the United States, most resident schemes have behavioural scientists attached to them who are often experienced in family therapy. It is my hope that before long all primary care teams will have clinical psychologists attached to them to serve not only as therapists but also as consultants to the team (Milne & Souter 1988, Deys et al 1989). I hope that they would also have family therapy skills.

CONCLUSIONS

It is my thesis that there are few formal screening procedures that are applicable to general practice except on a research basis. However, there are opportunities for increased suspicion of the possibility of sickness. It has been my experience that by understanding the 'family', and observing it one is able to anticipate problems and sometimes to ameliorate them.

The structure of the family, the family life cycle, life events and family functioning are important indicators of possible problems, both in individuals and the family. We could all be more aware of them. Many of the problems detected or anticipated are amenable to simple counselling of the family or individual. There is no easy way of ascertaining family function except in particular cases but there are methods of finding out about the structure, family life cycle and life events.

As yet there is no place for screening families in general practice in the United Kingdom but there is a definite place for surveillance. A family history *should* be taken from all newly registering patients and an opportunity found to update the family history of 'old' patients. It may be as important to learn the risk factors ascertained from this history as it is to find out about smoking and drinking. In one study twelve doctors each asked 10 consecutive patients about the morbidity or mortality of their parents and obtained information that changed their perception of the patient and the current problem in most of these consultations (Tomson 1989).

Whether or not a genogram or family history has been taken the implications for the family should be considered at every consultation.

If the consultation involves turning points in the family life cycle, acute or long-standing life events or lifestyle problems, the possibility of there being disturbances in the rest of the family should be strongly considered and some form of family enquiry made. This could be informal, a genogram, a family counselling session or the use of the APGAR.

My message is simple:

1. Somehow take a family history.
2. Be aware of the implications for the family in all consultations.
3. When appropriate, facilitate grieving for *all* members of the family.

REFERENCES

Papers that are important, as opposed to supporting the text, are marked with an asterisk.

Ancil R, Hilton S, Carr T et al 1986 Screening for antenatal and postnatal depressive symptoms in general practice using a microcomputer-delivered questionnaire. Journal of the Royal College of General Practitioners 36: 276–279

Arbogast R C, Scratton J M, Krick J P 1978 The family as patient: preliminary experience with a recorded assessment schema. Journal of Family Practice 76(6): 1151–1157

Beale N, Nethercott S 1988 The nature of unemployment morbidity. 1. Recognition. Journal of the Royal College of General Practitioners 38: 197–199

Beautrais A L, Fergusson D M, Shannon F T 1982 Life events and childhood morbidity: a prospective study. Pediatrics 70(6): 935–939

Berkman L F, Syme L 1979 Social networks, host resistance, and mortality: a nine-year follow-up study of Alameda County residents. American Journal of Epidemiology 109(2): 186–204

Blake R L, McKay D A 1986 A single-item measure of social supports as a predictor of morbidity. Journal of Family Practice 22(1): 82–84

Brown G W, Harris T 1978 Social origins of depressions. Free Press, New York

*Caplan G 1986 Preventing psychological disorders in

children of divorce: guidelines for the general practitioner. British Medical Journal 292: 1563–1566

*Caplan G 1986 Preventing psychological problems in children of divorce: general practitioner's role. British Medical Journal 292: 1431–1434

Carnwath T C M, Johnson D A W 1987 Psychiatric morbidity among spouses of patients with stroke. British Medical Journal 294: 409–411

Christie-Seely J 1984 Working with the family in primary care. Praeger Publishers, New York

Cogill S R, Caplan H L, Alexandra H et al 1986 Impact of maternal depression on cognitive development of young children. British Medical Journal 292: 1165–1167

Comley A 1973 Family therapy and the family physician. Canadian Family Physician 19: 81

Cox J, Holden J M, Sagovsky R 1987 Detection of postnatal depression by 10-item self-report questionnaire. British Journal of Psychiatry 150: 782–786

Davis J B 1977 Neurotic illness in the families of children with asthma and wheezy bronchitis: a general practice population study. Psychological Medicine 7: 305–310

Deys C, Dowling E, Golding V 1989 Clinical psychology: a consultative approach in general practice. Journal of the Royal College of General Practitioners 39: 342–344

Doherty W J, Baird M A 1983 Family therapy and family medicine. The Guilford Press, New York

*Epstein N B, Bishop D S, Levin S 1978 The McMaster model of family functioning. Journal of Marriage and Family Counselling 19–31

*Erstling S S, Devlin J 1989 The single session family interview. Journal of Family Practice 28(5): 556–560

Farmer A, Markus A 1986 Family influences on the development of psychological problems in teenagers. Journal of the Royal College of General Practitioners 36: 552–554

Furman B, Ahola T 1989 Adverse effects of psychotherapeutic beliefs: an application of attribution theory to the critical study of psychotherapy. Family Systems Medicine 7(2): 183–195

Gilleard C J, Belford H, Gilleard et al 1984 Emotional distress amongst the supporters of the elderly mentally infirm. British Journal of Psychiatry 145: 172–177

Gray D P 1988 Counsellors in general practice. Journal of the Royal College of General Practitioners 39: 118–120

Gropper M, Sadovsky R, Fraser Y, Weiner M 1987 Promotion of family enrolment in an urban family residency programme. Journal of Family Practice 24: 57–60

Hannay D R 1980 Religion and health. Social Science and Medicine 14a: 683–685

Henderson S, Byrne D G, Duncan-Jones P et al 1978 Social bonds in the epidemiology of neurosis: a preliminary communication. British Journal of Psychiatry 132: 463–464

Hilleard R, Gjerde C, Parker L 1986 Validity of two psychological screening measures in family practice: personal inventory and family APGAR. Journal of Family Practice 23(4): 345–349

Huygen F J A 1978 Family medicine. The medical history of families. Dekker and Van de Vegt, The Netherlands

Huygen F J A 1988 Longitudinal studies of family units. Journal of the Royal College of General Practice 38: 168–170

Jennings A J, Sheldon M G 1985 Review of the health of children in one parent families. Journal of the Royal College of General Practitioners 35: 478–483

Johnston I D A, Hill M, Anderson H R, Lambert H P 1985 Impact of whooping cough on patients and their families. British Medical Journal 290: 1636–1638

Kolvin I, Macmillan A, Nicol A R, Wrate R M 1988 Psychotherapy is effective. Journal of the Royal Society of Medicine 81: 261–266

Kumar R, Robson K 1978 Previous induced abortion and ante-natal depression in primiparae: preliminary report of a survey of mental health in pregnancy. Psychological Medicine 8: 711–715

Lanier D C 1984 Family alcoholism. Journal of Family Practice 18(3): 417–422

Lawrence D H 1915 The rainbow. Heinemann, London

Lieberman S 1979 Transgenerational analysis: the genogram as a technique in family therapy. Journal of Family Therapy 1: 51–64

*Like R C, Rogers J, McGoldrick M 1988 Reading and interpreting genograms: a systematic approach. Journal of Family Practice 26(4): 407–412

Marinker M 1976 The family in medicine. Royal Society of Medicine 69: 115–124

Markus A C, Murray-Parkes C, Tomson P, Johnston M 1989 Psychological problems in general practice. Oxford University Press, Oxford

*McGoldrick M, Gerson R 1985 Genograms in family assessment. Norton, New York

Medalie J 1976 Angina pectoris among 10,000 men. Psychosocial and other risk factors. The American Journal of Medicine 60: 910–921

Medalie J H 1979 The family life cycle and its implications for family practice. Journal of Family Practice 9(1): 47–56

Mengel M 1987 The Use of the family APGAR in screening for family dysfunction in a family practice centre. Journal of Family Practice 24(4): 394–398

Milne D, Souter K 1988 A re-evaluation of the clinical psychologist in general practice. Journal of the Royal College of General Practitioners 38: 457–460

Minuchin S 1974 Families and family therapy. Harvard University Press, Massachusetts

Murray M, Sydenham D, Westlake R 1974 A questionnaire as a data base in problem orientated records. Journal of the Royal College of General Practitioners 24: 572–575

Olsen D H, Bell R, Portner J 1978 FACES St Paul department of family and social science. Privately published

Orford J 1987 Coping with disorder in the family. Croom Helm, London

Playfair H R, Gowers J I 1981 Depression following childbirth - a search for predictive signs. Journal of the Royal College of General Practitioners 31: 201–206

Prince-Embury S 1984 The family health tree: a form for identifying physical symptom patterns within the family. Journal of Family Practice 18(1): 75–81

Rahe R H, Holmes T H 1967 Life change patterns surrounding illness experience. Journal of Psychosomatic Research 11: 341

Ramsay C N, Abell T D, Baker L C 1986 The relationship between family functioning, life events, family structure and the outcome of pregnancy. Journal of Family Practice 225: 521–527

Ransom D C, Vandervoort H E 1973 The development of family medicine: problem trends. Journal of the American Medical Association 225: 1098

Rogers J C, Cohn P 1987 Impact of a screening genogram on

first encounters in primary care. Family Practice 4(4): 291–301

Rogers J, Durkin M 1984 The semi-structured genogram interview I Protocol II Evaluation. Family Systems Medicine 2: 176–187

Romans-Clarkson S E, Clarkson J E, Dittmer I D et al 1986 Impact of a handicapped child on mental health of parents. British Medical Journal 293: 1395–1396

Rowland N, Irving J, Maynard A 1989 Can general practitioners counsel? Journal of the Royal College of General Practitioners 39: 118–120

Rutter M, 1972 Maternal reassessed. Penguin, Middlesex

Shapiro J, Neinstein L S, Barinovitz S 1987 The family APGAR: use of a simple family function screening test with adolescents. Family System Medicine 5(2): 220–227

Smilkstein G 1975 The family in trouble — how to tell. Journal of Family Practice 2(1): 19–24

Smilkstein 1978 The family APGAR. A proposal for a family function test and its use by physicians. Journal of Family Practice 6: 1231–1235

Stein A, Fairburn C G 1989 Children of mothers with bulimia nervosa. British Medical Journal 299: 777–778

Tarrier N 1989 Effect of treating the family to reduce relapse rate in schizophrenia: a review. Journal of the Royal Society of Medicine 82: 423–424

Textor M R 1989 The 'healthy' family. Journal of Family Therapy 11(1): 59–75

Tomson P R V 1989 General practitioners and family therapy-a dialogue. Journal of Family Therapy 11:

*Tomson P, Ineson N, Milton J 1986 Feasibility and usefulness of family record cards in general practice. Journal of the Royal College of General Practitioners 36: 506–509

Trepka C, Griffiths T 1987 Evaluation of psychological treatment in primary care. Journal of the Royal College of General Practitioners 17: 215–217

*Van Eijk J T 1985 Serious illness and family dynamics. 1. Changes in consulting patterns of the unafflicted family members. Family Practice 2: 61–69

Van Eijk J, Smits A, Huygen F, Van Den Hoogen H 1988 Effect of bereavement on the health of the remaining family members. Family Practice 5(4): 278–282

Widmer R B, Cadoret R J, North C S 1980 Depression in family practice: some hidden effects on spouses and children. Journal of Family Practice 10(1): 45–51

Williams P R 1989 Family problems. Oxford University Press, Oxford

Wirsching M, Stierlin H 1985 Psychosomatics 1. Psychosocial characteristics of psychosomatic patients and their families. Family Systems Medicine 3(1): 7–15

38. Occupational hazards and risks

A Ward Gardner

INTRODUCTION

This chapter outlines in principle some of the methods of screening that can be used in general practice to help to identify and assess occupational diseases/injuries/conditions. Examples are given of how some problems can be tackled. Sources of help are mentioned both in the text and in the references.

Screening for occupational risk factors is no different in principle from screening for other conditions: there must be a significant benefit; there should be little or no risk in the procedures; the cost–benefit ratio needs to be favourable and the results of screening should contribute to overall management by supplying useful information. It should not merely contribute to data overload (see Chapter 6). When considering whether screening is or may be appropriate to the condition presenting, the question of the occupational relationship of the condition may or may not cross the mind of either the doctor or the patient.

HOW TO DECIDE ON THE RELATIONSHIP BETWEEN OCCUPATION AND PRESENTING SYMPTOMS/DISEASE

The first and most important step in addition to normal clinical procedures is to take a *full* occupational history. This should begin with present work and should go back to the commencement of work. It is not

Table 38.1 Hazard exposure and risk

	Effect
Hazard	Intrinsic potential to cause injury/disease
Exposure	Circumstances of contact of person with hazard
Risk	Chance of injury/disease occuring
	Hazard x Exposure = Risk

Table 38.2 Risk at work

Risk factor	Effect
Work	Injure or cause disease
environment	Damage the physical and/or psychological health of the workperson
	Prejudice the safety of the workperson

sufficient to ask merely for job titles: an understanding of what the person actually does is essential. All substances contacted and handled *may* contribute to the aetiology. Are other people doing the same job(s) ill/affected? What is the emotional climate at work?

General practitioners may find themselves in difficulty in not knowing what conditions are like in the workplace(s) and may know little of the nature/toxicology/hazards and risks of any substance mentioned or of the hazards and risks of any particular type of work (Tables 38.1 and 38.2).

Without such knowledge of the workplace and its hazards, the practitioner will be reduced to guessing and speculation. How should this problem be tackled? Help is, fortunately, easily available and should always be sought.

Sources of help

The Health and Safety Executive (HSE) (or its equivalent in other countries) is very experienced in the assessment of workplace hazards and risks. The office addresses and telephone numbers are listed in the telephone book — so HSE can be contacted easily. Part of HSE is the Employment Medical Advisory Service (EMAS). This group of experts includes specialist occupational physicians, occupational health nurses and occupational (industrial) hygienists, who assess and measure workplace contaminants and are experts at quantifying workplace hazards and risks. It follows that in any case of doubt about occupational aetiology or problems, a vast resource is available via HSE and EMAS. In most cases the best first line of contact is with the EMAS occupational physician of HSE in your area or with a consulting occupational physician.

HSE has computerised databases about workplace hazards, toxicology, substance lists and so on. They are also able to call on a wide range of specialist skills in among other things, laboratory testing, epidemiology, toxicology, dermatology and chest disease. Should these skills and resources be needed, they are all freely available. Where difficulties may arise for doctor and patient alike is when this team help from HSE or from an occupational physician is not used. Unless the general practitioner thinks/suspects that an occupational aetiology may be of importance, and unless they take the necessary steps to find out about the occupational history and the workplace, little of use may be accomplished and, sadly, diagnosis of occupational problems will be missed. Occupational disease is believed to be underreported and underdiagnosed in the community.

The sentinel health event

A sentinel health event (SHE) is a preventable disease, disability or untimely death whose occurrence serves as a warning signal that the quality of preventive and/or therapeutic medical care may need to be improved (Rutstein et al 1984). We are all aware that in the management of pulmonary tuberculosis there are problems beyond the individual patient, e. g. there are others involved in transmitting and catching the infection. Measures may have to be taken to prevent spread and other possible cases must be identified. So *groups* of

people are involved. The presenting case is an example of a sentinel health event: further action is required in relation to other people and for preventive purposes. The alarm must be sounded: further action is necessary.

In relation to a new presentation of occupational disease, or suspected occupational disease, the wider implications encapsulated in the notion of the sentinel health event must be acted on. Others may be involved and may need help (Table 38.3).

CASE-FINDING AND SCREENING

In the section above, the discussion was mainly centred on *case-finding*, i.e. on the identification and detection of individual occupationally-related disease by means of medical procedures related to an *individual*, who is usually in a patient–relationship with the physician. *Screening* (see Chapter 2), on the other hand, looks at *groups* of people (a population, often a targeted one, but usually an unselected population) and, by various procedures, attempts to select out of this population individuals who are at greater risk than the rest.

This selection procedures may be very simple, e. g. selection into two groups — at risk, not at risk. The risks may be mortality, morbidity, overexposure or potentially higher risk people. Within the risks selected, the degree of risk can also be further categorised — as high, medium and low. The possibilities are therefore many and various.

Why screen at all?

In the first section of this chapter, and in Chapter 2, some of the broad principles of screening have been discussed. It is important to remember such principles so that any screening done can be defended as effective, efficient, ethically sound and safe. In addition to these general points, three useful questions of a management nature are usually worth asking:

1. Why do it at all?
2. Why do it now?
3. Why do it in this way?

When the answers to these questions are sought, systematically and honestly, much of interest will often emerge and subsequent decisions and choices can then be made on a basis of greater factual information than by rushing the fences or reacting to pressure. Many existing screening procedures, e.g. routine periodical medicals of fit people — often 'executives' — are still of unproven effectiveness and it still remains to be shown that mortality and morbidity among screened people

Table 38.3 Sentinel health events. Examples of occupationally related unnecessary diseases, disabilities and untimely deaths

Personnel	Condition
Medical/nursing/ dental/laboratory	Pulmonary tuberculosis
	Tetanus
	Hepatitis B
	Ionising radiation induced anaemia, skin cancer
	Cataract(s) (microwaves, ionising radiation)
	Sniffing anaesthetic gases
	Occupational asthma (instrument sterilising agents: formaldehyde, glutaraldehyde)
	Toxic neuropathy (inorganic mercury)

differ from those among people of similar age, sex, habits and so on doing similar work and living in the same community.

Finding cases of a medical condition does not per se lead to a benefit in a screened compared with a non-screened group (D'Souza 1979, Morgan 1979).

What procedures can be used in screening and case-finding in relation to occupational disease/hazards/exposures/suspected problems?

The general answer is that the list of possibilities is wide. Procedures range from questionnaires through clinical surveys to tests of all kinds and to epidemiological surveys.

The sensitivity and specificity and the margins of expected error in any tests and procedures must also be carefully noted. Without an understanding of this information the value of any procedure cannot be assessed properly.

The Office of Population Censuses and Surveys (OPCS) publish *Decennial supplements of occupational mortality* as part of the regular population census programmes, e.g. 1961, 1971, 1981. The occupational mortality figures can indicate high levels of mortality in certain occupations. Should screening be of benefit in the prevention of these conditions, a national basis for screening may be established. Simply knowing that a person of a certain occupation may be at special risk from this or that condition may also be useful information — to raise the index of suspicion about these diseases in persons of that occupation or to take further steps such as screening/surveillance to clarify what is going on.

Occupational morbidity

Good information in this field is less readily obtainable now on a national basis with the demise of medical certification of illnesses of short to medium duration. Local 'sickness' records can of course help.

Much 'sickness absence' — often called 'absenteeism' by those who attend work more regularly — is, of course, more properly called absence from work attributed to incapacity. Many short-term absences are not *due* to incapacity. The remedies for most short-term absences lie with managers and not doctors.

Screening people who have frequent short-term absences will usually reveal no significant medical condition. This, however, can help to strengthen the hand of any management trying to deal effectively with such problems. The best screen for future absence prediction is past absences.

Occupational asthma as an example of the need for screening

The prevalence of asthma is believed to be about 2% in the population of developed countries and that of occupational asthma is thought to be about 0.2%. Some causes of occupational asthma (the list is incomplete) are:

1. diisocyanates;
2. platinum salts;
3. formaldehyde;
4. acid anhydride and amine-hardening agents in epoxy resin mixes;
5. fumes from rosin and colophony used as a soldering flux;
6. proteolytic enzymes (*Bacillus subtilis*);
7. dusts from barley, oats, rye and wheat; and meal or flour made from such grain;
8. animal dander (cats, horses);
9. animal urine;
10. grain mites and weevils.

Apart from taking a history, is there any way in which the presenting asthma can be shown to be occu-

Observation Time	0200	0400	0600	0800	1000	1200	1400	1600	1800	2000	2200	2400
PEFR Record												
At work (Y or N)*												
Symptoms (Y or N)**												
Notes	* If at work but off your normal job put Y and then NE (not exposed) ** put down Y for cough, wheeze or chest tightness only. N for anything else.											

Fig. 38.1 Sample simultaneous daily record for PEFR, exposure and symptoms.

pational or non-occupational in origin? Fortunately there is — the method used is the 2-hourly recording of the peak expiratory flow rate (PEFR) in waking hours and the simultaneous recording of symptoms and location (Slovak 1987) (Fig. 38.1).

PEFRs in asthma of occupational origin will fall in relation to working times, although a lag period may occur. There is often a fall over the Monday–Friday period in those on day work. Significant rises in PEFRs occur during extended holidays and slighter rises at weekends. Non-occupational asthma will not show these work-related variations. A recording period of 4 weeks is usually sufficient to demonstrate or refute work-relatedness.

Occupational skin diseases

Occupational skin diseases are probably the most common occupationally-related conditions that will present to the general practitioner. Rycroft (1979) specified the need for diagnostic accuracy and posed three key questions:

1. Is it eczema (dermatitis) or not?
2. If eczematous (dermatitis) is it primarily caused by external factors in contact with the skin or not?
3. If contact eczema (contact dermatitis), is the contact factor a skin allergen (sensitizer) or a skin irritant or are factors of both types, or additional factors of sunlight, involved?

Allergic and irritant contact dermatitis are clinically alike: a careful personal and occupational history, a visit to the workplace and a careful examination may clarify the first two questions but the third can be answered definitively only by careful patch testing. This is best left to the specialist in the dermatological clinic both because of the possible risks and also on account of the difficulties of method and interpretation. So much for case-finding.

Is pre-employment screening of value in preventing occupational dermatoses? The short answer is not much. Any person who has obvious eczema or other skin disease that breaks the skin surface is at greater risk from irritants because the skin surface is already damaged. However, in the matter of skin allergies one allergy does not seem to predict another and a history of atopy does not appear to carry with it an increased risk of occupational allergic eczema. However, where diagnostic difficulties arise is in distinguishing one form of skin allergy from another. The medicolegal importance of this makes many employers who have potentially high levels of skin hazards and risks shy away from employing people with existing skin disorders and with any allergic history, including atopy.

A normal skin on the hands and forearms is a requirement in food handling to prevent the transmission of organisms that may inhabit dead skin or cracked and fissured areas. People with extensive psoriasis are often rejected for jobs that do not even require them to handle food but involve working in the area of wrapped foods, because of irrational fears that the condition is infectious or may result in food-borne disease. Accurate diagnosis and screening alone are not always the answer.

Occupational cancers and screening

Table 38.4 shows the established occupational risks of cancer.

There are many other suspected occupational cancer risks. Estimates of the prevalence of occupational cancer in the population of developed countries are usually in the region of 4–8% — so occupational cancers are not a large part of the total. Case-finding will be by the usual clinical method. The most useful screening methods are epidemiological (Coggon 1987) and are: analysis of occupational mortality and morbidity; analysis of cancer registrations by occupation studies involving detailed occupational data such as lifetime job histories and case-control studies, which compare occupations in people having specific cancers with controls; analysis by inferred occupational exposures and geographical analyses of mortality.

General practitioners are in a good position to develop 'hunches' in these matters if they see what are thought to be unusual cases (say an angiosarcoma of the liver, which may be related to vinyl chloride exposure at work) or a number of cases of a particular cancer (say nasal sinus cancer, which may be related to hardwood dust exposure at work). A 'hunch' may be a perfectly respectable hypothesis-generating mechanism. What needs to follow is a careful investigation by suitable methods to test the validity of the hypothesis. Here the non-epidemiologist should at once seek the help of colleagues who are expert in this specialty. In the example of nasal cancers, local hospital records of further cases of nasal cancers may be found with or without occupation being recorded in detail in the ENT department. Epidemiological investigations may then be commenced to sort out work-relatedness in people presumed at risk in similar jobs or with the same condition. Case/control studies would probably be the first method used to test hypotheses but longer-term prospective studies may also be needed.

No single method of screening/study is appropriate or ideally suited to all occupational cancers. The

Table 38.4 Established occupational risks of cancer

Agent or process	Site of tumour
Combustion products of coal, shale oil, polycyclic hydrocarbons (chimney sweeps, makers of coal gas, cotton mule spinners)	*Scrotum and other parts of skin, bronchus
Ultraviolet light (farmers, fishermen)	Skin
2-naphthylamine, benzidine (dye manufacturers, rubber workers, makers of coal gas)	Bladder
Mustard gas (makers of mustard gas)	Bronchus, larynx, nasal sinuses
4-amino-diphenyl (chemical workers)	Bladder
Vinyl chloride (manufacture of PVC)	Liver (angiosarcoma)
Arsenic (sheep dip manufacturers, copper smelters)	Bronchus, skin
Asbestos (asbestos workers, insulation workers, gas mask manufacturers)	Bronchus, pleura, peritoneum
Benzene (workers with glues, varnishes etc.)	Leukaemia
Ionizing radiation (haematite miners, fluorspar miners, luminizers, radiologists)	*Bronchus, skin, bone
Bischloromethyl ether (makers of ion exchange resins)	Bronchus
Chromate manufacture	Bronchus
Nickel refining	Bronchus, nasal sinuses
Furniture manufacture	Nasal sinuses
Manufacturer of isopropyl alcohol by strong acid process	Nasal sinuses
Boot and shoe manufacture	Nasal sinuses

* The site of the tumour depends upon the nature of the exposure. The occupations listed do not necessarily carry risks for all of these sites

method(s) selected must be finely and expertly tuned to the available information to give the best results.

New problems are often difficult to identify: here is a situation where the alert physician can contribute to finding new occupational causes for disease, including cancer.

A final word about the value of cancer prevention may be appropriate because cancers are seen as great killers: 'If all cancer was eliminated (in England and Wales) it would add less than three years to the average life expectancy of men and just over two and a half years to the life expectancy of women'. (Winter 1977).

What also matters, as the quotation shows, is the loss of years of survivable life. Deaths from injury in children and young adults result in much greater losses of life expectancy than cancer. The perceived importance of childhood injuries is, however, of a greatly reduced order by comparison. We should therefore look more closely at *loss of expectancy* coupled with *preventability* as measures of the importance that we should attach to any particular condition and as indicators of the amount of effort that should be put into its prevention.

MONITORING THE ENVIRONMENT

This method of screening is of great importance in relation to occupational exposures. Much is known about the levels of substances in air, water, food and so on which can be very unsafe/disease-producing, borderline, probably not disease-producing and unlikely to cause harm.

General practitioners are not normally trained in the use of these methods or in the interpretation of the numbers that are produced as a result of measuring. It is, however. very important to realise than working environments can be measured and assessed and to request, via HSE and EMAS or the employer, that this be done or, if it has been done, to know what the numbers are thought to mean.

We should also remember that environments can change and may have done so since measurements were made.

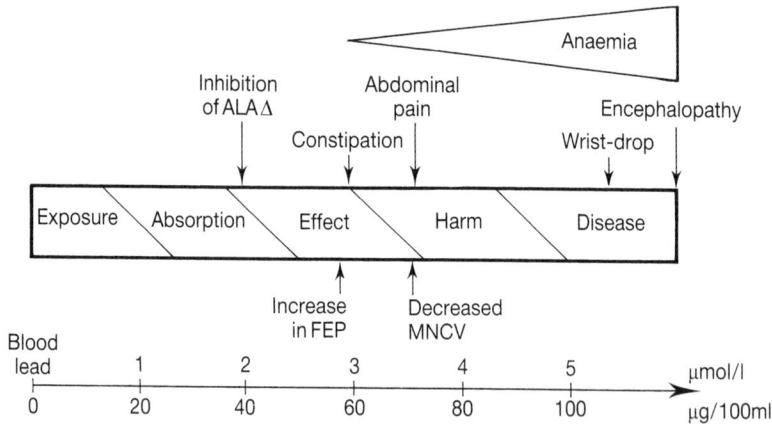

Fig. 38.2 Schematic representation of the relationship between the concentration of lead in blood and the onset of biochemical and clinical effects. The relationship between the concentration of lead in blood and the onset of biochemical and clinical effects (by kind permission of Dr David Gompertz.).

MONITORING THE INDIVIDUAL

The worst way of discovering occupational disease is to see a case of occupational disease or injury. It is also, usually, ethically less bothersome and more useful to measure environments — if this can be done in a meaningful way — than to attack the sufferer with a variety of medical tests, although both may be necessary. It should also be remembered that the risk from any toxic material in the working environment is related more directly to *uptake* than to environmental concentration (Gompertz 1980, 1981). Uptake is variable, for example:

1. Uptake of solvents will be greater in fat people than in thin ones.
2. Increased respiratory rates, e.g. from physical hard work, will increase the uptake of airborne toxins.
3. Patterns of uptake will vary with individuals. In any individual, uptake may vary with time of day, work practices, fitness, use of drugs/alcohol and so on.

The monitoring of an individual gives useful information about that person and his/her personal variability of uptake. In surveying individuals, we should also wonder about group levels of toxins in people doing similar work and remember the concept of the sentinel health event. What measures of uptake can be used?

1. Toxic material in body fluids such as blood, urine and breath.
2. Metabolites of toxic material in blood and urine.
3. Biochemical measurement of effect, e. g. inhibited enzymes and accumulated metabolites of inhibited pathways.

4. Indicators of early and reversible tissue damage, such as leakage of enzymes into blood or urine
5. Physiological changes such as motor nerve conduction velocity, tremor and behavioural effects.
6. Immunological changes, e.g. the induction of specific antibodies.
7. 'Genotoxic' indicators such as the Ames test.

An example of the relationship between the concentration of lead in blood and the onset of biochemical and clinical effects is given in Figure 38.2.

HSE publish guidance on environmental hygiene (EH series) and on medical matters (MS — medical series). Many of the MS notes relate to surveillance, e.g. MS8 is *Isocyanates: medical surveillance* and MS12 is *Mercury: Medical surveillance*. A catalogue of all HSE publications in the series is available from HSE Library and Information Services, Broad Lane, Sheffield S3 7HQ, Tel (0742) 752539.

CONCLUSION

In an occupational health context, there is considerable scope for screening and surveillance — both of the environment and of people. The screening must, however, be based on a proper appreciation of the hazards and the risks, and on a careful occupational and environmental history. Tests must always be aimed sharply at the problem(s). There is, in my view, no place for unspecific guessing, for hit-and-miss interventions or for other such blunt approaches. General practitioners who wish to become more familiar with occupational health problems could benefit from further training and from workplace visits in the company of a person who is familiar with workplace assessment.

Training in occupational health should, in my view, be included in vocational training schemes. Special introductory courses to occupational health are available for physicians and nurses at many centres throughout the UK. A list of these courses, which give a certificate of attendance, is available from the Faculty of Occupational Medicine, 6 St Andrew's Place, London NW1 4LB. These introductory courses usually last between 6 and 10 days. Applications should be made to the chosen postgraduate centre or department.

Workplace visits are especially valuable to help physicians to understand the work of their patients. Visits to local industries are especially valuable.

Workplace assessment is a skill which, like clinical assessment, can be learned best by doing or by following in the steps of people who have established competence in these matters.

When managing occupational health problems — whether involving screening and surveillance or other aspects of occupational health or disease — I would always recommend the approach that should be applied to any problem in medical practice: if you do not know how to handle it, refer the case or the problem to a colleague who is a specialist in that field. This should lead to better outcomes and solutions.

REFERENCES

Bailey A 1977 Health screening. Society of Occupational Medicine, London

Coggon D 1987 In: Ward Gardner A (ed) Monitoring for new occupational risks of cancer. Current approaches to occupational health, 2nd edn. Wright, Bristol, pp 27–42

D'Souza M 1979 Screening for all: excellence or extravagance. In: Ward Gardner A (ed) Current approaches to occupational medicine. Wright, Bristol pp 339–358

Gompertz D 1980 Solvents — the relationship between biological monitoring and metabolic handling — a review. Annals of Occupational Hygiene 23: 405–410

Gompertz D 1981 Assessment of risk by biological monitoring. British Medical Journal 38: 198–201

Kusnetz Z, Hutchison M K 1979 (eds) A guide to the work-relatedness of disease. Centres for Disease Control, National Institute of Occupational Safety and Health, Cincinnati, Ohio

Morgan P P 1979 The periodic health examination. Canadian Medical Journal 121: 1161–1162

OPCS Decennial supplements on occupational mortality (various years). HMSO, London

Rutstein D D, Mullan R J, Frazier T M, Halperin W E, Meruis J M, Sestito J P 1984 Sentinel health events (occupational): a basis for physician recognition and public health surveillance. Archives of Environmental Health 39: 159–168

Rycroft R J G 1979 Occupational serinatoses In: Ward Gardner A (ed) Current approaches to occupational medicine. Wright, Bristol, pp 124–136

Slovak A J M 1987 Occupational asthma In: Ward Gardner A (ed) Current approaches to occupational health, 3rd edn. Wright, Bristol, pp 14–26

Winter W M L 1977 In: Population trends. HMSO, London

FURTHER READING

Edwards F C, McCallum R I, Taylor P J 1988 Fitness for work. Oxford Medical Publications, Oxford

Gardner A W, Taylor P J 1975 Health at work. ABP, London

Harrington J M, Gill F S 1987 Occupational health. Blackwell Scientific Publications, Oxford

Health screening 1977 Society of Occupational Medicine, London

Lalonde M 1975 A new perspective on the health of Canadians. Information Canada, Ottowa

McGinty L 1979 The British way of death. New Scientist, 30 August Vol 83: 649–651

To measure or to take direct remedial action 1988 Swedish Work Environment Fund, Stockholm

Waldron H A (ed) 1989 Occupational health practice. Butterworths, London

World Health Organization 1985 Identification and control of work-related diseases. WHO, Geneva

World Health Organization 1986 Occupational Health as a component of primary health care. WHO Regional Office, Copenhagen

REFERENCE BOOKS

Parmegianni L (ed) ILO encyclopaedia of occupational health and safety, 3rd edn. ILO, Geneva

Clayton and Clayton (eds) Patty's industrial hygiene and toxicology, 3rd edn. Wiley, New York

39. Special problems of ethnic minorities

Bashir Qureshi

INTRODUCTION

General practice is as much the art of dealing with the realities of life as politics is the science of the possible. Fundamental changes in society, occuring in other countries by revolution, happen in the UK by evolution. A doctor who is willing to modify his or her attitudes and actions with time ensures a fair deal for himself or herself, the patient and society. Ethnic minorities are now an established part of the British nation. Ethnic minority patients — white and non-white — are British citizens but there is a world of difference in their needs when compared with the needs of the ethnic majority population. In the 1990s and thereafter, almost every GP is likely to see substantial, if varying, numbers of patients from ethnic minority groups.

Prevention is not only better but in the long run is cheaper than cure. Screening for conditions with sufficiently high prevalence that are easily detectable in their early stages by comparatively simple tests will become the hallmark of British general practice. Screening is also desired by 'The 1990 Contract' for general practice in the National Health Service, which the Government introduced on 1 April 1990. According to this contract, at the GP's discretion, information can be included in the local directories produced by the Family Health Services Authorities (Health Boards in Scotland) and in the GP's practice leaflets, showing whether a link-worker is available, what languages are spoken, and any particular clinical interests of the doctor such as screening and surveillance of ethnic minorities.

Traditionally, medical textbooks written by European authors describe a 'white European patient' model. Although applicable to white ethnic minorities to some extent, such books are not entirely appropriate for screening non-white ethnic minorities because of their different cultural customs, religious beliefs and ethnic origins. This chapter, based on my 25-year orig-

inal research, is aimed at bridging the gap, but it should be read in addition to, and not instead of, other chapters. Moreover, due to lack of space, the description of only common problems in many ethnic groups will be attempted. Readers should consult standard textbooks for details of diseases and diagnostic tests. Nevertheless, three questions will be specifically addressed:

1. What difficulties may arise when applying medical textbook knowledge to ethnic minorities screening, and how can these be tackled?
2. What specific conditions should be screened for in various ethnic groups and how should surveillance be carried out with available resources?
3. What plans to tackle such special problems can be devised for a practice team — where to begin, how far to go and where to stop — in ethnic minority screening and surveillance?

BRITISH ETHNIC MINORITIES

The ethnic majority in Britian comprises three groups — English, Scots and Welsh — as advised by the Commission for Racial Equality. All the rest are ethnic minorities, including the Irish and the Jews (Table 39.1). Broadly speaking, in Britain today there are citizens belonging to two cultures, six religions and four ethnicities (Table 39.2).

According to the results of the 1981 census, and assuming that there has been no significant change by immigration or emigration, there are 2.2 million people of the New Commonwealth, including Pakistan (which rejoined the Commonwealth in 1989), in the UK. Of these, 40% were born in the UK. Of the 2.2 million, 55% (1.2 million) are of Asian origin — 47% (1 million) from the Indian subcontinent and 8% (0.2 million) from East Africa — this includes 80 000 whites born in those countries; about 25% (0.55 million) are of African and Caribbean origin; approxi-

Table 39.1 British ethnic classification (from Qureshi 1989a)

Majority

    English, Scots and Welsh

Minorities

    1. Whites: Irish, Jews, Italians, Hungarians, Germans, Spaniards, Poles, White Americans, White South Africans, Australians, New Zealanders and other Europeans or Caucasians

    2. Non-white:

        a Asians or South Asians: Indians, Pakistanis, Bangladeshis, Sri Lankans and East African Asians

        b Middle Easterners: Cypriots, Greeks, Turks, Arabs, Israelis and Iranians

        c Blacks: Africans, Caribbeans and Black Americans

        d South East Asians: Chinese, Vietnamese, Indonesians, Malaysians, Filipinos and Japanese

mately 5% (0.1 million) are Hong Kong Chinese or other South-East Asians; about 2.5% (0.05 million) are Cypriots of Greek and Turkish origins; and 12.5% (0.25 million) are from other countries in the New Commonwealth (Qureshi 1989b).

The Commission for Racial Equality estimates that nearly 3.4 million people in the UK were born overseas. Out of these, 1.89 million are whites — 607 000 were born in the Republic of Ireland†; 153 000 in the Old Commonwealth (Australia, New Zealand and Canada); 1.13 million in other European countries, including Italy, Poland, Hungary, Germany, Spain and Portugal; and 1.41 million are non-whites born in the New Commonwealth and other Asian, African or South American countries.

The population of the UK has remained unchanged at around 56.5 million for the past 10 years and is expected to remain static for the next 10 years. The UK has lost more people through emigration that it has gained through immigration. Net migration figures from the Office of Population, Census and Surveys in 1982 showed that the UK gained 12 000 people in 1951–1961, lost 320 000 in 1961–1971 and again lost 306 000 in 1971–81. In the face of labour shortage, during the postwar era of economic expansion, immigration into the UK took place from 1953 to 1962 (when immigration controls were introduced) from the Republic of Ireland, West Indies and the Indian subcontinent. The 1971 Immigration Act has stringently controlled immigration and the stage of settlement has since been in progress.

To give effective medical advice to an individual, including screening and surveillance, requires an understanding of the patient's cultural habits, religious beliefs and ethnic characteristics. The difficulty that arises is that no two practices are the same. Some may have a high propotion of Pakistanis, others a high proportion of West Indians, and so on. Each practice will therefore have to decide on its own screening programme, according to the particular mixture of ethnic minorities and the resources available. Although this chapter is aimed at dealing with all ethnic groups, four major ethnic minorities require particular mention because of the complex nature of the problems they present: (i) Asians; (ii) Africans and West Indians; (iii) Chinese and South-East Asians; (iv) Cypriots.

Table 39.2 The British nation today (from Qureshi 1989a)

Cultures
    Western, Eastern, Westernised Eastern*

Religions
    Hinduism, Buddhism, Sikhism, Judaism, Christianity, Islam

Ethnicities
    Europeans (Caucasians), Asians (Asiatic), Africans (Negroids), Chinese (Mongoloids)

* A sizeable minority of British citizens are Westernised Easterners, e.g. Kenyan Asians and Caribbeans

Asians

'Asians' is the term used by the indigenous British population (for census purposes among other things) for immigrants from India, Pakistan, Bangladesh and Sri Lanka; this also includes their children and dependants. The English language, as with general pratice, is a living thing and is always changing. New

---

†Immigrants from the Republic of Ireland number 607 000, but it should be borne in mind that a large proportion of the 1.5 million people in Northern Ireland would regard themselves as being ethnically Irish.

Table 39.3   Qureshi's chart of Asian regional differences (from Qureshi 1989a)

Origin	Colour	Height	Weight	Food	Religion	Language
Pakistan						
Punjabis	Fair	Tall	Medium	Meat curry and chapati	Muslim	Urdu or Punjabi
Pathans	White	Tall and well built	Large	Tandoori meat and nan	Muslim	Pushtu or Persian
India						
Punjabis	Fair	Tall	Medium	Meat curry and chapati	Sikh or Hindu	Punjabi or Hindi
Gujaratis	Fair	Short	Light	Vegetarian or vegan	Hindu	Gujarati
Bengalis	Dark	Short	Light	Fish and rice	Hindu	Bengali
South Indians	Dark	Short	Light	Fish and Rice	Hindu or Christian	Tamil or Malyalam
Bangladesh						
Bangladeshis	Dark	Short	Light	Fish and rice	Muslim	Bengali
Sri Lanka						
Sri Lankans	Dark	Short	Light	Fish and rice	Buddhist or Hindu	Sinhalese or Tamil
Kenyan or Ugandan Asians						
Punjabis	Fair	Tall	Medium	Meat and wheat	Hindu or Muslim	Punjabi or Hindi/Urdu
Gujaratis	Fair	Short	Light	Vegetarian or vegan	Hindu	Gujarati

terms for this minority group are 'British Asians' or 'South Asians'. People in this ethnic group come from Eastern cultures, practice one of five main religions (Table 39.3) — Hinduism, Islam, Sikhism, Buddhism and Christianity — and are largely of Asiatic race. It should be remembered that, as in other ethnic groups, there are many subcultures, religious sects within each religion, and some people from other races among Asians. The first Asian language (Urdu/Hindi) radio in Europe began its broadcast from West London on 5 November 1989.

Africans and Caribbeans

Black people in Britian come mainly from the West Indies and Africa, and proudly believe that Black is Beautiful. They do not want to be called 'Afro-Caribbeans' and prefer separate terms such as 'West Indians' or 'Africans'. Whereas Africans have Eastern culture (reflected in their names, languages and music), Caribbeans have Western culture for historic reasons. West Indians have English or Scottish names and their mother tongue is English but their music is unique. Africans are either Christians — Catholics or Protestants — or Muslims and occasionally Jews, but West Indians are predominantly Christians — Catho-

lics, Protestants or Jehovah's Witnesses. The ethnicity of black people is described as 'Negroid' or 'Ethiopian'. It should be remembered that all classifications have to be flexible and other races, such as Caucasians or Asiatics, are also found among Caribbeans. Three-quarters of British black people are from Jamaica.

Chinese and South-East Asians

The Chinese in Britain have migrated from Hong Kong, mainland China, Taiwan island (Formosa), and other South-East Asian countries. Not only are there many kinds of Chinese food but also there are various dialects of the Chinese language. The Chinese have Eastern cultures based on centuries-old civilisation. The majority religion is Buddhism (which originated from Hinduism) but Christianity, especially Catholicism, is a close runner-up. Ethnicity is 'Mongoloid', which is a respectable term in China. Down syndrome should not be called 'mongolism' in today's multi-ethnic age. The Chinese should never be called 'slitty eyed' or 'yellow' but should be described as 'light-skinned'.

South-East Asians mainly come from Malaysia, the Philippines or Vietnam. They are Easterners by culture and have Buddhist, Christian, Muslim or Hindu religions. Ethnic origins may include Chinese (Mongoloid) or Asiatic (local or Indian).

Cypriots

Cypriots migrated from the Island of Cyprus in the Mediterranean, which is divided between the Greek Republic of Southern Cyprus and the Turkish Republic of Northern Cyprus.

Greek Cypriots have Western culture, their main religion is Greek Orthodox and ethnically they are Europeans. Turkish Cypriots also have Western culture but are Sunni Muslims; they too are Europeans by race. Notwithstanding differences in religion and political history, Greek and Turkish Cypriots have much in common. Recently, a commercial radio station for this ethnic minority has acquired a licence to broadcast from Islington (North London) in Greek and Turkish languages. Medical and health professionals should use local ethnic minority radios to advertise their campaigns for screening and surveillance so that their message can reach those people that the English media cannot reach.

TRANSCULTURAL PROBLEMS IN SCREENING AND SURVEILLANCE

The science of medicine is the same the world over but the art of medicine, i.e. a doctor's quality of care, is different as it is influenced by the distance between the doctor's and the patient's cultural customs, religious beliefs and ethnic characteristics. Whereas medicine is science, and we must use the knowledge in the current textbooks, general practice is very much an art. We should make allowances for a patient's individual needs and wishes. The following ten examples are given to emphasise this point briefly.

Concept of screening

In the West people are familiar with preventive aspects of medicine but in the East the concept of screening and surveillance, although accepted in principle, is very weak in practice. This is for a number of reasons, including scarce financial resources. An English or anglicised patient is happy to go along with the doctor's suggestion of screening for certain diseases for an early diagnosis and treatment. However, an Asian, African, Chinese or Malay needs to be talked into the idea of prevention. Assuming that all patients are not the same — in their thinking, behaviour, and social education — a GP should understand that an ethnic

minority patient may be clinging to the Eastern concept of demand-led consultation, i.e. a patient sees a doctor only in the case of an acute illness and expects an instant cure at any price. If this is the case, it is wise to provide some health education. This can be given by a member of the practice team or a health visitor and, where necessary, a local health education officer should be approached. The message should be in a language that the patient can understand.

Appointment system

As with time-keeping, or committees, appointment systems are a British custom. A Caribbean patient, familiar with Western culture, may keep an appointment but an Asian, African or Chinese patient may not keep an appointment for a GP's preventive clinic or surgery session. A patient may not realise the importance of keeping the appointment, may inadvertently not telephone to cancel it or apologise afterwards, may make an appointment for one person but consult the doctor for all the family members accompanying them, may see the doctor for him/herself and then ask for a number of prescriptions or investigation forms for other relatives at home, or may turn up without an appointment, even towards the end of a Friday evening surgery, and demand to see the doctor. A GP should not get annoyed by this cultural phenomenon, but should take the opportunity to educate the patient.

Screening organisation

Three problems are likely to arise in record keeping: naming customs, birth certificates and family data.

Naming systems differ throughout the world and are mostly related to a patient's religion. For example, Asians have three different naming systems, used by three main religious groups: Hindus, Muslims and Sikhs. They are fairly easy to identify and learn and must be correctly slotted in our record cards to avoid delays and errors (Henley 1979). Similarly, information about the naming systems of all ethnic minorities in the practice should be sought. Local community or religious leaders can not only recommend appropriate books but are also in a position to offer practical help.

Ethnic minority patients born before 1947 were colonial subjects of the British Empire and may not have a birth certificate. The registration of births, marriages and deaths of colonial subjects was not considered necessary by the administrators. A matriculation examination certificate is accepted as a substitute for a birth certificate in India, Pakistan, Bangladesh or Sri Lanka, for those who went to school. Because school education was not compulsory in colonial times, most people, particularly those in rural areas, remained illiterate, even in their native language, and immigrants merely made a guess at their date of birth when obtaining a passport before migrating to Britain. The age of such a mature patient will have to be estimated for the purpose of screening age-related diseases. Asking to see a passport is a sensitive matter and a GP should be content with checking the date of birth on a patient's medical card.

An ethnic minority patient may volunteer information about their family or relatives but may get very worried if asked about family data by a health professional. Perhaps this is due to lack of trust in strangers. A GP should obtain such information only if necessary, and with tactful reassurance.

Opportunistic screening

An ethnic minority patient may not appreciate any opportunistic screening, such as the checking of blood pressure, urine testing, or measurement of height and weight (even with clothes on) on an occasion when he attends the GP for the treatment of a chest infection or athlete's foot, because of his unfamiliarity with the concept. A non-European patient may even be afraid of becoming anaemic when some blood is taken for testing. It is essential to explain these procedures and allay any fears before obtaining informed consent.

Genetic risks

Cousin marriage is an old tradition among Muslims, Hindus and Sikhs. To preserve their heritage, Hindus often marry within the caste and Muslims often marry within the tribe. First cousin marriages are not uncommon and distant cousin marriages are common. Jews also prefer to marry within their race and some couples are distant cousins. With the exception of Christians, patients from all religions, particularly those practising the arranged marriage system, have the possibility of consanguinity of varying degrees. It is essential to remember this fact when screening by prenatal testing for many diseases related to cousin marriages, e. g. sickle-cell trait, thalassaemia trait and Hurler's syndrome.

Paediatric surveillance

Measurement of height and weight are important in the examination of children. It should be remembered that British height and weight charts do not apply to people from short and lightweight ethnic groups such as Chinese, Malays, Indonesians, and also Bangladeshis, Sri Lankans, South Indians and Gujaratis. Their normal children may fall below the 3rd centile and may be on the 1st centile of the British charts.

Immunisation

Four vaccines — measles, mumps, influenza and yellow fever — are made in egg or chick medium. Vegetarians, particularly vegans, who read about vaccines may not accept these immunisations. The majority of Hindus are vegetarians and many Europeans have chosen to become vegetarians. In a practice with vegetarian patients this problem should be identified and a compromise reached so as to promote compliance.

Adult screening

Language barriers can be overcome with the help of an interpreter or a linkperson (language and culture interpreter). The attitude of ethnic minority patients towards accepting screening and surveillance for conditions such as ischaemic heart disease and obesity can be improved by holding classes on health education and social education about the British health system. Such sessions could be held in a surgery or a nearby church hall.

Elderly screening

Mental illness is considered taboo in Eastern cultures. Some patients may attribute it to sins committed in this or a past life, and consult a traditional healer or a religious counsellor. But when they come to see a GP it is likely that psychological symptoms are presented in somatic language, e.g. pain in the chest or abdomen. GPs should consider such cultural factors in screening their elderly ethnic minority patients.

Cervical cytology

Ethnic minority women, particularly Asians or Arabs, may present three difficulties for a GP. First, the genitalia are considered to be an absolute taboo zone in Eastern cultures and an Eastern women may feel that a vaginal examination, except during the delivery of a baby, is very stressful, even if it is done by a female doctor. Secondly, because sex segregation is advised by all religions except Christianity, internal examination by a male doctor may be unacceptable. Moreover, an Asian or Arab husband may have feelings of jealousy if a male doctor were to carry out a vaginal examination on his wife. And finally, virgins will not allow a vaginal examination because virginity is a condition of an arranged marriage in Eastern cultures. Some nuns are of African and Asian origins. Under such circumstances a GP should use his or her skills of tact, counselling and compromise in meeting the patient's choice or needs.

SPECIFIC CONDITIONS AMONG VARIOUS ETHNIC GROUPS

One can never say 'never' or 'always' in medicine because there is an exception to almost every rule. While any disease can occur in every ethnic group, there are certain conditions to which a GP should be alerted by the fact that the patient belongs to a particular ethnic group. Some conditions are almost always confined to a particular ethnic group, e.g. Tay–Sachs' disease among Jews, sickle-cell anaemia among Africans or Caribbeans and glucose-6PD deficiency and thalassaemia, among Cypriots. However, other conditions are not confined to, although they are more common in certain groups, e.g. tuberculosis in the Irish and Asians, rickets or osteomalacia among Nothern Indians and leprosy among South-East Asians. It should be remembered that screening techniques will vary for the same conditions according to the customs, degree of literacy and whether an ethnic minority patient is a first-generation immigrant or a second- or third-generation, with a better command of English and adaptation to British customs. The proportion of first-generation immigrants relative to the other generations will vary from practice to practice, therefore provisions for screening and surveillance should be tailored to suit the ethnic mix of a practice.

The main areas to consider are haemoglobinopathies, inherited diseases, infectious diseases, skin problems, emotional and social problems, paediatric surveillance (especially centile charts) and special screening for newly-arrived immigrants, particularly those from tropical countries. The subject could make the text of a new book but a short list of specific conditions is mentioned here so as to raise the issues. The reader will find much further information in medical textbooks.

Ethnic Europeans

Pernicious anaemia

Pernicious anaemia is the most common cause of Vitamin B12 deficiency in the UK and occurs after the age of 30. It is rare in Africa and Asia (Swash & Mason

1984) and is therefore less likely to be encountered in Africans, Caribbeans and Asians in Britain. A sore tongue is a usual symptom and the tongue subsequently becomes reddened, smooth and shiny. The patient may complain of indigestion or diarrhoea and often has a moderately enlarged spleen. Mild jaundice is common. A blood test for auto-antibody studies in the serum will be positive for parietal cell antibodies in 95% of cases and for intrinsic factor antibodies in 60% of patients. Examination of a stained blood film shows a macrocytic blood picture. A low serum Vitamin B12 level is accompanied by a raised folate. A Schilling test will demonstrate that there is a failure of Vitamin B12 absorption due to a lack of the gastric intrinsic factor. Two things should be remembered in surveillance:

1. Patient compliance with treatment is vital. Regular doses of hydroxycobalamin must be given indefinitely (1000 micrograms i.m. every 3 months for pernicious anaemia or monthly in patients with subacute combined degeneration of the cord).
2. Gastric carcinoma is common among these patients and a GP should look out for early symptoms.

On these lines, other known ethnicity or culture-related conditions among Europeans can be screened and/or followed-up. Some examples include cystic fibrosis in all whites; congenital dislocation of the hip in those of Italian or Austrian descent — it is rare among Africans and Chinese — with a higher incidence among girls (Aston 1967); alcoholism in the Irish, Scots and French; paranoia among Poles and suicidal tendencies in Swedes, Hungarians and other East Europeans. The list is endless and deletions or additions will occur as research evidence accumulates. From the 1990s onwards, British GPs are likely to see more patients from European ethnic minorities because of the UK developing closer links with the European Economic Community and also as a result of the many political changes in Eastern Europe.

Ethnic Jews

Tay–Sachs' disease

Like Niemann–Pick disease, Tay–Sachs' is an autosomal recessive disorder and the patients are often Jewish (Jolly & Levene 1985). Previously termed 'Amaurotic familial idiocy', this disease is due to an accumulation of the ganglioside Gm2 in the nervous system as a result of a deficiency of hexosaminidase A. The infant is normal up to the age of 6 months and then develops mental retardation followed by spasticity, convulsions and blindness. There may be an increased startle reflex on examination at the age of 6 weeks because hyper-acusis is an early feature. Enlargement of the head is detectable in the majority of cases. On fundoscopy a cherry-red spot at the macula, the characteristic feature, can be found. A blood test will show hexosaminidase A in the serum of patients as well as carriers. Surveillance involves genetic counselling of carriers and parents. Further advice and help can be obtained from a local Jewish Rabbi or organizations such as the Tay–Sachs' Society (17 Sydney Road, Ilford Essex. Tel. 081 550 8989).

Ethnic Asians

Rickets

Biochemical vitamin D deficiency and clinical rickets occur predominantly in Asian children. The incidence is biphasic, occuring in toddlers and preadolescents. Biochemical osteomalacia is common among Asian women, especially in pregnancy (Williams & Qureshi 1988). Factors responsible include:

1. The high phytate content of chapatis impairs the absorption of calcium (and also of iron and zinc).
2. A dietary deficiency of vitamin D.
3. Increased requirement of vitamin D.
4. Lack of exposure to sunlight.
5. Cultural factors, such as 'purdah' in Muslim women.
6. A genetic predisposition.

An infant with rickets is restless, fretful and pale, floppy and prone to respiratory or gastrointestinal infections. The bony changes are charateristic features — craniotabes, enlargement of the epiphyses of the lower end of the radius and swelling of the costochondral junctions of the ribs (rickety rosary) are early signs. Later findings, such as 'bossing' of the skull, pigeon chest, and Harrison's sulcus may develop in infants and later still, in toddlers; bony deformities may develop, e. g. kyphosis, knock knees, bow legs and pelvic deformities (contracted pelvis). In addition to the detection of these clinical signs, assessment should involve radiological examination of the wrists, which may show a typical 'saucer' deformity, and a blood test for serum alkaline phosphatase (an increase is of diagnostic value). The treatment consists of a therapeutic dose of vitamin D (1000–5000 iu) daily and an ample intake of calcium (milk is the best source). It is advisable that all Asian children should receive daily vitamin D supplements of 400 iu up to the age of five. Routine supplements of 1000 iu daily have been recommended for pregnant Asian women to prevent fetal rickets. An untreated rachitic child is always at risk from respiratory infections, therefore an Asian child with recurrent chest infections should be investigated for rickets.

Other culture-related conditions for screening and surveillance include: haemoglobinopathy D disease in Punjabis from Pakistan and India, iron deficiency anaemia in vegetarians (most Hindus, particularly Gujaratis), tuberculosis and malaria. Constraint on space forbids me from describing these conditions here but I suggest books for further reading at the end of the chapter.

Ethnic Africans and Caribbeans

Sickle-cell disease

This genetic disorder has a high incidence among black people — Africans, West Indians, Black Americans — but to a lesser extent it occurs in other races, such as Asians and Chinese. It is caused by an abnormal haemoglobin, HbS and occurs in homozygous (sickle-cell anaemia) or in heterozygous (sickle-cell trait) forms. Sickle-cell anaemia is often fatal before adolescence, but with early diagnosis and management a patient may live for 40 years or longer. The condition is an autosomal recessive and, if both parents have the sickle-cell trait, 1 in 4 children may be born with sickle-cell anaemia. Paediatric surveillance of a 4-month-old (or older) infant will show chronic anaemia due to reduced red cell survival. This is resposible for fatigue, reduced exercise tolerance, increased susceptibility to infection, cardiomegaly, leg ulcers and cholelithiasis. The child may have 'bossing' of the skull, prominent malar bones and protruberant teeth. In a black child who has had symptoms of anaemia since infancy, sickle-cell anaemia should always be suspected. Infarction crises due to vascular occlusion of the spleen, kidneys, lungs, central nervous system, retinae and bones are common. Refractory ulcers of the lower legs and severe backache or joint pains are also common. At any age, mesenteric infarction may produce an acute abdominal emergency, which should not be mistaken for acute appendicitis. Four tests should be considered for children at high risk:

1. A stained blood film examination under a microscope will show some sickle-shaped red cells.
2. A qualitative tube test for detecting the presence of HbS has been developed. It is called 'Sickledex' and a reagent pack is available from Ortho Diagnostics (Raritan, New Jersey 08869, USA).
3. A small drop of blood diluted in saline may be incubated under a sealed cover slip overnight, when sickling will occur.

4. A family study to demonstrate inheritance should be carried out.

Key points in surveillance are (i) to treat the patient for haemolytic anaemia, infection and painful crises, and (ii) genetic counselling of a couple where both partners have the sickle-cell trait. Ideally all black people should be given the choice of having blood tests carried out and, where a person has the sickle-cell trait, he or she should be given premarital counselling. GPs and patients could benefit from the advice and help from the Sickle-Cell Society (c/o Brent Community Health Council, 16 High Street, Harlesden, London, NW10 4LX. Tel. 081 451 3293).

Similarly, attention should be paid to screening and following-through patients with other conditions specific to black people, e.g. haemoglobinopathy C and glucose-6PD deficiency (10% of African males are likely to have the less severe form).

Ethnic Mediterraneans

Thalassaemia

Beta thalassaemia is seen in its highest frequency among Mediterranean people — Cypriots, Greeks, Turks and Italians — and to a lesser extent it is found in Asians and Chinese. It is estimated that 15% of ethnic Cypriots may be heterozygous, i.e, have thalassaemia minor so 3% of marriages have a 1 in 4 chance of producing a child with thalassaemia major. The latter condition thus accounts for 6 in 1000 live births in ethnic Cypriots in Britian. Beta thalassaemia is the most common type and is due to a failure to synthesise beta chains. Thalassaemia minor, causes mild anaemia (not responding to iron therapy), but little or no clinical disability. A child with thalassaemia major presents with profound hypochromic anaemia, severe red cell dysplasia, erythroblastosis, reduction of haemoglobin A, and excess of haemoglobin F. A patient can survive only a few years without blood transfusion. Early clinical signs are profound anaemia, head bossing, prominent malar eminences, retarded growth and development, folate deficiency and splenomegaly. After screening and diagnosis, the child should be referred to the local hospital for treatment with blood transfusion and later for chelation therapy for haemosiderosis. Iron therapy is strongly contraindicated but folic acid supplements are given.

Three actions are important in screening and surveillance:

1. All single people from at-risk populations should be given a choice of a blood test and those who have thalassaemia minor should be offered premarital counselling.
2. Where both parents have thalassaemia minor, fetoscopy early in pregnancy may lead to the diagnosis of homozygous beta thalassaemia and the offer of a termination of pregnancy.
3. A GP should investigate every child who presents with anaemia and should not start iron therapy simply on clinical examination alone, particularly if the child belongs to an at-risk group.

Other conditions worthy of screening and surveillance among Mediterranean people include severe glucose-6PD deficiency and sensitivity to Fava beans (see also Chapter 10).

Ethnic Chinese and South-East Asians

Severe glucose-6PD deficiency

The ethnic link with a disease is clearly demonstrated in this condition. The most severe forms of glucose-6PD deficiency occur in Chinese, Vietnamese and South-East Asians. The severe variety occurs in Europeans and Mediterranean people. A less severe type, as mentioned earlier, occurs in Africans and West Indians (Macleod et al 1987). Favism — haemolytic anaemia from the ingestion of the broad bean, *Vicia faba* — is due to a deficiency of glucose-6PD of the severe European variety. A patient with this condition may also present with anaemia due to haemolysis from the ingestion of certain drugs, e.g. sulphonamides (in co-trimoxazole), antimalarials, chloramphenicol and aspirin. Anuria is an infrequent but serious complication. A GP should take the history from a screening angle and then confirm the diagnosis using blood tests, e.g.:

1. The Jacob and Jandle test, which is simple and cheap, is the ascorbate cyanide test to monitor the whole glutathione-regulating system, of which glucose-6PD is an essential part.
2. Spot tests employing either the fluorescence of NADPH, which is a bioproduct of glucose-6PD activity, or the reduction of soluble tetrazolium compounds to insoluble purple formazan.

In such cases a GP will benefit from close liaison with the local pathologist and also with hospital physicians.

Other conditions that may occur among these ethnic groups include: alpha thalassaemia, HbE disease, haemoglobinopathy H, rubella and leprosy.

Readers may remember hearing the news that when the Princess of Wales visited Indonesia in 1989, she shook hands with leprosy patients as a health education media exercise. The world has become a global village and no man is an island any more.

CONCLUSION

'The roots of education are bitter, but the fruit is sweet' (Aristotle). Every country in the world has been enriched by its ethnic minorities and Britain is no exception. It is estimated that ethnic minorities now constitute nearly 10% of the British population. Hindi/Urdu, for example, is probably the most commonly spoken language in Britain after English. What happens in Eastern Europe by revolution occurs in Britain by evolution. People from different cultural, religious and ethnic backgrounds have varying needs and there are many agencies in Britain today who are ready to offer help to health professionals almost free of charge (Table 39.4). In this chapter I have given an overview of the size of special problems among ethnic minorities so as to raise issues in relation to screening and surveillance in general practice. I suggest that every GP should consider the place of screening among ethnic groups in his or her practice, with particular attention to the top five ethnic categories. Additional funding may be obtained through the local Family Health Service Authority/Health Board. In

Table 39.4   Resources available (from Qureshi 1989a)

Local
Priest/Rabbi/Imam/Pandit/Guru
Community relations council
Interpreter/Linkperson/Relative
MP/Councillor/Leader/Friend

National
Commission for Racial Equality
Appropriate embassy/Department of Health
Voluntary organisations

addition, he or she should make use of local community resources and national agencies. This chapter can be used as a basis from which every primary care team can expand its own approach to ethnic screening. It should be remembered that differences are a respectable entity in science and 'classification' should neither be rigid nor be mistaken for 'stereotyping'. Similarly, 'distinction' should not be confused with 'discrimination'. Ethnic minority care is not only a humane challange, it can also be an enjoyable venture. The quality of care must include patients from all ethnic groups in Britain.

REFERENCES

Aston J N 1967 A short textbook of orthopaedics and traumatology. English Universities Press, London, pp 199–204
Henley A 1979 'Names' in Asian patients at hospital and at home. Kings Fund, London, pp 87–104
Jolly H, Levene M 1985 Diseases of children, 5th edn. Blackwell Scientific Publications, Oxford, p 524
Macleod J, Edwards C, Bouchier I (eds) 1987 Davidson's principles & practice of medicine, 15th edn. Churchill Livingstone, Edinburgh, p 512

Qureshi B 1989a Trancultural medicine: dealing with patients from different cultures. Kluwer, Lancester, UK
Qureshi B 1989b Multiethnic aspects of patient care: the scale of the problem. MIMS Magazine, 1 January: 27–28
Swash M, Mason S 1984 Hutchinson's clinical methods, 8th edn. Bailliere Tindall, London, pp 436–437
Williams C, Qureshi B 1988 Nutritional aspects of different dietary practices. In: Dickerson J W T, Lee H (eds) Nutrition in the clinical management of disease. Edward Arnold, London, pp 422–439

FURTHER READING

Cruickshank J K (ed) 1989 Ethnic factors in health and disease. Butterworths, London
Fuller J H S, Toon P D 1988 Medical practice in a multicultural society. Heinemann, London
Hart C Bain J (eds) 1989 Child care in general practice.

Churchill Livingstone, Edinburgh
Payer L 1989 Medicine and culture: notions of health and sickness in Britain, the US, France, and West Germany. Victor Gollancz, London

Index